Physical Disabilities Manual

Physical Disabilities Manual

Editor

Beatriz Colon Abreu, O.T.R.

Occupational Therapy Department
New York University
New York, New York

Raven Press ■ New York

Raven Press, 1140 Avenue of the Americas, New York, New York 10036

Made in the United States of America

Library of Congress Cataloging in Publication Data

Main entry under title:

Physical disabilities manual.

Includes bibliographical references and index.
1. Physically handicapped—Rehabilitation.
I. Abreu, Beatriz Colon. [DNLM: 1. Handicapped.
2. Rehabilitation. WB 320 P579]
RD797.P48 617 80-28205
ISBN: 0-89004-505-4

To Charles M. Houseman,
all individuals in search of knowledge, and
all my students at New York University

Preface

This unique manual fully incorporates theory with clinical practice. It describes evaluation and intervention techniques mostly in occupational therapy, but it can be used by students and practitioners in all the rehabilitation professions. Each chapter covers a particular system or dysfunction. Adult perceptual motor assessment, dysphasia, reflex testing and management, and apraxia are among the topics discussed. Occupational therapists, physical therapists, and speech pathologists—clinicians and educators with expertise in physical disabilities—have all contributed.

The volume's objectives are twofold: to define the theoretical and clinical basis for evaluation and intervention procedures, and to outline the multiple, and sometimes conflicting, procedures currently used in rehabilitation.

The text is extensively illustrated with original diagrams that add to its clarity. Chapter references provide guidance for those who wish to explore a particular topic in more detail.

The reader will find that the clinical material presented in this book is an important contribution to the field. Students and practitioners alike will benefit from this concise, well-organized manual designed to assist them in understanding the overall nature of the rehabilitation process.

Beatriz Colon Abreu

Acknowledgments

I would like to express my gratitude to Ralph Abreu for his contributions as art director, illustrator, photographer, consultant, and friend. He gave generously of his time and extraordinary talent. I also gratefully acknowledge the many colleagues and friends who provided editorial assistance; Kay Schwartz for her time and helpful comments on the original manuscripts; and Francis A. Acquaviva, Elaine Viseltear, Arthur Nelson, and Janice Gyuniecek for their review of the manuscripts.

I am also indebted to Lucy Hernandez who took responsibility for typing the manuscript and attending to the detail of preparing the final copy. She was assisted by Betsey Corwin.

I would like to thank Susan Ganz and Judy Grossman for their moral support, and, finally, Anne Cronin Mosey for her assistance, her advice, and her support as a colleague and friend.

All proceeds from this manual will be donated to the Metropolitan New York District, New York State Occupational Therapy Association. This money will be used to support other continuing education projects.

Contents

Contributors

Beatriz Colon Abreu, O.T.R.
Occupational Therapy Department
New York University
New York, New York 10003

S. Elaine Bennethum, M.S., O.T.R., R.P.T.
Occupational Therapy Department
Goldwater Memorial Hospital
New York University Medical Center
New York, New York 10017

Susan Miron-Bernstein, O.T.R.
Occupational Therapy Department
Institute of Rehabilitation Medicine
New York University Medical Center
New York, New York 10016

Annette Bieringer, O.T.R.
Occupational Therapy Department
Memorial Sloan-Kettering Cancer Center
New York, New York 10021

Sophia Chioteli M.A., O.T.R.
Occupational Therapy Department
Institute of Rehabilitation Medicine
New York University Medical Center
New York, New York 10016

Joanne De Scherer, R.P.T.
Physical Therapy Department
Long Island College Hospital
Brooklyn, New York 11201

Ruth E. Dickey, O.T.R.
Occupational Therapy Department
Institute of Rehabilitation Medicine
New York University Medical Center
New York, New York 10016

Elsie Dicmonas, M.A., O.T.R.
Occupational Therapy Department
Kingsbrook Jewish Medical Center
Brooklyn, New York 11203

Joyce Lawler, R.P.T.
Physical Therapist
Private Practitioner
175 Baltic Street
Brooklyn, New York

A. Damien Martin, Ed.D., L.S.P.
Speech Pathology and Audiology Department
New York University
New York, New York 10003

Anne Cronin Mosey, Ph.D., O.T.R., F.A.O.T.A.
Occupational Therapy Department
New York University
New York, New York 10003

Arthur J. Nelson, Ph.D., R.P.T.
Physical Therapy Department
New York University
New York, New York 10003

Peggy Strecker Neufeld, M.A., O.T.R.
Occupational Therapy Department
State University of New York
Downstate Medical Center
Brooklyn, New York 11203

Barbara E. Neuhaus, Ed.D., O.T.R.
Occupational Therapy Program
College of Physicians and Surgeons of Columbia University
630 West 158th Street
New York, New York 10032

Renee Okoye, MSHS, O.T.R.
Occupational Therapist
Private Practice
58 East Dover
Massapequa, New York 11758

Karen Prendergast, R.P.T.
Hand Rehabilitation Services
310 East 30th Street
New York, New York 10016

Laurie Kalb Ritter, O.T.R.
Occupational Therapy Department
Institute of Rehabilitation Medicine
New York University Medical Center
New York, New York 10016

Anne Hiller Scott, O.T.R.
Occupational Therapy Department
St. Vincent's Hospital
New York, New York, 10011

Cecilia Sattely Seiser, M.A., O.T.R., F.A.O.T.A.
Rehabilitation Medicine Service
Veterans' Administration Hospital
Bronx, New York 10468

Anita Simons, O.T.R.
Occupational Therapy Department
St. Vincent's Hospital
New York, New York 10011

Linda Stieritz, O.T.R.
Occupational Therapy Department
Institute of Rehabilitation Medicine
New York University Medical Center
New York, New York 10016

Joan Sullivan, M.A., O.T.R.
Occupational Therapy Department
Hospital for Joint Diseases
Orthopaedic Institute
New York, New York 10003

Pat Trossman, M.A., O.T.R.
Occupational Therapy Department
State University of New York
Downstate Medical Center
Brooklyn, New York 11203

Nina Wold-Tortelli, O.T.R.
Institute of Rehabilitation Medicine
New York University Medical Center
New York, New York 10016

Nancy Wasserman, M.S., L.S.P.
Speech Pathology Department
Long Island College Hospital
Brooklyn, New York 11201

G. Gordon Williamson, Ph.D., O.T.R.
Occupational Therapy Department
John F. Kennedy Medical Center
Edison, New Jersey 08817

Introduction: The Art of Practice

Anne Cronin Mosey

In our art
We touch,
If only for a moment,
The realness of each other.

Occupational therapy, in the course of its growth, has been defined in many and varied ways. But regardless of the time and particular orientation of its definers, most definitions begin with the phrase . . . "Occupational therapy is the art and science of . . ." And for good reason, for there is a considerable scientific foundation to our practice, and a definite art.

This manual outlines and defines a portion of the theoretical foundation of occupational therapy. This manual also describes, with care, how this theoretical foundation can be translated into practice that leads to decreased dysfunction and the enhancement of function for our patients and clients. This manual is rich in the articulation of scientific theory and its application. Our theoretical foundation is strong and in many respects, unique.

In the wealth of scientific information provided however, let us pause for a moment to consider our art. The art of practice may occasionally be submerged in the concern for verification and application of scientific theory. The purpose of this chapter is simply to remind the reader of our art.

The concept of art is derived from aesthetics. Philosophers concerned with aesthetics study artifacts and experiences contrived by individuals, groups, or by nature. There is art in painting, music, poetry and dance. There is art in the beauty of a perfect yellow rose and in the sound of the sea as it crashes against shore bound rocks. There is art in the gentle touch of a mother and in the joyous process of making love.

In the study of aesthetics, philosophers measure the artifacts of man, that which nature has provided and the interpersonal experiences of individuals according to a philosophical definition of art. Art is the composition of any artifact or interpersonal experience which diminishes the isolation of the individual; which reaffirms the power of the human mind, body and spirit; which assists the individual in discovering meaning in existence. That which is identified as art assists in fulfilling the universal need for kinship and relatedness to others and the need for a sense of individuality and selfness.

In the experience of involvement in art, we feel a sense of identification with others, with the human condition. We feel that someone, at last, understands and is able to give substance to our own unique ideas and concerns. In this experience we often have a flooding sense of our potentiality as an individual and as a participant in the comedy and tragedy of human life.

The study and appreciation of art is primarily focused upon the visual and performing arts. However, such a focus is narrow for it does not include the art in nature or in human interaction. As children we discovered some of the art of nature; we were astounded when we really understood that each snow flake was different, that every oak leaf had a similar design. As students of anatomy we discovered the art of the human body: the similarities and differences in the structure of each cell, the order of the nervous system. And if well taught, we stood in wonder and reverence.

The art of human interaction is frequently so much a part of experience that it is only perceived in retrospect or not at all. There are many people who influence our lives. Some people have a negative impact; others, a positive impact. And then there are those people who, in a short encounter or over a long period, provide us with direction. In illustration, the art of human interaction may be a father who explains the biblical parable of the talents; an individual we love who encourages growth, regardless of the consequences of that growth on the continuance of our relationship; the mentor who guides us in discovering and using our special skills in a way which enables us to leave this world a better place than it was at the moment of our birth.

The parents of the art of practice are the art of nature and the art of human interaction. The art of practice is an interaction between therapist and patient which assists in diminishing the isolation of a patient; reaffirms the power of the human mind, body and spirit; provides the means whereby the patient may discover meaning in existence. Through the art of practice we help individuals to grow in their relatedness to others, find significance in life, appreciate individuality, accept their limitations and discover their strengths.

The art of practice is difficult to describe. It is not the skilled application of scientific knowledge or a global sense of caring about and wanting to help others. The art of practice is something far greater; it is a mysterious mix of genetic inheritance, life experience, self-knowledge and a sense of universality.

The skilled practitioner is able to make fine discriminating choices of appropriate scientific knowledge and professional skills applicable to the individual problems presented by each client. Skilled practice is the ability to ask the right questions, to select suitable evaluative tools and to design activities to meet the current needs of each patient. Such discriminating use of knowledge may be combined with the art of practice, but the skilled application of knowledge per se is not art.

A practitioner can be concerned about the welfare of each individual client. Such an attitude is indeed important. However, practice only becomes an art when a therapist is able to transcend sympathy and translate empathy into a process which brings the individual to a state of renewed sense of self and a deeper understanding of one's place in the community of people in which we live.

The art of practice described in the negative is however not a good definition of art. And herein lies the mystery. We know little of how one becomes an artist; we know little about how to teach the art of practice. Most components of the creation of art are unknown both to the artist and the participant/observer. Thus it is as difficult to describe how one brings art to practice as it is to describe the impact of Titian's *Knight of Malta*.

And yet we all search for our art; for we know that it is our goal as practitioners.

Nevertheless, there are some aspects of the art of practice which are relatively known; which may provide some illumination of the continuing process of becoming a therapist who brings art to practice. The most basic component appears to be a personal philosophy which emphasizes the dignity and rights of the individual regardless of current circumstances. Although easily said, there are situations in which it is difficult to retain this philosophical orientation: the autistic child who violently rejects any human contact; the parent who has killed a child; the alcoholic derelict. The dignity and rights of the individual are often ascribed to in the abstract. The practitioner who affirms these ideas in daily interactions is an artist.

Another component of the art of practice is related to the perception of the individual as indivisible; as an integrated whole, not a collection of parts or systems. A person can not retain human qualities if divided or reduced to abstract elements. To even speak of the "mind, body and spirit'' denies individuality. It is true that in study we divide to understand more clearly. However, it is the art of practice which enables us to integrate and know each individual. Those who practice the art of occupational therapy are not concerned with encouraging a child to use both hands, assisting an individual to express feelings or helping a patient wash her face. Rather, the practitioner, as an artist, is concerned with the whole; hands, feelings and face belong to an individual. Each patient is special, unique and different from all other people. Each patient is an individual who can not be divided (1).

In addition, each individual is related to and embedded in a configuration of other individuals: family, culture and community. One component of the art of practice is to understand the individual in his relatedness to others and to the ideas, values and experiences of his culture. This component of art becomes especially difficult when the therapist and patient do not share the same cultural background, language or value systems. Thus, it is often difficult to comprehend parental rejection of a severely handicapped child, to describe a home-treatment plan to a relative who does not understand English, or to accept the fact that a person confined to a wheelchair is expected to remain in the role of a dependent invalid in some cultural groups. To be able to relate to individuals significant to the client and to accept the client's value system is one aspect of the art of practice.

Another component of the art of practice is an understanding and appreciation of a patient's relatedness to the nonhuman environment. Many patients are surrounded with nonhuman objects which have little or no meaning to them and by objects which they find offensive. Few patients are allowed to feel the rain upon their face, hear the sound of an outboard motor on a quiet lake, walk through newly fallen snow. Splints, crutches, braces and a vast variety of adaptive equipment can be threatening, ominous and violently rejected. The therapist who brings art to practice studies and accepts each individual's perception of the nonhuman environment.

Finally, the capacity to empathize with another individual is part of the art of practice. Empathy involves entering into the experience of another individual without loss of one's own sense of separateness as a unique and different individual. Empathy is the ability to feel the pain and joy of another individual, fully realizing it is not one's own pain and joy. To be separate from but with another individual requires a sense of relatedness to the human condition in all of its manifestations and a sense of one's own specialness. Understanding of one's self is basic to the empathetic process. To empathize, the therapist must have inner security, considerable knowledge of self, self-acceptance. In addition, the therapist must be open to the feelings, ideas and values of the many others with whom one interacts. The separateness of empathy is important for it allows the therapist to solve problems, make sound judgments and to interpret with objectivity. The togetherness of empathy is important for it allows the therapist to participate in maturation and development with many other individuals. (2)

But the mystery remains. The art of practice can not be defined, circumscribed or taught. It is an illusive quality conceived by recondite parents. Once discovered in ourselves or others we can only nurture its growth.

In summary, the art of practice is assisting another individual to learn and grow. It is the ability to guide others to know and use their potential, to be participants in a community, to love, to play, to find purpose in life.

With legitimate concern for our theoretical foundation, may we never forget our art.

REFERENCES

1. Magraw, R. M. (1973): Science and humanism. In: *Hippocratic Revisited,* edited by R. J. Bulger. Medcom Press, New York.
2. Blungart, H. L. (1973): The art and the science. In: *Hippocratic Revisited,* edited by R. J. Bulger. Medcom Press, New York.

BIBLIOGRAPHY

Axelrod, J. (1973): *The University Teacher as an Artist.* Jossey-Boss Publishers, San Francisco.

Cassidy, H. G. (1962): *The Sciences and the Arts: A New Alliance.* Harper & Brothers, New York.

Runes, D. D. (1962): *Living Schools of Philosophy.* Adams & Co., Paterson, N.J.

Sahakian, W. S. P. (1968): *Outline of the History of Philosophy.* Barnes & Noble, New York.

Searles, H. F. (1960): *The Nonhuman Environment.* International Universities Press, New York.

Evaluation 1

Beatriz Colon Abreu

This manual contains samples of evaluation systems and strategies used by experienced clinicians in their specialty areas. It outlines and defines certain aspects of dealing with physical disabilities that constitute a portion of the theoretical foundation of rehabilitation. The purpose of this chapter is to foster increased awareness to the evaluation feedback loop involving the patient, tests and measurements, and the therapist.

Evaluation is a process of examination by which the value and quality of a patient's behaviors are determined and judged. It is a necessary process and a prerequisite for the treatment plan. It helps to define the patient's problems, and it is the foundation for selecting treatment alternatives and training. Under the general heading of evaluation the therapist employs a variety of tests and methods to determine a patient's deficits and potentials and to measure progress as treatment proceeds. An ongoing process, evaluation is also used to determine at what point treatment is to be altered or discontinued.

Evaluation involves judgment on the part of the center, agency, school, physician, therapist, or other authority. The method or form used is determined by this authority and reflects its connections and preferences. Evaluation instruments employed by the therapist continue to be refined and updated. Many are not standardized. In evaluation, documentation is as important as the process. Inaccurate reporting can lead to legal and medical complications. The student will benefit each time an evaluation is performed by answering the following questions: Why is the evaluation procedure being used (e.g., to assist in diagnosis, to assist in disposition or placement, to serve as a base line for treatment planning)? What is the intended outcome (meaning, scores, form standards)? Who is the patient (age, degree of injury, stage of recovery, and degree of dysfunction)?

When patients are being evaluated, their behaviors are being observed, judged, and recorded. They may show changes or modifications in attention and behavior that are consciously or unconsciously, directly or indirectly, connected with the evaluation process. Impaired attention or disruption of the ability to remember instructions properly can result in low scores in performance skills tested, even though ability may be adequate. If the patient's level of attention is severely impaired, as in the case of coma, there will be limited use for evaluation tools. The evaluation may be temporarily limited to recording changes in postural muscle tone and reactions to stimuli. As the patient's attention level increases, the range of tools may be expanded, and specific aspects of mental and physical responses to the environment can be tested and recorded. One must remember that the degree of attention can fluctuate.

The degree of rapport between therapist and patient will facilitate or inhibit data gathering at the initial interview and evaluation. Figure 1 shows the important factors in the interview feedback loop. The patient's self-image and interaction with the therapist are equally important to motivation. The skills of the therapist in observing, questioning, and directing the patient will determine the degree of excellence of the evaluation. The tests the therapist uses are important, but no less important are the patient's reactions, limitations, and tolerance, the degree and stage of injury, and the patient's level of attention to the measurements.

In essence, the practice of occupational therapy is an exercise in problem solving. The therapist meeting a new patient is provided certain clues. Additional clues are uncovered by means of trained observation and skillful interaction. The therapist draws on professional knowledge to piece together the clues and develop a tentative definition of the problem. To confirm the definition, the therapist uses task analysis

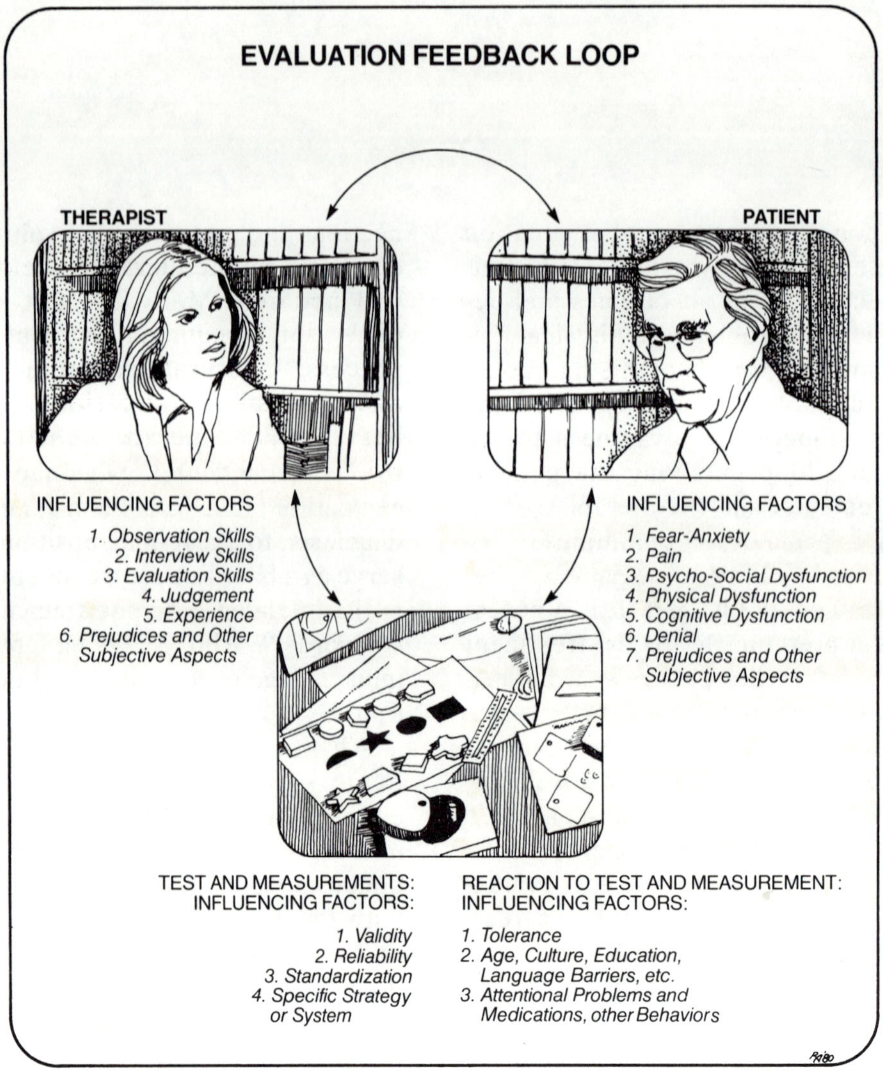

FIG. 1. Evaluation feedback loop.

with graduated activities. The therapist's observation skills, interview skills, evaluation skills, judgment, experience, prejudices, and other subjective aspects such as mood will influence the procedure.

Evaluation is a tool that is as good as the therapist using it. Methods of assessment should be standardized and should be continually reevaluated. If standard methods are not available, the therapist's ability to consistently and systematically observe and record behavior will provide base-line data on the patient's performance, as well as treatment and results.

The following chapters describe various evaluation and treatment strategies designed by specialized clinicians. They should give the student and clinician examples and ideas to use in treating the physically disabled.

Range of Motion 2

Joan Sullivan and Sally Poole

It is indeed a difficult task to shed new light on a topic that has been discussed in depth so many times in the past. Frequently, students are unnerved by the goniometer when asked to evaluate a patient. This may be the result of unfamiliarity with the tool and the process and their hesitancy to commit themselves to objective measurement. Our goal is to give the student or therapist a clear, concise presentation of the available literature. The range-of-motion chart includes not only goniometric placement but also prime movers and their innervations. This provides the reader with clear references to the structures that power the joint.

This presentation will be limited to the range of motion of the arm. However, this does not mean that the occupational therapist will never be required to measure lower extremity joint range of motion. We believe that once the therapist masters the techniques for upper extremity range of motion, this can be applied to lower extremity measurements, with the help of the appropriate literature.

This chapter will also deal with the concepts of total active motion and total passive motion. This is a fairly new method of recording and reporting range of motion of the hand.

The ability to accurately measure joint range of motion is an essential skill for the rehabilitation therapist. It enables the therapist to determine the extent of the limitation, set appropriate goals, and determine by reevaluation the effectiveness of the treatment employed.

The joint motions discussed here are those that occur around an axis/fulcrum perpendicular to one of three body planes: sagittal, frontal, transverse (3) (Fig. 1). Joint mobility and joint play are not discussed, since they are not measured objectively with a universal tool. The motions discussed are:

1. *True hinge motion:* Natural motion occurring away from (one direction only) the zero starting position, e.g., elbow and knee flexion. The *return* to the zero position is extension. Only when the motion opposite to flexion is unnatural should it be called hyperextension.
2. *Two-plane motion:* Natural motion occurring in two planes beginning at the zero starting position, e.g., wrist extension and flexion and radial and ulnar deviation.
3. *Ball-and-socket motion:* Natural motion occurring rotatorily, or in three planes, e.g., hip and shoulder movements.

Part of the responsibility of the occupational therapist to help patients return to their highest

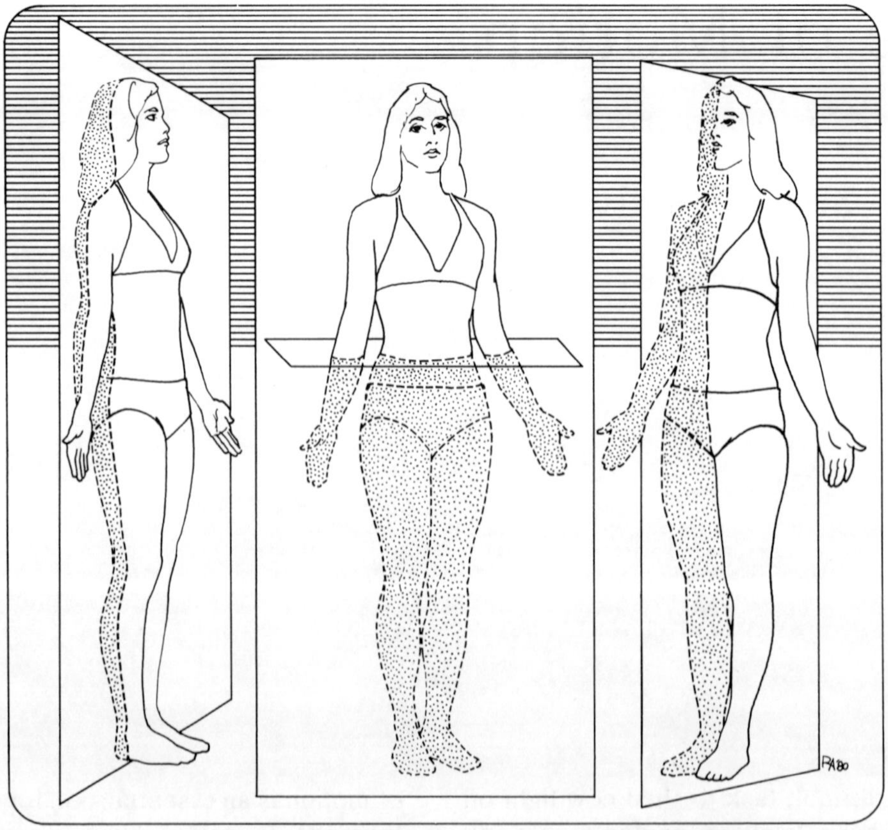

FIG. 1. Planes of motion—frontal, transverse, and sagittal.

possible levels of functioning involves evaluation and treatment of joint limitations. Limitations can occur after disease or trauma to the joint itself or to soft-tissue structures that power the joint (nerve, tendon, muscle); they can also result from prolonged immobility.

MEASUREMENT TOOLS

In order to obtain accurate measurements in a range-of-motion evaluation, care must be taken to use appropriate tools and to use them correctly. When evaluating any system in the human body, the many variables can cause even the most experienced therapist's findings to differ slightly from day to day. What follows is a discussion of the tools used to measure range of motion and how to select and use them appropriately.

Goniometry

The goniometer is the standard tool used to measure joint motion, i.e., the angles produced at the joint during movement. It consists of two calibrated arms attached to a protractor, the center of which is the axis of movement. One arm is fixed to the protractor (stationary arm); the other is free to follow the movement at a given joint (movable arm).

Goniometers are available in various sizes and various materials (Fig. 2). Although some goniometers are calibrated to measure the full 360° circle, the most common method of joint measurement employs the 180° half-circle method. The starting or anatomic position (the point at which we begin to measure degrees of movement) has been designated as 0° (zero starting position); therefore the degrees of movement are added in the direction *away* from the zero starting position (4). Care must be taken to stay within the correct plane of motion.

The goniometers shown in Fig. 2 are those most commonly used by therapists today. The large goniometers (#1 and #2) are excellent for measuring large joints (hip, knee, shoulder); the others (#4 and #5) are better used on smaller joints (ankle, wrist, elbow). Naturally the clear plastic goniometers (#5) allow for easy reading by the therapist. The smallest "finger" goniometer (#6) has been an enormous success in measuring the small joints of the hand, since they are measured dorsally rather than laterally. An im-

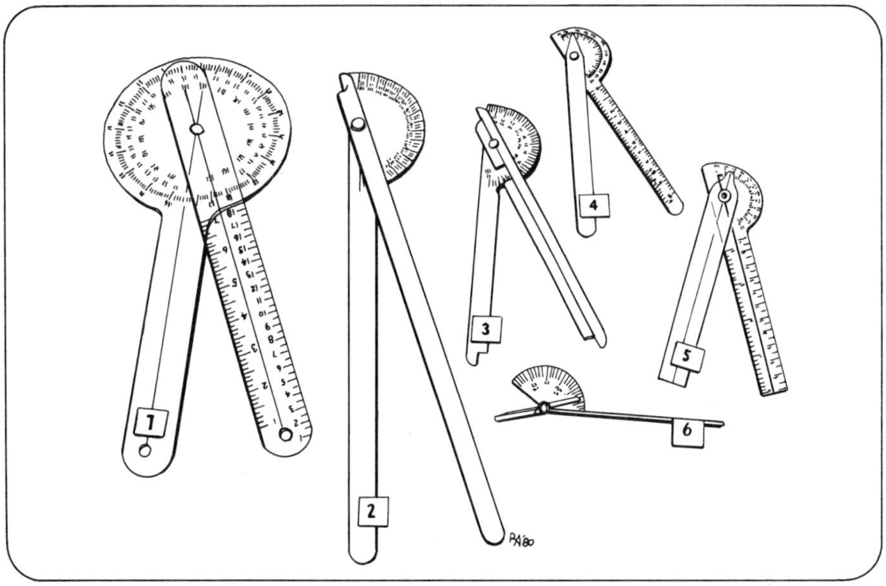

FIG. 2. Standard goniometers.

portant feature of goniometer #3 is that it can be recorded on X-ray. Choosing the appropriate goniometer is a key factor in accurate and reliable joint measurement.

Guidelines for Measuring Joint ROM

1. Explain the purpose of the evaluation to the patient.
2. Take care not to fatigue the patient, as this may affect the results. If possible, the evaluation and reevaluation should be done by the same therapist at the same time of day.
3. Place the joint to be measured in the proper test position, and place the goniometer as follows: (a) the axis/fulcrum of the goniometer over the axis of the joint, (b) the stationary arm parallel to the longitudinal axis of the part proximal to the joint, (c) the movable part parallel to the longitudinal axis of the part distal to the joint (8).
4. Instruct the patient to move the joint through the desired motion, and be sure that the patient is not deviating out of the correct plane or using substitute motions.
5. Indicate whether the measurement is passive or active, and record the findings on the appropriate evaluation form.

Evaluation/Recording Form

Each institution or rehabilitation department has its own form for recording range-of-motion (ROM) findings that may or may not be included in the patient's medical chart. Although many experienced therapists do not use a form, this practice is not recommended for students or beginning therapists. Various forms differ somewhat, but in addition to the degrees of movement, each should include the following: therapist's name, date of evaluation or reevaluation, active or passive ROM, right or left extremity, limitations, and pain. (Fig. 3).

Total Active Motion/Total Passive Motion

When evaluating ROM of the digits in the hand, the therapist can use a method advised by the Clinical Assessment Committee of the American Society for Surgery of the Hand. This method is known as total active motion/total passive motion (TAM/TPM).

TAM/TPM is measured individually for each digit (6). TAM is a measure of tendon excursion, and it equals the sum of the angles formed by the metacarpophalangeal (MP), proximal interphalangeal (PIP), and distal interphalangeal (DIP) joints in maximum active flexion, minus total extension deficit at MP, PIP, and DIP joints with active finger extension (Figs. 4a, 4b).

TAM = active flexion
(MP + PIP + DIP)
− incomplete active extension
(MP + PIP + DIP)

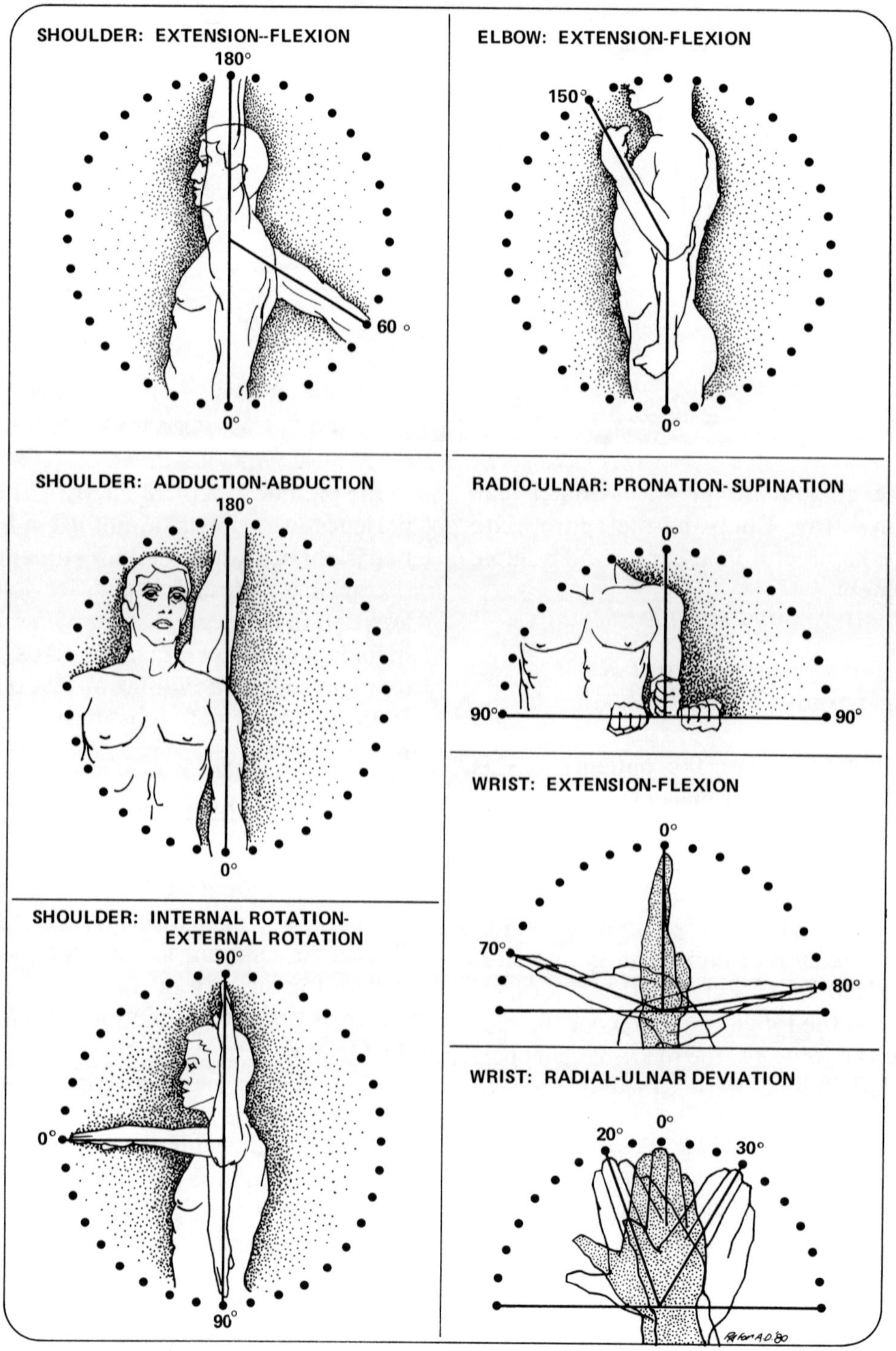

FIG. 3. A type of Rom form.

NORMAL

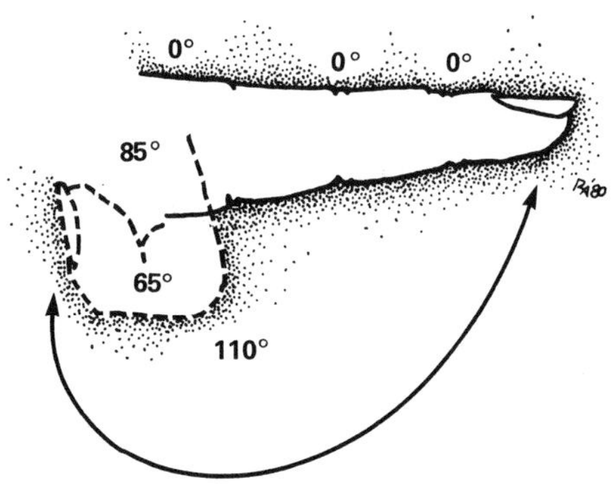

For example:

Normal

Active	Flexion	Extension Lack
MCP	85°	0°
PIP	110°	0°
DIP	65°	0°
Totals	260°	0°

Total Active Motion (TAM)
260° - 0° = 260°

FIG. 4a. TAM. Reprinted with permission from The American Society of the Hand.

STIFF MCP +
LIMITED PIP EXTENSION

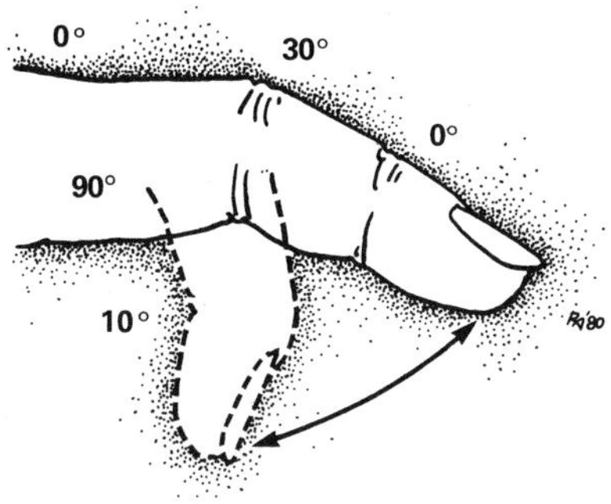

Stiff MCP + Limited PIP Extension

Active	Flexion	Extension Lack
MCP	0°	0°
PIP	90°	30°
DIP	10°	0°
Totals	100°	30°

Total Active Motion (TAM)
100° - 30° = 70°

LIMITED MCP + PIP FLEXION
WITH GOOD EXTENSION

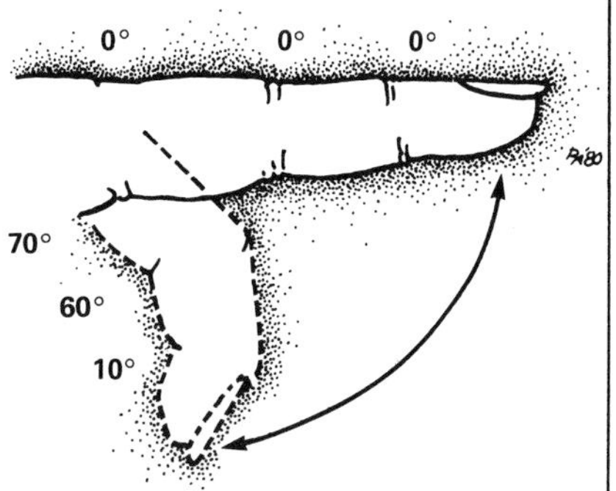

Limited MCP + PIP FLEXION
with Good Extension

Active	Flexion	Extension Lack
MCP	70°	0°
PIP	60°	0°
DIP	10°	0°
Totals	140°	0°

Total Active Motion (TAM)
140° - 0° = 140°

FIG. 4b. TAM. Reprinted with permission from The American Society of the Hand.

SWAN NECK DEFORMITY

BOUTONNIERE DEFORMITY

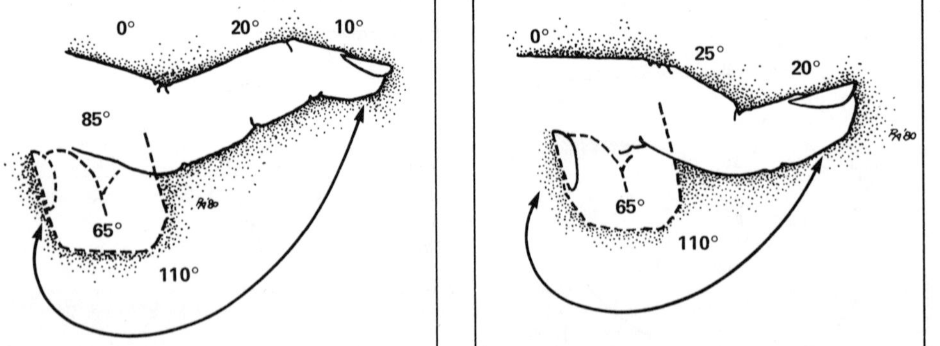

Swan neck deformity: Hyperototension of PIP + Flexion of DIP

Active	Flexion		Extension Lack
MCP	85°		0°
PIP	110°	(Hyperext.)	20°
DIP	65°		10°
Totals	260°		30°

Total Active Motion (TAM)
260° - 30° = 230°

Boutonniere deformity: Flexion of PIP Hyperextension of DIP

Active	Flexion		Extension Lack
MCP	85°		0°
PIP	110°		25°
DIP	65°	(Hyperext.)	20°
Totals	260°		45°

Total Active Motion (TAM)
260° - 45° = 215°

FIG. 4c. TAM.

TAM/TPM

		Active Ten.		Tot.	Passive Jt.		Tot.
Thumb	MP	10	35	25	0	50	50
	IP	0	80	80	0	90	90
		TAM		105	TPM		140
Index	MP	0	40	40	0	85	85
	PIP	25	60	35	20	70	50
	DIP	10	30	20	10	35	25
		TAM		95	TPM		160
Long	MP	15	45	30	15	60	45
	PIP	5	55	50	0	55	55
	DIP	0	20	20	0	30	30
		TAM		100	TPM		130
Ring	MP	20	60	40	20	70	50
	PIP	10	55	45	10	55	45
	DIP	0	45	45	0	50	50
		TAM		130	TPM		145
Small	MP	30	35	5	25	40	15
	PIP	25	30	5	15	40	25
	DIP	15	45	30	10	45	35
		TAM		40	TPM		75

Hyperextension at any joint, particularly the PIP and DIP joints, is to be recorded as a deficit in extension and is included in the total extension deficit, except for nonpathological MP hyperextension. Hyperextension is to be considered an abnormal value, as in swan neck (PIP) and boutonniere (DIP) deformities (Fig. 4b). Normal values for TAM are 240° to 270°.

TPM is a measure of joint mobility, and it equals the sum of the angles formed by the MP, PIP, and DIP joints in maximum passive flexion minus the sum of the angles of deficit from complete passive extension at each of the three joints.

$$\text{TPM} = \text{passive flexion} \; (\text{MP} + \text{PIP} + \text{DIP}) - \text{incomplete passive extension} \; (\text{MP} + \text{PIP} + \text{DIP})$$

The TAM/TPM method is a standardized evaluation procedure used by both therapists and surgeons. It provides the members of the hand rehabilitation team an objective language that can be used to report results of surgery or therapy.

For ease of recording, the evaluation form shown in Table 1 was devised. Extension or extension lag is subtracted from flexion both actively and passively, and a total is determined for each joint motion. These are added for each digit, with TAM/TPM being the sum. Table 1 shows an initial evaluation of a patient with multiple fractures of the right hand.

REFERENCES

1. Brunstrom, S. (1972): *Clinical Kinesiology*. F. A. Davis, Philadelphia.
2. Daniels, L., Williams, M., and Worthingham, C. (1956): *Muscle Testing Techniques of Manual Examination*, ed. 2. W. B. Saunders, Philadelphia.
3. Esch, D., and Lepley, M. (1971): *Evaluation of Joint Motion: Methods of Measurement and Recording*. University of Minnesota Press, Minneapolis.
4. AAOS (1965): *Joint Motion Method of Measuring and Recording*. American Academy of Orthopedic Surgeons, Chicago.
5. Rasch, P., and Burke, R. (1971): *Kinesiology and Applied Anatomy: The Science of Human Movement*, ed. 4. Lea & Febiger, Philadelphia.
6. ASSH (1978): *The Hand Examination and Diagnosis*. American Society for Surgery of the Hand, Aurora, Colorado.
7. Thompson, C. (1973): *Manual of Structural Kinesiology*. ed. 7. C. V. Mosby, St. Louis.
8. Trombly, C. A., and Scott, A. D. (1977): *Occupational Therapy for Physical Dysfunction*. Williams & Wilkins, Baltimore.

APPENDIX

TABLE 1. *ROM Comprehensive Chart—Compiled from the Available Literature* (2, 3, 8)

Motion	Plane[a]	Prime movers and Innervation[b]	Goniometer placement[c]		Expected range
Shoulder flexion	S	Deltoid (anterior fibers)	TP:	Arm at side in midposition	0–180°
		N: Axillary	A:	Center of the shoulder joint just below the acromion process	
		Coracobrachialis	S:	Parallel to the lateral midline of the trunk	
		N: Musculocutaneous	M:	Parallel to the long axis of the humerus along the lateral side	
			EP:	Arm directly overhead in midposition	
			Beware:	Trunk extension, shoulder abduction	
Shoulder extension	S	Latissimus dorsi	TP:	Arm at side	0–60°
		N: Thoracodorsal	A:	Center of shoulder joint just below the acromion process	
		Teres major N: Low Subscapular	S:	Parallel to the lateral midline of the trunk	
		Deltoid (posterior fibers)	M:	Parallel to the longitudinal axis of the humerus along the lateral side	
		N: Axillary	EP:	Arm stretched backward to the limit	
			Beware:	Trunk flexion, scapular elevation, rotation, shoulder abduction	

[a] S: sagittal. F: frontal. T: transverse.
[b] N: nerve.
[c] TP: test position. A: axis of movement. S: stationary arm. M: movable arm. EP: end position.

TABLE 1—*Continued*

Motion	Plane[a]	Prime movers and Innervation[b]	Goniometer placement[c]		Expected range
Shoulder abduction	F	Deltoid (middle fibers) N: Axillary Supraspinatus N: Suprascapular	TP: A: S: M: EP: Beware:	Arm at side in external rotation A point through the anterior or posterior aspect of the glenohumeral joint Parallel with the midline of the body Parallel to the longitudinal axis of the humerus Arm overhead with palm facing opposite side Lateral flexion of trunk, scapular elevation, shoulder flexion or extension	0–180°
Horizontal abduction	T	Deltoid (posterior fibers) N: Axillary	TP: A: S: M: EP: Beware:	Arm internally rotated and at 90° of shoulder flexion A point on top of the acromion process Parallel to the long axis of the humerus, perpendicular to the body Parallel to the long axis of the humerus Arm at 90° shoulder abduction Trunk rotation	0–90°
Horizontal adduction	T	Pectoralis major N: Medial and lateral anterior thoracic	TP: A: S: M: EP: Beware:	Arm internally rotated and at 90° of shoulder flexion A point on top of the acromion process Parallel to the long axis of the humerus perpendicular to the body Parallel to the long axis of the humerus Arm across trunk to the maximal motion Trunk rotation	0–45°
Internal rotation	T	Subscapularis N: Upper and lower subscapular Pectoralis major N: Medial and lateral anterior thoracic Latissimus dorsi N: Thoracodorsal Teres major N: Lowest subscapular	TP: A: S: M: EP: Beware:	The arm is supported in 90° abduction with elbow flexed 90° and palm down Olecranon process of ulna Perpendicular to the floor with goniometer reading 90° Parallel to long axis of the ulna Arm in 90° abduction and 90° elbow flexion with hand pointing to floor to the maximal motion Scapular elevation and downward rotation, trunk flexion and elbow extension	0–90°

TABLE 1—*Continued*

Motion	Plane[a]	Prime movers and Innervation[b]	Goniometer placement[c]		Expected range
Forearm supination	T	Biceps brachii N: Musculocutaneous Supinator N: Radial	(1) TP:	Humerus adducted, elbow flexed to 90°, forearm in midposition	0–90°
			A:	Parallel to the long axis of the forearm displaced toward the ulna	
			S:	Perpendicular to the floor	
			M:	Across the distal radius and ulna or the volar surface	
			EP:	Forearm rotated so that the palm faces up	
			Beware:	Shoulder adduction and external rotation	
			(2) TP:	Humerus adducted, elbow flexed to 90°, forearm in midposition with subject holding pencil in closed fist with the pencil protruding from the radial side of the hand	
External rotation	T	Infraspinatus N: Suprascapular Teres minor N: Axillary	TP:	The arm is supported in 90° abduction with elbow flexed 90° and palm down	0–90°
			A:	Olecranon process of ulna	
			S:	Perpendicular to the floor with goniometer reading 90°	
			M:	Parallel to long axis of the ulna	
			EP:	Arm in 90° abduction and 90° elbow flexion with hand pointing toward ceiling to the maximal	
			Beware:	Scapular depression and upward rotation, trunk extension, elbow extension	
Elbow flexion-extension	S	Flexion: Biceps brachii N: Musculocutaneous Brachialis N: Musculocutaneous Extension: Triceps N: Radial	TP:	Arm in anatomic position or to the limit of rotation; this measurement is recorded as the limit of extension	0–150°
			A:	Lateral epicondyle of humerus	
			S:	Parallel to the long axis of the humerus on the lateral aspect	
			M:	Parallel to the long axis of the radius	
			A:	Head of the third metacarpal, which coincides with the longitudinal axis of the forearm	
			EP:	Forearm has moved toward the humerus so that the hand is near the shoulder to the maximal motion	

TABLE 1—*Continued*

Motion	Plane[a]	Prime movers and Innervation[b]	Goniometer placement[c]		Expected range
			A:	Head of the third metacarpal coinciding with longitudinal axis of forearm	
			S:	Perpendicular to floor	
			M:	Parallel to pencil	
			EP:	The forearm is rotated so that the palm faces up; the pencil is still held tightly	
			Beware:	Movement of the pencil, shoulder adduction and external rotation	
Forearm pronation	T	Pronator teres N: Median Pronator quadratus N: Median	(1) TP:	Humerus abducted, elbow flexed to 90°, forearm in midposition	0–90°
			A:	Long axis of forearm displaced toward ulnar side	
			S:	Perpendicular to floor	
			M:	Across the distal radius and ulna on the dorsal surface	
			EP:	Forearm rotated so that palm faces down	
			Beware:	Abduction and internal rotation of shoulder	
			(2) TP:	Humerus adducted, elbow flexed to 90°, forearm in midposition with subject holding pencil in closed fist with the pencil protruding from the radial side of the hand	
			A:	Head of the third metacarpal, which coincides with the long axis of the forearm	
			S:	Perpendicular to floor	
			M:	Parallel to pencil	
			EP:	Forearm rotated so that palm faces down; the pencil is still held tightly	
			Beware:	Movement of pencil, wrist flexion or deviation, abduction and internal rotation of shoulder	
Wrist flexion	S	Flexor carpi radialis N: Median Flexor carpi ulnaris N: Ulnar	TP:	Arm at side, elbow flexed, wrist in neutral position, fingers relaxed	0–80°
			A:	Centered at ulnar styloid	
			S:	Parallel to long axis of ulna	
			M:	Parallel to long axis of the fifth metacarpal	
			EP:	Hand moves toward volar forearm to the maximal motion	

TABLE 1—*Continued*

Motion	Plane[a]	Prime movers and Innervation[b]	Goniometer placement[c]		Expected range
Wrist extension	S	Extensor carpi radialis longus N: Radial Extensor carpi radialis brevis N: Radial Extensor carpi ulnaris N: Radial	TP: A: S: M: EP:	Arm at side, elbow flexed, wrist in neutral position, fingers relaxed Centered at ulnar styloid Parallel to long axis of ulna Parallel to long axis of the fifth metacarpal Hand moves toward dorsal forearm to the maximal motion	0–70°
Ulnar deviation	F	Extensor carpi ulnaris N: Radial Flexor carpi ulnaris N: Ulnar	TP: A: S: M: EP: Beware:	Elbow flexed, forearm pronated, wrist in neutral position, fingers relaxed On the dorsal aspect of the wrist joint in line with the base of the third metacarpal Along the midline of the dorsal surface of the forearm Along the midline of the third metacarpal The hand moves to the ulnar side so that the fifth finger approaches the ulnar to the maximal motion Wrist extension and flexion	0–30°
Radial deviation	F	Extensor carpi radialis longus N: Radial Flexor carpi radialis N: Median	TP: A: S: M: EP:	Elbow flexed, forearm pronated, wrist in neutral position, fingers relaxed On the dorsal aspect of the wrist joint in line with the base of the third metacarpal Along the midline of the dorsal surface of the forearm Along the midline of the third metacarpal The hand moves to the radial side so that the thumb approaches the radius to maximal motion	0–20°
MP extension and flexion	S	Flexion: Interossei N: Ulnar Extension:	TP: A: S:	Wrist in neutral position, MP to be tested is held at 0° (extension) Centered over the MP joint On the dorsal surface along the midline of the metacarpal of the finger being tested	0–100°

TABLE 1—*Continued*

Motion	Plane[a]	Prime movers and Innervation[b]	Goniometer placement[c]	Expected range
		Extensor digitorum communis N: Radial Extensor indicis proprius N: Radial Extensor digiti quinti N: Radial	M: On the dorsal surface along the midline of the proximal phalanx EP: The volar surface of the proximal phalanx approaches the palm to the maximal motion	
PIP extension-flexion	S	Flexion: Flexor digitorum sublimis N: Median Extension: Lumbricales N: Median, ulnar Interossei N: Ulnar Extensor digitorum N: Radial	TP: Wrist in neutral position; PIP to be tested is held at 0° (extension) A: Centered over the PIP joint S: On the dorsal surface along the midline of the proximal phalanx of the finger being tested M: On the dorsal surface along the midline of the middle phalanx EP: The volar surface of the middle phalanx approaches the volar surface of the proximal phalanx to maximal motion	0–90°
DIP extension-flexion	S	Flexion: Flexor digitorum profundus N: Ulnar and median Extension: Lumbricales N: Median ulnar	TP: Wrist in neutral position; DIP to be tested is held at 0° (extension) A: Centered over the DIP joint S: On the dorsal surface along the midline of the middle phalanx of the finger being tested M: On the dorsal surface along the midline of the distal phalanx EP: The volar surface of the distal phalanx approaches the volar surface of the middle phalanx to maximal motion	0–90°
Thumb MP extension flexion	F	Flexion: Flexor pollicis brevis N: Median (lateral portion) N: Ulnar (medial portion) Extension: Extensor pollicis brevis N: Radial	TP: Hand in neutral position; MP joint is held in extension A: On the dorsal aspect of the MP joint S: On the dorsal surface along the midline of the first metacarpal M: On the dorsal surface along the midline of the proximal phalanx of the thumb EP: The thumb moves across the palm toward ulnar side of the hand to the maximal motion	0–50°

TABLE 1—*Continued*

Motion	Plane[a]	Prime movers and Innervation[b]	Goniometer placement[c]		Expected range
Thumb IP extension-flexion	F	Flexion: Flexor pollicis longus N: Median Extension: Extensor pollicis longus N: Radial	TP: A: S: M: EP:	Wrist in neutral position; IP joint is held in extension On the dorsal aspect of the IP joint On the dorsal surface along the proximal phalanx On the dorsal surface along the distal phalanx The volar surface of the distal phalanx approaches the volar surface of the proximal phalanx to the maximal motion	0–90°

Sensory System Structure and Function

3

Elsi Dicmonas

The senses are the means by which the brain is informed of events and processes that are happening in the environment and within the body. Understanding the intricacies of sensory dysfunctions depends on knowledge of the anatomic organization and functional relationships of the structures within the sensory systems.

FRAMEWORK FOR ANALYSIS

The various sensory systems convey to the brain visual, auditory, gustatory, and olfactory information. The somesthetic sensations convey bodily experiences such as touch, pressure, pain, temperature, head and body positions, and movements. The various sensory systems have similar structural organizations and operate basically through the same functional processes. Thus each of these systems can be studied by means of the approach outlined in the following sections. As one studies and analyzes the sensory systems and compares their structures and functions, it becomes obvious that the outstanding phenomena of the substructures of the sensory systems are the functions of detecting and extracting informational features. With these functions the peripheral and central nervous systems are able to receive, analyze, synthesize, code, store, and retrieve a multitude of environmental and internal signal-impulse activities without crisscrossing, blurring, or confusing simultaneous and successive sensory information of various characteristics derived from various sensory systems.

STRUCTURES AND THEIR FUNCTIONS

Structures Contributing to Signal Transmission

Receptors and Modality Specificity

Receptor structure and neurophysiological activity may differ from one sensory receptor to another, but the overall function remains the same for each sensory system. Receptors are sensory end-organs that function as minute transducers that convert stimulus into energy that has specific characteristics (1,2). Each of these complex structures is highly sensitive to only one type of stimulus application, either physical or chemical in nature (3). The sensitivity lies in the receptor's lowest level or threshold level at which a stimulus is recognized. Surrounding receptors of different morphologies may also be acted on by the same stimulus, but their thresholds for the particular stimulus may be too high to permit triggering of receptor activity. Each type of stimulus that conveys specific sensory information is called a modality (4). Thus the sensory system, through its receptors' various sensitivities to stimuli, can detect the modality specificity of the various environmental and internal information.

For each sensory stimulus characteristic or modality, a chemical or physical signal composition is generated, called the receptor potential (5). This, in turn, generates an action potential at the nerve endings of those fibers sensitive to the characteristics of the particular stimulus-impulse composition.

Neurons and Sensory Pathways

In addition to the feature detection capability, the structural organization of the sensory system allows for spatial detection of stimulus application or the localization specificity of stimulus application. The receptor area, its related pathways over which sensory information travels, and the corresponding cortical area are topographically organized. This means that there is a point-to-point relationship and physical continuity from the receptor area of a particular body part to the cortex that represents that body area.

Signals travel within the sensory pathway over several synaptic junctions, the connections of neurons that are the substructures of the sensory pathway. These neurons are numbered in sequential order: first-order neurons (1° neurons), second-order neurons, third-order neurons, etc. Their axons, combined in a bundle, are sometimes called tracts; again, they are numbered as 1° tracts, 2° tracts, etc. At each neuronal interconnection or synaptic junction, sensory impulses are analyzed, modified, and converged with related signals or diverged. In addition, collateral fibers emerge from sensory pathways to convey information to subcortical integration and modulation centers such as the cerebellum, reticular formation, cranial nuclei, and thalamus. Regardless of these interneuronal connections and signal modulation processes, the precise signal flow remains intact from the point of origin to the cortical innervation. This point-to-point signal transmission continuity accounts for the ability to localize the stimulus application. Two-point discrimination, double-tactile recognition, and finger identification and its related activities such as typing, playing instruments, and reading braille are all activities and experiences that are dependent on the intactness of localization of sensory stimuli. When studying the directions of pathways, it is helpful to be aware of the neighboring structures of other nervous systems and the source of blood supply to a regional anatomic area through which a sensory pathway passes as it ascends to the cortex. This knowledge will assist the clinician in understanding symptom constellations of diseases or injuries.

Primary Cortex

It will be remembered from neuroanatomy lectures that the cortices reflect a morphological organization of six horizontal layers. These layers are the stratification of interrelated cortical cells that are vertically aligned to form cell columns (6,7). Every sensory cortex is composed of three fields of sensory interpretation functions. The primary cortex or interpretation field contains innumerable vertical cell columns, each of which responds only to one specific sensory signal composition that carries messages of single characteristics of environmental events or bodily experiences (e.g., in the visual cortex, a cell column may be sensitive only to signals representing a 1-inch vertical line). The cell columns that interpret one small detail of one sensory modality are called simple cell columns and are the functional units of the primary cortex. Knowledge of the theory of cell column specificity is helpful in observing and evaluating performance as a patient relates sensorily and perceptually to the environment.

Signal Modification and Feedback Control

We are bombarded continuously by innumerable sensory stimuli from the environment and from within. We are able to ignore most of them and give selective attention to those sensory events that are important for achieving our goals. The ability to deal with the competing foreground-background sensory infringement (called by clinicians figure-ground perception) is not necessarily dependent on willpower or self-control and attention span. The ability to disregard or tune down certain groups of sensory stimuli and simultaneously recognize other types of sensory information is dependent on neuronal mechanisms that are responsible for signal modification at the receptor level and at every neuronal junction (synapse) over which the impulses travel. Not only are the sensory impulses modulated before they reach the sensory cortex, but also certain pathways give off collateral information to the reticular formation and other subcortical structures. These structures alert and inform the cortex of the incoming sensory information composition.

Cortical Afferentation

The intrasensory cortex (in the somatosensory system, the motor cortex) in turn sends impulses through its centrifugal fibers to those sensory substructures (nuclei, synapses, receptor fields) that act as signal transducers and/or signal modulators. Hence the sensory signal modification system works through a feedback loop mechanism. In the receptor field, the impulse modulation occurs in the form of lateral inhibition (8). On stimulus application, the surrounding receptors are inhibited from simultaneous stimulus-impulse transduction. Therefore, the activity of the facilitated receptor can be perceived as a distinct sensory modality, and the site of the stimulus application can be localized.

Another sensory modulation mechanism was described by Elliott (9): the approach of drowning out painful sensations on stumps (neuromas) by superimposing pressure (tapping) on the area. This procedure, it is assumed, activates the larger and faster-conducting A fibers, which in turn inhibit the slower-conducting C fibers that mediate pain and temperature sensation. This approach of stimulus-impulse modification at the receptor level is applied by the therapist in the form of sensory desensitization; the stimulus modulator, besides tapping, can be brushing, rubbing, or vibration.

Sensory modulation, according to Elliott (9), may also occur through relegation of an unpleasant sensory experience to the subconscious level by drawing the attention of the patient to other, perhaps more pleasurable, stimuli. This emphasizes the neurophysiological value of diversional occupational therapy.

As mentioned earlier, morphological structures, the centrifugal fibers, have been found to originate in the cortices and extend to nuclei in the brainstem and spinal cord, as well as to the dorsal horn, in which sensory synaptic junctions of the somatosensory system lie (9–11).

This knowledge, combined with an understanding of sensory signal modification, "gate control" mechanisms (12), functioning at various levels along the signal transmission path and the signal interpretation area (cortex), helps give an appreciation of the underlying causes of such processes as hyperesthesia, tactile defensiveness, referred pain, seizure-proneness to certain sensory stimulation, inability to precisely localize stimulus application.

Sensory-Motor Integration

Reticulothalamic feedback loops are corticofugal fibers projecting from most cortices to the thalamus and activating the reticular formation. Nuclei of these subcortical structures project reciprocal fibers to almost all cortical areas. Multisensory feedforward and feedback information is analyzed and integrated in these nuclei, and the "result" is relayed to cortical and subcortical motor control centers, which in turn modulate the motor signal outflow. This reciprocal cortical-subcortical exchange of information is the underlying mechanism for precise coordinated movements while interacting with the environment (13,14).

Corticostriate and corticopontine fibers project to the basal ganglia and the cerebellum, respectively. These fibers originate from motor cortices as well as from sensory cortices. Without these sensory feedback control mechanisms, our movements would be clumsy and uncoordinated, a symptom that is described clinically as sensory ataxia.

Cortices project centrifugal fibers to the hippocampus and limbic system. These structures contribute to modulation of the emotional state with respect to sensory experiences. This accounts for individual differences in sensitivity to stimuli, especially those for kinesthetic, tactile, and pain sensations (15).

Intrasensory and intersensory motor coordination is achieved through corticofugal fibers of specific sensory systems. These fibers relay signals to nuclei of the brainstem that coordinate motor activity in conjunction with and in response to specific sensory information. The following description is an example of an important cortical-subcortical sensory-motor coordination feedback loop: Efferent fibers project from the visual primary and association cortex to the superior colliculi, which coordinate and integrate unilateral and bilateral oculomotor activities of the related cranial nerves. The colliculi also receive corticofugal fibers from the frontal eye field. Through this feedback loop, the individual moves the eyes on verbal command and inhibits these movements in response to visual stimuli not pertinent to an activity. Visual cortical fibers project to the cerebellum via corticopontine fibers (16).

Secondary and Tertiary Analysis and Synthesis

Association Areas

The various sensory association areas border the primary sensory cortex. Certain areas are demarcated by sulci or are described as areas of gyri.

The functional units are the complex cell columns, also vertically arranged. These receive axons from several simple cell columns of the corresponding primary cortex. Thus isolated information bits converge on a complex cell column, which synthesizes these information bits to a whole, a gestalt of an environmental or internal experience (17). Through this integrative function of these complex cell columns, one can recognize and differentiate objects, space, and events such as music and language. The cell columns of secondary interpretation fields integrate mainly intrasensory information. The tertiary interpretation field receives its fibers from the primary and the secondary sensory fields. Its cells are hypercomplex and are capable of interpreting and integrating a multitude of intrasensory and intersensory modalities, e.g., objects of various shapes and colors. This understanding of sensory functions at various levels of complexity enables the clinician to analyze and evaluate the patient's level of sensory perception and integration. The patient's strategies of performance when dealing with environmental information and the verbalization of the procedures by which the patient attempts to deal with the various characteristics of events and objects will reveal to the evaluator the degree of recognition of single characteristics of sensory events and the ability to deal with the totality of multisensory information that characterizes events and objects. The perception of part-part interrelatedness, as well as part-whole relationships of objects and events (even if their reference points of form and orientation change), reflects the intactness of the hierarchical information exchange between primary, secondary, and tertiary cortical interpretation fields. This exchange is mediated through the association fibers, which are dendrites and axons of interneuronal cells of the primary, secondary, and tertiary sensory cortices.

Intrahemispheric Connections

Association fibers exchange information between association areas of neighboring sensory systems, thus contributing to multisensory perception and integration (e.g., integration of visual-tactile sensory experiences starts earlier in a child's development than does visual-auditory integration). When a child is ready for learning speech, occipitotemporal sensory integration will develop; with progressing growth and maturation, visual-tactile integration and sensory awareness will be subordinated to subconscious experiences.

Association fibers connect the various sensory cortices and the motor cortex of the same hemisphere. These association fibers account for eye-hand coordination, movement to music, and the kinesthetic motor function imperative to coordinated postural and unilateral limb movements (18).

Interhemispheric Connections

All cortices receive association fibers from the prefrontal cortex. Cognition is the initiating and guiding force for successful performance of all of our life tasks, each of which requires selective specific sensory-perceptual-motor function (19).

The primary sensory cortices do not exchange information through the interconnecting commissures; however, there are morphological connections between the bilateral visual association areas. It is this evidence of interhemispheric exchange of visual information that should encourage the therapist to use functional activities for brain-damaged patients, even if only the noninvolved extremity can be used. There is no sensory information exchange occurring for the two hands; the right hand does not know what the left is doing, from a neurophysiological point of view. Much has been written about the functional phenomena of the bisected brain (20,21).

Interhemispheric sensory-motor connections are related to visual motor tasks. The fibers of the corpus callosum provide for sensory-motor signal transmission between the two hemispheres. Patients with left-hand dominance are extremely dependent on this interhemispheric exchange of sensory-motor information when engaged in skills that require simultaneous use of language or its representation and motor performance (e.g., visual motor tasks of writing and other visual motor activities that depend on verbal instruction). A left-handed person functions through the integration of both visual cortices, the left temporal lobe for language processing and the right somatesthetic and motor cortices for control of hand activity. Since there is no known commissural fiber connection for cortical sensory-motor hand representation, interhemispheric information exchange occurs through a network of reticulo thalamic and other subcortical feedback loops and the sensory perceptual integrative centers of the overlapping occipital-parietal-temporal association areas (Brodmann's areas 39 and 40 in the supramarginal and angular gyri) (22–25). This background information is very important when training a patient in nondominant left-handed writing following a cerebrovascular accident in the left hemisphere, especially if the thalamus is also involved.

Commissural fibers contribute to motor coordination for bilateral rhythmic or complementary movements and integration of postural movements and controls, as well as oculomotor control. These control mechanisms of integration of the two body halves contribute to the development of laterality, directionality, and space perception through space-related kinesthetic feedback of movement patterns that cross body midlines or lead away from either body half (26).

Interhemispheric transmission of information regarding the activities of the two hemispheres that enables the brain to establish bilateral memory traces (27) is very important for bilateral representation of cognitive-sensory-perceptual-motor engrams of previously learned functional movements. This accounts for the ease with which a patient can perform gross motor activities with the nondominant extremity but cannot easily accomplish fine movement coordination with the hand that had not been trained to do the task, since there is only interhemispheric information exchange from the somatosensory-motor cortices representing the limb parts proximal to the foot and hand.

Effector System and Adaptive Responses

Every major sensory system has its own effector system that modulates sensory signals before they reach the cortex that is to analyze and synthesize sensory information. The signal modulation processes are very important to the development and continuous functioning of the highest order of sensation: perception. Centrifugal fibers from the sensory cortices make connections with structures of the brainstem and spinal cord for the purpose of directly or indirectly affecting signal transmission by influencing presynaptic and postsynaptic activities of the ordered neurons that constitute a particular sensory pathway. Cortical motor controls also influence the receptor fields contributing to the phenomenon of lateral inhibition.

It is interesting that the sensory systems use motor responses through intrasensory and intersensory motor feedback loops for modulating the amplitude and frequency of signal transmission. The visual system, through centrifugal fibers to autonomic nervous system nuclei, facilitates smooth-muscle activity to control pupil dilation and constriction and lens accommodation. In addition, centrifugal fibers synapse bilaterally with the superior colliculi, which in turn coordinate the oculomotor nuclei activity for bilateral focusing and convergence of eye muscles. This assures integration of the anteroposterior signal projection from the bilateral retinal field to the visual cortex.

The auditory system uses the motor activity of two small skeletal muscles (the tensor tympani, innervated by the trigeminal nerve, and the stapedius, innervated by the facial nerve) for signal modulation. These muscles control the vibration of ossicles, and they, in turn, control the tympanic membrane for the purpose of influencing the amplitude and frequency of auditory signal transmission. This is an example of how additional sensory-motor systems are used for quality control of signal transmission and hence precision of sensory perceptual experiences.

The somatosensory system sends its signal control impulses to the topographically related motor cortex area, which transmits signals through centrifugal fibers running along the pyramidal tract to the synaptic junctions of the somatosensory neurons of the dorsal column and the spinothalamic tract. These motor impulses facilitate or inhibit presynaptic or postsynaptic activity, as well as the receptor field signal transduction, through lateral inhibition. The signal modulation in this sensory system occurs contralaterally.

In summary, precision of stimulus-impulse generation, signal transmission, and analysis, synthesis, and intrasensory and intersensory integration is a prerequisite to successful functioning in the environment, for adaptation and accommodation to life situations through precise coordinated environment-oriented motor responses. One can plan these responses appropriately only if the innumerable varieties of environmental signals are perceived accurately. Therefore, motor planning and motor performance are intrinsically dependent on the function of every substrata of each sensory system and the information exchange and integration of the various sensory systems' activities. Feedforward and feedback of information play equal roles in the achievement of smooth coordinated movements. Intrahemispheric and interhemispheric sensory-motor signal processing is necessary for both unilateral and bilateral movement coordination (e.g., visual motor tasks require simultaneous bilateral and contralateral sensory-motor integration of cortical and subcortical activities, whereas kinesthetic tactile tasks depend on contralateral signal processing). Both variations of sensory-motor task performances are neurophysiologically mediated through structures and functions located along and within the longitudinal axis (midline) of the brain. The blood supply to this area derives mainly from the vertebral-basilar artery circulatory system. The occipital lobe and the vestibulo-cerebellar integrative system receive their blood supply from this source. The laterally and anteriorly situated cortices and the reticulothalamocortical fiber connections depend on the supply from the carotid arteries.

From an analysis of the organization of the sensory systems and their structural and functional relationships it can be seen that the precision of sensory perceptual function is dependent on the integrity of motor systems. Sensory-motor interdependence is reflected in environment-oriented movement performance and its consequent sensory feedback. Motor systems contribute directly to the experiences of modality specificity and stimulus localization specificity that are the results of the feature detection and feature extraction functions of the sensory systems' substructures. The functional reciprocity of the sensory and motor systems is the neurophysiological substratum to movement coordination and integration. Guyton described this sensory-motor interdependence (28): "There is no known mechanism by which the motor cortex can conceive the entire sequential pattern that is to be achieved by the motor movements. . . . Therefore, we are left with an unanswered question: What is the locus of the initiation of voluntary motor activity? . . . We will learn that the reticular formation of the brainstem and much of the thalamus play essential roles in activating all other parts of the brain. Therefore, it is very likely that these areas provide the initial signals that lead to subsequent activity in the motor cortex, basal ganglia, and the cerebellum at the onset of voluntary movement. Here again, we come to circular question: What is it that initiates the activity in the brainstem and the thalamus? We do know part of the answer to this: The activity is initiated by continual sensory input into these areas, including input from the peripheral receptors from the body and from the cortical sensory storage, or memory, areas. Much of motor activity is almost reflex in nature, occurring instantly after an incoming sensory signal from the periphery. But so-called voluntary activity occurs minutes, hours, or even days after the initiating sensory input—after analysis, storage of memories, recall of the memories, and finally initiation of a motor response. . . . The control of motor activity is strongly influenced by these prolonged procedures of cerebration. Furthermore, damage to the essential areas of the cerebral cortex for analysis of sensory information leads to serious deficits and abnormalities of voluntary muscle control."

SOMATIC SENSATIONS

Somatic sensation refers to the sensory information that arises from the body (soma), its walls, deep structures, and limbs.

Classifications of Somatic Sensations

A brief listing of various classifications will be given to illustrate the many frames of references from which receptor characteristics and sensory experiences can be analyzed. Note that some descriptions of receptors and sensations may be grouped under several classifications.

Conscious and Unconscious Sensory Experiences

Sensory classification can refer to the level of awareness at which one experiences sensations: (a) Two sensations that are not consciously experienced are those from muscle spindles and Golgi tendon organs. They are analyzed and integrated with the structures of the motor control system on the subcortical level. (b) Conscious sensations are those that are processed, analyzed, synthesized, coded, and stored cortically. Usually, types of sensations that one becomes aware of and hence that can be evaluated are clinically referred to as being of the sensory modality.

Clinical Classifications

Sensations can be grouped according to the depth of their receptor sites within the body wall: (a) superficial sensations: light touch, temperature, pain, cutaneous vibration sensation; (b) deep sensations: pressure, pain from muscles, joints, and internal organs, position and movement sensation, vibration from bony structures.

Sensations may be classified with respect to their sites within body organs: (a) cutaneous sensation; (b) visceral sensations of internal organs, such as pain, pressure, hunger, thirst, and nausea.

Sensations may be classified with reference to the subjective experience that one encounters: (a) Diffuse sensations: dull pain, aches, pressure or touch from clothing, the touch of another's hand. These sensations are often linked with an emotional state: a warm feeling, a cold shoulder, a frightening experience causing cramps in the stomach. These diffuse types of sensations have been described as protopathic sensations (29). They are to a great extent preanalyzed in the thalamus. Therefore it is assumed that these sensations are common to most animal species and have developed phylogenetically. (b) Localized discriminatory sensations. Their characteristics are well differentiated and specific and are precisely localized, especially in the hand and face. These specific sensations have been called epicritic experiences. They account for the ability to identify objects by touch (stereognosis), the experience of graphesthesia, double tactile localization, laterality, and other intersensory perceptions. Epicritic sensations are developed in higher species and require cortical processing. They make modality specificity and localization specificity possible.

Sensations may be classified according to their pathways. Clinicians often speak of dorsal column sensations as opposed to spinothalamic sensations. They group these sensations in reference to the signal transmission patterns and the pathways over which their impulses travel. There are structural and functional relationships of pathways and the sensory experiences described previously that are mediated through these two major sensory pathways: (a) Dorsal column sensations are epicritic discriminatory sensations. (b) The spinothalamic sensations are the protopathic diffuse sensory experiences.

Sensations may be classified with respect to type and distribution of receptors: (a) General sensations are those whose receptors are distributed all over the body: pain, pressure, joint receptors, etc. (b) Special sensations are experienced through only one kind of receptor located in one specific area: vision, hearing, taste, smell, equilibrium.

Classifications of Receptors

Functional Classification

Receptors are sensory end-organs that have the ability to detect the characteristics of stimuli and extract their neurophysical and neurochemical properties for the purpose of producing an electrical signal, an impulse. The types of features or modalities these receptors can detect are (a) light touch or tactile sensation, (b) deep touch or pressure sensation, (c) pain sensation, (d) temperature sensation, (e) kinesthetic (proprioceptive) sensation, and (f) vibration sensation.

Morphological Classification

There are three morphological types of receptors: free ending types, those with encapsulated tips, and encapsulated organs. Some examples from among these types are as follows: (a) Meissner's corpuscles identify touch sensation. (b) Ruffini's end-organs recognize differences in warmth. (c) Krause's end-bulbs detect differences in cold sensation. (d) Pacini's corpuscles are sensitive to pressure application. (e) Golgi tendon organs recognize stretch of muscle-tendon fibers. (f) Muscle spindles are sensitive to length distortion of spindle fibers, as well as the velocity at which the length is being distorted.

Sensitivity Classification

Receptors may be classified with regard to sensitivity to stimulus characteristics: (a) Mechanoreceptors: A physical event that deforms the tissue is the stimulus (touch, pressure, pain, equilibrium). (b) Thermoreceptors: Sensitive to degrees of temperature levels. (c) Chemoreceptors: Chemical changes surrounding the receptor field cause the formation of a receptor potential (smell, taste). (d) Electromagnetic receptors: Rods and cones of the retina. (e) Nocireceptors: Sensitive to either physical or chemical distortion of tissue, producing pain.

Origin or Site Classification

Receptors may be classified according to origin or site of stimulus: (a) Telereceptors: Stimuli originate at a distance from the body (light rays, sound waves, smell). (b) Exteroceptors: Stimuli are applied to the exterior of the body wall (pain, touch, temperature). (c) Proprioceptors: Stimuli originate within the body and give information on the positions of body parts in space (kinesthesia, which includes position and motion sense, equilibrium). (d) Interoceptors: Stimuli are within the body cavity (internal organs, internal body walls).

SENSORY EVALUATION

Knowledge Required

The therapist must know the following: structures and functions of the various sensory systems; the importance of sensory function to performance; the terminology of sensory irritations and deficits; symptoms related to lesions of the peripheral nervous system; symptoms related to lesions of the central nervous system (CNS): (a) spinal cord lesions involving the dorsal funiculi, gray horn, central gray matter surrounding the spinal canal, or anterlateral funiculi; (b) supraspinal lesions (brainstem and somatosensory cortex) involving the medulla, pons, mesencephalon, thalamus internal capsule, or sensory-motor cortex; symptom clusters related to lesions of regional areas of the CNS; variations of blood supply to regional areas.

The therapist must know evaluation techniques specific to diagnoses of peripheral nerve lesions (peripheral nerve distribution pattern), dorsal root and spinal cord lesions (segmental dermatomal distribution), and supraspinal lesions (dissociated modality specificity pattern in the brainstem and body part representation in the cortex).

The therapist must be able to deduce from observations and evaluation data the deficiencies within other functional systems whose structures are located in the area of a lesion.

Principles

Sensory testing must be appropriate to the patient's level of functioning. In order to achieve reliable results, it is most important that the therapist be able to communicate with the patient through verbal or nonverbal language. Therefore, it is essential that the patient be alert and be able to communicate and understand instructions. Children less than 4 years of age cannot be reliably tested for sensation.

Individual differences in sensitivity to stimulus application are related to the intellectual ability and emotional state of the patient: (a) tolerance to stimulus application, (b) attention span, (c) the need to conform, (d) ability to follow instructions. The therapist must take into consideration the fact that data from sensory evaluation are responses to the patient's subjective experiences, conveying to the therapist what the patient feels, making distinctions in degrees of stimulus intensity, and identifying the location of stimulus application. The analytical process takes place on the cortical level.

Individual differences in sensory experiences are related to life-styles and age; possible variations in "normal limits" are related to the aging process, to life-style, and to vocational experiences.

Variations in responses may be related to secondary diagnoses of which the patient may not be aware (e.g., median nerve injury with a wrist fracture, spinal spondylosis and diabetes).

The therapist must determine the relationship of sensory impairment to motor control dysfunction. The therapist must differentiate causes of decreased muscle strength, atrophy, and incoordination and must be aware that sensory deficiencies can lead to decreased muscle tone "recruitment" because of lack of sensory feedforward that results normally from proprioceptors of joints, muscles, fascia, and stretched skin. Incoordination can be caused by sensory ataxia because of lack of proprioceptive feedback during movements.

There are some factors to be considered in evaluating sensations with various involvements of substructures of the somatosensory pathway and cortex.

Peripheral Nerves

It is suggested that patients be tested with limbs in anatomic positions so that the peripheral nerve distribution pattern can be easily identified. Stimulus should be applied over the smallest receptor field possible to prevent spread of stimulus application to surrounding receptors. Therefore, for testing fine tactile sensation, a fine sable brush should be used, applied as lightly as possible. For testing deep pressure, the head of a straight pin should be used to achieve the best possible localization specificity response. In comparing deep pressure sensation and pain sensation, it is advisable to alternate the tip and head of the pin.

It is preferable to test all modalities, despite the fact that a peripheral nerve is a mixed nerve fiber bundle that transmits all modalities to the CNS. Patients diagnosed as having neuropathies, neuritis, or injured nerves in a state of regeneration may have symptoms of (a) irritations (paresthesia, which may be hypersensitivity to one or another sensory modality, e.g., hyperalgesia) or (b) deficiencies (giving evidence of impairment of threshold values to stimulus application, so that the patient may not perceive light tactile sensation but will clearly experience stronger stimuli such as pressure or pain).

Dorsal Root and Spinal Cord

Extremities should be in anatomic positions during testing so that the dermatomal distribution pattern can be easily identified.

Dorsal Root Ganglion. The symptoms of dorsal root involvement are as follows: Dorsal root ganglion: All modalities are involved. Dorsal root: (a) Irritative symptoms are caused by traction compression, inflammation, extramedullary tumors, and fiber injury. The patient may experience the following: (a) root pain (radicular pain), with spreading of symptoms over the dermatome belonging to the affected root; (b) paresthesias (sensations of numbness, pricking, tingling, especially burning) and other peculiar sensory experiences; (c) hyperesthesias (very low threshold of pain). The deficiencies are losses of all modalities, with destruction of dorsal root fibers.

Dissociated sensory impairment gives indication of lesions in the spinal cord and brainstem; this is because on entering the spinal cord, the fibers separate, and the impulses conveyed by them take different courses up to the thalamus.

Overlappings of dermatomes differ for the various modalities. Fibers of pain sensation, on entering the spinal cord, ascend by spanning over one segment above the entry level, whereas the other modalities span over two to three levels. This accounts for the overlapping of dermatomes and their variations in the distribution pattern. Pain sensation is most likely confined to one dermatome. Therefore, to determine the level of lesion through sensory evaluation, one must carefully observe pain experiences with respect to the dermatomal distribution pattern.

Groups of sensory modalities must be tested in reference to the funiculi (tracts) in which they are ascending; this is important for differential diagnosis and precautions to be considered with loss of pain and temperature sensations, as well as treatment approaches in reference to loss of kinesthetic, tactile, and pressure sensations.

The site of the sensory impairment is related to the level of crossing of fibers within the spinal cord and brainstem. In the posterior column (dorsal funiculi), the fibers ascend ipsilaterally and do not cross before the medulla. Therefore, symptoms of sensory involvement will occur on the same side of the body where the lesion is located, with involvement of tactile, deep pressure, proprioceptive, and vibration sensations.

Dorsal Horn. Fibers of the anterolateral funiculi or anterolateral spinothalamic tract come from the dorsal root and enter the dorsal horn, synapse with interneurons, and cross in front of the central canal to the contralateral side of the spinal cord entry before they ascend in the spinothalamic tract. Lesions of the dorsal horn show ipsilateral symptoms of loss of pain and temperature sensations (modalities mediated via the spinothalamic tract). The area around the central canal causes bilateral symptoms, since fibers from both sides of the spinal cord (dorsal horn) overlap while crossing in front of the canal. Lesions within the spinothalamic tract cause contralateral symptoms. These fibers ascend on the contralateral side up to the cortex. Therefore, loss of pain and temperature sensations related to lesions of the spinal cord, brainstem, thalamus, internal capsule, and somatosensory cortex can be identified on the contralateral side of the body.

Medulla

Nuclei Gracilis and Cuneatus. The fibers of the dorsal columns (epicritic, discriminative) synapse in the nuclei gracilis and cuneatus, where signals are modulated through the motor fibers from the sensory-motor cortex. The axons of these nuclei extend to the medial lemniscus in the middle brainstem, where they cross to the opposite of the medial longitudinal fasciculus. A lesion caudal to the decussation causes ipsilateral deficiencies of epicritic sensations and contralateral deficiencies of pain and temperature sensations.

A lesion of the vertebral artery or its branches can produce the following symptoms because of dysfunction of cranial nerves and other structures (a) vagus nerve (X) motor dysfunction of swallowing, dysphonia, and other impairment of pharynx and larynx; (b) cranial nerves XII, XI, and IX contributing to dysfunctions of the tongue, neck muscles, pharynx, and larynx; (c) olivocerebellar fibers and vestibular substructures causing motor ataxia and equilibrium dysfunction; (d) sensory dysfunctions of the lower part of the face caused by descending trigeminal peripheral fibers.

Upper Medulla and Pons. There will be contralateral sensory impairment of all modalities or bilateral epicritic sensory impairment if the lesion is small and confined around the brainstem midline. Associated symptoms may include the following: (a) cranial nerve involvement of VI (abducens), V (trigeminal), and VII (facial) (facial paralysis, facial sensory involvement, and impairment of lateral gaze are ipsilateral if the lesion is affecting the peripheral fibers of these cranial nuclei); (b) ataxia caused by lesions of the pontocerebellar fibers; (c) diplopia (optic radiation fibers sweep around the fourth ventricle). Hyperpathias that may occur with lesions of the medulla include hypersensitivity to application of pain stimulus (painful sensation lasts long after stimulus has been removed). The causes of these impairments may include vascular accidents of the basilar artery and its branches, as well as tumors.

Mesencephalon

Symptoms of sensory impairment usually involve all modalities contralaterally by hyperesthesia caused by lack of sensory input modulation through corticofugal fibers. Associated symptoms include (a) oculomotor impairment (III and IV cranial nerves); (b) hyperkinesia caused by impairment of the nuclei of basal ganglia, substantia nigra, and/or red nucleus and impaired reticular formation function. The blood supply is from the basilar artery and its branches (posterior cerebral artery).

Thalamus

The therapist should evaluate the patient's body parts with respect to their thalamic and cortical representation (face, hands, forearms, arms, etc.), testing all modalities. Although all fibers of the somatosensory pathways terminate in the ventral-posterior-lateral (VPL) thalamic nuclei and maintain their topographic representations, the structures are anatomically so closely confined within a small space that lesions in the area may not spare the sensations of specific areas of the body segments. Therefore, a lesion in this area leads to loss of localization specificity. Because of the spreading of diffuse pain sensation, the patient may not be able to distinguish sensory modalities or localize the stimulus application precisely. There is intense hypersensitivity to any stimulus application. Pain continues after removal of the stimulus. Intense pain may also appear spontaneously, without peripheral facilitation. Recovery usually remains incomplete. The patient may regain diffuse tactile, temperature, and pain sensations, but will not regain discriminative sensations (these need cortical analysis and synthesis for appreciation).

Internal Capsule

The symptoms of sensory impairment are contralateral losses of all modalities. Associated symptoms may include hemianopsia contralaterally; the optic radiation fibers intermingle with fibers of the posterior limb of the internal capsule. With lesion of this brain structure, the fibers of the optic tract may also be damaged.

Sensory-Motor Cortex

The postcentral gyrus of each hemisphere receives all somatosensory fibers originating from every body part contralateral to the hemisphere in which these body segments are represented. Deficits of sensory modalities, especially discriminative sensations, are caused by lesions in the cortex (protopathic sensations of pain, temperature, and crude touch are analyzed and synthesized preliminarily in the thalamus). This may cause impairment of somatosensory integration and cause a sensory rivalry; e.g., a patient may be able to hold a utensil in the hand, but when the utensil is used, it may fall out of the hand unless the patient gives this hand visual attention (heightening conscious awareness of the goal to be achieved). This lack of synthesis prevents the "chaining" of tactile and kinesthetic sensations that can be experienced as isolated modalities.

Patients may have difficulties in eye-hand coordination because they cannot integrate visual sensation with simultaneous tactile-kinesthetic sensation. Patients may handle tools clumsily when performing tasks and may prefer to close their eyes during performance of known tasks. Coordination improves without visual guidance of movements. Therefore, the incoordination is not caused by apraxia or primary sensory loss but rather by impaired information exchange and/or integration of dual sensory experiences of two adjacent hemispheres. It may also be caused by sensory rivalry between the nonimpaired and the recovering synthesis mechanisms.

As mentioned previously, irritation symptoms and decreased localization specificity may be caused by impairment of the sensory modulation control fibers that send their signals to the synaptic junctions of all neurons in the sensory pathways.

SUMMARY

This framework for analyzing structures and functions of the sensory systems can be used as a guide for the formulation of observation strategies, evaluation principles and techniques, and treatment approaches. The therapist must remember that sensory impairment and perceptual deficits may have various origins: (a) inability to perceive or interpret sensory stimuli; (b) decreased function or inability to transmit impulses over the pathways, so that too little sensory information reaches the cortex; (c) bombardment by sensory noises that cannot be turned off because of malfunction of signal modulation mechanisms of the motor cortex and its subcortical control centers; (d) impairment of the primary sensory cortices, so that specific identifying characteristics of external and internal events are not recognized or are received with distortion; (e) impairment of the intrasensory association fibers because of malfunction in clustering and synthesizing of related sensory information, leading to acquisition of splinter knowledge of environmental objects and events and self; (f) dissociation of functional connections between various sensory systems within one hemisphere and/or lack of information exchange between the two hemispheres, so that bilateral memory traces cannot be established.

By using this background knowledge of the structures and functions of the sensory systems, the therapist can develop the skills necessary for observing and listening to patients' verbal and nonverbal behavior. After all, their responses are the clinical mechanisms by which the therapist collects and verifies data concerning the information skills by which patients perceive themselves and the world around them.

REFERENCES

1. Truex, R. C., and Carpenter M. B. (1969): *Human Neuroanatomy,* ed. 6. Williams & Wilkins, Baltimore, p. 174.
2. Guyton, A. C. (1976): *Organ Physiology, Structure and Function of the Nervous System,* ed. 2. W. B. Saunders, Philadelphia, pp. 88–89.
3. Truex and Carpenter, op. cit., p. 188.
4. Guyton, op. cit., p. 87.
5. Ibid., p. 89.
6. Truex and Carpenter, op. cit., p. 555.
7. Favreau, O. E., and Corballis, M. C. (1976): Negative aftereffects in visual perception. *Sci. Am.* 235:42–48.
8. Guyton, op. cit., pp. 103, 259.
9. Elliott, F. A. (1971): *Clinical Neurology.* W. B. Saunders, Philadelphia, pp. 8–9.
10. Brodal, A. (1969): *Neurological Anatomy in Relation to Clinical Medicine.* Oxford University Press, New York, p. 58.
11. Truex and Carpenter, op. cit., p. 580.
12. Ayres, J. A. (1977): *Sensory Integration and Learning Disorders.* p. 214. Western Psychological Services, Pasadena, California.
13. Truex and Carpenter, op. cit., pp. 577–580.
14. Guyton, op. cit., p. 106.
15. Ayres, op. cit., pp. 49–52, 133.
16. Glickstein, M., and Gibson, A. R. (1976): Visual cells in the pons of the brain. *Sci. Am.* 235:90–98.
17. Brodal, op. cit., p. 477.
18. Ibid., pp. 649–650.
19. Ibid., p. 650.
20. Ibid., pp. 88, 651.
21. Eccles, J. C. (1977): *The Understanding of the Brain,* ed. 2. McGraw-Hill, New York, pp. 209–222.
22. Truex and Carpenter, op. cit., p. 552.
23. Brodal, op. cit., pp. 677–678.
24. Luria, A. K. (1966): *Higher Cortical Functions in Man.* Basic Books, New York, pp. 123–124.
25. Guyton, op. cit., pp. 191–193, 201, 203.
26. Howard, I. P., and Templeton, W. B. (1966): *Human Spatial Orientation.* John Wiley & Sons, New York, Chapter 11.
27. Guyton, op. cit., pp. 196–200, 202–203.
28. Ibid., p. 174.
29. Brodal, op. cit., p. 41.

BIBLIOGRAPHY

Barsch, R. H. (1968): *Achieving Perceptual Motor Efficiency, A Space-oriented Approach to Learning, Vol. 1.* Special Child Publications, Seattle.

Bernstein, B. (1967): *The Coordination and Regulation of Movements.* Pergamon Press, New York.

Bossy, J. (1970): *Atlas of Neuroanatomy and Special Sense Organs.* W. B. Saunders, Philadelphia.

Carpenter, M. B. (1972): *Core Text of Neuroanatomy.* Williams & Wilkins, Baltimore.

Cohen, L. A. (1961): The role of the neck receptors for the maintenance of dynamic body equilibrium. *J. Neurophysiol.* 24:2–11.

Critchley, M. (1953): *The Parietal Lobes.* Arnold, London.

Curtis, B. A. (1972): *An Introduction to Neurosciences.* W. B. Saunders, Philadelphia.

Denny-Brown, D., and Chambers, R. (1958): The parietal lobe and behavior. *Res. Publ. Assoc. Res. Nerv. Ment. Dis.,* 36:35–117.

Denny-Brown, D. (1966): The cerebral control of movements. In: *The Sherrington Lectures VIII.* Charles C. Thomas, Springfield, Ill.

Denny-Brown, D. (1962): The midbrain and motor integration. *Proc. R. Soc. Med.,* 55:527–538.

Escourolle, R. and Poirier, J. (1973): *Manual of Basic Neuropathology.* W. B. Saunders, Philadelphia.

Everett, N. B. (1971): *Functional Neuroanatomy.* Lea & Febiger, Philadelphia.

Ford, D. H., and Schade, J. P. (1967): *Atlas of the Human Brain.* Elsevier, New York.

Ford, D. H., and Schade, J. P. (1973): *Basic Neurology, An Introduction to the Structure and Function of the Nervous System,* ed. 2. Elsevier, New York.

Ganong, W. F. (1965): *Review of Medical Physiology.* Lange Medical Publications, Los Altos, Calif.

Gazzaniga, M. (1970): *The Bisected Brain.* Appleton-Century-Crofts, New York.

Gentile, A. M. (1972): A working model of skill acquisition. Quest XVII monograph.

Gibson, E. J. (1970): The development of perception as adaptive process. *Am. Sci.,* 58:98–107.

Hausman, L. (1961): *Illustrations of Nervous System, Atlas III.* Charles C Thomas, Springfield, Ill.

Hochberg, J. E. (1964): *Perception.* Prentice-Hall, Englewood Cliffs, N.J.

Konorski, J. (1967): *Integrative Activity of the Brain, An Interdisciplinary Approach.* University of Chicago Press, Chicago.

Langworthy, O. (1970): *The Sensory Control of Posture and Movement*. Williams & Wilkins, Baltimore.

Legge, D. (1970): *Skills*. Penguin, Baltimore.

Members of the Department of Neurology, University of Minnesota (1971): *Clinical Examinations in Neurology*. W. B. Saunders, Philadelphia.

Miller, G., Galanter, E., and Pribram, K. H. (1960): *Plans and the Structure of Behavior*. Holt, Rinehart and Winston, New York.

Mysak, E. (1971): *Speech Pathology and Feedback Theory*. Charles C Thomas, Springfield, Ill.

Noback, C. R. (1975): *The Human Nervous System*. McGraw-Hill, New York.

Netter, F. N. (1962): *The Ciba Collection of Medical Illustrations, Vol. 1. Nervous System*. Ciba Pharmaceutical Company, Summit, N.J.

Penfield, W. R. (1959): *Speech and Brain Mechanisms*. Princeton University Press, Princeton, N.J.

Piaget, J. (1963): *The Origin of Intelligence in Children*. W. W. Norton, New York.

Rose, J., and Mountcastle, V. (1959): Touch and kinesthesis. In: *Handbook of Physiology,* edited by J. Field and H. W. Magoun, *Vol. 1*. Field & Magoun, Washington, D.C.

Ruch, T. C., and Patton, H. D. (1966): *Physiology and Biophysics*. W. B. Saunders, Philadelphia.

Somjen, G. (1972): *Sensory Coding in the Mammalian Nervous System*. Appleton-Century-Crofts, New York.

Sperry, R. W. (1974): The great cerebral commissure. *Sci. Am.,* 210:42–57.

Welford, A. T. (1968): *Fundamentals of Skills*. Methuen, London.

SENSORY SYSTEM

KINGSBROOK JEWISH MEDICAL CENTER — DEPARTMENT OF REHABILITATION MEDICINE

EVALUATION of PERIPHERAL SOMATOSENSORY FUNCTION — OCCUPATIONAL THERAPY

Patient's Name ________ Address ________ Telephone ________

Hospital Unit ________ Chart ________ Diagnosis ________

Disability ________ Age ________

Precautions ________

Handedness ________ Date of Onset ________ Date of Prescription ________ / ________

Referring M.D.s ________ Therapist ________

Prescriptions: PT ________ OT ________ Speech ________ EMG ________ Orthotic/prosthetic device ________

RIGHT SIDE

Key:
P = present, I-1 or I-2 = impaired
A = absent

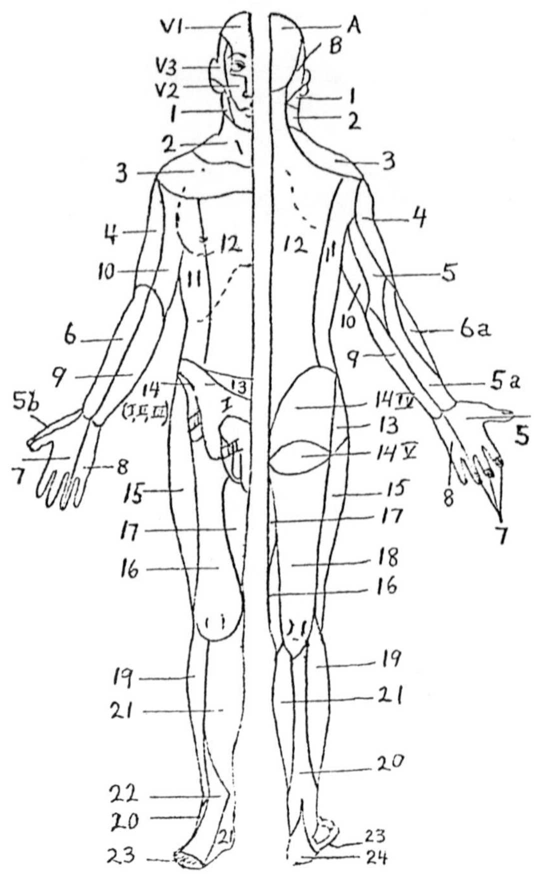

	Anterior Side				Posterior Side			
	LIGHT TOUCH	DEEP TOUCH	TEMP.	PAIN	LIGHT TOUCH	DEEP TOUCH	TEMP.	PAIN
V I Trigeminal					XXXXXXXXXXXXXXXXX			
V II Trigeminal					XXXXXXXXXXXXXXXXX			
V III Trigeminal					XXXXXXXXXXXXXXXXX			
A Greater occipital	XXXXXXXXXXXXXXXXX							
B Lesser occipital	XXXXXXXXXXXXXXXXX							
1 Greater auricular								
2 Transverse colli								
3 Supraclavicular								
4 Axillary								
5 Rad. post. brach. c.	XXXXXXXXXXXXXXXXX							
5a R. dors. antibr. c.	XXXXXXXXXXXXXXXXX							
5b Radial								
6 Musculocutaneous					XXXXXXXXXXXXXXXXX			
6a MuCu. lat. antibr.	XXXXXXXXXXXXXXXXX							
7 Median								
8 Ulnar								
9 Med. antibrach. c.								
10 Med. brach. cut.								
11 Lat. intercost. br.								
12 Med. thoracic nn.								
13 Ilio-hypogastric								
14 I Ilio-inguinal					XXXXXXXXXXXXXXXXX			
14 II Genito-femoral					XXXXXXXXXXXXXXXXX			
14 III Genito-femoral					XXXXXXXXXXXXXXXXX			
14 IV Sup. clunical	XXXXXXXXXXXXXXXXX							
14 V Inf. clunical	XXXXXXXXXXXXXXXXX							
15 Lat. femoral cut.								
16 Ant. cut. femoral								
17 Obturator								
18 Post. cut. femoral	XXXXXXXXXXXXXXXXX							
19 Lat. sural c. peron.								
20 Sural (tibial)								
21 Saphenous, femoral								
22 Superficial peron.					XXXXXXXXXXXXXXXXX			
23 Plantar tibial								
24 Med. calcan. (tibial)								

KINGSBROOK JEWISH MEDICAL CENTER | DEPARTMENT OF REHABILITATION MEDICINE

EVALUATION of PERIPHERAL SOMATOSENSORY FUNCTION | OCCUPATIONAL THERAPY

Patient's Name ______________________ Address ______________________ Telephone __________

Hospital Unit __________ Chart __________ Diagnosis ______________________

Disability ______________________ Age __________

Precautions ______________________

Handedness ______ Date of Onset __________ Date of Prescription __________/__________

Referring M.D.s ______________________ Therapist ______________________

Prescriptions: PT ______ OT ______ Speech ______ EMG ______ Orthotic/prosthetic device __________

LEFT SIDE

Key:
P = present, I-1 or I-2 = impaired
A = absent

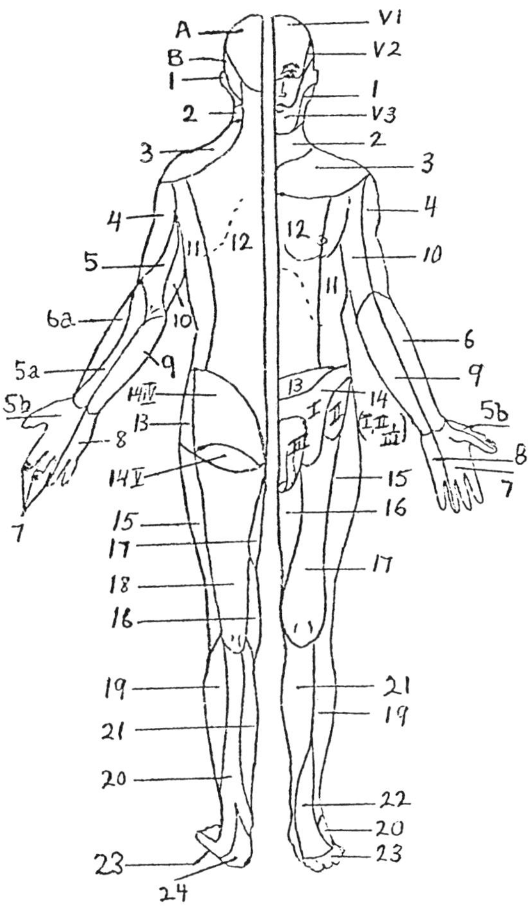

	Posterior Side				Anterior Side			
	LIGHT TOUCH	DEEP TOUCH	TEMP.	PAIN	LIGHT TOUCH	DEEP TOUCH	TEMP.	PAIN
V I Trigeminal	XXXXXXXXXXXXXXXX							
V II Trigeminal	XXXXXXXXXXXXXXXX							
V III Trigeminal	XXXXXXXXXXXXXXXX							
A Greater occipital					XXXXXXXXXXXXXXXX			
B Lesser occipital					XXXXXXXXXXXXXXXX			
1 Greater auricular								
2 Transverse colli								
3 Supraclavicular								
4 Axillary								
5 Rad. post. brach. c.					XXXXXXXXXXXXXXXX			
5a R. dors. antibr. c.					XXXXXXXXXXXXXXXX			
5b Radial								
6 Musculocutaneous	XXXXXXXXXXXXXXXX							
6a MuCu. lat. antibr.					XXXXXXXXXXXXXXXX			
7 Median								
8 Ulnar								
9 Med. antibrach. c.								
10 Med. brach. cut.								
11 Lat. intercost. br.								
12 Med. thoracic nn.								
13 Ilio-hypogastric								
14 I Ilio-inguinal	XXXXXXXXXXXXXXXX							
14 II Genito-femoral	XXXXXXXXXXXXXXXX							
14 III Genito-femoral	XXXXXXXXXXXXXXXX							
14 IV Sup. clunical					XXXXXXXXXXXXXXXX			
14 V Inf. clunical					XXXXXXXXXXXXXXXX			
15 Lat. femoral cut.								
16 Ant. cut. femoral								
17 Obturator								
18 Post. cut. femoral					XXXXXXXXXXXXXXXX			
19 Lat. sural c. peron.								
20 Sural (tibial)								
21 Saphenous, femoral								
22 Superficial peron.	XXXXXXXXXXXXXXXX							
23 Plantar tibial								
24 Med. calcan. (tibial)								

KINGSBROOK JEWISH MEDICAL CENTER — DEPARTMENT OF REHABILITATION MEDICINE

EVALUATION of CUTANEOUS SOMATOSENSORY FUNCTION — PHYSICAL and OCCUPATIONAL THERAPY

Patient's Name ______________ Address ______________ Telephone ________

Hospital Unit ________ Chart No. ________ Diagnosis ______________

Disability ______________

Precautions ______________ Age ________

Handedness ________ Date of Onset ________ Prescription ________/________/________

Referring M.D.s ______________ Therapist ______________

Prescriptions: PT ________ OT ________ Speech ________ Orthotic/prosthetic device ________ other ________

LEFT — RIGHT

LIGHT TOUCH: Use sable brush; ask the patient "Where do you feel the touch of the brush?" and point to the spot with a finger of the opposite hand.

Grade:see key	Comments	I.1*	I.2*	A	P		P	A	I.1*	I.2*	Comments
Med. border											
Lat. border						ARM					
Post. surface											
Med. surface											
Med. border											
Lat. border						FOREARM					
Post. surface											
Ant. surface											
Thumb											
Finger 1						HAND					
F.3/rad. side											
Finger 4											

DEEP TOUCH: Use an eraser tip of pencil or head of straight pin; give the same instruction.

	Comments	I.1*	I.2*	A	P		P	A	I.1*	I.2*	Comments
Med. border											
Lat. border						ARM					
Post. surface											
Ant. surface											
Med. border											
Lat. border						FOREARM					
Post. surface											
Ant. surface											
Thumb											
Finger 1						HAND					
F.3/rad. side											
Finger 4											

PAIN: Use a straight pin; tell the patient to distinguish between the two stimuli (sharp/dull), and to point to spot of stimulus application.

	Comments	I.1*	I.2*	A	P		P	A	I.1*	I.2*	Comments
Upper 1/3											
Middle 1/3						ARM					
Lower 1/3											
Med. border											
Lat. border											
Post. surface						FOREARM					
Ant. surface											
Palmar surf.											
Dorsal surf.											
Thumb						HAND					
Finger 1											
Finger 4											

TEMPERATURE: Use two metal spoons, tips in hot/cold water before application to the skin; ask the patient to distinguish between temperature changes.

	Comments	I.1*	I.2*	A	P		P	A	I.1*	I.2*	Comments
Arm surface											
Forearm surf.											
Dorsum/hand						HAND					
Palm											

* I.1: impairment of modality specificity; I.2: Impairment of localization specificity; A: absent; P: present.

KEY TO INTERPRETATION OF SENSORY IMPAIRMENT

I.1	Impairment of modality specificity
I.1a	Inability to identify sensory modalities clearly
I.1b	Confusion in identifying sensory modalities
I.1c	Type of irritative sensations to testing modality
I.1d	Perception of stimulus strength above normal (hypersensitivity)
I.1e	Vague perception of stimulus strength indicating impairment of threshold value
I.1f	Delayed timing of response to stimulus application of specific sensory modalities
I.1g	Perception of pain sensation after stimulus has been removed
I.2	Impairment of place or localization specificity
I.2a	Inability to identify the place of stimulus application in relation to:
I.2a.1	Body segments
I.2a.2	Segmental or dermatomal cutaneous sensory distribution
I.2a.3	Peripheral nerve distribution
I.2a.4	Joint sensation distribution pattern
I.2b	Confusion of place specificity
I.2c	Diffuse localization specificity within the correct body segments
I.2d	Type of irritative symptoms over a certain area of stimulus application
I.2e	Vague perception of stimulus strength over a specific area indicating impairment of threshold value over a certain area
I.2f	Delayed timing of response to stimulus application over specific sensory distribution patterns

SUMMARY OF SENSORY EVALUATION REPORTING

Normal Sensory Perception

1. Patient's normal sensations in reference to modality specificities
2. Patient's normal sensations in reference to localization specificities related to (a) body segments, (b) segmental-dermatomal sensory distribution pattern, (c) joint receptor distribution pattern, or (d) peripheral nerve sensory distribution pattern

Impairment of Sensory Perception

1. Impairment of modality specificity related to the distribution patterns mentioned earlier
2. Impairment of threshold value in relation to modality specificity and/or place specificity
3. Timing of responses in relation to modality specificity and/or place specificity
4. Patient projecting irritative symptoms

Sensory Losses

1. Loss of sensibility specific to sensory modalities
2. Loss of sensation in relation to place specificity

Biomechanical Assessment in Clinical Practice 4

Anita Simons and Pat Trossman

This chapter will describe a plan for comprehensive biomechanical assessment of the upper extremity in patients with musculoskeletal dysfunction, secondary to disease or trauma, which can be used to determine the structure or structures interfering with normal movement. The assessment involves evaluation of joints and their surrounding tissues by means of a systematic physical examination emphasizing concepts of joint mobilization and tissue healing. These methods will assist the occupational therapist in localizing the patient's problem and directing treatment to the site of dysfunction. Joint dysfunction is defined as a "pain-producing pathological condition that causes loss of movement" or "loss of normal joint play movement" (1).

The biomechanical assessment described here integrates concepts basic to traditional occupational therapy assessment with newer concepts emphasizing current knowledge of joint function. The biomechanical approach to occupational therapy evaluation and treatment, as described by Trombley and Scott, applies the mechanical principles of kinetics and kinematics to therapeutic exercise to restore movement in the human body. The evaluation emphasizes examination of muscles, joints, tendons, ligaments, skin, and peripheral nerves. Treatment focuses on such processes as increasing the strength and endurance of muscles, increasing joint ranges of motion of joints, restoring proper alignment of bones and joint structures, restoring the gliding function of tendons, and managing pain. The biomechanical approach to assessment and treatment is appropriate for patients with dysfunction of any part of the musculoskeletal system. This approach assumes that the patient has an intact central nervous system and that the patient's musculoskeletal impairment is not the result of central nervous system dysfunction (2).

This biomechanical assessment involves a problem-solving approach using a four-step process: (a) data collection, including both subjective and objective information, (b) data analysis and interpretation, (c) treatment, and (d) reassessment. The therapist records data gathered from interview and observation of the patient, inspection and palpation of all structures of the upper extremity and, evaluations of active, passive, resistive, and accessory movements, hand function, and ability to perform functional activities. Reassessment determines whether or not treatment is appropriate and identifies new treatment priorities. The process of physical examination, treatment, and reassessment is repeated throughout the treatment phase.

Restriction of movement in conjunction with pain experienced during movement are frequent sequelae to upper extremity trauma. If the site of restricted movement is a finger, the occupational therapist must determine if the cause is an adherent tendon, a tight intrinsic muscle, or a tight joint capsule. The same analytical process is used to determine the causes of restricted movement in the shoulder, elbow, forearm, and wrist. Many previously described occupational therapy assessments that have not used an analytical approach emphasizing accurate identification of underlying problems have led to ineffective treatment planning. In the clinic we have often observed patients who have achieved adequate self-care independence yet remain with limited range of motion, pain and stiffness. In this chapter we will describe how the causes of dysfunction can be accurately identified by detailed examination of joint structures and how this can lead to more effective treatment planning.

The assessment described here incorporates principles derived from several sources: the biomechanical diagnostic methods of Cyriax, the mobilization evaluation techniques described by Paris and others, physical examination of the extremities as described by Hoppenfeld, and the biomechanical approach of Trombley and Scott (2–6). In addition, the documentation involved in evaluation of the hand is based on recommendations of the American Society of Hand Surgeons and the American Society of Hand Therapists (7). The references cited will provide more detailed information on specific subject matter.

Normal arm function requires that many complex structures work interdependently. It is important that the occupational therapist have a basic knowledge of the normal anatomy, neurology, and kinesiology of all joints of the upper extremity. The kinesiologic concepts of osteokinematics, the study of bone movements, and arthrokinematics, the study of movements within the joints, are particularly relevant (8). An understanding of pathology and the biological process of wound healing is also important (9).

CONCEPTS IN ANATOMY AND KINESIOLOGY

Movements of body parts take place at joints. The joints that provide the greatest range of motion are the synovial joints (Fig. 1), whose characteristic features are lubricated articular hyaline cartilage, synovial membrane, a fibrous articular capsule, and a potential joint cavity (10–12).

The smoothness of the articular surfaces of the apposed bones is due to their hyaline cartilage covering. This thin avascular cartilage appears to

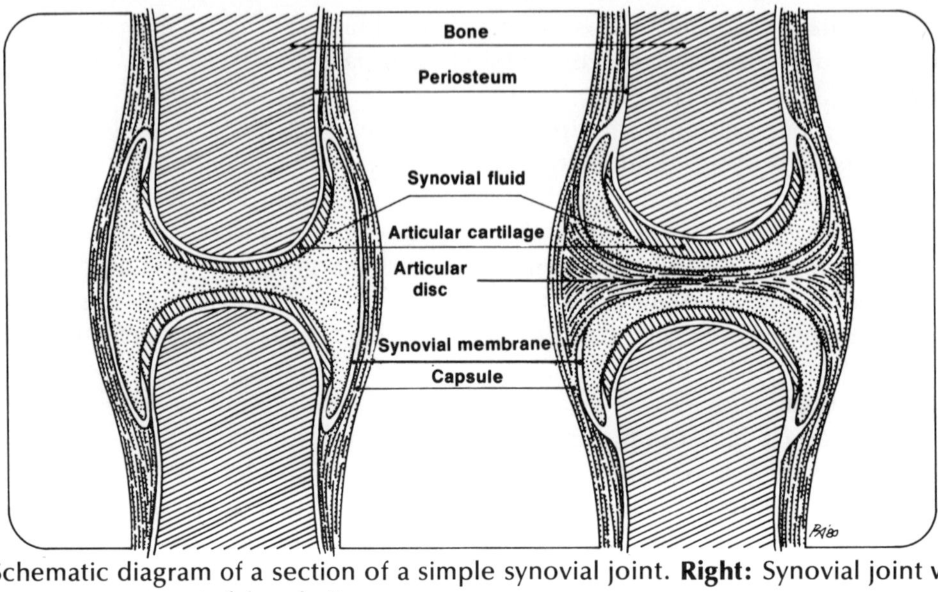

FIG. 1. Left: Schematic diagram of a section of a simple synovial joint. **Right:** Synovial joint with an articular disk. Joint spaces are exaggerated for clarity.

be nourished by synovial fluid, a clear viscous liquid that is present in small quantities. The joint surfaces are lubricated by the synovial fluid, which reduces friction and erosion. It is believed to be produced by the synovial membrane, a sheetlike specialization of connective tissue that covers all structures within the joint except for the articular surfaces themselves. Synovial folds and fringes project into the joint (10–13).

The articular capsule of the joint is composed of fibrous connective tissue. It attaches to bones just beyond the limits of the joint cavity, usually enclosing the joint completely. Two or more joints may share the same capsule and still retain their separate functions, as in the case of the elbow joint and the proximal radioulnar joint. The articular capsule may be strengthened by localized thickenings called ligaments. If these are separate from the capsule, they are called accessory ligaments. Ligaments have a protective role, preventing movements in undesired planes and checking movements at the extremes of the range of motion (10–13).

Some synovial joints have a fibrocartilaginous articular disk or meniscus (Fig. 1B). This can act as a shock absorber; it can also increase the congruity of articular surfaces and facilitate combined motions. The disk may divide the joint into two separate synovial joints, each performing separate actions, as in the case of the temporomandibular joint (10–13).

The nerve supply to joints is derived from the same nerves that innervate muscles acting on the joints and their overlying skin. Proprioception is an important type of sensation from joints. There are numerous specialized endings of myelinated fibers in the articular capsule and ligaments that carry proprioceptive stimuli to the brain via the spinal cord. Free nerve endings are also numerous. These terminal endings of nonmyelinated and finely myelinated fibers are believed to mediate pain sensation. They respond particularly to stretching and twisting (12,13).

Bone is a framework of fibrous connective tissue in which inorganic salts, primarily calcium and phosphates, are deposited. The typical long bone consists of a hollow shaft of compact bone with expanded ends for articulation with adjacent bones. These ends have a thin shell of compact bone and an internal zone of spongy or cancellous bone. The spongy bone is laid down in thin plates or lamellae, arranged as struts that will resist both compressive and tensile forces. These become rearranged whenever abnormal sets of stresses and strains are present, such as after a fracture that did not heal properly or after the development of deformity. Bone is covered with periosteum, except at its articular surfaces. The inner surface of periosteum is available to form new bone in the event of fracture or disease (10,12,13).

Skeletal muscle has a contractile component that allows it to shorten and thus produce movement at joints. Its connective-tissue components constitute a noncontractile framework through which the contraction forces of muscle fibers are transmitted to bone. Muscles attach firmly to bones by means of tendons. The dense connective-tissue fibers of tendons blend with and penetrate the periosteum. Cyriax classified muscle, tendon, and periosteum as contractile tissues, because a pathological process in any one of these will cause pain on resisted movement;

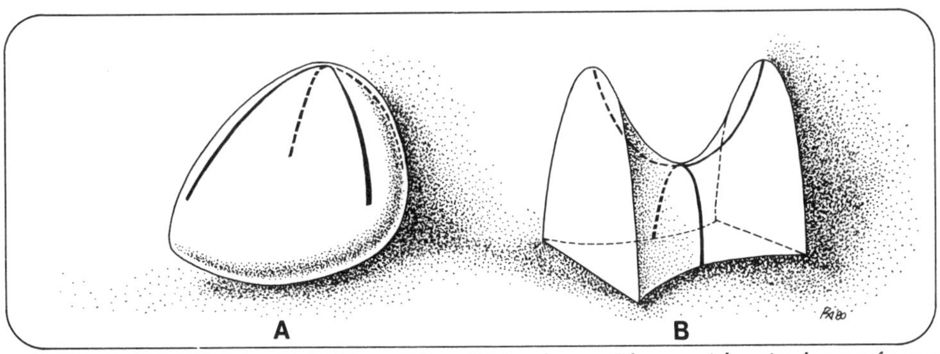

FIG. 2. A joint surface may be either ovoid **(A)** or sellar **(B)** in shape. The ovoid articular surface may be convex, as shown, or concave. The sellar or saddle-shaped articular surface is concavoconvex. Gray's Anatomy, edited by Warwick and Williams, 35th British edition, 1973, adapted with permission from Churchill Livingstone, Edinburgh, Scotland.

however, only muscle fibers have the ability to actively contract (3,10,12).

In most joints the contact or weight-bearing surfaces change with changes in the position of the joint. At any point in the range of motion the area of contact is small, but this area changes as the joint position changes. Joint movement takes place around constantly shifting axes of rotation. In this way the stress of contact or weight bearing is distributed to all parts of the articular surfaces.

Articular surfaces of synovial joints can be classified as either ovoid or sellar in shape (Fig. 2). The ovoid surface is either concave in all directions or convex in all directions. Each synovial joint contains one or more mating pairs of articular surfaces. When the articular surfaces are ovoid in shape, the convex surface is considered the male surface, and the concave surface is considered the female surface. The female surface is always smaller in area than the male. The sellar surface is saddle-shaped (concavoconvex). It has a convex surface in one plane, with a concave surface at right angles to this. When two sellar surfaces articulate, the larger of the two surfaces is considered the male and the smaller the female (8,13).

The most stable position of a joint is called the close-packed position (Fig. 3B, Table 1). In this position the articulating joint surfaces are perfectly congruent, and the tension on the articular capsule and ligaments is maximal. The joint surfaces are usually temporarily locked together. The locking together is frequently performed by a screw-home movement, which is a movement with a small rotary component. The close-packed configuration usually occurs at a position that is the extreme of the most habitual position of the joint. For example, the close-packed position for the wrist joint is full extension. The other extreme position of the joint that is less commonly assumed is also very congruent, and it is called the potential close-packed position (8,11,13).

In any other position of the joint the articular surfaces are not congruent, and some part of the joint capsule is lax; in these positions, the joint is said to be loose-packed (Fig. 3A). In many cases there is sufficient laxity in midrange to allow separation of the joint surfaces by an externally applied distractive force. The laxity of the capsule in the loose-packed position allows for the elements of spin, roll, and glide, which are present in most joint movements. The ideal position for evaluation and treatment procedures used in joint mobilization is the maximum loose-packed position (Table 1) (8,11,13).

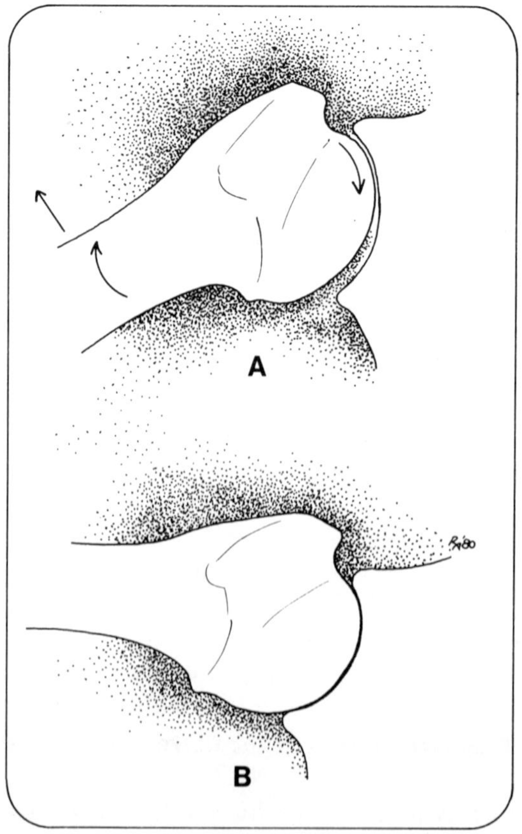

FIG. 3. Glenohumeral joint. **A:** In the loose-packed position the articular surfaces are not congruent. This is exaggerated here for clarity. **B:** In the close-packed position the articular surfaces are maximally congruent. Note that the head of the humerus abducts, rotates laterally, and descends into the lower portion of the glenoid cavity as it comes into the close-packed position.

Concepts of bone motions (spin and swing) and their relationships to intraarticular motions are significant for joint examination. During spin, the bone is rotated around its stationary mechanical axis. A concave articular surface can spin on a convex joint partner, or a convex surface can spin on a concave joint partner. During swing, a roll-glide takes place in the joint. A concave articular surface can roll on a convex joint partner, or a convex surface can roll on a concave joint partner. Roll and glide are always found together but not always in equal proportions. During roll, new points on one joint surface come in contact with new points on the

TABLE 1.

Upper extremity joint	Close-packed position (19, 22, 25)	Loose-packed position (19, 22, 25)
Glenohumeral	Abduction and external rotation, combined or in sequence	Semiabduction
Humeroulnar	Maximum extension and supination	Semiflexion
Humeroradial	90° flexion and semipronation	Extension and supination
Radioulnar	Halfway between pronation and supination	Slight supination
Radiocarpal	Full extension	Semiflexion
Most intracarpal joints	Full extension	Semiflexion
First carpometacarpal	Full opposition	Neutral position
Metacarpophalangeal (1)	Full extension	Semiflexion
Metacarpophalangeal (2-5)	Full flexion	Semiflexion and ulnar deviation
Interphalangeal joints	Full extension	Semiflexion

other joint surface; during glide, the movement does not change direction, and one constant point on one surface glides on new points on the other joint surface (8,14).

CONCEPTS IN WOUND HEALING

Musculoskeletal trauma is defined as injury to skin, muscles, tendons, nerves, blood vessels, bones, or joints. What happens when one or more of these structures are traumatized? Most tissues have a common response to trauma that includes the process of inflammation and repair. The therapist must be knowledgeable about the normal stages of wound healing that occur, since this will affect outcome. Normal wound healing is a three-stage process. The inflammatory phase of vasodilation and edema occurs immediately and lasts 48 hr. This is followed by the fibroblastic phase, during which wound stabilization occurs (2–5 days after trauma). During this phase the wound space is filled with collagen fibers laid down in random fashion. As collagen fibers appear, the scar begins to gain strength, with the collagen fibers uniting all surrounding structures (between 5 days and 2 months). During the remodeling phase the collagen fibers reorganize and become oriented along lines of normal tension, the scar matures, and the tissue regains tensile strength; this occurs between 2 months and 1 year after injury (9).

At any time during the early stages and on through the later stages of collagen production and wound remodeling the tissue may react. Recurrent edema or prolonged edema may contribute to a vicious cycle: Trauma produces inflammation and pain; the inflammation contributes to edema; the patient postures the arm in a protected position, which leads to further immobilization, muscle spasm, and more edema, inflammation, and pain. The process occurs rapidly and is slow to recede. The patient is left with pain, which interferes with joint mobility, ultimately resulting in joint dysfunction, stiffness, and adhesions or contractures.

In cases involving surgical repair of tissues, consideration of the processes of wound healing will help the therapist determine the critical period for mobilizing structures. Depending on the type of tissue involved and its particular healing time, the therapist must initiate movement of the part appropriately. For example, following a flexor tendon repair in the finger, controlled movement may be started 1 week after repair to prevent adhesions and preserve flexor tendon gliding (15).

To illustrate the relationship between wound healing and joint dysfunction, consider the sequence of events that occurs when a patient sustains trauma to the wrist resulting in a fracture with dorsal displacement of the distal radius. The patient is examined, X-rays are taken, a closed reduction of the fracture is performed, and a long arm plaster-of-paris cast is applied. Typically the wrist is positioned in slight flexion and ulnar deviation and immobilized for 4 to 6 weeks, until satisfactory bone healing occurs (15). During the period of immobilization the patient is subject to the initial inflammatory response and subsequent tissue healing process, affecting both the bone and the surrounding joints. Within 2 to 3 days adhesions form. Collagen fibers are quickly deposited, producing scar tissue that restricts movement between radiocarpal, radioulnar, and midcarpal joints, seriously impeding wrist flexion, extension, and ulnar and radial deviation, as well as forearm supination and pronation. When the hand remains immobile during healing, edema will develop, particularly beneath the dorsal skin. Inactivity leads to stiffness, muscle spasm, and pain as the tissue fluids stagnate and develop into thick unyielding fibrotic tissue. The extent of dysfunction depends on the extent of the initial trauma and the degree of inflammation; the greater the inflammatory response, the longer the repair process and the greater the amounts of pain and muscle spasm. Frequently, long after the initial problem is resolved, the patient remains with disability. This example illustrates the mechanisms that produce joint dysfunction following a primary pathological process such as a fracture (inactivity, edema, fibrosis, collagen alteration, and anatomic derangement) (16).

PAIN

Pain is produced by various noxious stimuli, and it serves a protective function by warning of a threat to the body. Pain is often the symptom that brings a patient for treatment. Knowledge of the characteristics of various types of pain can be useful in determining the cause and in planning for treatment.

Pain can be divided into a number of subcategories on the basis of its site of origin and its characteristics. Somatic pain that results from stimulation of pain receptors (nociceptors) in the skin is called superficial pain. It is usually a sharp and easily localized pain that fades away rapidly after the noxious stimulus is removed, but it may be followed by a delayed pain that is characteristically dull and burning and slow to recede. An example of superficial pain is the pain felt when the surface of the skin is pricked with a pin. Pain that results from stimulation of nociceptors in the bones, joints, muscles, and connective tissue is called deep pain. It tends to be dull in nature and poorly localized, radiating to surrounding areas (17). Pain resulting from stimulation of nociceptors in the viscera is called visceral pain. Visceral pain resembles deep pain in that it is dull and diffuse in nature (17).

Some special forms of pain commonly observed are referred pain and projected pain. Referred pain results when pain signals from the viscera are experienced at a superficial location distant from the primary source. There may or may not be accompanying pain at the internal organ itself. The referred pain is always experienced in a peripheral area supplied by the same spinal nerve segment as the affected internal organ. In other words, the pain is referred to the somatic area whose dermatome is supplied by the spinal nerve segment that supplies the visceral organ. A familiar example is that pain originating in the heart during angina pectoris or myocardial infarction may be felt in the axilla and inner aspect of the left upper extremity. This is the dermatome supplied by spinal nerve segments from T1 and T2, which also supply the visceral afferent terminations for the coronary arteries (17,18).

Projected pain is another special form of pain. When an afferent fiber is stimulated along its course, the stimulus is transmitted to the brain via the lateral spinothalamic tract, giving rise to sensation in the cutaneous area supplied by the afferent fiber. For example, a sharp blow to the ulnar nerve at the elbow produces tingling sensations in the ulnar distribution of the forearm and the hand. The central nervous system (CNS) evidently projects the activity elicited in the afferent nerve fibers at the elbow to the cutaneous regions innervated by these fibers. This type of projected pain is transitory, but there are other types of projected pain of greater clinical significance. A herniated intervertebral disk may compress a spinal nerve as the nerve enters the spinal cord, generating pain sensations that are projected into the cutaneous area supplied by the stimulated nerve (17).

Whether pain is superficial or deep, projected or referred, once it is felt in a specific area the muscles in that area will respond in a protective manner by going into spasm. When pain is felt in the arm and shoulder, the shoulder muscles may go into spasm and prevent the accessory motions that are part of normal shoulder motion. If the spasm continues for any length of time, these component motions may be lost. This explains how a frozen shoulder can be one of the sequelae of myocardial infarction (1,17).

Pain, restricted movement, and decreased function are the factors that can cause the patient to seek treatment. Pain is a subjective symptom, and therefore it is difficult to assess, particularly as the intensity and duration of pain that can be tolerated will vary among patients. Information regarding the patient's pain can be obtained by a series of questions designed to elicit information about the location and nature of symptoms and by an examination of active, passive, and resisted movements. Analysis of these data will help the therapist determine the cause of the pain (6).

BIOMECHANICAL ASSESSMENT

The biomechaical assessment should begin with the collection of data, including subjective and objective information. In addition to the diagnosis from the referring physician, the therapist will need additional definitive information for treatment planning.

Subjective History

A subjective history will provide information about the patient's symptoms, specifically pain, impaired movement, and loss of function. The history should be taken from the patient in a structured interview designed to elicit specific data.

The patient's age, sex, occupation, and hand dominance should be noted. Then the problem should be stated in the patient's own words. The date of onset should be noted, and the patient should be asked to describe the nature of the onset (traumatic, gradual, unknown). If the onset was traumatic, the patient should narrate the incident: how, where, and when it occurred, the sequence of emergency care, surgical treatment, postoperative course, and treatment received thus far. In cases of disease, relevant past history must be documented, including medical and surgical treatment and postoperative care. The patient's home therapy program should be described or demonstrated. Is the program of the patient's own devising? Or is it a prescribed home program of active exercise and elevation?

Information regarding the location and nature of symptoms is needed. The patient should be asked to describe current symptoms of dysfunction, including localization of symptoms, duration of symptoms (constant or intermittent), factors that exacerbate symptoms, factors that interrupt or suppress symptoms, and how these symptoms interfere with the patient's functional activities (19).

Some typical interview questions regarding pain and function are as follows: Where is your pain? What type of pain is perceived? Dull, tingling, sharp, aching? Pain associated with regenerating peripheral nerves may be described as hypersensitive. What is the effect of activity on the pain? Is the pain aggravated or relieved? What is the effect of rest on the pain? Is it relieved, or does the upper extremity become more stiff? At what time of day or night is the pain worst? What activities are you able to perform? How does the pain interfere with your daily life in terms of household and vocational tasks?

If the patient is currently employed, the therapist must obtain a description or demonstration of the physical requirements of the job, including the motor and sensory components, hand function and type of grasp, and dexterity and coordination required to perform the tasks. This information will help the therapist determine if the patient is stressing the affected part (possibly exacerbating symptoms), if the patient is performing tasks by using compensatory movements or substitutions, or if further testing is needed to determine when the patient can return to employment. Also to be considered are the patient's motivation, psychological state, and life goals, all of which influence performance. The daily activities of living, such as household and leisure activities, must be similarly analyzed.

Objective Information

Objective information is obtained by inspection and palpation, assessment of movement, circumferential and volumetric measurements, sensory evaluation, assessment of circulation, grip and pinch strength tests, and assessment of coordination.

Inspection

Inspection includes those observations that can be made by looking at the patient. Abnormalities detected during this part of the evaluation warrant more comprehensive evaluation of the involved component.

Posture and Symmetry. The patient must be observed from the back, front, and sides for asymmetry of posture. Postural deviations may be indicative of muscle imbalance, compensatory positions assumed to relieve pain, alignment problems, and other pathological processes. When the patient is walking, the arm should swing in tandem with the opposite lower extremity.

Skin Appearance. The skin must be observed for evidence of discoloration, trophic changes, calluses, and scars. Discoloration may be an indication of increased or decreased circulation to the limb. A white or blue color is symptomatic of decreased circulation; a red color suggests increased circulation. Trophic changes may include the following: smooth glossy skin; absence of sweating or reduced or increased sweating; excess hair or loss of hair; brittle ridged nails; trophic ulcers. Such changes may have a neurological, nutritional, endocrine, or circulatory basis. Calluses provide information about hand and upper extremity use. External scars should be noted and examined further as possible sites of adhesions (20).

Shape and Size. The upper extremity should be inspected for changes in shape and size. If atrophy or edema is noted, circumferential and volumetric measurements must be taken and compared with those for the intact upper extremity. These procedures will be described in some detail later. The arches of the hand and creases of the hand, wrist, and elbow should be observed and compared with those on the intact side. Joints must be inspected for proper bony alignment. Bony contours must be observed for signs of subluxation or dislocation. For example, in evaluating a patient with rheumatoid arthritis, the examiner must be alert for typical signs of deformation such as ulnar drift of the metacarpophalangeal (MP) joints of the fingers, volar subluxation of the carpal bones on the radius, or dorsal subluxation of the distal ulna on the radius (21).

Palpation

During palpation to detect abnormalities, contact with the patient should be gentle but firm.

Skin Temperature. The skin temperature of the affected upper extremity must be compared with that on the intact side, using the fingertips. The examiner's hand should be capable of detecting a difference of several degrees between two areas. Increased skin temperature may be a sign of inflammation or infection. This may be particularly important in an insensitive hand or arm in which the usual warning signal of pain is lacking. Decreased skin temperature may be a sign of autonomic or circulatory dysfunction. Day-to-day variations in hand temperature can be substantial; therefore it is important to make a comparison with the intact side or with other normal tissue. If a pathological process is suspected, an electronic or glass skin thermometer will give a more accurate measurement (22).

Skin, Subcutaneous Tissue, and Tendons. Skin and subcutaneous tissues must be palpated for thickening, loss of pliability, and adherence to underlying structures. Tendons must be palpated for thickening, tenderness, and the presence of nodules. Audible or palpable crepitus during tendon motion should be noted, as well as the motion that elicited it. Tendon sheaths and bursa also must be palpated for thickening and tenderness.

Tendon adherence in the hand produces deficits in active movement that are greater than the deficits in passive movement in one direction, as well as slight but equal deficits in active and passive movements in the opposite direction. The location of tendon adherence in the hand is determined by adjusting the positions of the surrounding joints. For example, in testing a proximal interphalangeal joint (PIP) joint (assuming no contracture of PIP joint capsule), if full flexion of the MP joint permits PIP extension, the adhesion is proximal to the MP joint. If it does not, the flexor tendon is adherent to the proximal phalanx. Tendon adherence to the skin is tested by active contraction of the muscle or by passive stretch; dimpling of the skin will occur at the site of the adhesion (23).

Joints. Joints should be palpated for swelling, bogginess, loose bodies, crepitus, tenderness, positional faults, subluxation, and laxity or tightness of joint structures. For example, in testing the integrity of joint structures at the PIP joint, the joint is held in full passive extension. The proximal phalanx is stabilized, and an attempt is made to move the middle phalanx from side to side, followed by gliding in an anteroposterior direction. If the motion from side to side is more than a few degrees, this is indicative of collateral ligament laxity. Excessive anteroposterior motion without excess lateral motion indicates laxity of the joint capsule rather than the collateral ligaments (21).

Assessment of Movement

Examination of movements is used to detect joint dysfunction. Joint movements may be active (accomplished by the patient voluntarily) or accessory (normally occurring joint movement that cannot be reproduced by the patient, but must be performed by the therapist). Thus a comprehensive assessment of movement must include evaluation of both classic movements (active and passive motion) and accessory movements (joint play and component motions). Throughout the examination the patient must be encouraged to state which movements reproduce the pain symptom (6).

Active Movements. Active joint movements, also known as physiological movements, are those movements that take place as a result of voluntary muscle action, e.g., movement at the glenohumeral joint in shoulder flexion. The patient should be asked to raise the affected arm in the sagittal plane; the response will provide information regarding range of motion, muscle function, crepitus (state of gliding surfaces), and the patient's willingness to move. Following hand trauma, assessment of active movement will reveal the status of tendon glide and permit determination of the integrity of the musculotendinous unit and restriction of tendon motion. Assessment of active movement provides specific information about muscles and tendons and their insertions. During the examination of active joint movements, the therapist must take into account both range of motion and pain and determine the range of motion through which pain is felt. Reproduction of symptoms aids the therapist in determining the status of these tissues (6,10,14).

Resisted Movements. Resisted movements provide additional information about muscles and tendons and their insertions. Examination of resisted movement is used to test contractile structures for pain or weakness. Resistance must be applied selectively to ensure that only one group of muscles is tested at a time. If pain is felt and/or weakness is detected, differentiation must be made between muscles in the group. The joint should be positioned in midrange to ensure capsular and ligamentous laxity, and the muscles should then be tested isometrically, allowing no joint movement. For example, the patient may be asked to hold the arm in shoulder abduction while the therapist applies resistance. Then the presence of pain or weakness is recorded. Four combinations are possible in resisted movements: (a) strong and painless (contractile tissues are normal); (b) weak and painless (either a complete rupture of tendon or muscle or a neurological lesion); (c) weak and painful (major lesion of muscle or tendon); (d) strong and painful (minor lesion of muscle or tendon) (3).

The manual muscle test described by Daniels and Worthingham (24) may be used to assess muscle strength.

Passive Movements. In addition to recording objective data about muscle function, the therapist must assess passive joint movement to obtain information about the noncontractile tissues, specifically joint capsule, ligaments, bursae, fascia, and nerves. It is extremely important that the patient relax so that the therapist can move the extremity through the available range of motion. To assure maximum relaxation, passive movements should be tested in a reclining position. As passive physiological movements are performed, the therapist should note the presence of pain and resistance during the movement. At the end of the range, the therapist should apply slight additional pressure to the joint, noting the "end feel." All joints have characteristic end feels distinctive to the tissues being stressed and differing for the various movements tested. Five normal end feels can be identified (Table 2). As clinical experience is gained, the therapist will begin to distinguish between these normal end feels and abnormal end feels. Some abnormal end feels that have been categorized are muscle

TABLE 2. *End feel*

Normal end feels	Description
Tissue approximation	Soft arrest of movement as muscles contact each other (e.g., extreme of elbow flexion)
Muscular	Elastic reflex resistance with discomfort (e.g., shoulder abduction with external rotation)
Capsular	Hard arrest of movement with a slight give (e.g., shoulder external rotation at end of range)
Nonelastic (cartilage)	Sudden stop to movement (e.g., extension of the elbow)
Ligamentous	Firm arrest of movement with no give, (e.g., abduction of PIP joint of extended finger)

Adapted from Cyriax (3) and Paris (6).

spasm, bony block, pannus, and capsular-pattern end feel. An abnormal end feel gives a clue to the cause of restricted range of motion, thus contributing to treatment planning. For example, if muscle-spasm end feel is detected, treatment may include techniques of muscle relaxation. A loose end feel with ligamentous laxity and hypermobility of the joint capsule, as seen in rheumatoid arthritis, calls for activities that will not lead to further joint capsule stretching (6,19).

Comparison between active and passive movement restrictions, according to Cyriax, leads to the following conclusions: Active and passive movements that are restricted or painful in the same direction indicate a problem in the noncontractile structures, since active joint motion involves both contractile and inert surrounding tissues (e.g., when the joint capsule is stretched at the end of the active range of motion). Active and passive movements that are restricted or painful in opposite directions indicate a problem in muscles or tendons or their insertions. For example, if active movement in one direction produces pain and passive stretch of the musculotendinous unit in the opposite direction produces pain, this indicates a problem in contractile structures (e.g., active or resisted pronation of the forearm and passive stretch of the pronator teres into supination produces pain). Relative restriction of passive range of motion in various directions indicates a capsular pattern. A capsular pattern of restricted motion is caused by irritation of the joint capsule or the synovium (arthritis) that produces characteristic proportionate limitation of movement in the joint. It does not indicate what type of arthritis is present, only that the capsule or synovium is involved. Each joint has its own capsular pattern (Table 3). A typical capsular pattern of movement for the shoulder joint may be abduction limited by 45 degrees, external rotation limited by 60 degrees, and internal rotation limited by 10 degrees. Arthritis of the elbow joint is likely to limit flexion more than extension. Limitations of motion not in the same proportions as the capsular pattern indicate that arthritis is not the cause of restriction. This suggests that a ligamentous or localized capsular adhesion, internal derangement in the joint, or an extraarticular lesion (bursitis) may be present (3,6).

Active and passive ranges of motion can be measured in degrees with a goniometer and recorded using the method developed by the American Academy of Orthopedic Surgeons (31). To assess active and passive motions in the impaired hand, a computation of total active movement and total passive movement (TAM and TPM) is used, as described by the American Society for Surgery of the Hand (7). For additional information, refer to Chapter 2.

Accessory Movements. Accessory movements are involuntary movements of the joint that cannot be reproduced by the patient. They accompany classic movements and are necessary for

TABLE 3. *Capsular pattern of upper extremity joints*

Joint	Proportion of limitation
Shoulder	Limited abduction, external rotation more restricted than internal rotation
Elbow	Flexion more limited than extension
Wrist	Limitation is equal in flexion and extension
Fingers	Flexion more limited than extension
Thumb CMC joint	Limited abduction and extension, no limitation of flexion

Adapted from Cyriax (3).

normal full range of motion. Loss of accessory movement results in joint dysfunction. Examination will reveal whether accessory movements are normal, hypermobile (more range than normal), or hypomobile (less range than normal). Determination of accessory movement, traditionally part of the joint mobilization examination, is necessary if the therapist is to restore the normal roll-glide action that takes place during joint movement. There are two types of accessory movements: joint play and component motions. Additional reading is available for details on testing individual joints (6,14,25).

Joint play motion is not under voluntary control; it occurs only in response to an outside force. It is the normal movement available in each joint. In testing joint play, the joint is held in the loose-packed position, and the therapist applies a small amount of traction to unload the joint surfaces. For example, to test PIP joint play, the therapist stabilizes the proximal phalanx just above the joint space and applies longitudinal traction, decreasing the friction in the joint between the proximal and middle phalanges. Depending on the response, different amounts of traction may be applied. Stage 1 traction ("piccolo") and stage 2 traction ("taking up the slack") are joint distractions using, respectively, a small amount of force to unload the joint surface and force sufficient to distract a joint partner as far as the soft tissues allow (6,14,19).

Component motions are joint motions taking place in the joint complex or related joints that accompany and are necessary for full active range of motion. For example, gliding the head of the humerus into the lower portion of the glenoid fossa during active movement of the shoulder is a component motion. While the arm is by the side of the body, the head of the humerus occupies the upper part of the glenoid cavity. As the arm is raised above the head, the muscle action will move the head of the humerus downward into the glenoid cavity, changing the joint surface relationships. The therapist must know which joints are ovoid and which are sellar and the loose-packed position of the joint. In testing for component motions in the ovoid joint, the therapist must also know whether the shape of the articular surface of the joint partner to be moved is convex or concave in order to determine the direction in which gliding takes place. If a bone motion takes place in one direction, the gliding in the joint that accompanies that motion takes place in the opposite direction if the moving joint surface is convex and in the same direction if the moving joint surface is concave (Fig. 4). The convex/concave rule states that if the joint partner is convex, the test movement is in the opposite direction to the restriction, and if the joint partner is concave, the test movement is toward the restriction. For example, in testing for limitation in shoulder abduction, the therapist should depress the head of the humerus in the direction opposite to the limitation, since the humeral joint surface is convex. If the limitation is in PIP joint flexion, the therapist should glide the middle phalanx in the same direction as the limitation, since the joint surface is concave. This rule applies to component motions in ovoid joints (14,19,25).

Mennell's nine rules (1) for examination of accessory motion may be condensed as follows: (a) The patient must be relaxed with joints supported so that pain and muscle spasm will not prevent the performance of examining movements for

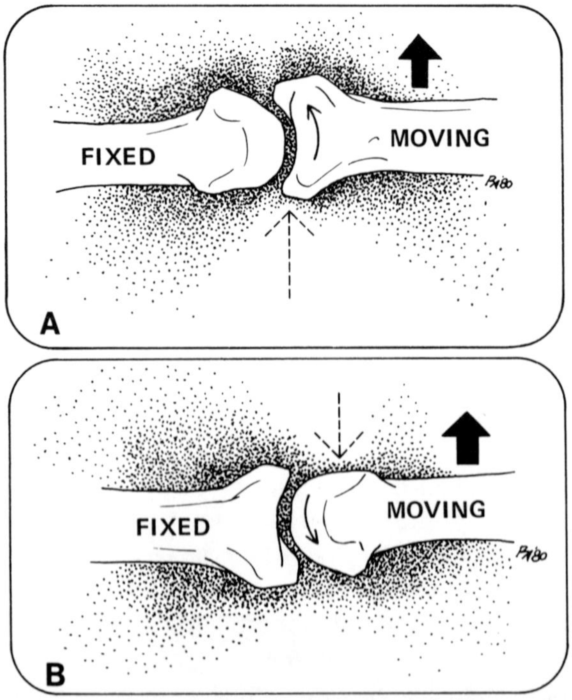

FIG. 4. A: Concave rule: concave joint surface moving on convex joint surface. Example: If the metacarpophalangeal joint is limited in extension, mobilization will glide the proximal phalanx in the direction of extension. **B:** Convex rule: convex joint surface moving on concave joint surface. Example: If the glenohumeral joint is limited in abduction, mobilization will depress the head of the humerus in the direction opposite the limitation. Adapted with permission from Kaltenborn (14).

joint play. (b) The examiner must be relaxed. (c) The examination must be conducted one joint at a time. Examination of the wrist, for example, includes the radiocarpal joint, the midcarpal joint, the ulnomeniscocarpal joint, and the inferior radioulnar joint. (d) Each joint must be examined one movement at a time. (e) During examination, one mobilizing force and one stabilizing force must be used. (f) To determine joint play, comparison is made with the uninvolved arm. (g) No forceful or abnormal movement should be used. (h) Examining movements must be stopped at the onset of pain. (i) Examination must not be attempted during active joint disease.

Application of Accessory Movement Examination to Clinical Practice. Following this method of peripheral joint examination, the therapist can set about restoring normal movement in the involved structures. For example, if examination reveals that wrist movement is restricted in flexion and extension, and if further accessory movement examination reveals that anterior and posterior glide is limited at the radiocarpal joint, the therapist can apply mobilization movements that will help restore normal accessory movement to the joint (Fig. 5). For specific techniques of mobilization, the occupational therapist is directed to courses available that deal with mobilization techniques. If an attempt is made to increase passive range of motion without taking into account these accessory joint movements, the results may be increased pain, inflammation, and compression of joint surfaces, joint range of motion will not be adequately affected, and the patient can be left with pain and stiffness. Joint mobilization movements must be followed by active movement of the part within the newly acquired range, as well as functional activities to maintain the range of motion.

Circumferential and Volumetric Measurements

Circumferential measurements of the arm should be taken and compared with those for the intact arm to determine the amount of edema present. A Gulick anthropometric tape is recommended for accurate measurement. A spring attachment permits constant tension on the tape so that the conditions of measurement will be the same in successive examinations. Recommended measurement sites are the upper arm (7 cm proximal to the elbow flexion crease), the forearm (11 cm proximal to the distal wrist flexion crease), the wrist (at the level of the distal flexion crease), the hand (at the level of the distal palmar crease), and around the PIP and DIP joints. Arm and forearm sites can also be used to determine loss of muscle bulk due to atrophy (26,27).

Volumetric measurement of the hand may also be used to determine the amount of edema or atrophy. The volumeter designed by Brand measures the volume of water displaced by the hand. The difference in volume between the involved hand and the intact hand may be attributed to either edema or atrophy. It should be kept in mind that there is some size difference between the hands for all individuals. Successive measurements of the same hand must be compared to show changes (26,28).

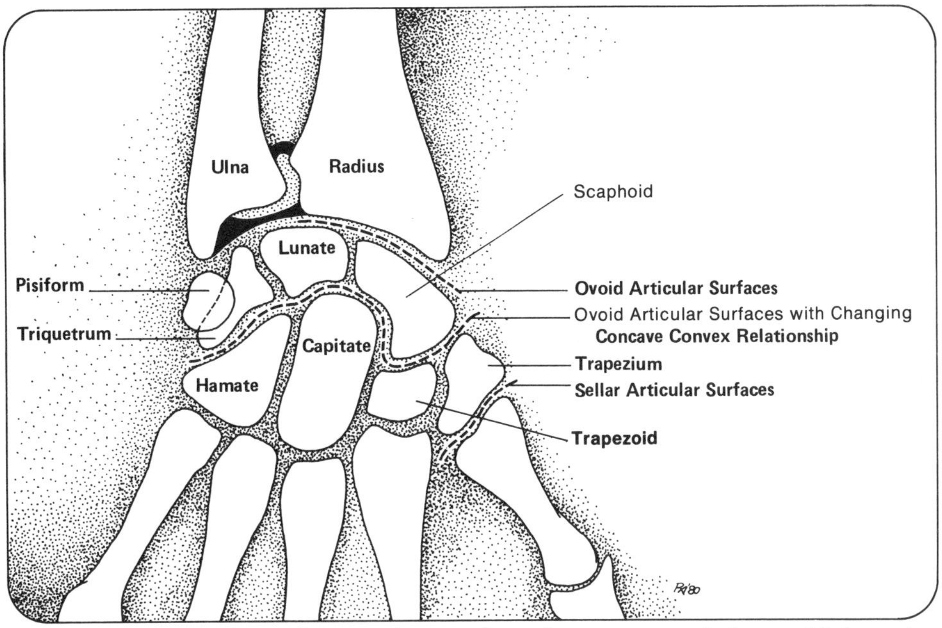

FIG. 5. Coronal section through the radiocarpal, carpal, and metacarpophalangeal joints showing ovoid and sellar articular surfaces.

Sensory Evaluation

The sensory evaluation of the arm may be subdivided into three areas: exteroception, proprioception, and cerebral sensory function (13,18,20). *Exteroception* involves the stimulation of receptors in the skin and mucous membranes, and the central processing of these signals. This is sometimes called the sense of touch. This includes light touch or tactile sensation, pain (sharp dull discrimination) and temperature discrimination (18). *Proprioception* involves sensations perceived as a result of the stimulation of receptors in the deeper tissues of the body (muscles, ligaments, joint capsules, and tendons). Proprioception includes position sense, motion sense (kinesthesia) and vibration sense. There are also receptors for vibration stimuli in some of the more superficial tissues (13,18,20). *Cerebral sensory functions* require a combination of exteroception and cognitive ability. If exteroceptive sensation is absent or severely impaired, cerebral sensory functions cannot be tested. If cognitive ability is limited because of brain damage or intellectual deficit, it will be difficult to test cerebral sensory functions (13,18,20). All sensory evaluation must be carried out in a quiet, non distracting environment with the patient's vision occluded.

Exteroception. Tactile sensation (light touch) is most accurately tested by means of Semmes-Weinstein nylon monofilament sets in lucite rods (Table 4). These are calibrated to bend when specific pressures are reached and thus are able to measure levels of sensation from light touch to deep pressure. These monofilaments have four levels of stiffness: those that test normal levels of sensation, those that measure diminished light

TABLE 4. *Interpretation of Semmes-Weinstein test*[a]

Filament marking	Sensory level
1.65–2.83	Normal
3.22–3.61	Diminished light touch
3.84–4.31	Diminished protective sensation
4.56–6.65	Loss of protective sensation
Greater than 6.65	Untestable

[a] Adapted from Fess et al. (26).

touch, those that measure diminished protective sensation, and those that test loss of protective sensation. Testing is begun with the lighter filaments first. The patient is asked to state when a touch has occurred and then point to the spot touched (precise point localization is a cerebral sensory function). The entire upper extremity may be tested in this manner (26,29). Sensory impulses travel from receptors in the skin and mucous membranes via the peripheral nerves to spinal root ganglia, then ascend to the cortex via the ipsilateral dorsal columns and the opposite ventral spinothalamic tract (20).

Testing the range of light touch/deep pressure with these monofilaments has been found to correlate with information about the presence of protective sensations in patients with peripheral nerve injuries (29). Some authorities recommend that testing of pain and temperature sensations not be carried out in these patients; one may wish to test these sensations in patients with other diagnoses.

Pain (sharp/dull discrimination) is tested using the sharp and blunt ends of a safety pin. Stimuli are presented randomly, and the patient indicates when something is felt and whether it is sharp or dull. Pain-producing stimuli are carried from receptors in the skin and mucous membranes via the peripheral nerves through spinal root ganglia synapsing with second-order neurons in the dorsal gray columns. The axons of these cross immediately to the lateral spinothalamic tract on the opposite side and proceed to the sensory cortex (2,20,26).

Temperature sensation is evaluated using two test tubes of warm and cool water. A person with normal sensation should be able to distinguish a temperature difference of 1°C to 5°C. Therefore the water should not be excessively hot or cold. The stimuli are randomly applied, and the patient indicates "hot" or "cold." Temperature stimuli are carried to the sensory cortex by the same route as pain stimuli (2,20,26,29).

Proprioception. Position sense is tested by passively moving the joints through their ranges of motion. At various points each motion is stopped, and the patient is asked to describe the position or to duplicate it with the other arm (2,20,26). Motion sense (kinesthesia) is tested by moving each joint in flexion or extension and asking the patient to state whether it is moving up or down (2,20,26). Vibration sense is tested with a tuning fork whose frequency is 30 cps. Vibration stimuli are carried from peripheral receptors via peripheral nerves through the dorsal root ganglia and ascend to the cerebral sensory cortex via the posterior columns (2,20,26).

Cerebral Sensory Functions. Stereognosis is tested by placing an easily recognized object in the hand. The patient must manipulate the object and identify it by touch alone. If necessary, the patient may be given assistance in manipulating the object. Objects ordinarily used are a coin, a key, a safety pin, a small sponge, etc. (2,26,29).

Two-point discrimination is tested with a vernier caliper adapted for sensory testing (the points of the caliper are blunted to prevent the introduction of pain stimuli during testing). The level of two-point discrimination is considered to correlate highly with the quality of useful sensation, particularly in patients with nerve repair. The palmar surfaces of the hand and digits are tested. The area tested is touched by either one point or two points of the instrument applied to the longitudinal axis of the digit. The pressure applied should not blanch the skin. The patient is asked to state whether one point is felt or two points are felt. The smallest distance between the two points that the patient can still perceive as being two points is recorded for each area tested (2,26,29). The norms (26) for the palmar surface of the hand are as follows: normal, 6 mm or less; fair, 6 to 10 mm; poor, 11 to 15 mm; protective, one point perceived; anesthetic, no point perceived.

Circulation

The Allen test is used to determine radial and ulnar arterial supply to the hand. Both arteries are occluded at the wrist by the therapist's middle and index fingers of both hands. To expel residual blood, the patient closes the hand firmly. When the hand is again relaxed, with occlusion continued, the hand appears pale. Removal of occlusion from one artery, while maintaining occlusion of the other, should rapidly produce a pink blush. If obstruction is suspected, the test should be repeated. The other vessel is tested similarly, and the opposite hand is tested for comparison (5).

Grip and Pinch Strength

Grip strength is evaluated using the Jaymar dynamometer. The handle of the dynamometer should be in the second position, unless the patient is unable to grasp it in that position. If the position is changed, the new position must be noted. If several dynamometers are in use in the clinic, the serial number of the dynamometer must be recorded, because calibration varies from one dynamometer to another. The same instrument is then used for reevaluation (26).

The dynamometer is grasped with the most forceful grip possible, with care being taken not to bring the instrument or the arm in contact with the patient's body. Kellor recommended giving the patient two chances to grip the dynamometer. The highest score of the two should be recorded as the patient's grip strength. This may be compared with the norms published by Kellor and associates (30). The American Society for Surgery of the Hand suggests taking three successive measurements and recording the average (7). Kellor's method would seem to be more closely related to the standard definition of muscle strength (the maximum force muscles can apply in a single voluntary contraction).

Pinch strength is evaluated with a standard commercial meter such as the Osco pinch meter. As with the dynamometer, the serial number must be noted and the same instrument used for reevaluation. Kellor recommended evaluating palmar pinch (between pads of thumb and index and middle fingers), three point pinch (between tips of thumb and index and middle fingers), and lateral or key pinch (between pad of thumb and radial side of middle phalanx of index finger). The forearm should be pronated, and the patient should be given only one opportunity to perform each type of pinch. These values may be compared with norms published by Kellor and associates (30). The American Society for Surgery of the Hand recommends evaluating lateral (key) pinch; three successive efforts are made, and the average is recorded. Tip pinch, defined as pinch between the tips of the index finger and thumb, may be recorded in a similar fashion (7).

For the very weak, painful, or arthritic hand, an adapted sphygmomanometer or bulb dynamometer may be used to measure grip strength. The smallest bulb of the bulb dynamometer may also be used to measure pinch. The size of the bulb used should be recorded for the purpose of retesting (21,26).

Coordination

Gross coordination of the upper extremities is evaluated simply by having the patient throw and catch a large nerf ball or by having the patient stack cones.

Fine coordination or manual dexterity is tested using the beaded peg test described by Kellor and associates. A 100-hole pegboard is divided in half using colored tape. The patient fills the right half of the pegboard with beaded pegs using the right hand and the left half using the left hand. The two sides are timed separately with a stopwatch, and the scores are compared with norms (30). If more detailed information is needed, either the Purdue pegboard test or the O'Connor dexterity test may be used.

SUMMARY

This brief introduction to a system for examination of joint dysfunction has stressed the importance of subjective history and assessment of movement, including active and passive range of motion, joint hypermobility and hypomobility, joint play, and component motions. Analysis of data helps determine whether restricted movement and pain are caused by joint problems or soft-tissue problems. With experience, the therapist will become skilled in analyzing joint problems. On the basis of this system of joint examination, the occupational therapist can select treatment techniques of joint mobilization, therapeutic exercise, functional activities, and splinting that correlate with specific examination findings and that are most appropriate for restoration of normal movement.

REFERENCES

1. Mennell, J. (1964): *Joint Pain,* pp. 1–11. Little, Brown, Boston.
2. Trombley, C. A., and Scott, A. D. (1977): *Occupational Therapy for Physical Dysfunction.* Williams & Wilkins, Baltimore.
3. Cyriax, J. (1973): Diagnosis of soft tissue lesions.

In: *Textbook of Orthopedic Medicine,* Vol. I. Williams & Wilkins, Baltimore.

4. Cyriax, J. (1971): Treatment by manipulation, massage and injection. In: *Textbook of Orthopedic Medicine,* Vol. II. Williams & Wilkins, Baltimore.
5. Hoppenfeld, S. (1976): *Physical Examination of the Spine and Extremities,* pp. 1–104. Appleton-Century-Crofts, New York.
6. Paris, S. V. (1979): Introduction to Extremity Dysfunction and Mobilization (course notes). Institute of Graduate Health Sciences, Atlanta.
7. American Society for Surgery of the Hand (1973): *The Hand, Examination and Diagnosis.* ASSH, Aurora, Ill.
8. MacConaill, M. A., and Basmajian, J. V. (1977): *Muscles and Movements, A Basis for Human Kinesiology,* ed. 2. R. E. Krieger Publishing, Huntington, N.Y.
9. Bryant, M. W. (1977): Wound healing. CIBA, *Clin. Symp.,* 29: 2–15 Summit, N.J.
10. Basmajian, J. (1976): *Primary Anatomy,* ed. 7, pp. 76–78. Williams & Wilkins, Baltimore.
11. Barnett, C., Davies, D., and MacConaill, M. A. (1961): *Synovial Joints, Their Structures and Mechanics.* Charles C Thomas, Springfield, Ill.
12. Jobst Institute (1972): Instructions for measuring: The Jobst glove and web spacer, pp. 388–407. Jobst Institute, Toledo.
13. Warwick, R., and Williams, P. (editors) (1973): *Gray's Anatomy,* ed. 35. W. B. Saunders, Philadelphia.
14. Kaltenborn, F. (1976): *Manual Therapy for the Extremity Joints.* Olaf Norlis Bokhandel, Oslo.
15. Flynn, E. J. (1975): *Hand Surgery,* ed. 2, p. 112. Williams & Wilkins, Baltimore.
16. Curtis, R. M. (1978): Management of the stiff hand. In: *Rehabilitation of the Hand,* edited by J. M. Hunter, L. H. Schreider, E. J. Mackin, et al. C. V. Mosby, St. Louis.
17. Schmidt, R. F. (editor) (1978): *Fundamentals of Sensory Physiology,* pp. 81–125. Springer-Verlag, New York.
18. Woodburne, R. T. (1978): *Essentials of Human Anatomy,* ed. 6, pp. 34–42. Oxford University Press, New York.
19. Maitland, G. D. (1977): *Peripheral Manipulation,* pp. 7–43. Butterworth, Boston.
20. Chusid, J. G. (1976): *Correlative Neuroanatomy and Functional Neurology,* ed. 16. Lange Medical Publications, Los Altos, Calif.
21. Melvin, J. L. (1977): *Rheumatic Disease: Occupational Therapy and Rehabilitation,* pp. 97–127; 143–144. F. A. Davis, Philadelphia.
22. Blakeney, A., Bergholdt, H. T., and Wood, H. L. (1978): Injury splinting and temperature assessment of the insensitive hand. In: *Rehabilitation of the Hand,* edited by J. M. Hunter, L. H. Schreider, E. J. Mackin, et al., pp. 613–614. C. V. Mosby, St. Louis.
23. Lister, G. (1977): *The Hand, Diagnosis and Indications,* pp. 58–59. Churchill-Livingstone, New York.
24. Daniels, L., and Worthingham, C. (1972): *Muscle Testing, Techniques of Manual Examination.* W. B. Saunders, Philadelphia.
25. Cookson, J. C., and Kent, B. E. (1979): Orthopedic manual therapy—an overview. Part I: The extremities. *Phys. Ther.,* 59: 135–146.
26. Fess, E. E., Harmon, K. S., Strickland, J. W., et al. (1978): Evaluation of the hand by objective measurement. In: *Rehabilitation of the Hand,* edited by J. M. Hunter, L. H. Schreider, E. J. Mackin, et al., pp. 70–93. C. V. Mosby, St. Louis.
27. Baker, A. B. (ed.) (1955): *Clinical Neurology,* Vol. 1, pp. 3–13. Paul Hoeber Inc., New York.
28. Hunter, J. M., and Mackin, E. J. (1978): Edema and bandaging. In: *Rehabilitation of the Hand,* edited by J. M. Hunter, L. H. Schreider, E. J. Mackin, et al. C. V. Mosby, St. Louis.
29. Bell, J. (1978): Sensibility evaluation. In: *Rehabilitation of the Hand,* edited by J. M. Hunter, L. H. Schreider, E. J. Mackin, et al., pp. 273–291. C. V. Mosby, St. Louis.
30. Kellor, M., Kodrasuk, R., Iverson, I., et al. (1971): Technical Manual, Hand Strength and Dexterity Tests. Sister Kenny Institute, Minneapolis.
31. Heck, C. V., Hendryson, I. E., and Rowe, C. R. (1965): *Joint Motion, Method of Measuring and Recording.* American Academy of Orthopedic Surgeons. Chicago.
32. Nissenbaum, M. (1978): *Early Care of Flexor Tendon Injuries: Application of Principles of Tendon Healing and Early Motion,* edited by J. M. Hunter, L. H. Schneider, E. J. Macklin, et al., pp. 187–195. Mosby, St. Louis.

Basic Concepts in Hand Therapy: A Biological Approach

5

Karen Prendergast

In the last 10 years there has been increased interest in improving therapy for disability of the hand. This has resulted in part from increasing recognition that hand disability has considerable economic significance on society and in part from the new possibilities opened up by advances in microsurgery techniques. These new developments have made possible new standards of patient care. The surgical procedure is only the first step on the road to recovery. Optimum therapy demands equal attention to postoperative therapy. It has been clearly demonstrated that skilled hand therapists, working directly with the surgeon in a team effort, can provide a higher level of therapeutic care than has yet been achieved.

Undergraduate programs in therapy cannot provide sufficient background to make it possible for the therapist to fulfill the necessary responsibilities at the optimum level of skill and competence. It has become necessary that the graduate therapist seek out advanced training in hand therapy based on biological principles. The hand therapist must learn to make decisions based on knowledge of the latest developments in hand care or reconstruction and therapy, thorough investigation of a patient's needs and capacities, and good judgment developed through extensive experience in working with hand disabilities. The therapist cannot rely on a cookbook approach to therapy. The therapist must remember that any protocol only provides a base line from which to deal with the exceptions, which are in the majority (12).

Hand therapists must have considerable knowledge of both surgical and surface anatomy. They must understand surgical procedures and the goal of any particular procedure. Too often the therapist expects too much of the surgical procedure and too little of the patient. The therapist must also have a thorough knowledge of functional anatomy. Knowledge of anatomy without knowledge of functional applications is practically useless to the therapist.

The goal that the therapist and patient try to achieve is comfortable sensibility combined with strength and coordinated with refined precision. Loss of any one of these components can leave the patient with a severe functional deficit.

Littler (19), in 1956, pioneered this awareness of the importance of sensibility: "An anaesthetic hand is a blind hand. . . . The insensible hand is in a constant state of jeopardy with respect to

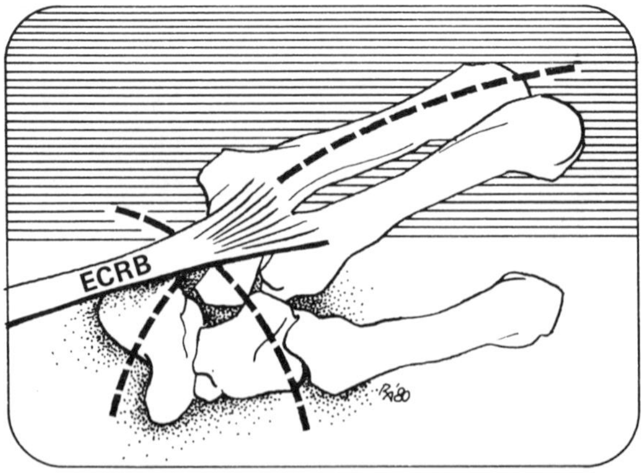

FIG. 1. Wrist stability is provided by the extensor carpi radialis brevis as it inserts in the base of the fixed second and third metacarpals; it has the ability to control both arches affecting the wrist. The volar approach necessitates a strong dorsal wrist strap to secure the splint. The dorsal approach affords counter pressure along the entire length of the splint, thereby preventing buckling into flexion.

trauma, and contributes to the individual only when it is under constant surveillance (16)."

The functional objectives of hand and arm rehabilitation may be said to begin proximally and proceed distally, from shoulder to elbow to hand, preserving the ability to reach out and return. The forearm must perform supination and pronation. The wrist must be a strong stabilizer factor, enabling the patient to adjust the hand in space. The hand must have the ability to manipulate and grasp. Each component has a role affecting the functioning of the others, except possibly the forearm rotation. Proper functioning is dependent on all the component parts working synergistically. A good example of this is the bimanual act of wringing out a wet cloth. In the extremes of wrist range of motion, the muscles become inefficient because of their reduced mechanical advantage. Wrist stability (accomplished primarily by the musculus extensor carpi radialis brevis) is one of the most important functional priorities to be preserved or regained in postoperative therapy (Fig. 1) (22).

Another important functional priority is the strength of the intrinsic muscles. True balance between the flexor and extensor extrinsic muscles can be established only with the cooperation of the intrinsic lumbrical and interosseous muscles. No motion of the hand nor contraction of muscle is exclusive. It is important to remember this principle in developing any type of postoperative therapy program.

Classification of muscles into separate kinesi-

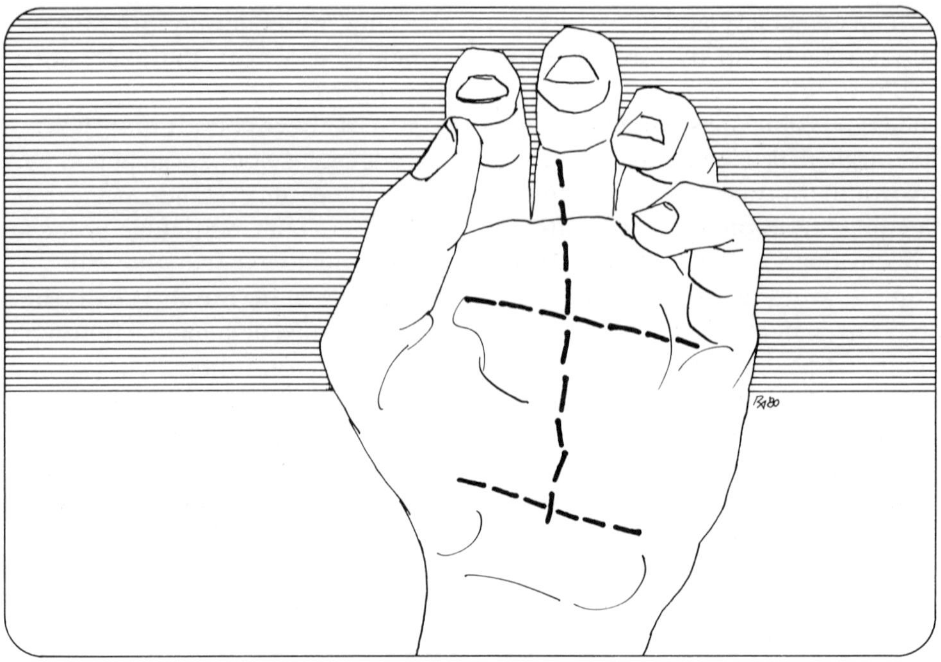

FIG. 2. The hand has three arches: the two transverse arches are formed by the distal carpal row and the metacarpal heads. The longitudinal arch runs from the capitate distally through the tips of the index and middle fingers.

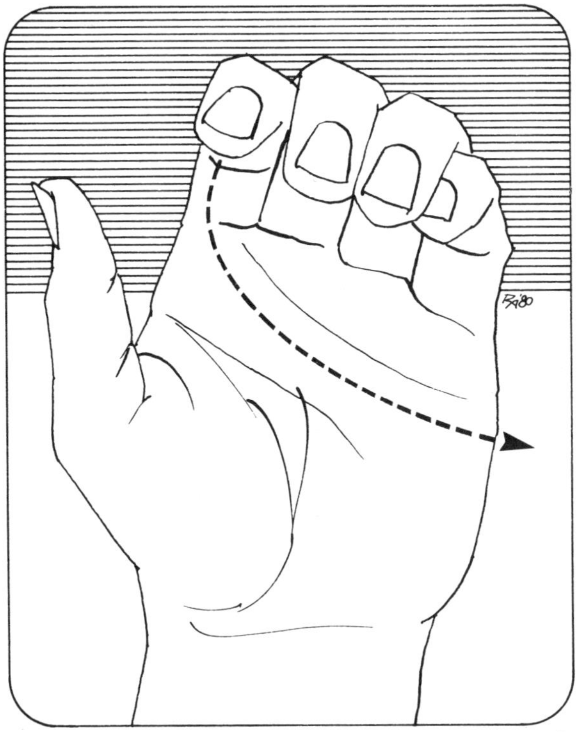

FIG. 3. The function of the index is relatively independent of power grasp. It typically exhibits a strong first dorsal interossei muscle, an independent digital extensor and a tendinous connection between the index digitorum profundus and the flexor pollicis longus tendon. The index is thus adapted to facilitate pinch independent of the other fingers.

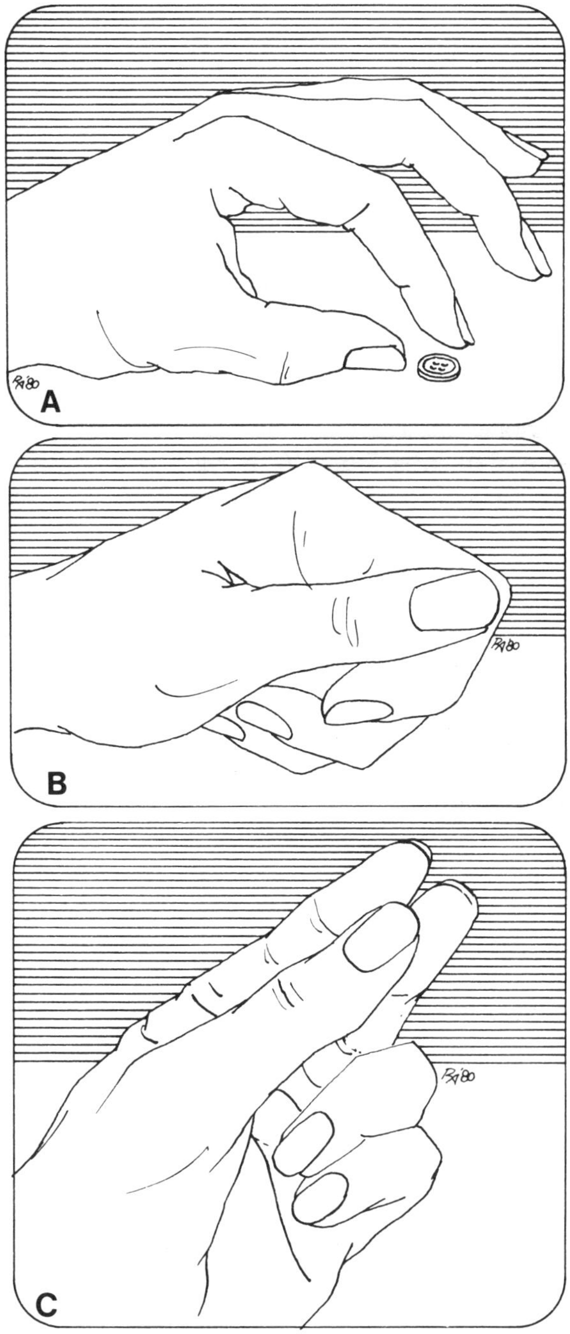

FIG. 4. A. Pulp to pulp pinch. **B.** Key pinch. **C.** Three jaw chuck pinch.

ological groups as described in undergraduate textbooks should be viewed with reservation. These classifications do not permit a complete picture of muscular activity. Such an incomplete picture shows only limited motions that may vary considerably under various conditions, especially injury. Every voluntary motion that is executed with precision must be moderated by the antagonist muscles and stabilized by synergist muscles.

KINESIOLOGY; FUNCTION AND ANATOMY

The hand has three arches, two transverse and one longitudinal. The two transverse arches form the cupping mechanism: Proximally there is the transverse arch across the carpal bones; distally there is the transverse arch running through the heads of the metacarpals. The longitudinal arch starts in the carpal bones in the capitate and runs through an axis between the second and third carpals and up through the center line between the index and middle fingers (Fig. 2). These arches permit the hand to be molded around various objects. These arches as described are anatomic reference points.

The hand may also be divided into three functional units. The thumb is linked with the trapezium and scaphoid to constitute the first functional unit; the index and middle fingers, acting mainly in precision activities with the thumb, compose the second unit; the ring and small fingers, providing mainly power grasp and cupping, form the radial functional unit. Disability in any one of these functional units produces a major functional deficit for the patient. Among the characteristic features of the human hand are the comparatively long thumb and the presence of the musculus flexor pollicis longus. The long thumb permits better opposition. The musculus flexor pollicis longus provides the element of stability. Another characteristic is the relative independence of the index finger (16). In Fig. 3, note that the distal palmar crease terminates in the web between the index and middle fingers. The design of these two digits allows a variety of pinch movements. There are several ways to categorize various types of pinch movements, as well as subclassifications of the various categories. For simplicity, they will be broken down here into three major types of pinch (Fig. 4A): (a) pulp-to-pulp pinch, as though one were picking up a pin from a table surface (Fig. 4B); (b) key pinch, as the thumb presses against the radial border of the index finger when one holds a key to turn in a lock (Fig. 4C); (c) three jaw chuck, the opposition between the thumb pulp, index, and middle finger pulp.

Although there is relative independence of the functional units, the four fingers act as a team. A limitation in one of the digits interferes with the functioning of the others; because of this, every effort must be made to restore a damaged hand to its preinjury status. Thus far we have been discussing the capabilities of the normal hand. When one is considering the hand in the context of deformity, injury, disease, or postoperative condition, one must determine the various attitudes that the hand will assume and distinguish between those that are detrimental to the progress of the therapy and those that will tend to preserve its structures. The position of rest, as seen in Fig. 5, shows that the tendon lengths are influential because the muscles are relaxed, not under tension. However, the position of function is quite different (Fig. 6). This position is assumed in preparation for grasping or releasing an object. Here the wrist is stabilized (Fig. 7). Figure 3 shows a trauma posture that a hand assumes after injury. This position is characterized by dorsal edema and a taking up of the slack of the musculus extensor digitorum communis tendons, which creates hyperextension at the metacarpophalangeal (MP) joint. The musculus extensor pollicis longus also pulls the thumb into adduction. The position of the MP joint puts extra tension on the flexor tendons, thus creating flexion at the proximal interphalangeal (PIP) and distal interphalangeal (DIP) joints, as well as flexion of the interphalangeal (IP) joints of the thumb from the musculus flexor pollicis longus tendon. It is dangerous for the hand to remain in this position for any length of time, as it is detrimental to maintenance of the resting length necessary for full active joint mobility of the IP joints of the digits. The position of safety (Fig. 8) for a hand following an injury is a position opposite to the posture that results from trauma. This position keeps the wrist in a neutral position and flexes the MP joints to 70 degrees, thus putting the collateral ligaments on full stretch and producing full abduction of the thumb and extension of the IP joint of the thumb. By putting the collateral ligaments on stretch and stretching out the web space of the thumb, one will preserve the lengths of these structures and prepare the way for a shorter recovery period. It is far easier to mobilize a lengthened structure than it is to elongate a shortened structure, such as the collateral ligaments.

Next we shall consider what happens to these mechanisms in the presence of disease or trauma.

BIOLOGICAL PRINCIPLES OF RECONSTRUCTIVE SURGERY AND THERAPY

Littler stated that "joint mobility with tendon gliding and muscle contractility are all highly essential functions which deserve every surgical effort to preserve and restore" (21). It is fundamental that the therapist must understand the physiology of tissue repair in order to be able to care for the traumatized hand, to know what constitutes a properly healing wound, and to know how to promote more rapid healing. Control of edema is one of the first priorities in caring for wounds, and an understanding of tissue repair processes will reveal why edema control is so important. Selection of an appropriate therapeutic exercise program must be governed by the

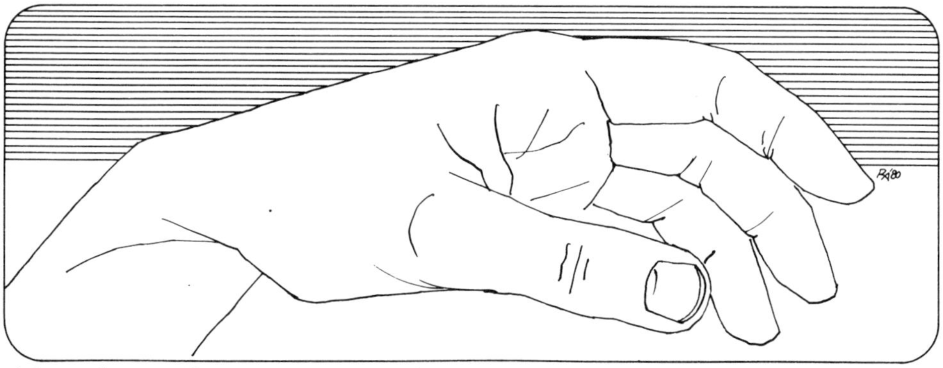

FIG. 5. The position of rest: The nontraumatized hand assumes this position when the forearm muscles are relaxed. The digital resting position is determined by the length tension of the extrinsic tendons as they stretch across the wrist joint.

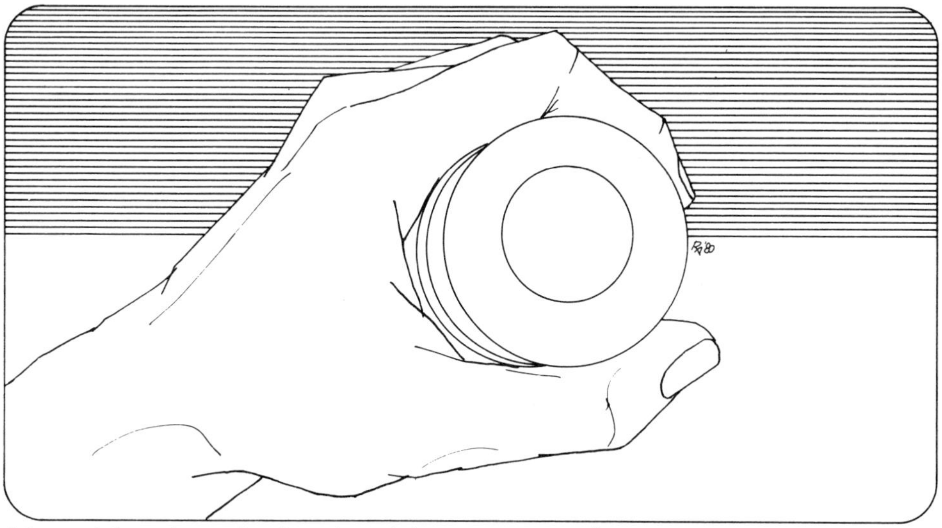

FIG. 6. The position of function: the hand and forearm musculature is in a preparatory posture, the wrist muscles contract providing wrist stability for action of the digits.

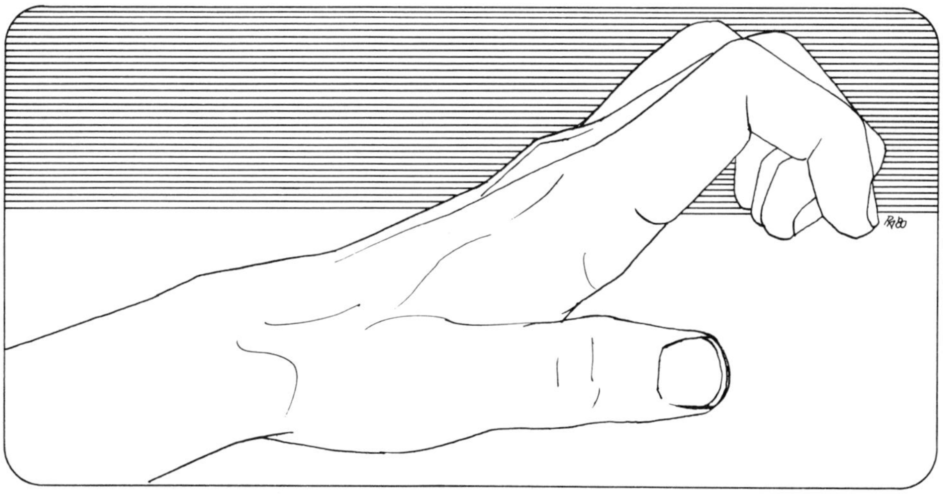

FIG. 7. The trauma posture: the traumatized hand at rest is under the influence of tendon length. Dorsal edema and fibrosis acts on the digital extensors hyperextending the MP joints and adducting the thumb. The MP position then creates extra pull on the IP joints by the extrinsic digital flexor muscles.

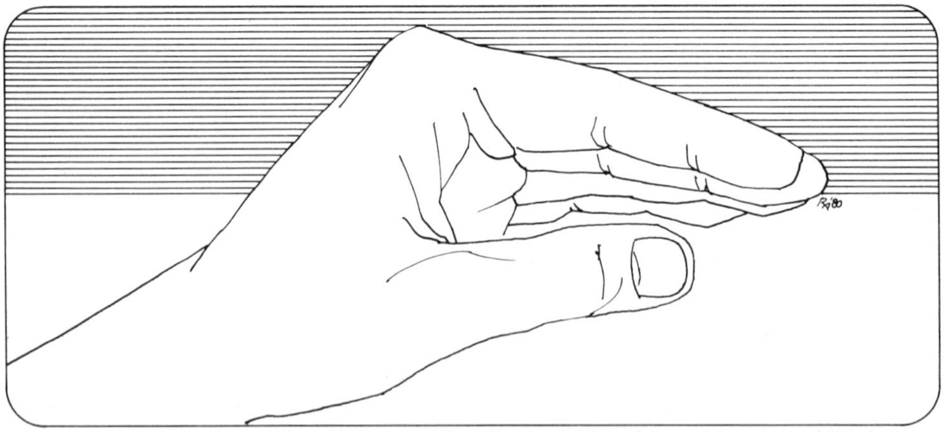

FIG. 8. The position of safety: when the traumatized or immobilized hand is placed in this position the joints are safely preserved for future function. The length of the collateral ligaments is maintained and the thumb web is stretched to preserve thumb opposition and abduction.

strength of the tissues involved. The therapist must learn to choose a therapy program according to the principles of tissue healing. The therapist works with scar tissue and its process of maturation in every case; the structural organization of collagen depends on the forces applied to it. Peacock stated that "it is almost axiomatic that injury is followed by inflammation. Vascular and cellular response is designed to defend the body against alien substances and to dispose of dead and dying tissue preparatory to the repair process" (32). What this means to the therapist is that every time an inflammatory response occurs, whether because of disease or trauma or because of a heavy-handed therapy program, that inflammatory response will be followed by the full cycle of the repair process, which means that there will be scar formation.

Wound Healing

There are three phases of wound healing. First there is the exudative phase, which lasts approximately 5 days to 10 days. Following that, the fibroblastic phase lasts from approximately the 5th day after injury to the 25th day. Finally, the maturation phase follows the ending of fibroplasia, beginning about the 25th day and going on for several years.

During the exudative phase, cells modulate into migratory fibroblasts. The inflammatory exudate contains large amounts of fibrinogen, from which fibrin is formed and laid down as a hemostatic barrier. The migratory fibroblasts later use the strands of fiber as a scaffold on which to lay down collagen fibers. At the end of a surgical procedure, the macrophages or phagocytes in the exudate area and the spindle-shaped polymorphonuclear leukocytes are in close proximity to the wound. By 24 to 48 hr after the operation the macrophages gather at the base of the wound, and the fibrin has clotted into the exudate area. Escaped fluid from local blood vessels combines with migrating leukocytes and dead tissue to produce what is called the inflammatory exudate. This inflammatory exudate and lysed polymorphonuclear leukocytes constitute pus. The presence of pus does not necessarily mean that there is bacterial infection. What it does mean is that there is inflammation. Destructive inflammation is fostered by the presence of dead tissue, bacteria, and blood clots and by poor circulation. In such instances the therapist can contribute to wound healing by removing dead tissue and blood clots and applying techniques designed to augment the circulation.

Local vasodilation, leakage of fluid into the extravascular space, and cessation of lymphatic drainage are the signs of inflammation. The symptoms include redness, swelling, heat, and pain that may result from pressure or chemical stimuli.

During fibroplasia, the second phase of wound healing, there will be significant change in the tensile strength of the wound tissue. The fibrin provides a framework for the fibroblasts. Capillary formation follows, with endothelial budding. The fibrin network is lysed and removed, and collagen synthesis then predominates. It is during this phase that the internal area of the wound is becoming more dense and viscous, and the patient may notice decreased mobility in the involved digits. It is because of this change in viscosity in the wound during fibroplasia that one can make a good case for early mobilization of structures following injury, if structural strength permits. Fibroplasia begins at 5 to 8 days postoperatively, with predominance of spindle-shaped polymorphonuclear leukocytes. At 10 to 15 days postoperatively there is giant cell formation and an increase in the production of collagen fibers, with the fibrin clot being separated from the endothelium.

When collagen production and collagen degradation reach a balance, this is considered the beginning of the maturation phase of wound healing. This lasts for months, sometimes even years, after the initial wound. For example, studies have shown that skin wounds reach approximately 75% of their ultimate tensile strength at 150 days after the initial wounding.

Reconstructive Principles

Every tissue that has been traumatized through injury or surgery will undergo fibroblastic proliferation. This is the basis of all repair in all connective tissues (32). Although the skin is the organ of first contact, every structure beneath the skin that is involved in the trauma will be involved in the healing process and subject to fibrosis. Since there is no differentiation between specialized parts, there exists a common bed of scar tissue. Independent function of the structures within the common bed is lost; thus, one of the principles of reconstructive surgery is to introduce only normal tissue into a bed of scar tissue in order to prevent adherence of one to the other.

It is essential to ensure that functional units be preserved intact; then they must be mobilized, taking advantage of the available power and sensibility efforts must be concentrated on those areas where the best functional result can be achieved. It is much like a banking system; one places assets where they will produce the highest return (21).

Role of the Therapist

The therapist must examine the hand at rest and during function and carry out postoperative treatment. Treatment usually begins with some form of thermotherapy. Thermotherapy provides analgesia, increases peripheral blood flow, increases the suppurative process, and provides a sedative effect. Thus its contraindications would include impaired arterial blood supply, chronic venous insufficiency, and edema associated with venous disease. Edema itself is not an indication for thermotherapy. It was previously noted that edema is one of the body's first responses to trauma and is also one of the first treatment priorities for the therapist. The indications for cryotherapy include severe pain and acute inflammation; it is also used when the therapist wishes to provide a counterirritant. The contraindications to cryotherapy include retardation of wound healing and hypersensitivity to cold (17).

Therapeutic Massage

Unless there is adequate skin elasticity, hand mobility and function are restricted. One way to preserve and restore skin elasticity is through therapeutic massage. Massage will not directly increase the strength of normal muscle, nor will it increase muscle tone. Most important, it will not prevent muscle atrophy. However, massage can lessen fibrosis, help maintain muscle nutrition, loosen and flatten scar tissue, and desensitize sensory receptors through mechanical stimulation. Massage produces mechanical stimulation of tissues by means of rhythmically applied pressure and stretching. By changing the lumina of the blood vessels and lymph spaces, it affects capillary, venous, arterial, and lymphatic circulations. Massage is an excellent mode of preparation for therapeutic exercise (2).

Therapeutic Exercise Program

Control of edema is the first priority. As stated earlier, edema is a precursor to the formation of scar tissue. Lymph can move in any direction; its course is determined by gravity, muscle contraction, joint movement, and massage. We have discussed massage. Gravity is self-explanatory, and it is used by most physicians to help control stasis edema or edema of dependency after trauma or a surgical procedure. Muscle contraction has a strong influence in reducing lymphedema, and in this light we shall emphasize therapeutic exercise and muscular stimulation.

There are other methods to control edema. Examples include increasing the distal pressure through the use of an elastic garment such as a Jobst custom-fitted glove or sleeve, wrapping with increasing pressure from distal to proximal using either string wrapping or elastic bandage wrapping, and electrotherapeutic stimulation of the muscles. Edema can be controlled by applying alternating current stimulation to force muscle contraction. Alternating current can be used circumferentially around a digit (19). Another form of electrostimulation is high-voltage galvanic stimulation, using either pad electrodes or electrodes under water.

Therapeutic exercise is the mainstay of the treatment program. It helps to reduce edema, restore tissues to their working lengths, and build the strength required for functioning. Exercise producing a rhythmic alternation between sustained contraction and relaxation produces a milking action in the deep veins to enhance venous return. Joint stability is enhanced if balance is maintained in the program for rebuilding muscle strength. These are all reasons for concentrating on the exercise phase of the treatment program.

Building muscle balance is not the same as building muscle bulk. Simply building muscle bulk is not in keeping with the goal of rehabilitating patients for their formal life-styles or professions. Muscle strength is related to the ability to develop tension in muscle fibers under full voluntary control, as well as to the number of motor units that can be activated by a voluntary effort. Thus strength is dependent on two factors: cross section of muscle fiber and its innervation. Work is defined as force times the distance through which the force acts. The force is, of course, related to the muscle's strength; the distance is determined by the anatomic placement of the muscle and the ability for these tendon to glide during the execution of a movement. Power is work capacity or work per unit of time. Therefore, the ability to develop power is dependent on normal tendon excursion and on muscle strength. In order to perform work in a vocational setting, one must have stamina or endurance. Stamina is related to metabolic turnover. This will be influenced by physical well-being in terms of nutrition of the patient's entire organic system, as well as by metabolism in the muscle and tissues within the extremity. Another very important aspect of daily living and vocational success is the development of skill. Skill is a matter of central nervous system involvement with the structures of the arm. This requires a learning process, for skills are easily lost after trauma or disease. The ability to work over a period of time, and to develop the stamina to continue to function, is an essential component of daily living. Maintenance of muscle strength is not sufficient in a rehabilitation setting. The therapist must encourage the patient to work to capacity over increasing periods of time; this will increase the metabolic capacity of the muscles and structures of the arm and facilitate relearning the skills involved in daily living and in vocational accomplishment. Power, endurance, and skill are the goals necessary for carrying out the activities of daily living and preparing for a vocation. (17).

The exercise program must be designed to enchance the metabolic capacity of the muscles. The general effects are most beneficial when the exercise involves multiple large muscle groups and is sufficiently prolonged and strenuous to induce metabolic and circulatory stress. Thus the severity of the exercise must be continually readjusted. The therapist must continually reevaluate to determine if the muscle groups are being adequately challenged.

Exercise can take many forms. The therapist must be sure to focus on the desired functional action or muscle group. Arm rehabilitation includes shoulder strength, wrist stability, coordination, and digital power, not only in the five digits working together but also in the fingers working individually. In many cases it is necessary to establish proximal stability before developing distal power. This is most frequently seen in the wrist, where one must achieve wrist stability before grasp strength can be developed.

The best exercises are those that develop not only strength but also power and stamina. The ideal situation is to have a workshop right in the therapy office, but in many cases the therapist can assign tasks for the patient to do at home using hand tools, such as using a hammer or screwdriver, as well as specific activities of daily living.

Splinting

The small joints between the bones of the hand have been highly developed for grasp and manipulation. Proper motion of the joints is essential for performing even routine tasks, but the elasticity of the small collateral ligaments and joint capsules can be easily lost through injury, immobilization, or disease. Small amounts of shortening in these soft tissues interfere with motion to a greater extent than do similar changes in the larger joints of the arm and leg.

Preservation of joint function is a key concern of the therapist. With immobilization, even nontraumatized joints exhibit changes in their lubricating mechanisms and changes in collagen (1). Traumatized joints become distorted by edema, with resultant formation of scar tissue. Regardless of the specific change within the joint, it is essential that mobilization begin as early as possible, within the structure's strength limitations.

When preservation of joint function has not been accomplished during the early stage of rehabilitation, it becomes necessary to think in terms of restoring collagen and stretching ligamentous structures to resting lengths that will be compatible with the full range of motion of the joint. This is most often accomplished through prolonged gentle stretching of the structures by means of splinting techniques.

Splint by Objective

Since there is a zigzag relationship among the joints in this multiarticulated system, each joint will affect the position of the joint proximal or distal to it. With just a small alteration in the delicate balance between the flexor and extensor tendon systems, the abnormal forces acting on the joints will cause them to buckle in a predictable manner. The MP joint affects the PIP joint. As the MP joint flexes, there is a tightening of the forces on the musculus extensor digitorum communis tendon that creates an overpull on the PIP joint (Fig. 9). In the opposite situation, where the MP joint is hyperextended, again it is a tendon that is overpulled, this time that of the musculus flexor digitorum sublimis, which overpulls on the PIP joint, creating PIP flexion. Thus if there is capsular tightness of the MP joint, one will have to splint the PIP joint in the reciprocal position in order to have a permanent effect on the capsule of the MP joint, because of the forces exerted on the joint by the tendons.

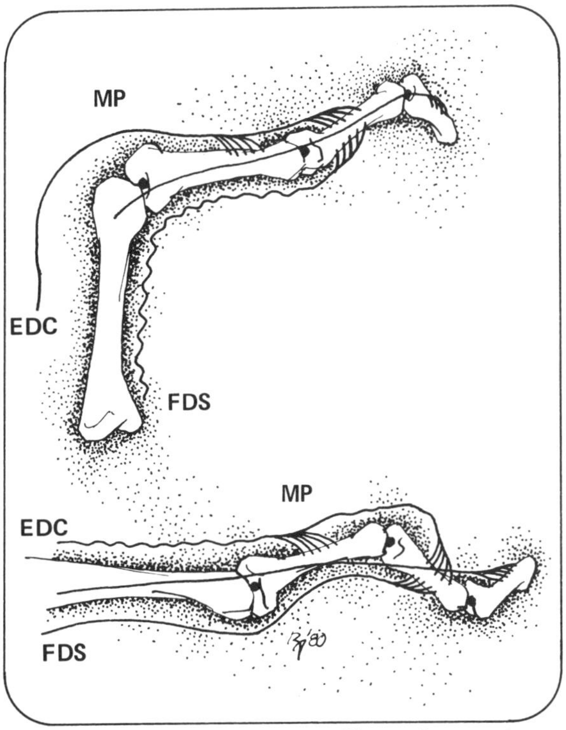

FIG. 9. The MP joint position affects the tendon and ligament pull on the distal joints. When the MP joint rests in flexion, the slackened flexor digitorum sublimus allows the extensor digitorum communis muscle to dominate. With the MP resting in hypertextension the slackened extensor digitorum communis allows flexor digitorum sublimus dominance.

In the normal relationship between the lateral bands of the PIP joint and the musculus digitorum profundus of the PIP joint, the lateral bands lie dorsal to the axis, and the profundus lies volar to the axis of the joint. If there is capsular tightness in PIP flexion, there will be an overpull on the lateral bands and a slackening of the profundus tendon, thus creating hyperextension at the DIP joint as a reciprocal effect to the flexion contracture at the PIP level.

Reciprocally (Fig. 10), if the PIP joint has been tightened or stiffened in hyperextension, the lateral bands will be loose change or rather add after loose, the force of the lateral bands acts dorsal to the joint axis and the flexor digitorum profundus is free to overpull. The result will be flexion deformity of the DIP joint in addition to the

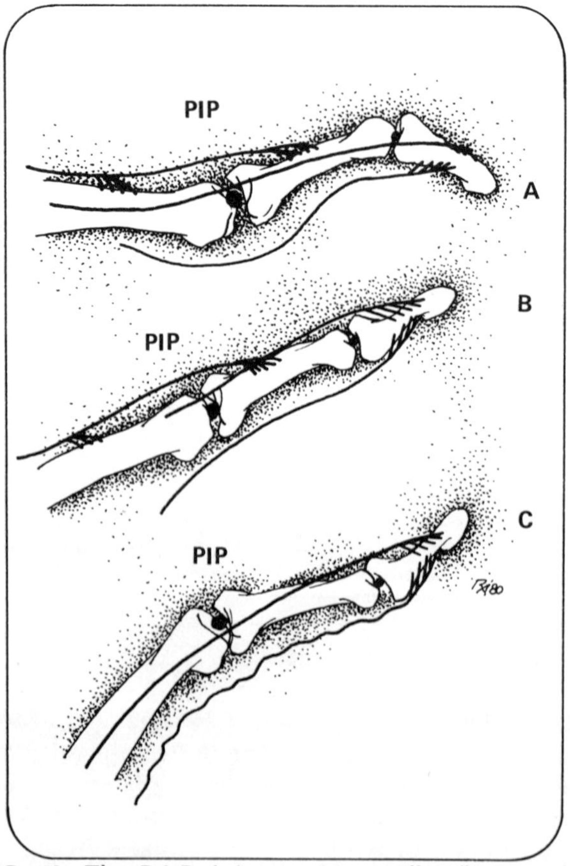

FIG. 10. The P.I.P. joint position will influence the resting position of the D.I.P. joint. **A.** Hypertension of the P.I.P. allows the distal insertion to slip volarly enough to exert a flexor force on the D.I.P. joint creating the swan neck deformity. **B.** The natural forces of the extensor digitorum communis central slip and the lateral bands opposing the flexor forces of the flexor digitorum sublimus and flexor digitorum profundus acting on the P.I.P. joint. When this equilibrium is altered through trauma the resting positions will depend on the forces in relation to the axis at the P.I.P. joint. **C.** Lateral bands have shifted volarly creating excessive flexor forces on the P.I.P. joint and facilitating on overpull on the D.I.P. joint.

hyperextension deformity of the PIP. In splinting, to restore the appropriate range of motion of a PIP joint, one must either splint the DIP joint in the opposite direction or leave the DIP joint free to be exercised by the patient. But under no circumstances, when there is capsular tightness in the PIP joint, should the DIP be forced in the same direction (Fig. 11).

Consider the DIP joint. In various injuries the DIP joint is left to tighten in joint flexion, thus creating a shift in the lateral bands to an extreme dorsal position at the PIP level. This extreme causes an imbalance of the extensor forces at the PIP joint and creates a severe hyperextension deformity. In the case of a fixed boutonniere deformity, which affects both the PIP and DIP joints, the DIP joint will be in severe hyperextension. The lateral bands will have drifted volar to the axis of the PIP joint, creating an extreme pull of the lateral bands at the distal insertion. To correct this deformity, one must splint one joint at a time to change the position of the lateral bands in relation to the axis at the PIP joint. In an attempt to correct a mallet deformity, again, one must not splint the two joints, PIP and DIP, with the forces acting volarly. One must support the DIP joint by lifting the distal phalanx in relation to the middle phalanx, at the same time allowing the PIP joint to flex and giving the lateral bands a chance to drift volarly (Fig. 12).

Splint Design

It would take an entire book to discuss the intricacies of biomechanics and bioengineering involved in splint design. Here there is room only for a few principles to serve as basic guidelines. There are three things to consider when designing a splint. First, one must think in terms of curves. A curve is structurally stronger than a straight line or straight edge, and any splint built on a curve will provide more support (Fig. 12). When the edges are rolled or curved, such as at the distal palmar crease or at the base of the forearm, there is a comfort factor, for the curved edge provides a ledge on which the tissue can roll. The second principle is that of building the splint on a diagonal. Since the venous circulation runs longitudinally from distal to proximal, it makes sense to place pressures diagonally so that not all venous return will be blocked at the same level. This may apply to the basic structure of the splint with thermoplastic materials, and it may also apply to the strap materials used for closure. The third principle is that of pressures (Fig. 13). Pressures must be considered in every aspect of splint design. The amount of pressure exerted is derived from the formula P = mass/area. In keeping with this formula, one can adjust the pressure on any area, either dispersing the pressures by increasing the area over which pressure is applied or increasing the pressure by decreasing the area over

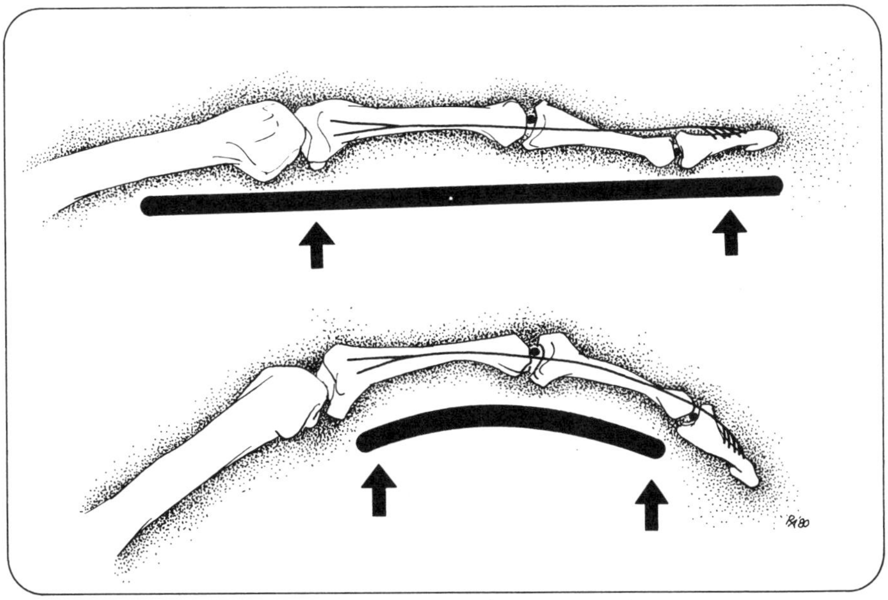

FIG. 11. In the case of PIP capsular tightness, the two volar points of pressure must act on the proximal and middle phalanges only. **Top:** the distal pressure on the DIP joint will hyperextend it, thus perpetrating the flexion deformity. **Bottom:** the pressure points act appropriately and allow the DIP joint free to flex.

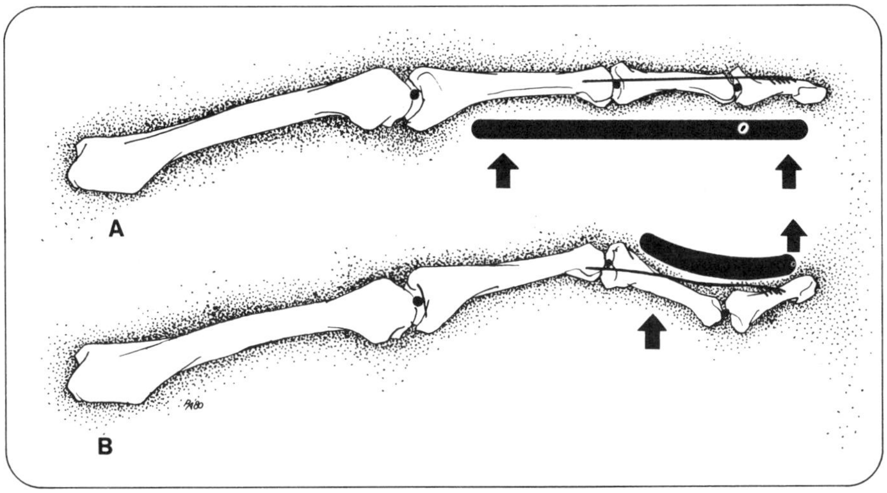

FIG. 12. Splint one joint at a time to allow the lateral bands to slip above or below the axis of the PIP joint. In the case of the mallet deformity in order to permit reapproximation of the distal insertion by hyperextension the PIP must be free to flex. In the case of PIP capsular tightness the two volar points of pressure must act on the prox and middle phalanges only. In **A** the distal pressure on the DIP joint will hyperextend it, thus perpetrating the flexion deformity. In **B** the pressure points act appropriately and allow the DIP joint free to flex.

which the pressure is applied (decreasing the area of the material applied over a given point). An example of an area that always presents a problem in splinting is the dorsal aspect of the hand. If a wide area is covered by thermoplastic material, the pressure is dispersed sufficiently to provide comfort. However, if the therapist should leave a small tight band that concentrates the pressure over the metacarpal bones, there will be complaints about the comfort of the splint. This situation can also occur when splinting the IP joints. If one carefully contours the volar surface of the splint, thus creating a large area for pressure dispersion, the volar surface will be comfortable and

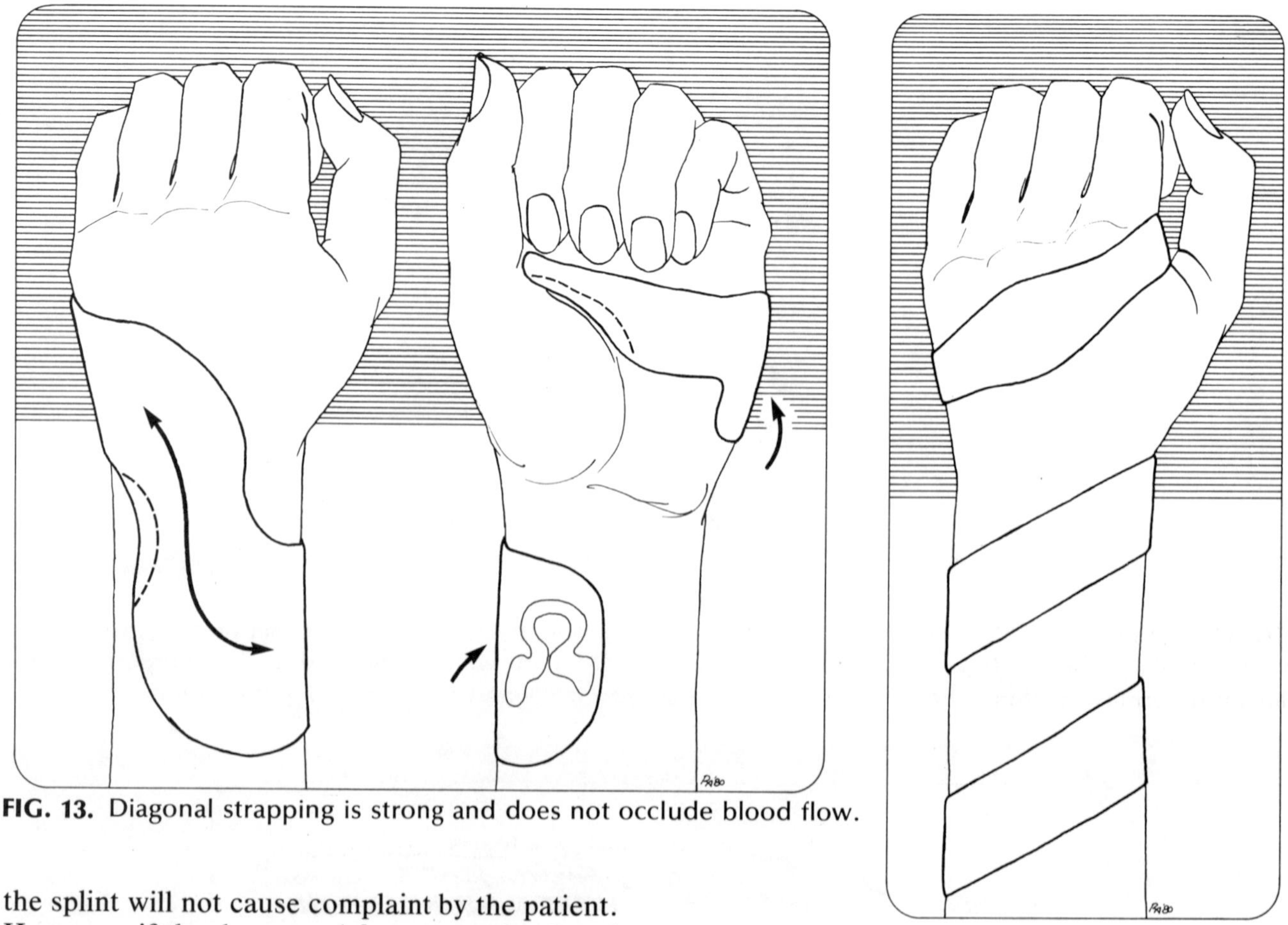

FIG. 13. Diagonal strapping is strong and does not occlude blood flow.

the splint will not cause complaint by the patient. However, if the downward force over the dorsal surface is simply a tiny strap or a flat piece of plastic, there will be point pressure over the highest point of the bony structure, which will cause tissue breakdown under the dorsal tab of the splint (Fig. 13).

Splints must be designed to incorporate other basic principles. In designing a splint, one must allow sufficient length from the fulcrum (normally the wrist joint) to provide a lever arm long enough so that the splint can support the weight of the hand at the opposite end from the fulcrum. This becomes a less crucial measurement with the newer thermoplastic materials, which have greater structural strength than the older Orthoplast™. Another structural consideration is the possibility of a spine placed on the surface of the splint to create greater structural strength. This is especially useful in splints that support the entire weight of the hand, as in the case of radial nerve paralysis or median ulnar difficulties where the wrist joint is unstable.

All splints must contour exactly to the surface anatomy of the patient. If this principle is not observed, the splint will not serve to best advantage, as contact will be concentrated at fewer points, and the pressures will become greater at those points. But if the splint is properly contoured, the pressure will be dispersed and the splint will be more comfortable. Another reason for contouring the splint to the skin surface is to preserve the natural arches of the hand. The two transverse and one longitudinal arches were mentioned earlier; these three arches must be considered in splint design. The ligamentous structures supporting these arches need to be supported. This is accomplished by contouring the splint on the volar surface. Finally, one must always remember that the arcs of flexion of the MP joints are different. Thus the volar surface of the palm necessitates a slanted transverse portion at the distal end of the splint to allow complete flexion of the MP joints, including the small finger. The distal palmar crease must be followed in the pattern of the splint, and one must actually be able to see the distal palmar crease when the

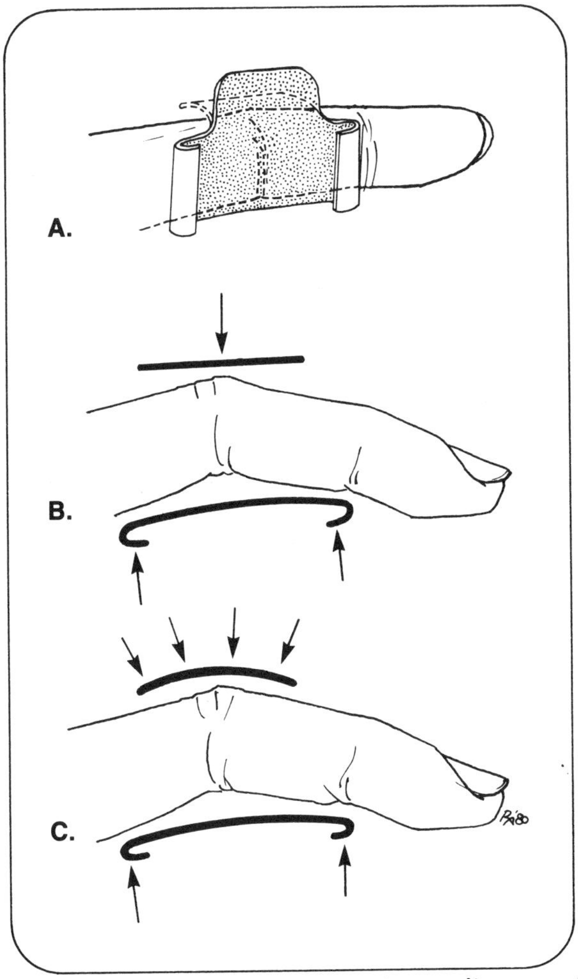

FIG. 14. A standard PIP extension splint can be made strong by curling edges. **A.** direct pressure over the bony prominence of the PIP joint can be avoided by contouring the dorsal tab. By pressure dispersion tissue trauma is avoided (**B** and **C**).

splint is applied and test whether or not the small finger is able to complete its full excursion. This is also true of the thenar eminence, which should not be blocked under most circumstances. The thenar eminence should be free to complete opposition, and thus the edge of the splint on the radial aspect will need to be rolled away sufficiently to allow the thenar eminence appropriate mobility.

Approach

In creating a wrist support splint, one has the choice of a dorsal or volar approach. Naturally, the choice may be influenced by the need to cover and thus render insensible one surface or the other.

The dorsal approach is preferable when possible. The weight of the hand exerts a considerable flexion force on the fulcrum of the wrist. The moment arm from this fulcrum to the distal end of a volar splint is too short to effectively push the hand dorsally. Its effectiveness lies in its ability to bow away at its center, remaining fixed at the palmar strap and forearm strap (Fig. 14). This greatly increases the pressures of these two areas as the wrist bucks away. In order to prevent further wrist flexion one is forced to supply a strong strap across the joint itself. This strap not only can occlude venous return from the hand but places great pressures on the ulnar styloid as it changes contour from pronation to supination (Fig. 14).

The dorsal approach is more successful at maintaining wrist extension (Fig. 15). The moment arm from the wrist fulcrum is still short but the convex shape of the splint against the convex shape of the dorsum of the hand helps to maintain the convexity. The fixed palmar and forearm straps provide a force to maintain this relationship. The dorsal contour in total contact with the skin prevents any bucking collapse of the wrist into flexion. Any excessive pressures on the ulnar are alleviated by a well beveled foam disc molded into the splint. The strap pressure is easily handled by the well padded palmar fascia (Fig. 15). The dorsal wrist extension splint is strong, secure, and comfortable. Naturally, with problems of spasticity or open wounds, one very often does not have a choice in this matter.

A few comments are in order regarding prefabricated splints. It is difficult to modify most prefabricated splints. As there is no such thing as a universal hand, there is no splint that fits all hands, or even A, B, C, and D sizes. Considering the time it takes to modify a prefabricated splint for comfort and effectiveness, it may be better to spend the same amount of time fabricating a splint of thermoplastic materials. A second consideration is that prefabricated splints, almost without exception, are more expensive than splints fabricated in the office or hospital setting. Many prefabricated splints, because of the attempt at a universal fit, never quite achieve the desired action. As in the case of the prefabricated flexion cuff, it always seems that the joint that is stiffened does not receive the forces, and the effects of the traction are concentrated on the joints

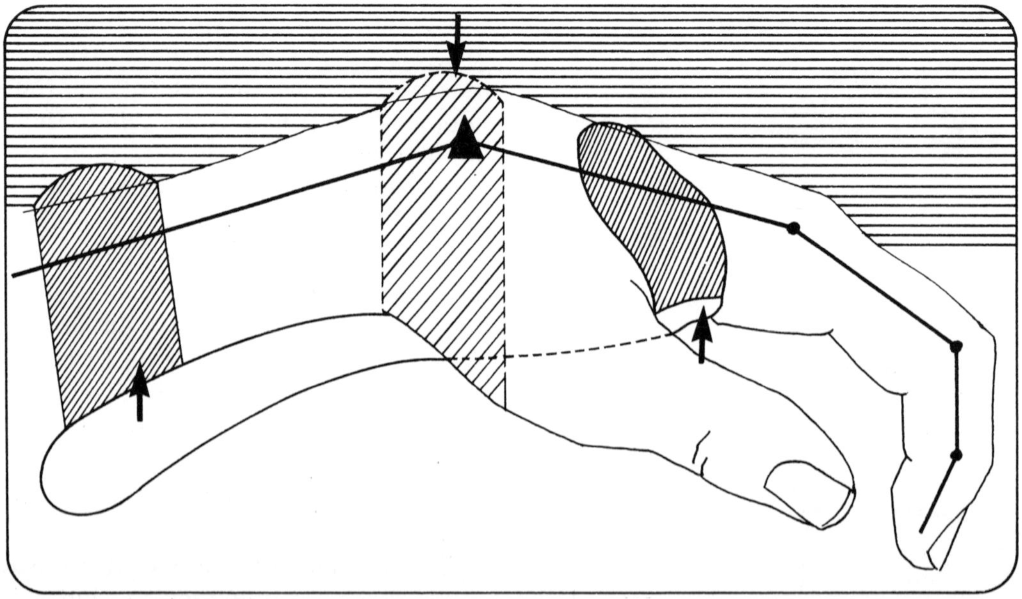

FIG. 15. The volar approach necessitates a strong dorsal wrist strap to secure the splint.

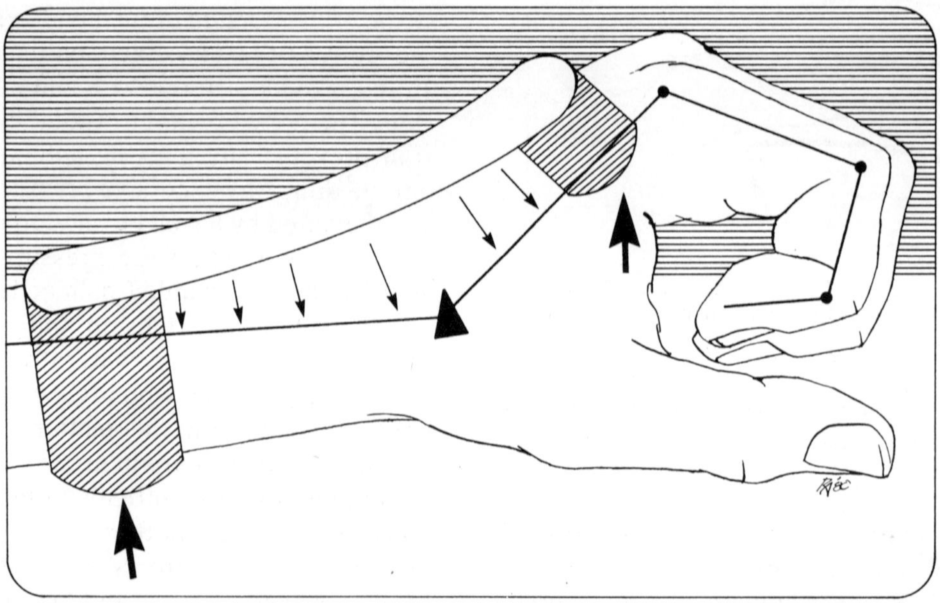

FIG. 16. The dorsal approach affords counter pressure along the entire length of the splint thereby preventing buckling.

that are mobile enough to flex with the traction. There is also the element that the wrist position has a strong influence on the potential excursions of the MP and IP joints. Since the flexion cuff does not include a wrist stabilization factor, one must accept the fact that there will be tenodesis action of the extensor tendons as the wrist flexes, as it often does in sleep, or one must build yet another splint to go underneath the flexion glove to stabilize the wrist in a neutral position (Figs. 16, 17).

These few comments on the basic ideas of splinting derive from experience. They by no means constitute a complete list or a complete guide to splint fabrication. It is unfortunate that undergraduate schools have so little time to devote to the bioengineering concepts of splinting. It will be necessary for the student of hand

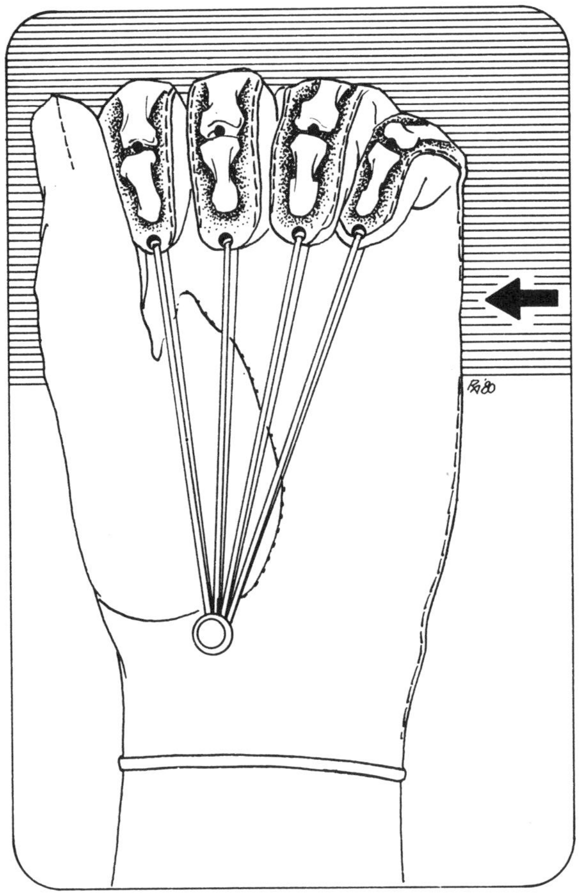

FIG. 17. Prefabricated exercise devices often lack the ability to control unwanted joint motion. In the case of the flexion glove the pull of the elastic bands yields flexion of the more supple I.P. joints while not concentrating forces on the stiffened M.P. joints.

therapy to refer to one of the more complete texts on the subject to become properly knowledgeable, in addition to spending years in practice with the various materials. Dynamic splinting is a topic too complex to be approached in this limited space.

OCCUPATIONAL KINESIOLOGY AND BIOMECHANICS

The hand therapist must understand the patient's needs in the work environment. One must understand the implications and effects of doing repetitive work within a fixed environment. It makes no sense to carry out a rehabilitation program and then return the patient to the same dangerous work situation or work pattern. In most occupational situations, workers are doing repetitive types of work using universal tools within a fixed environment. The design of the hand is such that it is able to cope with many changing pressures and stresses. However, in a situation where the same exact pressures are applied over an 8-hr day for several years, there are consequences to this repetitive stress. One should be familiar with the key points and key areas of stress, especially when they affect structures that lie deep to the surface. We have stated that there is no such thing as a universal hand, and therefore tools that are designed to be used by all workers will undoubtedly affect that population of workers who fall above or below the median anthropometric measurements of hand size and dimensions. The worker works within a fixed environment, partially surrounded by desk or machinery. This environment does not change throughout the 8-hr day. As a result, the torsion movements that the body completes repetitively will have an effect, not only on the hand but also on the arm, the curvature of the neck, and the stresses on the spine. This is an entire field of study, but one that the hand therapist should be aware of in rehabilitating a worker who will have less adaptability and less ability to handle stress on the tissues after an injury has been sustained or a disease has taken its toll on the structures (35).

PSYCHOLOGY

The hand therapist must become familiar with the fundamentals of enhancing the psychological readjustment of the patient to self and society. The therapist must try to understand what makes the patient tick. We cannot say that the physically disabled are not well adjusted, any more than we can say that the physically normal are always well adjusted. Attitudes vary widely and appear to have little relation to the degree of disability sustained. The ability to adjust and the patient's attitude appear to be related to personality characteristics that existed before the injury, and acceptance appears to be predicated on one's ability to change one's personal value system (39). An example of inability to change the value system and accept a disability is seen in the patient who is overly zealous about the therapy program. There is a discrepancy between the desired gain and the gain that may realistically be expected.

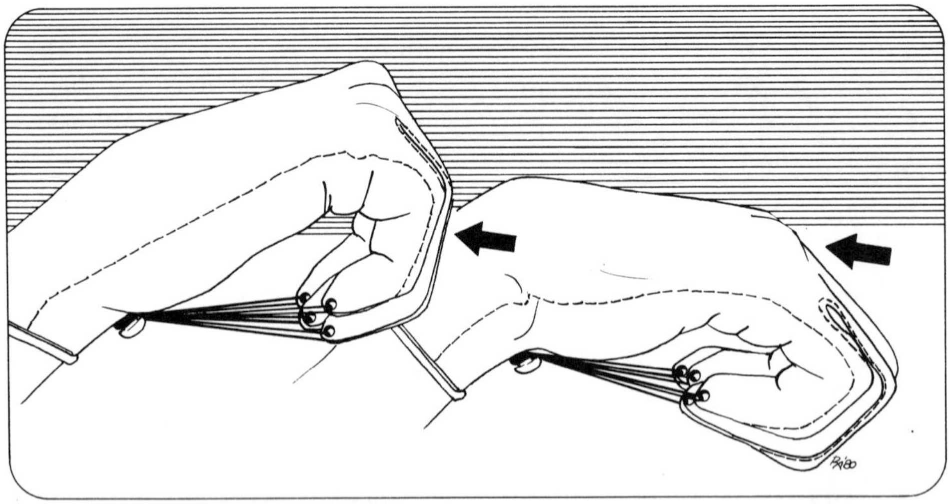

FIG. 18. When the wrist is maintained in extension by voluntary control the glove is effective in passively flexing both M.P. and P.I.P. joints, however as soon as the wrist is allowed to flex tenodesis of the digital extensors dominates and the objective is lost.

All too often this results in patients being disappointed by the final results of their hard work in rehabilitation, and there is resentment against the therapists and doctors who were not able to convey realistic goals. Patient interaction, as in groups, is an excellent means of influencing patients to accept realistic goals following trauma or illness.

The therapist must learn the various patient responses to pain and trauma. There will be inhibition patterns that are characteristic and stand out as warning signals to the therapist. An example of this is extreme extension of the index finger, sometimes called extensor habitus, with the patient reporting inability to flex the digit. At the same time there may be extreme contraction of the musculus extensor digitorum communis and musculus extensor indicis proprius; if relaxation does not occur, there may be muscle spasm. The patient will have to learn how to relax the muscles prior to relieving the pattern and gaining index flexion. The protective postures are also characteristic warning signals of secondary problems. One common protective posture is that of bracing the arm against the trunk, with the shoulder held in tight adduction and elevated, the arm internally rotated, and the forearm pronated. This protective posture may be effective in preventing contact between the arm and surrounding objects, but it results in a pattern of muscle spasm and pain, as well as capsular tightness for the shoulder joint. Another response that the therapist should learn to recognize is the diathesis involving propensity to reflex sympathetic dystrophy. Certain patients have a low threshold for pain and tend to exaggerate it beyond what one would consider realistic norms. These patients often complain of nonspecific pain and tend to regard the pain as an overwhelming factor in their lives. If the therapist can recognize this diathesis early, it may be possible to change the patient's attitude. This is usually accomplished by proving to the patient that motion and activity do not necessarily create further pain and discomfort.

It is difficult to make generalizations about patients' personalities; however, there are four types of patients that should be mentioned, not from the viewpoint of the professional psychologist but from the viewpoint of one who observes personalities during one's career. First, there is the patient of a certain personality or mentality who will begin therapy with the attitude that the insurance compensation following an accident will more than make up for a poor rehabilitation result. Often this attitude is promoted by lawyers or by friends; it is totally counter-productive to the patient's rehabilitation goals. Such patients often do not realize the rehabilitation possibilities of which they are capable, and many of them are also disappointed in their court settlements.

Another situation that is detrimental to rehabilitation goals involves the patient who, for some reason, gets into a position such that the injury provides a secondary gain. It often happens that all the family members change their life patterns to accommodate the patient, and the situation becomes so comfortable that the patient doesn't want to change things by getting better. Often it is the case that a worker was at a job he did not like, and the injury allowed him to be on temporary vacation, but the financial situation forced the wife to go to work, very often with the children being responsible for taking care of the "invalid." Such a new life pattern can easily get out of hand. The wife may find herself a rewarding career. The children may feel useful and may receive appropriate affection and reward from the father. The father may be very comfortable occupying center stage and receiving attention from the children; he may even enjoy the tranquil pace of being away from a job that was not desirable to begin with. It is at this point that it might be suggested to the patient that perhaps by means of vocational rehabilitation he might find a more desirable and rewarding profession. It often comes as a shock to the patient, after medical therapies are withdrawn and disability compensation no longer comes in the mail, that the situation has gone too far, and yet the hand has not been rehabilitated to its original potential.

Some patients feel that the hand therapy office is more like a dry cleaning establishment than a place for hard work. They do not accept the fact that hand rehabilitation is their own responsibility. Patients must learn from the beginning that the hand therapist is a teacher or a guidance counselor who is there to teach patients how to take responsibility on themselves for working a hand back to its full potential. And then there is the heartbreaker. Certain patients feel that deformity has so interfered with body image that they withdraw from all social contact. This is a difficult situation, one that requires professional psychological help. However, the therapist can assist these patients not only by demonstrating acceptance of them but also by introducing them to others in a group setting. If the patient can be convinced to expose the hand to other patients and discuss with them the difficulties of social interaction, the patient may be able, with the support of the group, to express underlying disappointment and vent frustrations, perhaps gaining the courage required to focus attention on things other than the injured hand.

Co-management is an essential part of patient management. Co-management is achieved through patient education. Wright stated that "inner strength and self-respect grow in a relationship where the person feels that he has an important role in planning his life and that what he says and feels is respected." Only after patients are taught the essential parts of their anatomy and the workings of that anatomy, and after their problems with that anatomy are discussed, will they be able to communicate as peers with the therapist. Only when they feel that they can ask intelligent questions about the disabled member will self-respect grow and rapport be established between the professional and the patient. Patient education should begin with initial orientation to the setting and to the professional therapy staff. It is dangerous to allow stratification between professional staff and patients. This can undermine the goals of building self-esteem and a strong body image, and it can undermine the patient's motivation to get well. Motivation can also be improved through co-management. Co-management allows for personal adjustments by the patient who has gained self-respect. There is less tendency to dissipate energies on minor complaints and to focus on certain small problems. The patient will begin to assume responsibility for their own treatment. Patient education will facilitate personal motivation, and this motivation will enable the patient to work to the potential of which the hand is capable.

SUMMARY

The therapist must be able to evaluate the patient, develop short-term and long-term goals for the patient, and educate the patient. The therapist must be capable (39) of adapting and being flexible within the treatment approach. The therapist must know methods of therapeutic exercise and activity, including activity analysis. The therapist must be able to instill patient motivation and assist the patient in adapting psychosocially and vocationally. The therapist must not expect the impossible. There are a few suggestions that come to mind: (a) Don't expect the patient to remember your instructions; write them down in a language the patient can understand. (b) Don't expect a foreign-born patient to obey English commands. (c) Don't expect a child to stick to a regimented exercise program. Play exercises are fun for everyone. (d) Don't expect an apartment-dweller with a family to concentrate on an involved sensory reeducation program three times a day. You will not see the results of your treatment program. (e) Don't expect an apartment-dweller to have a hammer and saw to build a bookcase in the name of therapy. (f) Don't expect a person who was used to being waited on to take responsibility for the exercise program. If it is important enough, enforce intensive therapy within the therapy office. (g) Don't expect the surgeon to be Superman. Medical science, sophisticated as it is, still does not have all the answers and all the solutions. (h) Finally, don't expect the patient to report the same complaints to the physician and to the therapist. Teamwork is a must, involving the therapist, the patient, and the physician. Isolated encounters between any two members of the team, leaving out the third member, will almost certainly result in misinterpretation at some point.

Finally, in therapy, try to expect the unexpected. Remember Murphy's law: "Whatever can go wrong will go wrong." One should try to be flexible enough to adapt to the situation, whatever it may be.

REFERENCES

1. Akeson, W. H. (1961): Experimental study of joint stiffness. *J. Bone Joint Surg.* (*Am*), 43A:1022–1034.
2. Beard, G. and Wood, E. (1965): *Massage Principles and Techniques,* W. B. Saunders, Phila.
3. Beasley, R. W.: The Orthopedic Clinic of North America: Surgery of the Hand, Nov. 1970, Vol. 1, No. 2 (whole book).
4. Bechtrol, C. (1954): Grip test—use of a dynameter with adjustable hand spacings. *J. Bone Joint Surg.* [*Am.*], 36:820.
5. Boyes, J. H. (editor) (1970): *Bunnell's Surgery of the Hand,* ed. 5. J. B. Lippincott, Philadelphia.
6. Burman, M. (1943): Kinetic disabilities of the hand and their classification. *Am. J. Surg.*, 61:167.
7. Cannon, B. and Peacock, E. (1967): Plastic surgery: The hand. *N. Engl. J. Med.*, 263:238.
8. Cleland, A. (1878): On the cutaneous ligaments of the phalanges. *Journal of Anatomy and Physiology,* 12:526–527.
9. Cotton, F. J. and Sawyer, E. J. (1921): Stiff fingers. *Boston Medical and Surgical Journal,* 186:183.
10. Cutler, C. W., Jr. (1942): *The Hand: Its Disabilities and Diseases.* W. B. Saunders, Philadelphia.
11. Dickson, J. A. (1920–21): Treatment of stiff metacarpophalangeal joints where there is no cross bony alterations. *Br. J. Surg.*, 8:272.
12. Hunter, J., Schneider, L., Mackin, E., and Bell, J. (editors) (1978): *Rehabilitation of the Hand.* C. V. Mosby, St. Louis.
13. Kaplan, E. (1939): Pathology and operative correction of finger deformities due to injuries and contractures of the extension digitorum tendon. *Surgery,* 6:35.
14. Kaplan, E. (1936): Extension deformities of proximal interphalangeal joints of the fingers. *J. Bone Joint Surg.* [*Am.*], 18:781.
15. Kaplan, E. (1940): Mallet or baseball finger. *Surgery,* 7:784.
16. Kaplan, E. (1965): *Functional and Surgical Anatomy of the Hand.* J. B. Lippincott, Philadelphia.
17. Licht S. (editor) (1965): *Therapeutic Exercise, Vol II,* Physical Medicine Library, Waverly Press, Baltimore, Maryland.
18. Licht, S. (editor) (1965): *Therapeutic Heat and Cold, Vol 2,* Physical Medicine Library. Waverly Press, Baltimore, Maryland.
19. Licht, S. (1967): *Therapeutic Electricity and Ultraviolet Radiation,* Vol IV, Physical Medicine Library. Waverly Press, Baltimore, Maryland.
20. Littler, W. (1949): Tendon transfers and arthrodesis in combined median and ulnar nerve paralysis. *J. Bone Joint Surg.* [*Am.*], 31:225–234.
21. Littler, W. (1956): Principles of reconstructive surgery of the hand. *Am. J. Surg.*, 92:88.
22. Littler, W. (1960): The physiology and dynamic function of the hand. *Surg. Clin. North Am.*, 40:259.
23. Little, J. W., and Eaton, R. G. (1967): Redistribution of bones in the correction of the Boutonniere deformity. *J. Bone Joint Surg.* [*Am.*], 49:1267–1274.
24. Lyle, H. (1923): Treatment of disabilities of the hand. *Ann. Surg.*, 78:822–844.
25. Madden, J., and Peacock, E. (1968): Studies on the biology of collagen during wound healing. *Surgery,* 64:288.
26. Manhold, J. H. (1977): Extension of a hypothesis, psychosomatic factors in wound healing. *Psychosomatics,* 19:143.
27. Nordzeh, B. (1977): Reimplantation of an amputated hand. *Scand. J. Plast. Reconstr. Surg.*, 11:251.

28. Peacock, E. (1959): A study of the circulation in normal tendons and healing grafts. *Ann. Surg.*, 149:415–428.
29. Peacock, E. (1959): Morphology of homologous and heterologous tendon grafts. *Surg. Gynecol. Obstet.*, 109:735–741.
30. Peacock, E. (1959): Some problems in tendon healing. *Surgery,* 45:415–423.
31. Peacock, E. (1966): Some biochemical and biophysical aspects of joint stiffness. *Ann. Surg.*, 164:1–12.
32. Peacock, E., and Van Winkle, W. (1970): *Wound Repair.* W. B. Saunders, Philadelphia.
33. Rank, B. K., Wakefield, A. R., and Hueston, A. (1953): *Surgery of Repair as Applied to Hand Injuries,* ed. 3. E. & S. Livingstone, Edinburgh.
34. Steindler, A. (1935): *Mechanics of Normal and Pathological Motion in Man.* Charles C Thomas, Springfield, Ill.
35. Tichauer E. R. (1970): *Ergonometric and Occupational Biomechanics.*
36. Weckester, E. C. (1974): *Treatment of Hand Injuries.* Year Book Publishers, Chicago.
37. Weeks, P. M., and Wary, R. C. (1973): *Management of Acute Hand Injuries: A Biological Approach.* C. V. Mosby, St. Louis.
38. Williams, D. F., and Harrison, I. D. (1977): The variation of mechanical properties in different areas of a healing wound. *Biomechanics,* 10:633.
39. Wright, B. A. (1960): *Physical Disability: A Psychological Approach.* Harper & Row Publishers, New York.

Pediatric Overview 6

G. Gordon Williamson

In this chapter we shall present some basic concepts for evaluation and treatment of children with developmental disabilities. The discussion will focus on sensorimotor dysfunction that interrupts the normal sequence and rate of growth and development. Such disabilities may be related to various etiological factors: birth defects, traumatic injuries, psychomotor retardation, and associated neurobehavioral disorders. This chapter is not intended to be a comprehensive survey of the special needs of exceptional children or the diverse roles of occupational therapists in the pediatric field. Information provided in other parts of the book are directly relevant to this population.

The functions of the occupational therapist in pediatrics vary widely depending on the types of children served and the clinical setting. The work environment has expanded greatly from the original hospital-based milieu to include rehabilitation centers, residential facilities, school systems, social welfare agencies, and the client's home. Each setting requires specialized competencies for the provision of services (1).

Developmental concepts form the basis of intervention within the realms of habilitation and rehabilitation. Habilitation is the process of developing new skills and abilities that have never been part of the child's learned behavior. Rehabilitation is the redevelopment or relearning of skills that have been lost because of trauma or disease. The process of habilitation is frequently the most common component of pediatric practice, and it is always part of the rehabilitative process.

This chapter is divided into four sections: normal sensorimotor development, abnormal sensorimotor development, evaluation, and principles of treatment. Normal development and atypical development receive special attention because knowledge in these areas is critical to pediatric intervention.

NORMAL SENSORIMOTOR DEVELOPMENT

Because therapy is founded on an understanding of human growth and development, it is important to highlight some of the major factors that influence the sensorimotor processes leading to adaptive skills. The development of goal-directed movements does not occur spontaneously in a vacuum. Rather, it reflects interaction between neurological maturation and environmental experience. This section will examine the nature of sensorimotor adaptation, the development of controlled movement patterns, and the acquisition of stability and mobility functions.

Sensorimotor Adaptation

The child's ability to organize and plan purposeful movements is dependent on morphologic, biomechanical, and environmental constraints imposed on the movements (2,3). Morphologic constraints include the structure of the musculoskeletal system and the other characteristics of the child, such as shape, age, and sex. The structural morphology of any individual changes dramatically from infancy to adulthood, and these changes have profound impact on motor performance. Movement patterns must continually accommodate changes in size, height, weight, and strength of the child. It is common, for instance, for children to exhibit temporary deterioration in motor skills during periods of rapid linear growth (4).

Biomechanical constraints are the physical forces that influence the organization of movements, such as gravity, mass, and inertia. The child must overcome these external forces to accomplish functional tasks. A prime example is the progressive attainment of antigravity positions (from lifting the head while lying prone, through sitting and quadripedal creeping to standing); the child applies physical and mechanical principles of movement acquired through experience.

The environment imposes constraints of space and time to which the child's movement patterns must be accommodated in order to attain a goal (3,5). These spatial and temporal elements are important in the monitoring of motor planning and performance. A typical example is tossing a beanbag at a stationary target. The spatial characteristics of the movement pattern are determined by the size of the target and the size, weight, and shape of the beanbag. With accurate processing of exteroceptive and proprioceptive sensory information, the child's movement pattern will match these environmental characteristics, and the beanbag will hit the target. If the movement pattern does not conform exactly to these conditions, the target will be missed. In the situation of popping soap bubbles in the air, the child must accommodate to the speed of the descending bubbles (a temporal condition) as well as the spatial dimensions of the bubbles. In this sense, movement is regulated by the environment as well as by the influences of morphology and biomechanics.

Sensory and motor systems are so intimately related that the development of movement and posture can be considered a sensory-motor-sensory process of adaptive integration (6,7). The child receives and organizes sensory stimuli in a manner that allows for the planning of purposeful movements. The proprioceptive, tactile, and visual receptors are particularly important sources of information for correcting and reorganizing motor programs (8). Some motor acts, however, are less dependent on afferent monitoring than others. Experience is cumulative in the sense that each new encounter is handled in terms of previous experience, and each new experience modifies what is carried to subsequent encounters (9).

Learning depends on this processing of sensory information (Appendix A). The lower neurological centers of the brain stem, thalamus, and cerebellum are especially important in sorting out relevant stimuli and integrating inputs from two or more sensory systems (10). The child's adaptive skills depend on this ability to associate sensory modalities at the subcortical level as well as the cortical level.

As sensations are integrated into meaningful units, they become part of the child's conceptual makeup, allowing increasingly sophisticated abstract imagery or symbolism. Therefore, intersensory integration facilitates the development of perceptual skills that constitute the foundation for organized thought and language. As a result, one can see sandpaper and know that it feels rough; with eyes closed, one can smell a flower and identify it.

The tactile, proprioceptive, and vestibular systems are phylogenetically older modalities that mature first to act as substrata for the younger visual and auditory systems (11,12). Touch, considered to be the oldest of all the senses, governs many early neonatal reflexes and contributes profoundly to the perception of other types of sensation. Praxis, the ability to motor plan, is dependent on the tactile system (13). Proprioception through receptors in the muscles, tendons, joints, and viscera provides the sense of body position and movement. The vestibular system is a type of proprioceptor that consists of the semicircular canals and vestibules in the inner ear and their connections to the vestibular nuclei in the brain stem. This system detects changes in the position of the head in space through sensitivity to gravity and any rotary or linear movement of the head.

Somatosensory feedback provides the basis for establishing a body schema, an inner awareness of body parts, of their relationships to the whole, and how they move through space. During discovery of the physical self, the child concomitantly develops a sense of laterality, an awareness of two distinct sides of the body, and bilaterality, the coordination of the two sides of the body together. The body schema thus becomes the reference point for self-to-object or I-to-it relationships. Objects are viewed in relation to the child (behind, in front of, or to the right of me). Mental projection of self into space culminates in object-to-object or it-to-it relationships in which objects are seen as they spatially relate to each other (e.g., the cup is on the table and next to the plate) (14,15).

It is within this broad framework that sensorimotor development must be viewed: complex integration of maturational and learning processes as the child interacts with and adapts to the environment. Coordination is the critical concern in motor development, not the acquisition of new movements (16). From the start the neonate has a diverse repertoire of motor activities, including rooting and sucking behaviors, crying, head turning, hand-to-mouth patterns, thrashing movements of the limbs, and wiggling of the fingers and toes. However, these movements reflect a low level of neurological operation and are primarily automatic and reflexive in nature.

Gradually the infantile reflexes are modified within a hierarchy of controlled behaviors to function as the basic substrata for willed movement (17,18). Coordination results from a complex interactive process that involves integration of experience, central nervous system activity (memory, planning, and information processing), biomechanical factors, and conditions of morphology and the environment (3). As the child develops skill in postural stability and limb manipulation, each of these ingredients comes under increasing control.

Control of Movement Patterns

Motor development progresses from head to foot (a cephalo to caudal direction) and from the central axis of the body to the limbs (proximal to distal). Thus the infant develops control of the head, trunk, shoulder girdle, and pelvic girdle before refined coordination of the extremities. Postural stability of the head and trunk provides the foundation for skilled distal movements of the hands and feet (19). Consequently, therapy stresses the attainment of central control as a prerequisite for limb transport and manipulation.

The development of controlled movement follows a characteristic sequence: extension, flexion, lateral flexion, and rotation (20). A cephalocaudal progression is first seen in the development of controlled extension. Extension occurs at the neck by 2 months, progresses to the midback at 3 months, to the low back by 4 months, crosses the hips by 5 months, and continues through the lower extremities during the next few months. Controlled flexion follows behind the caudal progression of extension by 1 or 2 months. Only after extension is counterbalanced by flexor control can lateral flexion appear. Rotation is the most sophisticated motor component. It is the last pattern to develop in infancy and the first to be lost as a result of trauma.

Therapy is founded on an understanding of the manner in which these movement patterns come together as components of a new skill or "milestone." Motor development during early infancy provides an illustration (Fig. 1). The 3-month-old infant lying on the abdomen has controlled extension through the midback, and this causes the scapulae to retract and the upper limbs to assume an abducted, internally rotated posture. This initial extension is facilitated by optical and labyrinthine righting reactions acting on the head.

As the flexor component develops, the upper extremities are brought toward shoulder flexion and adduction. This counterbalance of flexion allows the infant to assume a puppy propping position, and an elongated neck begins to appear. At this time no lateral flexion is present to allow for coordinated weight shifting. If the child looks to the side, the body weight is displaced in that di-

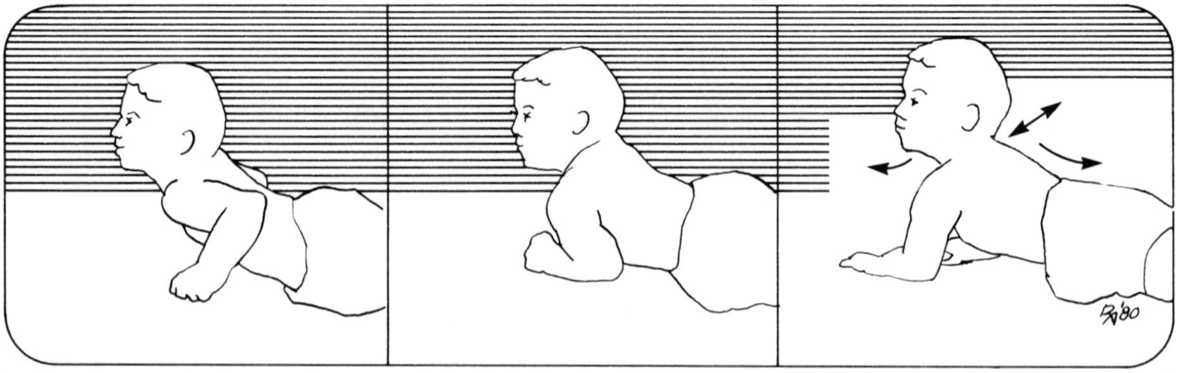

FIG. 1. Development of scapular control. **Left:** Extension dominates, retracting the scapulae. **Center:** Extension counterbalanced by flexion for puppy propping. **Right:** Lateral flexion achieved with weight shifting in the prone-on-elbows position.

rection (weight shift toward the face side), and an asymmetrical tonic neck reflex may cause the child to collapse.

By the age of 4 months extension has progressed to the low back, and playful "bottom lifting" may be observed when the infant is lying prone (repetitive anterior tilting of the pelvis by the low back extensors). Flexor patterns are practiced in the infant seat or while lying supine as the child develops midline-oriented skills such as bringing the hands together or to the mouth. This increased control of shoulder flexion and adduction allows the infant to assume a true prone-on-elbows position. With patterns of extension and flexion as a base, righting reactions acting on the head facilitate the emergence of controlled lateral flexion. By the fifth month the child can turn the head toward one side and automatically shift weight toward the other side for postural security (weight shift toward the skull side).

This ability to shift weight from side to side requires lateral flexion of the head and upper trunk. With this development of controlled lateral flexion, the child can maintain a side-lying position during play for the first time. Upper trunk rotation is gradually experienced during these activities and is reinforced as the child begins to reach out for toys. Righting reactions acting on the body facilitate further development of trunk rotation as segmental rolling patterns appear.

The child initially develops control of movement in weight-bearing postures. The increased joint compression, resistance, stretch, and tactile input seem to reinforce proximal stability and coordination of the extremities (21). Only later are the coordinated patterns noted when reaching freely in space.

In the prone-on-elbows position, for example, the child experiences stabilization and dissociation of the shoulder girdle mechanism while bouncing up and down, shifting weight from side to side, and beginning to push up on extended arms. A weight shift onto the left elbow facilitates adduction and external rotation of the left shoulder, supination of the forearm, and pressure on the ulnar border of the hand. The left (weight-bearing) side tends to elongate through the head and trunk, and the right side laterally flexes. As the child shifts the weight back toward the midline, the left limb undergoes abduction and internal rotation of the shoulder and pronation of the forearm, and the pressure rolls onto the radial aspect of the palm.

The degree of weight shifting when propped on the elbows seems directly related to the amount of supination that the child demonstrates in the hand-to-mouth pattern. Likewise, the practice of pushing up on extended arms appears related to the child's ability to achieve an extended forward reach into space for an object. Lively weight-bearing activities provide increased sensory feedback from the vestibular system, the cutaneous receptors, and the proprioceptors that aid the development of coordination.

This example of movement organization in infancy has implications for clinical practice. Treatment planning is guided by task analysis of the sensory, perceptual, cognitive, and motor processes required to achieve proficiency in a new adaptive behavior. The therapist recognizes the importance of central control and follows a developmental progression in the attainment of coordinated movement patterns. Somatosensory input is stressed through movement in weight-bearing postures.

Stability and Mobility Functions

Organization of movement can be further analyzed within the context of mobility and stability functions. In reality, these dual motor components cannot be separated into distinct categories; however, it is helpful to analyze movement from a functional perspective to determine if motor activity is assisting the body in meeting stability needs or mobility needs.

Mobility responses are characterized by quick initiation, wide range of motion, and fast speed (19). Mobility is the dynamic component of movement that gives the child the means of changing position and interacting with the environment. In contrast, stability involves movements that maintain the position of the body against gravity and keep the range of movement in check so that the posture can be held. In this context, body stability is considered the adaptive background for voluntary movement.

Posture is based on continuous subtle changes in muscle tone as well as more overt compensatory movements. It is supported by postural reflex mechanisms such as righting and equilibrium reactions. Coordinated movement and postural functions are complementary in nature. Mobility and stability are essential components of any motor act (22).

With each new position that an infant assumes, there is a developmental progression in acquiring motor control. The child first learns stability in order to maintain the antigravity posture. However, very quickly a mobility component is introduced on the developing stable base. Rocking and weight-shifting activities are practiced, and later reaching patterns of the arms bring in more active trunk rotation. Only after the child is able to combine the stability and mobility elements is locomotion in the position possible (20).

This developmental cycle is repeated in every new position during the first year of life. As the infant assumes the prone-on-elbows posture, proximal stability is the first goal in order to maintain the position, but soon the child introduces mobility patterns in a predictable order. Movements are first performed in symmetrical alignment, such as bouncing and rocking in the sagittal plane, which requires flexion and extension in an anterior-posterior direction. Next, an asymmetrical displacement of the center of gravity allows weight shifting from side to side, which requires lateral flexion. Gradually the infant reaches out with one extremity while supported on the other. The rotary action of the trunk associated with the reaching pattern enables the infant to combine movements of flexion and extension into more fluid purposeful activity.

Finally the child has the postural control required to locomote in the prone position by pushing backward with the arms, by pivoting in a circle, or by crawling forward on the abdomen. In this latter task the reciprocal movements of the arms and legs provide counterrotation to the trunk, and this aids proximal stability (the shoulder girdle rotating in one direction and the pelvis in the other).

Another example of this developmental progression is seen in the quadrupedal position (Fig. 2). As the baby develops stability in the posture, controlled mobility skills are acquired through rocking back and forth, bouncing up and down, shifting weight in all directions, unilateral play in the position, and free swinging of one or more limbs while bearing weight on the other limbs. These are preparatory events for locomotion when the infant can move an arm and opposite leg simultaneously and achieve reciprocal creeping. The necessary stability is gained through counterrotation of the trunk. The acquisition of stability, mobility based on stability, and then locomotion occurs in all developmental positions: propping on elbows, sitting, quadruped, kneeling, and standing.

Children with sensorimotor problems fail to develop proper integration of stability and mobility functions. Children with learning disabilities and mentally retarded children often have poor proximal stability related to low muscle tone, inadequate bilateral coordination, and immature righting and equilibrium reactions. Spastic children have rigid nonadaptive stability and limited mobility patterns. The aim of the therapeutic process is to establish a balance between these vital components of functional performance.

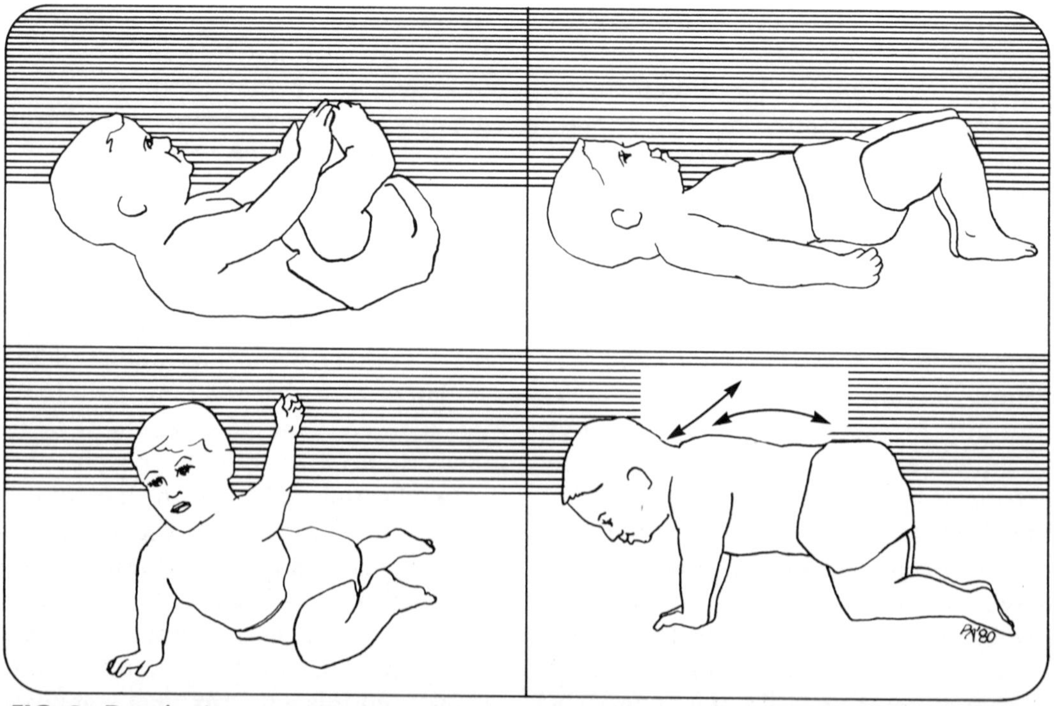

FIG. 2. Developing prerequisite stability and mobility skills for quadrupedal creeping.

ABNORMAL SENSORIMOTOR DEVELOPMENT

This section will be concerned with issues related to abnormal sensorimotor development that are directly applicable to evaluation and treatment procedures. First, a distinction will be made between primitive and pathological movements. Next, the sequential nature of abnormal motor development will be described. Finally, disorders in sensory integration will be presented.

Primitive and Pathological Movements

Children with dysfunction of the central nervous system exhibit two types of movement patterns: primitive and pathological (6). Primitive patterns represent arrested or delayed motor development and are characteristic of lower-level behaviors seen in younger children. Infantile synergies may be retained, such as early mouthing patterns noted during feeding, primitive kicking, or reaching patterns with internal rotation and pronation. Primitive performance is seen in children with Down's syndrome, who tend to use a palmar grasp excessively and who exhibit limited prehensile patterns during manipulative play. Primitive movements are typically described as immature and awkward, reflecting poor adaptation to the spatial and temporal demands of the environment.

Inadequate reflex maturation and postural stability are also considered primitive. Children may have delays in developing head and trunk control, rotation within the body axis, and ability to assume or maintain antigravity positions. Reflex integration is intimately related to this emergence of functional motor skills. Molnar (23) conducted a study of children under 3 years of age who had mental retardation and delayed motor development but no evidence of neuromuscular disability. These children were delayed in the appearance of postural adjustment reactions, such as propping and equilibrium responses. However, once specific automatic reactions emerged, appropriate motor tasks followed within 1 to 4 weeks. Although they were slow for chronological age, motor development in these retarded children was consistent with reflex maturation and illustrated primitive behavior.

In contrast, pathological movement patterns reflect defective sensorimotor integration or disinhibition resulting in the domination of tonic reflex activity over other patterns of coordination (24). Pathological patterns are usually associated with abnormal muscle tone, whether hypertonic, hypotonic, or hyperkinetic, such as the disorganized fluctuating tonus of the child with athetosis. Examples of pathological signs are opisthotonos (marked arching of the body into extension), spastic adduction and extension of the lower extremities, and asymmetrical responses in the parachute or Moro reactions (25).

Pathological development is often subtle in the beginning and is seen as deviations from primitive movement patterns. The child may fail to demonstrate a wide variety of independent random movements, such as wiggling the wrists and ankles. On close observation, the quality of movement will be seen to be too stereotyped and obligatory. For instance, abduction of the hips always occurs with flexion, never with hip extension. The ankles are inverted and plantar flexed, never everted and dorsiflexed. Internal rotation of the shoulder is always associated with elbow extension. Kicking is unilateral and not reciprocal (26).

Unless they are severely handicapped, young infants with neuromotor dysfunction of central origin do not have spasticity, pathological movement patterns, or orthopedic complications such as joint contractures and spinal column deformities (27). Behavior tends to be primitive. As the damaged nervous system matures, alterations in movement patterns gradually emerge. By careful analysis of these subtle changes, an early diagnosis can be made before muscle tone disorders are evident and abnormal patterns are established and habituated (28).

Sequential Nature of Abnormal Development

Abnormal motor development occurs in a sequence similar to the cephalocaudal progression in the nonhandicapped child (25). Low muscle tone and primitive movement patterns are usually present at birth. Against the background of low postural tone, the atypical infant begins to fix or tense the muscles to achieve motor control. For example, elevation of the shoulder girdle may be used to stabilize the head. These fixing patterns may become so strong that they block the development of more sophisticated movement components such as lateral flexion and rotation required for righting and equilibrium reactions.

The typical development of the cerebral palsied infant with spastic diplegia serves as a case in point. From an initial status of low muscle tone, the child's movement becomes blocked at characteristic points as extension progresses from head to foot (26). As noted in Fig. 4, the first block is hyperextension of the neck, normal for the infant of 2 months, but deviant when not counterbalanced over time with flexion of the head and upper extremities. The second block occurs at the shoulder girdle, with scapular retraction. When lying in the prone position, the infant adducts the scapulae to reinforce the spinal extension needed to lift the head farther off the supporting surface. When the infant is lying supine, scapular retraction is reinforced by the tonic labyrinthine reflex (29).

This retraction of the scapulae causes the upper extremities to pull back into a W posture, thus preventing midline-oriented play such as bringing the hands together and plucking the clothes. The fixing in extension prohibits the development of controlled flexion and adduction of the upper limbs for attaining the prone-on-elbows position. Therefore free dissociated movement of scapula and humerus fails to develop. The scapular-humeral angle becomes fixed, and the segment slides as a unit on the thorax in a typical winged fashion.

The third block occurs in the extensor muscles of the low back, causing increased lordosis of the spine. This muscular pull tilts the pelvis anteriorly and leads to hip flexion, the site of the fourth block. With inadequate activity of the abdominal muscles, the child fails to develop isolated control of the pelvis. Eventually the lower extremities become blocked in hip adduction and internal rotation, with plantar flexion of the feet.

The diplegic child gradually learns to compensate for these original motor blocks. When propped in a sitting position, for example, the child is pulled backward by extensor tone. To prevent falling, the child flexes the upper trunk forward with excessive effort. Flexor spasticity is then superimposed on the original problem of too much extensor tone. The resulting clinical picture (Fig. 5) becomes clear: the pelvis is locked in midrange as the child sits on partially flexed hips, with marked rounding of the spine; the legs tend to scissor in adduction and internal rotation; the head hyperextends on the flexed trunk to view the surroundings. The stress of maintaining this unstable position can increase abnormal flexor patterns in the arms (humeral adduction and internal rotation, elbow flexion, forearm pronation, and wrist flexion, with ulnar deviation).

The atypical movement patterns become habit with repetition, and they severely limit the child's repertoire of adaptive behaviors. Conspicuously absent or diminished in the presence of aberrant postural tone is the integrated component of rotation. Because of overuse, spasm, or poor positioning, muscle shortening occurs, and this promotes joint contractures and deformities.

Intervention is necessary to break this cycle of motor blocks that leads to compensatory movements that become habit over time to create contractures and deformities. Ideally the infant should be treated early to prevent fixing and to prevent compensatory patterns from becoming habits through use. In therapy, one carefully analyzes the child's motor performance to ascertain the nature of the original problem, as well as the compensation. In the case of the older diplegic child, spastic flexion may appear to dominate, but the original block was abnormal extension. Thus treatment must inhibit hypertonus and elongate shortened muscles in both flexor and extensor groups as a foundation for balanced movement.

Disorders in Sensory Integration

The tactile, proprioceptive, and vestibular systems have critical influences on posture, muscle tone, motor planning, ocular control, auditory-language functions, and academic achievement (30–32). Deficits in somatosensory and vestibular processing are seen in a wide variety of diagnostic categories, such as learning disability (33,34), mental retardation (35,36), behavioral disorders (37–39), communication handicaps (40), and spina bifida (41). Recent research has indicated that therapy that emphasizes the integration of these sensory modalities significantly improves reflex and motor development in certain populations of normal and atypical children (42–45).

The professional literature reflects controversy regarding a neurobehavioral basis for learning disabilities (46,47). Research generally suggests no significant effect of traditional perceptual-motor training programs on reading achievement (48). However, current intervention studies emphasizing a sensory integrative approach with specific types of learning-disabled children indicate improvement in auditory-language skills and academic learning (31,49–52). It is increasingly evident that learning disabilities represent more than one clinical entity. Greater diagnostic precision is required to identify specific syndromes and relate them to etiology, prognosis, and treatment (53).

Ayres discussed two broad sensory integrative syndromes of learning-disabled children (10,54). The "vestibular and bilateral integration syndrome" reflects lack of coordinated function between the two sides of the body. It is hypothesized that inadequate maturation of postural reactions mediated by the brain stem interferes with interhemispheric integration at this neurological level, which results in limited lateralization of function by the cerebral hemispheres (30).

Clinical findings in this disorder include hyporesponsivity to vestibular stimulation (depressed or attenuated postrotary nystagmus), poorly integrated tonic neck and tonic labyrinthine reflexes, immature righting and equilibrium reactions, muscular hypotonia, and irregular ocular pursuit. Frequently there is difficulty in establishing hand dominance and crossing the midline of the body with the extremities, as well as incoordinated bilateral use of the hands.

The "developmental dyspraxia syndrome" is a deficit in planning and executing skilled or nonhabitual motor tasks. The disorder is associated with dysfunction in the processing of somatosensory or vestibular information. The child fails to develop an adequate body schema to serve as the basis for motor planning. Consequently, there are postural control problems, inability to sustain motor acts, and difficulty in anticipating required responses. The child typically has poor oral-motor and extraocular coordination, decreased tactile discrimination, and labored development of manipulative skill.

Associated deficits are noted, such as auditory-language problems, social-emotional immaturity, distractibility, and tactile defensiveness. This latter condition is an oversensitivity to tactile stimulation in which the child has a sympathetic nervous system fight-or-flight response.

Low tolerance for texture, taste, and temperature may be noted in the oral area, as well as general defensiveness to sound and smell.

A disorder in form and space perception is seldom seen independent of other sensory integrative disturbances (54). Characteristic signs include inability to identify forms, difficulty in interpreting the spatial relationships between objects, and impaired figure-ground perception (ability to select and attend to relevant visual stimuli from a rival background).

EVALUATION

Evaluation is a process of collecting relevant information about the child's performance so that a base line is established on which to plan and implement a therapeutic program. Careful initial evaluation and ongoing reassessment of the child during treatment are imperative for effective intervention. Pertinent information can be obtained through free observation of behavior, interviews with the family, and written or verbal reports from other professionals in the health, psychosocial, and educational fields.

Many factors influence the nature and content of the evaluation. This section will be concerned with issues related to child assessment in the areas of development, physical status, sensory-perceptual-motor processing, and psychosocial and play skills.

Developmental Assessment

Comprehensive assessment is important in all areas of development: movement, cognition, communication, emotional well-being, and adaptive behavior. Developmental testing provides essential information during each stage of the therapeutic process. During the initial screening and evaluation period, the tests help to identify the child with special needs and to determine the degree of functional ability and impairment. Next, the developmental appraisal provides guidelines for setting goals and planning treatment. Finally, by means of frequent reevaluation, progress can be documented and the therapeutic program updated.

The assessment process can employ a standardized formal instrument or an informal scale, checklist, or functional profile improvised by a treatment center to meet individual needs. These center-produced tools are usually compilations of test items taken from established standardized scales and from the professional literature in child development. These two groups of assessment measures serve different purposes (55). The standardized tests are appropriate for determining the motor, mental, or developmental age at which a child is functioning or comparing the child's performances with those of peers. Administration of such tests requires strict adherence to the standard procedures described in the test manual. In contrast, the center-made measures are constructed by the staff of the treatment center to yield specific information concerned with the ordering of target behaviors to assist treatment planning.

Published developmental instruments frequently used in the field include the Bayley Scales of Infant Development (56), the Denver Developmental Screening Test (57), the Functional Developmental Assessment of the Children's Hospital at Stanford (58), and the Gesell Developmental Schedules (59). Of particular concern to occupational therapists are areas related to gross motor performance (rolling, sitting, athletics), fine motor and adaptive skills (manipulation of blocks, puzzles, pencils), activities of daily living (feeding, dressing, toileting), and personal-social skills (emotional expression, self-esteem, social interactions). If a child shows a delay in any performance area, further evaluation is required to ascertain the nature of the problem. For instance, difficulty in feeding would necessitate detailed investigation of oral-motor functioning with additional assessment tools (60).

Before using a standardized test, the clinician should determine the quality and appropriateness of its psychometric properties from the perspective of the developer and the perspective of the user of the scale. Berk and De Gangi (61) presented a checklist for evaluating the validity and reliability of pediatric motor scales. The major limitations of center-made tests should also be appreciated. Misuse and misinterpretation of formal and informal instruments are common in the field of rehabilitation (62).

A number of concerns and precautions in the use of developmental batteries should be kept in mind. In most tests the age level assigned to developmental tasks reflects the age at which 50%

of children in the normative sample passed a given item. It is critical to recognize the wide variability among children in the time of acquisition of new skills. The Bayley Scales of Infant Development list a median age of 9.7 months to demonstrate an ability to play pat-a-cake in the midline of the body (56). However, 5% of children in the standardization sample accomplished the task by 7 months of age, and 5% passed the item after 15 months.

Individual variation is also seen in the sequence in which skills are obtained. Frequently a child emphasizes one area of development at the expense of another. For example, during a time of major gains in gross motor skills, speech development may plateau or even regress. Children may skip a motor act entirely or may demonstrate that behavior later after having progressed to more sophisticated activities (63). For instance, some children avoid creeping in the quadrupedal position; from scooting on the floor in a sitting position as a means of locomotion, they pull directly up to standing to cruise along furniture and walk.

The various developmental instruments often show inconsistencies in the ages at which similar tasks are accomplished (55). Age norms should be viewed as general indicators within a continuum of normal behavior. Overinterpretation of the scales may lead to a narrow view of development as discrete milestones appearing in static time frames. Appreciation of the overlapping and interrelated nature of the developmental process may be lost. For example, while mastering a certain task, a child may already be experimenting with component movement patterns of so-called more advanced skills. Around 8 to 9 months an infant may concurrently learn to pull to the sitting, kneeling, and standing positions. The child 4 to 5 years of age runs, walks, jumps, and climbs with proficiency, has nearly mastered hopping, and attempts unsuccessfully to skip and gallop. These abilities are practiced simultaneously and are not attained in exclusive steps or stages.

Most developmental appraisals are limited to a quantitative measure—the child has or has not achieved a certain number of tasks. From a therapeutic perspective, one is interested not only in task accomplishment but also in the qualitative nature of the performance. Relevant issues include the degree of coordination and timing, the presence of primitive or abnormal patterns of movement, the state of muscle tone, and the extent of reflex integration. A distinction must be made between a "log roll" using the neck righting reaction, a roll using spastic hyperextension of the head and trunk, and a mature roll with segmental rotation of the torso. Likewise, in the evaluation of feeding skills, distinctions must be made between a primitive suckling pattern of the tongue (rhythmic extension-retraction) and a mature sucking pattern (series of tongue elevations to the hard palate) and between a primitive phasic bite reflex (rhythmic opening and closing of the jaw) and a pathological tonic bite reflex (strong closure of the jaw when the teeth or gums are stimulated).

There are two critical therapeutic questions: How does the child perform? Why does the child organize movements in this manner? These are qualitative concerns that are not typically addressed in developmental batteries. Solid knowledge of the processes and principles of normal and abnormal development is required in order to use the scales appropriately. Otherwise, intervention may consist in teaching isolated, splintered skills.

Physical Assessment

Physical evaluation assesses joint range of motion, reflex integration, sensory status, muscle strength, coordination, and endurance. Movement patterns are examined according to quality (age-appropriate, primitive, or pathological) and related to the degree of muscle tone during activity and at rest. The original patterns of dysfunction are determined, as well as resultant compensatory patterns, in order to understand fully the motor behavior. The functional balance between stability and mobility skills is also noted. Special attention is directed to factors that contribute to joint and spinal column deformities, such as pathological reflexes, abnormally shortened muscles, and asymmetries of movement and posture.

Functional use of the upper extremities is evaluated according to the level of manipulative skill, the development of hand dominance, and the degree of bilateral coordination. Reach, grasp, and release patterns are assessed for quality and age-appropriateness. The Erhardt Developmental Prehension Assessment (64) provides helpful descriptions and norms for skill development in limb transport and manipulation. The instrument can also be used to evaluate the development of pencil grasp through 6 years of age.

The evaluation of reflexes warrants additional discussion. Fiorentino (65,66) described a popular method of testing reflexes that represent spinal and brainstem levels of integration as well as the neurologically more advanced righting and equilibrium reactions of the midbrain and cortex. Frequently in clinical practice, reflex maturation and motor skill development are tested separately. As a result, the inherent relationship between reflex integration and the acquisition of adaptive motor abilities may not be appreciated.

The Milani-Comparetti Motor Development Screening Test (67,68) is a unique instrument that is designed to correlate reflex behavior with gross motor skills from birth to 2 years of age. The display chart is divided into two sections. The upper section lists motor skills in a developmental sequence of increasing complexity of movement patterns and postural control. The skills include head control in various positions, sitting balance, assuming the quadrupedal and standing postures, and locomotion. The lower section of the form presents primitive reflexes and the righting, parachute, and tilting reactions that underlie antigravity control of the body axis.

The chart is designed so that the reflex patterns necessary for each motor task are in vertical alignment with the functional skill. Therefore, one can ascertain which reactions must be present before a motor behavior is achieved, as well as the reactions that must be suppressed to allow a new behavior to occur. For example, the influence of the Moro reaction on the upper extremities must be inhibited before parachute and tilting reactions appear. In turn, the forward parachute reaction prepares the child for weight bearing on the upper limbs in the quadrupedal posture. Whereas the symmetrical tonic neck reflex aids stability in maintaining the quadrupedal position, it must be integrated before reciprocal creeping is possible.

Hoskins and Squires (69) constructed a similar instrument combining the reflex and gross motor evaluations. It is modeled after the Milani-Comparetti format, but it includes more specific items requiring volitional behaviors. The child is asked to perform such voluntary activities as pivoting in the prone position, squatting in play, ascending and descending stairs, kicking, jumping, riding a tricycle, and hopping on one foot. A qualitative measure of performance is also incorporated into the grading system to indicate poor coordination caused by abnormal muscle tone.

Assessment of Sensory-Perceptual-Motor Processing

Numerous formal and informal evaluation procedures are available to assess sensory integration and perceptual-motor processing in children. The Southern California Sensory Integration Tests (70) developed by Ayres are 17 tests that examine somatosensory perception (touch, kinesthesia), form and space perception (visual figure-ground, stereognosis, design copying), and motor control (bilateral motor coordination, imitation of postures, standing balance). The Southern California Postrotary Nystagmus Test (71) is a companion tool that taps one facet of vestibular functioning.

A standardized instrument is available for assessing sensorimotor integration in preschool children (72). The 21 items that compose the test measure postural control, reflex integration, bilateral motor coordination, and vestibular processing. The Bruininks-Oseretsky Test of Motor Proficiency (73) has norms for examining gross motor performance (running speed and agility, balance, strength) and fine motor abilities (response speed, visual-motor control) in children from 5 to 14 years of age. The Purdue Perceptual-Motor Survey (74) is a general nonstandardized tool for observing skills in balance, coordinated movement, ocular pursuit, and visual perception.

Common pencil-and-paper tests require drawing the human figure (75) or copying geometric forms (76). The Motor-Free Test of Visual Perception (77) is particularly useful for children with movement disorders. A popular instrument is the Frostig Developmental Test of Visual Perception (78), which reportedly taps five separate perceptual factors, such as form constancy and spatial relations. However, factor analysis studies have indicated that the Frostig test assesses a single common perceptual function related to visual-

Child's Name ____________ Birthdate ________ Form completed by ________ Relationship ____________ Date ________
After each category add any comments you feel may be helpful. Responses are 1 (yes), 2 (sometimes), 3 (no).

AUDITORY: Does your child:
Respond negatively to unexpected or loud noises? ____
Have difficulty paying attention when there is other noise? ____
Miss hearing some sounds? ____
Seem confused as to the direction of sounds? ____
Seem to enjoy strange noises and/or make loud noises? ____
Enjoy music? ____
Have a diagnosed hearing loss? ____
Has your child had a hearing test? If so, give date and name of physician.
List any sounds your child particularly likes and/or dislikes:

VESTIBULAR: Does your child:
Rock while sitting or on play equipment more than other children? ____
Jump a lot? ____
Like being tossed in the air? ____
Seem fearful of space, i.e., going up and down stairs, riding teetertotters? ____
Like merry-go-rounds? ____
Spin and whirl more than other children? ____
Get car sick? ____
Between the ages of 6 months to 2 years, did your child tend to arch back when held or moved? ____
Did your child enjoy being rocked as an infant? ____

VISUAL: Does your child:
Blink at bright lights? ____
Make reversals when copying? ____
Appear to be happier in the dark? ____
Pick picture or object and look very closely and carefully at it? ____
Have difficulty discriminating shapes, colors, etc.? ____
Resist having eyes covered? ____
Become excited when there is a variety of visual objects? ____
Squint often? ____
Can you get your child to look at something far away? ____
Can you get him to look at something close? ____
Has your child had an eye examination? If so, give physician, diagnosis, and date.

PROPRIOCEPTIVE: Does your child:
Hold his hands in strange positions? ____
Hold his body in strange positions for periods of time? ____
Have good motor coordination with small things, i.e., using pencil, buttons? ____
Walk on toes, or did when younger? ____
Did your child:
Go from sitting to standing with little or no crawling? ____
Creep on tummy rather than hands and knees? ____

GUSTATORY-OLFACTORY-ELIMINATION: Does your child:
Act as though all food tastes the same? ____
Explore by tasting? ____
Chew on non-food objects? ____
Have unusual craving for certain foods? ____
Dislikes foods of certain texture? ____
Explore by smelling? ____
Discriminate odors? ____
React negatively to smell? ____
Ignore unpleasant odors? ____
Have trouble with constipation? ____
Did your child:
Wet the bed after 3 years of age? ____
Have trouble learning urinary control? ____
Have trouble learning bowel control? ____

TACTILE: Does your child:
Avoid playing in "messy" things, i.e., finger paint, paste, mud, sand, etc.? ____
Appear to be irritated by cloth of certain textures? ____
Object to being touched? ____
Dislike being cuddled? ____
Prefer to touch rather than being touched? ____
Avoid using hands for extended periods? ____
Bang his head on purpose, or has he in the past? ____
Pinch, bite, or otherwise hurt himself?
Examine objects by exploring them thoroughly with his hands? ____
Examine objects by putting them in his mouth? ____
Tends to feel pain less than others? ____
Isolate self from other children? ____
Frequently bumps and pushes other children? ____
Avoid certain textures of food? ____
List any textures your child particularly likes or dislikes:

FIG. 3. Sensory history form. (Courtesy of Jo Murphy Hyland, O.T.R., adapted from forms of A. J. Ayres, Pat Wilbarger, Patricia Montgomery, and Eileen Richter.)

motor organization (79,80); it does not measure discrete abilities or serve as a good predictor of reading achievement.

Informal procedures are most valuable in the evaluation process. A sensory history completed by the parents helps to relate sensory integrative dysfunction to behavior (see Fig. 3). Special clinical observations are conducted to determine muscle tone, integration of brainstem reflexes, equilibrium reactions, diadochokinesia (rapid forearm rotation), eye preference, and ocular pursuit. The flexor postural pattern is very difficult to assume and maintain for children with developmental dyspraxia (a curled-up position while lying supine). In contrast, the prone extension postural pattern is particularly demanding for children with dysfunction in vestibular and bilateral integration (lifting the head, shoulders, and extended legs off the surface when lying prone).

Assessment of Psychosocial and Play Skills

Critical to a comprehensive evaluation is assessment of the child's performance in work, play, and leisure activities. Such occupational performance reflects the integration for purposeful action of the sensory, motor, cognitive, and psychological systems. The child is thus viewed as an integrated whole in the process of doing and becoming (81). The child acquires a sense of mastery and competence through adaptation and learning during daily tasks (82).

Play behavior is unique in several ways. It is a spontaneous and voluntary involvement initiated and regulated by the child. The acts of play are performed for their own intrinsic reward, rather than as means to an end. Since the child is in command, the constraints of reality can be ignored for free expression of fantasy and imagination (83). The three dominant theories of play are those of Freud, Piaget, and Ellis (84). It is hypothesized that play serves a critical role in sensorimotor, social, and cognitive development.

Assessment of the child's play and leisure skills is aided by interest checklists (85), classification systems of play development (86), and measures of occupational roles (87). The exceptional child frequently has a delayed and restricted repertoire of play behaviors. Intervention may require special positioning of the child to allow for motor exploration, adaptation of the physical surroundings to achieve a play milieu, or careful selection of appropriate toys, materials, and equipment (88–90). Additionally, play serves as a major medium in occupational therapy practice for remediation of specific physical, mental, and emotional deficits.

According to Chess (91), individual differences are most notable in eight behavioral areas. They include the child's general activity level, regularity in daily schedules, adaptability to routine changes, tolerance to sensory stimulation, bias toward positive or negative mood, typical energy level or intensity of response, distractibility, and persistence. An assessment along these parameters by the therapist and parent assists the planning of treatment and guides the home management program. Since each family member contributes to the emotional climate of the home, the social and physical needs of the entire family must also be considered.

PRINCIPLES OF TREATMENT

Many principles and suggestions for treatment have already been discussed in this chapter. The cornerstone for intervention is sound knowledge of normal and abnormal development combined with strong evaluation skills. This section will further examine the developmental framework for therapy, the management of muscle tone and facilitation of movement, and the grading of the treatment program.

Developmental Progression of Treatment

Treatment follows a developmental progression, with one skill serving as a constituent part of a more complex skill. However, the latitude and diversity seen in normal development are reflected in therapeutic intervention with physically disabled children. The developmental sequence is not followed in a dogmatic fashion and rigidly imposed on the children. Some children may be encouraged to skip certain developmental tasks if the activity reinforces abnormal movement patterns. Bridging, W sitting, and creeping in quadruped are three examples of common motor behaviors that may be damaging to certain handicapped children (26).

When lying on a mattress in the supine position, children often push down on the feet and lift the pelvis from the mattress in a practice referred to as bridging. For the child with athetosis this activity facilitates abnormal extension of the neck and retraction of the scapulae, thus preventing forward reach of the arms and lift of the head to initiate sitting up. For many children with cerebral palsy, the W sitting position (resting on the buttocks between the heels of the feet) fosters exaggerated internal rotation, flexion, and adduction of the lower limbs which may undermine a proper gait pattern and lead to subluxation of the hips. Likewise, creeping on all fours may be contraindicated for diplegic and quadriplegic children if it increases flexor spasticity and promotes contractures and deformities of the spine, hips, and knees. It is the responsibility of the clinician to provide alternative means of positioning and locomotion that are therapeutically beneficial and also allow the child the freedom to explore and play.

A child should not be expected to attain perfect control over one activity before progressing to the next. Therapy emphasizes many different skills at the same time. There are occasions when the therapist may introduce an activity that is ordinarily considered too advanced for the child's developmental age. For instance, the athetotic

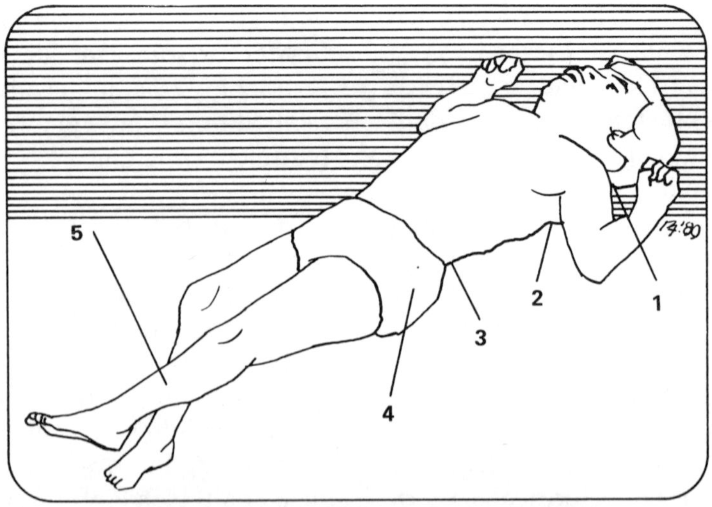

4

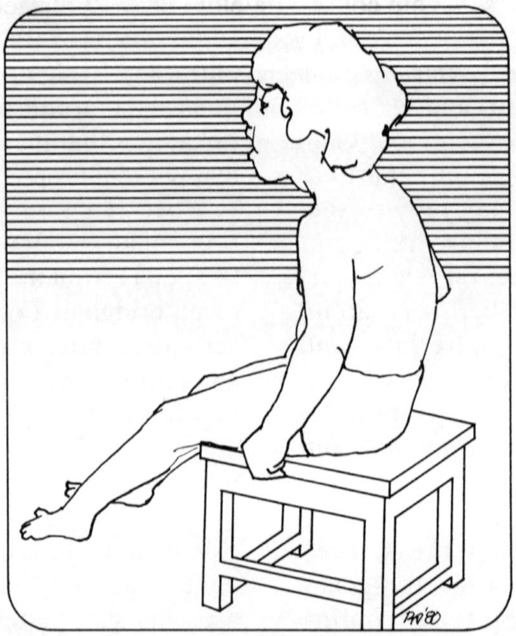

5

FIG. 4. Motor blocks in spastic diplegia: (1) hyperextension of neck; (2) retraction of scapulae; (3) anterior pelvic tilt; (4) hip flexion; (5) scissoring of legs, with ankle plantar flexion.
FIG. 5. Spastic child sitting with inadequate flexion of hips, rounded spine, hyperextended neck, and scissored legs.

child may be placed quite early in sitting, kneeling, and standing positions in order to develop head and trunk control. The prone position may be deemphasized. The more upright positions provide weight bearing through the body axis, and this seems to increase proximal stability and limit flailing motions (20).

In treatment planning based on a developmental frame of reference, the clinician needs to know the underlying components of movement, the prerequisite behaviors that are necessary for the attainment of a new skill. For example, it is important to identify the movement patterns and activities in the prone and supine positions that specifically prepare the infant for independent sitting with arm support. Such activities as pushing up on extended arms while lying prone or playing with the feet while lying supine should be analyzed in terms of developing control of extension, flexion, lateral flexion, and rotation in preparation for sitting. A task analysis of each motor skill should include (a) the components of

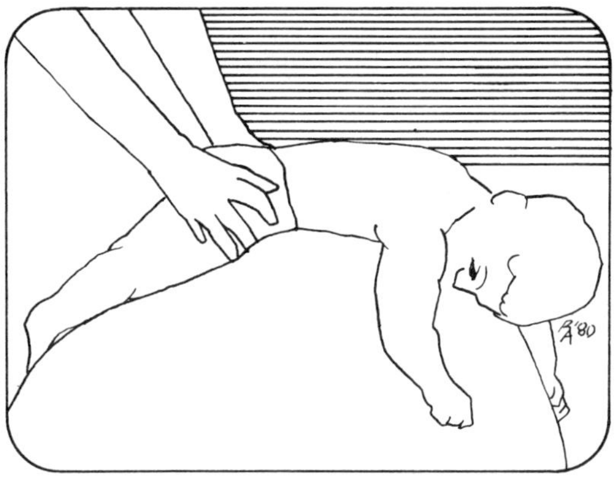

FIG. 6. To reduce spasticity, apply gentle pressure on alternate sides of the pelvis while rocking the ball. With the reduction of tonus, an activity is introduced to elicit desired movement patterns.

movement required to master the skill, (b) the future skills to which this act can be considered an important contribution, and (c) the cognitive and social abilities likely to be facilitated by this motor accomplishment (20).

Management of Tonus and Facilitation of Movement

Children with cerebral palsy and related neurological disorders typically have a mixture of primitive and pathological patterns of movement. In treatment it is important to delineate which movement behaviors are fairly normal but reflect delayed development and which represent pathological postural reflex activity. The therapeutic concern is more than general stimulation of motor development; it is more than a question of achieving the next milestone by filling in developmental gaps. Instead, therapeutic intervention attempts to counteract the development of pathological movement and muscle tone while simultaneously facilitating more coordinated patterns of movement and posture (92).

The child cannot superimpose normal movement on a background of abnormal muscle tone (22). In disorders of postural tone, inadequate or distorted proprioceptive feedback from the muscles and joints is sent to the central nervous system for processing. This defective sensory information leads to further aberrant movement. Thus a faulty reafference through the feedback circuit or servomechanism perpetuates the motor deviance (93). Therapeutic handling procedures are applied to inhibit abnormal tonus and tonic reflexes and encourage righting and equilibrium reactions necessary for orientation of the body against gravity. By normalizing postural mechanisms, more accurate movement-produced feedback may be available for control of body stability and limb transport (94). Normalization of tonus is inferred when movements appear more selective and are not bound by stereotyped patterns.

The techniques of inhibition and facilitation are used concurrently to increase the possibility and probability of higher integrated patterns of adaptive performance. Key points of control, such as the neck, spine, shoulder girdle, and pelvic girdle, are emphasized, since central control has a determining influence on distal coordination (95). For example, passive flexion at the neck and hips diminishes the spastic extensor patterns of arched spine and extended adducted legs. Likewise, the pelvis functions as the key point of control in sitting. With a posterior tilt of the pelvis, the spine rounds into a kyphotic curve. As the pelvis assumes more of an anterior tilt, the trunk tends to straighten into extension.

Numerous clinicians have made contributions to a sensorimotor approach to treatment based on neurodevelopmental and neurophysiological principles. The various methods have areas of commonality and divergence. However, they share a basic concept that sensory stimuli influence the motor system and can be employed therapeutically to activate or inhibit responses (96). The professional literature provides detailed descriptions of specific therapeutic procedures and their applications (10,21,22,92,97–101).

Child with Hypertonicity

The child with spasticity has an exaggerated degree of stability and inadequate development of mobility skills. Hypertonus prevents full expression of righting and equilibrium reactions as well as protective extension responses of the limbs. Consequently, the rotary component of movement is diminished, and the child maintains static postures, with a paucity of movement, for fear of falling. Movements are slow, labored, and within restricted patterns of coordination. Voluntary efforts to deviate markedly from the stereotyped synergies usually result in an increase in spasticity and reinforcement of the unwanted pattern. The child is unable to use the same muscles in different synergic combinations.

The degree of muscle tone may vary according to environmental stimulation, demands of an activity, affect, and other diverse conditions. If a child becomes overly excited or irritable, associated reactions cause involuntary tensing of muscles within pathological patterns (97). In addition, different parts of the child's body may exhibit varying levels of tonus. For instance, it is common for children to be more involved on one side of the body than the other. This asymmetrical distribution may lead to a scoliosis, a tendency to fall laterally to one side, and overutilization of the less affected side (29). Treatment stresses inhibition of the associated reactions and development of a flexible midline orientation.

Spasticity is reduced by movement (102). Therefore, handling techniques guide the child into postural patterns that counteract the spastic reflexive ones. For inhibitory purposes, handling procedures are applied rhythmically with the tempo graded to the child's tolerance level. The velocity of stretch can be monitored so that the body part can be taken through its full range of motion without eliciting hyperactive stretch reflexes (103,104).

Rotation of the trunk is a major means for decreasing overall spasticity of the body (22). With muscle tone inhibited, the rotational component of the trunk becomes available for postural support and balance. Treatment of the spastic child is often on a mobile surface, such as an inflatable beachball, bolster, or even the therapist's lap. With graded movement of the support surface, hypertonicity can be controlled and mobility skills practiced (Fig. 6).

Usually the inhibitory pattern is opposite to the spastic posture that the child tends to assume (105). Thus elevation of the extended and externally rotated arm over the head of the child inhibits a spastic flexor pattern of the limb. At the same time, selective movements are encouraged that deviate from the abnormal synergies. The components of a total pattern must be dissociated so that the child can gain voluntary control of isolated motions and joints.

Child with Hyperkinesis

Since the athetotic child has excessive mobility and insufficient proximal stabilization, therapy for hyperkinesis is quite different than therapy for spasticity (19). Since postural control is unreliable, distal movements are disorganized, erratic, and in extremes of range. Marked asymmetry is often noted, with the right side usually more involved than the left. Consequently the head is turned to the side, limiting the use of vision to direct upper extremity movement (29).

The goal of therapy is to achieve sustained postural tone with graded control of movement. Treatment focuses on the development of stability through weight bearing in antigravity positions. As the child is able to maintain positions, slow graded weight shifting is introduced. This intervention prepares the extremities for coordinated movement in midrange. Therapy stresses body symmetry and the ability to maintain and independently move the head in the midline (dissociation of the head on the trunk). Thus the influence of the asymmetrical tonic neck reflex is to be inhibited.

Since extreme effort increases hyperkinesis, demands on the child must be carefully monitored. If the activity requires fine manipulation, proper positioning should be assisted by the therapist or by the use of adaptive equipment. On the other hand, if the emphasis of the task is to maintain a desired body posture, activities should be presented that require mostly observation. Therefore a balance is maintained between postural requirements and limb manipulation so as to avoid overtaxing the child's ability and eliciting involuntary movement.

Child with Hypotonicity

The hypotonic child with cerebral palsy or Down's syndrome primarily lacks stability, but mobility skills are also delayed. The child may be passive and quiet, with little spontaneous motion, or may demonstrate rather active squirming movement. Children with low tone tend to assume a froglike position at rest (flexion, abduction, and external rotation of the limbs). Maintaining this static posture for extended periods of time can lead to deformities such as hip dislocations (106). With age, some hypotonic children develop extensor spasms, ataxia, or a mixture of tonal features.

The intent of treatment is to develop stability against gravity with head, trunk, and extremities in proper alignment. Postural tone is carefully increased through cutaneous, vestibular, and proprioceptive stimulation, such as therapeutic use of stretch, resistance, vibration, and joint compression (21,100). For example, bouncing a properly positioned child on an adult's lap increases holding contractions of the trunk musculature for proximal stability (co-contraction patterns). The bouncing provides joint compression through the spine, vestibular and visual stimulation for postural righting against gravity, and the cutaneous feel of weight bearing equally on both buttocks. Caution is in order to avoid overstimulation, which can produce intermittent or persistent hypertonus.

The "floppy" athetotic or ataxic child may achieve stability by fixing, locking, or tensing the muscles in characteristic patterns. For example, the child may stabilize the head by extreme elevation of the shoulder girdle, develop stiffness in the trunk to aid postural control, or hyperextend the knees to maintain stance. Reliance on these compensatory tensing postures is to be avoided. The aim of treatment is a complementary development of movement and posture.

In summary, the goal of neuromotor intervention is to achieve maximal function with minimal abnormal movement (107). Therapeutic activities, proper positioning, and adaptive equipment are employed to normalize muscle tone, decrease the influence of pathological reflexes, increase joint range of motion, reduce the tendency to deformities, expand postural control, and facilitate components of normal movement in a developmental sequence.

Grading the Therapeutic Experience

Effective treatment requires close grading of the therapeutic program according to the degree of sensory input, the use of activity, and the role of parents in the treatment process. The therapeutic experience should be systematically monitored to assure that the child is not bombarded with sensory stimulation. Children vary greatly in their capacity to control their states of alertness, their capacity to habituate to disturbing or novel events, and their capacity to perform integrated motor acts in response to their surroundings (108).

The autonomic nervous system helps to maintain the constancy, or homeostasis, of the internal environment of the body. The sympathetic division becomes active during stress to produce fight-or-flight responses. For example, heart and respiratory rates increase, pupils dilate, and the skin vasoconstricts. The parasympathetic division serves as a functional balance to inhibit and calm the system (blood pressure decreases, breathing slows, musculature relaxes).

Young children, especially those with developmental delay or disability, have precarious equilibrium between these autonomic functions. They demonstrate bias toward the sympathetic, and they can readily overload with multisensory stimulation (109). Behavioral responses to unpleasant or inappropriate stimuli include active withdrawal through physical escape (arching, running away), tuning out (staring into space, yawning), rejection (pushing the stimulus away with hands or feet), or signaling distress (crying, verbalizing). When a child is in such an emotional state, pathological movement patterns are reinforced, and skilled motor performance is restricted. Likewise, the ability to solve problems and learn is severely limited. During treatment, the clinician must regulate sensory input (environmental demands) in order to influence the motor, cognitive, and affective behaviors of the child.

In therapy for sensory integrative disorders, gross motor activities are provided that enhance cutaneous, vestibular, and proprioceptive processing at subcortical levels (such as scooter board, barrel, and climbing tasks). Therapeutic procedures facilitate the maturation of postural responses, develop the capacity for motor planning, and encourage bilateral integration of body and space (10,30). The choice, intensity, and variety of treatment activities are based on the child's changing ability to organize sensory information and produce an adaptive purposeful response.

As a general rule, concerted "cortical" effort by the child increases abnormal muscle tone and incoordination. Therefore activities are employed to elicit desired sensorimotor behavior on an automatic integrated basis. The child's attention is directed to the meaningful activity, not to the movement patterns per se (98). Therapeutic handling procedures should lead directly into functional skills and should not operate as fragmented isolated exercises.

Parents have an important contribution to make to the planning and implementation of the therapeutic program, particularly in the home management component. Consequently, intervention is oriented toward the family, with caregivers viewed as authoritative and knowledgeable. Active parent involvement encourages the incorporation of therapy into activities of daily living in the home.

However, the home management program must not place the parenting role under stress and thereby jeopardize parent-child attachment. Research by Tyler and Kogan (110–112) compared the interactions of mothers and their children with cerebral palsy during therapeutic and play sessions. When the mothers performed therapy, they became excessively controlling, and greater amounts of negative behaviors were noted. They tended to interpret the children's inability to perform as demonstration of their inadequacy as caregivers. The presence of a handicapping condition makes special demands on the child, the parents, and the family. It is a challenge to the therapist to foster an environment in which all may prosper.

ACKNOWLEDGMENTS

The author wishes to thank Lois L. Bly, R.P.T., and Joan Day Mohr, R.P.T., for their contributions to pediatric rehabilitation and concepts presented in this chapter, Jo Murphy Hyland, O.T.R., and Virginia Scardina, O.T.R., for their willingness to share charts, and Patricia E. Gilchrist, O.T.R., for encouragement and helpful suggestions.

REFERENCES

1. Gilfoyle, E. M., and Hays, C. (1979): Occupational therapy roles and functions in the education of the school-based handicapped student. *Am. J. Occup. Ther.*, 33:565–576.
2. Gentile, A. M., and Nacson, J. (1976): Organizational processes in motor control. In: *Exercise and Sport Sciences,* Vol. 4, edited by J. Keogh and R. S. Hutton, pp. 1–33. Journal Publishing Affiliates, Santa Barbara.
3. Higgins, J. R. (1977): *Human Movement: An Integrated Approach.* C. V. Mosby, St. Louis.
4. Cratty, B. J. (1967): *Movement Behavior and Motor Learning.* Lea & Febiger, Philadelphia.
5. Gentile, A. M., Higgins, J. R., Miller, E. A., and Rosen, B. M. (1975): The structure of motor tasks. In: *Movement,* edited by C. Bard, M. Fleury, and G. Salmela, pp. 11–28. Canadian Psycho-motor Learning and Sports Psychology, Quebec.
6. Gilfoyle, E. M., and Grady, A. P. (1978): Posture and movement. In: *Willard and Spackman's Occupational Therapy,* edited by H. L. Hopkins and H. D. Smith, pp. 58–81. J. B. Lippincott, Philadelphia.
7. Fitts, P. M., and Posner, M. I. (1967): *Human Performance.* Brooks/Cole, Belmont, Calif.
8. Higgins, J. R. (1972): Movements to match environmental demands. *Res. Q. Am. Assoc. Health Phys. Educ.*, 43:312–336.
9. Welford, A. T. (1968): *Fundamentals of Skill.* Methuen, London.
10. Ayres, A. J. (1972): *Sensory Integration and Learning Disorders.* Western Psychological Services, Los Angeles.
11. Carmichael, L. (1970): The onset and early development of behavior. In: *Carmichael's Manual of Child Psychology, Vol. 1,* edited by P. H. Mussen, pp. 447–563. John Wiley & Sons, New York.
12. Fox, M. W. (1970): Reflex development and behavioral organization. In: *Developmental Neurobiology,* edited by W. Himwich. Charles C Thomas, Springfield, Ill.
13. Henderson, A., and Coryell, J. (editors) (1973): *The Body Senses and Perceptual Deficit, Proceedings of the Occupational Therapy Symposium on Somatosensory Aspects of Perceptual Deficit.* Boston University Press, Boston.
14. Daffner, C. (1977): An occupational therapy model for treating learning disabilities. *N. J. Speech Hear. J.*, 15:(1)14–15, 35–36.
15. Kephart, N. C. (1971): *The Slow Learner in the Classroom,* ed. 2. Charles E. Merrill, Columbus, Ohio.
16. Kay, H. (1969): The development of motor skills from birth to adolescence. In: *Principles of Skill*

Acquisition, edited by E. A. Bilodeau, pp. 33–57. Academic Press, New York.

17. Easton, T. A. (1972): On the normal use of reflexes. *Am. Sci.,* 60:591–599.
18. Zelazo, P. R. From reflexive to instrumental behavior. In: *Developmental Psychobiology: The Significance of Infancy,* edited by L. Lipsitt, pp. 87–104. Lawrence Erlbaum, Hillsdale, N.J.
19. Stockmeyer, S. A. (1972): A sensorimotor approach to treatment. In: *Physical Therapy Services in the Developmental Disabilities,* edited by P. H. Pearson and C. E. Williams. Charles C Thomas, Springfield, Ill., pp. 186–222.
20. Connor, F. P., Williamson, G. G., and Siepp, J. M. (editors) (1978): *Program Guide for Infants and Toddlers with Neuromotor and Other Developmental Disabilities.* Teachers College Press, New York.
21. Griffin, J. W. (1974): Use of proprioceptive stimuli in therapeutic exercise. *Phys. Ther.,* 54:1072–1079.
22. Voss, D. E. (1972): Proprioceptive neuromuscular facilitation: The PNF method. In: *Physical Therapy Services in the Developmental Disabilities,* edited by P. H. Pearson, and C. E. Williams, pp. 223–282. Charles C Thomas, Springfield, Ill.
23. Molnar, G. E. (1974): Motor deficit of retarded infants and young children. *Arch. Phys. Med. Rehabil.,* 55:393–398.
24. Twitchell, T. E. (1966): Sensation and the motor deficit in cerebral palsy. *Clin. Orthop.,* 46:55–61.
25. Saint-Anne Dargassies, S. (1972): Neurodevelopmental symptoms during the first year of life. *Dev. Med. Child Neurol.,* 14:235–246.
26. Bobath, B., and Bobath, K. (1975): *Motor Development in the Different Types of Cerebral Palsy.* W. Heinemann, London.
27. Samilson, R. L., and Perry, J. (1975): The orthopaedic assessment in cerebral palsy. In: *Orthopaedic Aspects of Cerebral Palsy,* edited by R. L. Samilson, pp. 35–70. Spastics International Medical with W. Heinemann, London.
28. Milani-Comparetti, A., and Gidoni, E. A. (1967): Pattern analysis of motor development and its disorders. *Dev. Med. Child Neurol.,* 9:625–630.
29. Bobath, B. (1971): *Abnormal Postural Reflex Activity Caused by Brain Lesions,* ed. 2. W. Heinemann, London.
30. Ayres, A. J. (1975): Sensorimotor foundations of academic ability. In: *Perceptual and Learning Disabilities in Children, Vol. 2,* edited by W. M. Cruickshank and D. P. Hallahan, pp. 301–358. Syracuse University Press, Syracuse, N.Y.
31. de Quiros, J. B., and Schrager, O. L. (1978): *Neuropsychological Fundamentals in Learning Disabilities.* Acad Therapy Publications, San Rafael, Calif.
32. Weeks, Z. R. (1979): Effects of the vestibular system on human development. Part 1. Overview of functions and effects of stimulation. *Am. J. Occup. Ther.,* 33:376–381.
33. de Quiros, J. B. (1976): Diagnosis of vestibular disorders in the learning disabled. *J. Learn. Dis.,* 9:50–58.
34. Ottenbacher, K. (1978): Identifying vestibular processing dysfunction in learning-disabled children. *Am. J. Occup. Ther.,* 32:217–221.
35. McCracken, A. (1975): Tactile function of educable mentally retarded children. *Am. J. Occup. Ther.,* 29:397–402.
36. Weeks, Z. R. (1979): Effects of vestibular stimulation on mentally retarded, emotionally disturbed, and learning-disabled individuals. *Am. J. Occup. Ther.,* 33:450–457.
37. Bauer, B. A. (1977): Tactile-sensitive behavior in hyperactive and nonhyperactive children. *Am. J. Occup. Ther.,* 31:447–453.
38. Ornitz, E. M. (1970): Vestibular dysfunction in schizophrenia and childhood autism. *Compr. Psychiatry,* 11:159–173.
39. Ritvo, E., Ornitz, E., Eviatar, A., Markham, C., Brown, M., and Mason, A. (1969): Decreased postrotary nystagmus in early infantile autism. *Neurology,* 19:653–658.
40. Stilwell, J. M., Crowe, T. K., and McCallum, L. W. (1978): Postrotatory nystagmus duration as a function of communication disorders. *Am. J. Occup. Ther.,* 32:222–228.
41. Grimm, R. A. (1976): Hand function and tactile perception in a sample of children with myelomeningocele. *Am. J. Occup. Ther.,* 30:235–240.
42. Chee, F. K. W., Kreutzberg, J. R., and Clark, D. L. (1978): Semicircular canal stimulation in cerebral palsied children. *Phys. Ther.,* 58: 1071–1075.
43. Clark, D. L., Kreutzberg, J. R., and Chee, F. K. W. (1977): Vestibular stimulation influence on motor development in infants. *Science,* 196:1228–1229.
44. Kantner, R. M., Clark, D. L., Allen, L. C., and Chase, M. F. (1976): Effects of vestibular stimulation on nystagmus response and motor performance in the developmentally delayed infant. *Phys. Ther.,* 56:414–421.
45. Montgomery, P., and Richter, E. (1977): Effect of sensory integrative therapy on the neuro-

motor development of retarded children. *Phys. Ther.*, 57:799–806.
46. Mann, L. (1971): Perceptual training revisited: The training of nothing at all. *Rehabil. Lit.*, 32:322–327, 335.
47. Vellutino, F. R., Steger, B. M., Moyer, S. C., Harding, C. J., and Niles, J. A. (1977): Has the perceptual deficit hypothesis led us astray? *J. Learn. Dis.*, 10:54–64.
48. Hammill, D. D., and Bartel, N. R. (1975): *Teaching Children with Learning and Behavior Problems*. Allyn & Bacon, Boston.
49. Ayres, A. J. (1972): Improving academic scores through sensory integration. *J. Learn. Dis.*, 5:24–28.
50. Ayres, A. J. (1976): *The Effect of Sensory Integrative Therapy on Learning Disabled Children*. Center for Study of Sensory Integrative Dysfunction, Pasadena, Calif.
51. Ayres, A. J. (1978): Learning disabilities and the vestibular system. *J. Learn. Dis.*, 11:18–29.
52. Frank, J., and Levinson, H. N. (1976): Dysmetric dyslexia and dyspraxia. *Acad. Ther.*, 11:133–143.
53. Denckla, M. B. (1972): Clinical syndromes in learning disabilities: The case for "splitting" vs. "lumping." *J. Learn. Dis.*, 5:26–32.
54. Ayres, A. J. (1976): *Interpreting the Southern California Sensory Integration Tests*. Western Psychological Services, Los Angeles.
55. Meisel, J. (1977): *Guide to Program Evaluation*. United Cerebral Palsy Associations, New York.
56. Bayley, N. (1969): *Bayley Scales of Infant Development*. Psychological Corp., New York.
57. Frankenburg, W. K., and Dodds, J. B. (1970): *Denver Developmental Screening Test*, rev. ed. La Doca Foundation, Denver.
58. Brower, C. (1975): Functional developmental assessment. In: *Physically Handicapped Children: A Medical Atlas for Teachers*, edited by E. E. Bleck and D. A. Nagel, pp. 69–87. Grune & Stratton, New York.
59. Gesell, A., and Amatruda, C. S. (1947): *Developmental Diagnosis*, ed 2. Paul B. Hoeber, New York.
60. Morris, S. (1977): *Program Guidelines for Children with Feeding Problems*. Childcraft Education Corp., Edison, N. J.
61. Berk, R. A., and De Gangi, G. A. (1979): Technical considerations in the evaluation of pediatric motor scales. *Am. J. Occup. Ther.*, 33:240–244.
62. Lewko, J. H. (1976): Current practices in evaluating motor behavior of disabled children. *Am. J. Occup. Ther.*, 30:413–419.
63. McGraw, M. B. (1966): *The Neuromuscular Maturation of the Human Infant*. Hafner, New York.
64. Erhardt, R. P. (1980): *Erhardt Developmental Prehension Assessment*. R. P. Erhardt, Fargo, N.D.
65. Fiorentino, M. R. (1963): *Reflex Testing Methods for Evaluating C.N.S. Development*. Charles C Thomas, Springfield, Ill.
66. Fiorentino, M. R. (1972): *Normal and Abnormal Development: The Influence of Primitive Reflexes on Motor Development*. Charles C Thomas, Springfield, Ill.
67. Milani-Comparetti, A., and Gidoni, E. A. (1967): Routine developmental examination in normal and retarded children. *Dev. Med. Child Neurol.*, 9:631–638.
68. Trembath, J. (1977): *The Milani-Comparetti Motor Development Screening Test*. Meyer Children's Rehabilitation Institute, Omaha.
69. Hoskins, T., and Squires, J. (1973): Developmental assessment: A test for gross motor and reflex development. *Phys. Ther.*, 53:117–126.
70. Ayres, A. J. (1972): *Southern California Sensory Integration Tests*. Western Psychological Services, Los Angeles.
71. Ayres, A. J. (1975): *Southern California Postrotary Nystagmus Test*. Western Psychological Services, Los Angeles.
72. De Gangi, G. (1979): *Assessment of Sensorimotor Integration in Preschool Children*. Georgetown University Child Development Center, Washington, D.C.
73. Bruininks, R. H. (1979): *Bruininks-Oseretsky Test of Motor Proficiency*. American Guidance Service, Circle Pines, Minn.
74. Roach, E., and Kephart, N. (1966): *The Purdue Perceptual-Motor Survey*. Charles E. Merrill, Columbus, Ohio.
75. Goodenough, F. L., and Harris, D. B. (1963): *Goodenough-Harris Drawing Test*. Harcourt, Brace & World, New York.
76. Berry, K. E., and Buktenica, N. A. (1967): *Developmental Test of Visual-Motor Integration*. Follett, Chicago.
77. Colarusso, R., and Hammill, D. (1972): *The Motor-Free Test of Visual Perception*. Acad Therapy Publications, San Rafael, Calif.
78. Frostig, M., LeFevre, W., and Whittlesey, J. R. B. (1966): *Administration and Scoring Manual, Marianne Frostig Developmental Test*

of Visual Perception, rev. ed. Consulting Psychologists Press, Palo Alto, Calif.

79. Olson, A. V. (1968): Factor analytic studies of the Frostig Developmental Test of Visual Perception. *J. Spec. Educ.,* 2:429–433.
80. Smith, P. A., and Marx, R. W. (1972): Some cautions on the use of the Frostig test: A factor analytic study. *J. Learn. Dis.,* 5:42–47.
81. Fidler, G. S., and Fidler, J. W. (1978): Doing and becoming: Purposeful action and self-actualization. *Am. J. Occup. Ther.,* 32:305–310.
82. King, L. J. (1978): Toward a science of adaptive responses. *Am. J. Occup. Ther.,* 32:429–437.
83. Gunn, S. L. (1975): Play as occupation: Implications for the handicapped. *Am. J. Occup. Ther.,* 29:222–225.
84. Wehman, P., and Abramson, M. (1976): Three theoretical approaches to play: Applications for exceptional children. *Am. J. Occup. Ther.,* 30:551–559.
85. Rogers, J. C., Weinstein, J. M., and Figone, J. J. (1978): The interest check list. *Am. J. Occup. Ther.,* 32:628–630.
86. Florey, L. (1971): An approach to play and play development. *Am. J. Occup. Ther.,* 25:275–280.
87. Black, M. M. (1976): Adolescent role assessment. *Am. J. Occup. Ther.,* 30:73–79.
88. Michelman, S. (1974): Play and the deficit child. In: *Play as Exploratory Learning: Studies of Curiosity Behavior,* edited by M. Reilly, 157–207. Sage, Beverly Hills, Calif.
89. Wehman, P. (1975): Establishing play behaviors in mentally retarded youth. *Rehabil. Lit.,* 36:238–246.
90. Wehman, P., and Marchant, J. A. (1978): Improving free play skills of severely retarded children. *Am. J. Occup. Ther.,* 32:100–104.
91. Ames, L. B. (1970): *Child Care and Development.* J. B. Lippincott, Philadelphia.
92. Bobath, B., and Bobath, K. (1972): Cerebral palsy. In: *Physical Therapy Services in the Developmental Disabilities,* edited by P. H. Pearson and C. E. Williams, 31–185. Charles C Thomas, Springfield, Ill.
93. Fischer, E. (1967): Factors affecting motor learning. *Am. J. Phys. Med.,* 46:511–519.
94. Goff, B. (1972): The application of recent advances in neurophysiology to Miss M. Rood's concept of neuromuscular facilitation. *Physiotherapy,* 58:409–415.
95. Manning, J. (1972): Facilitation of movement: The Bobath approach. *Physiotherapy,* 58: 403–408.
96. Huss, J. (1969): Controversy and confusion in physical dysfunction treatment techniques: Clinical aspects. In: *Expanding Dimensions in Rehabilitation,* edited by L. J. Zamir, pp. 68–72. Charles C Thomas, Springfield, Ill.
97. Brunnstrom, S. (1970): *Movement Therapy in Hemiplegia: A Neurophysiological Approach.* Harper & Row, New York.
98. Farber, S. D., and Huss, A. J. (1974): Treatment. In: *Sensorimotor Evaluation and Treatment Procedures for Allied Health Personnel,* ed. 2, edited by S. D. Farber, pp. 39–51. Indiana University Foundation, Indianapolis.
99. Stockmeyer, S. A. (1967): An interpretation of the approach of Rood to the treatment of neuromuscular dysfunction. *Am. J. Phys. Med.,* 46:900–956.
100. Till, D. (1969): The uses of reflexes in the restoration of normal movement. *Physiotherapy,* 55:2–8.
101. Trombly, C. A., and Scott, A. D. (1977): *Occupational Therapy for Physical Dysfunction.* Williams & Wilkins, Baltimore.
102. Williamson, G. G. (1978): Effect of Therapeutic Handling on Reaction Time and Movement Time of Forward Limb Movement in Spastic Children with Cerebral Palsy. Doctoral dissertation, Columbia University. Dissertation Abstracts International, 1978, 39, 2190A (University Microfilms No. 7819466).
103. Bishop, B. (1977): Spasticity: Its physiology and management. *Phys. Ther.,* 57:371–401.
104. Lance, J. W., and Burke, D. (1974): Mechanisms of spasticity. *Arch. Phys. Med. Rehabil.,* 55:332–337.
105. Finnie, N. R. (1975): *Handling the Young Cerebral Palsied Child at Home,* ed. 2. E. P. Dutton, New York.
106. Twitchell, T. E. (1965): Variations and abnormalities of motor development. *J. Am. Phys. Ther. Assoc.,* 45:424–430.
107. Bergen, A. (1974): *Selected Equipment for Pediatric Rehabilitation.* Blythedale Children's Hospital, Valhalla, N.Y.
108. Brazelton, T. B. (1973): *Neonatal Behavioral Assessment Scale.* William Heinemann, London.
109. Brazelton, T. B., Koslowski, B., and Main, M. (1974): The origins of reciprocity: The early mother-infant interaction. In: *The Effect of the Infant on Its Caregiver,* edited by M. Lewis and L. A. Rosenblum, pp. 49–76. John Wiley & Sons, New York.
110. Tyler, N. B., and Kogan, K. L. (1972): The so-

cial by-products of therapy with young children. *Phys. Ther.*, 52:508–513.

111. Tyler, N. B., Kogan, K. L., and Turner, P. (1974): Interpersonal components of therapy with young cerebral palsied. *Am. J. Occup. Ther.*, 28:395–400.

112. Kogan, K. L., Tyler, N. B., and Turner, P. (1974): The process of interpersonal adaptation between mothers and their cerebral palsied children. *Dev. Med. Child Neurol.*, 16:518–527.

APPENDIX A: HYPOTHESIZED SEQUENCES IN HUMAN DEVELOPMENT RELATED TO SENSORY PROCESSING AND INTEGRATION[a]

The inherent function of the nervous system and the organization of the information of the sensory receptors of:

Touch	Vision	Smell
Movement	Hearing	Pain
Gravity	Body chemical changes	Temperature

are used to develop:

Reflex maturation	Motor planning ability
Body scheme	Postural balance
Center of gravity awareness	Bilateral body use

These sensorimotor patterns enhance the development of:

Motor skills	*Emotional stability*	*Perceptual skills*
Oral	Mastery of environment	Visual spatial relations
Ocular	Feelings of adequacy	Kinesthesia
Body	Behavioral control	Auditory-language
Hand		

These skills provide the foundation for:

Reading	Number work	Independent work
Writing	Problem solving	Spontaneous play
Spelling	Ability to conceptualize	Creativity

Ability to form meaningful personal relationships

FIG. 1. Sensory integration as the foundation of normal development (Developed by Virginia Scardina, OTR).

[a] Courtesy of Virginia Scardina, O.T.R., F.A.O.T.A., 1979; adapted from A. J. Ayres, 1961.

Testing Reflexes

7

Joyce Lawler

Methods of testing reflexes for evaluation of motor development have been well documented by Barnes et al. (1), Bobath (3–5), and Fiorentino (5,6). Besides describing a particular reflex and methods for its evaluation, they have reported the appearances of the different reflexes, their development and frequent integration by the higher centers of the central nervous system, and their actual purpose in the maturation of the central nervous system.

The purpose of this chapter is to show the value of reflex testing in relation to treatment of children who have developmental disabilities caused by central nervous system impairment. We shall briefly describe some reflexes or reactions whose inhibition or development plays an important role in motor development. Next there are some ideas on treatment procedures that will enhance or, in the case of primary reactions, inhibit some of these developmental reflexes.

These treatment ideas are only outlined to give the student an indication of their use in a treatment program. Basic muscle tone, joint contractures or deformities, and the emotional and mental status of the patient must be considered before an effective treatment program can be planned.

PRIMARY REFLEXES

The primary reflexes are present at birth or earlier. They become integrated during the first few months of life because they are total patterns of response dealing only with flexion and extension, ignoring the third dimension of movement (rotation). Integration modifies these total reflex patterns but does not extinguish them, using their components to expediate development of normal gross motor patterns.

During treatment, the therapist should not try to evoke primitive responses in a child with central nervous system damage, these reflexes should be inhibited. The goal is to promote free motor patterns that exhibit the three dimensions of movement rather than the stereotyped reactions of the primary responses.

The primary responses that will be described are those that usually require the most frequent inhibition during treatment. These are the tonic labyrinthine reflex in supine and prone, the asymmetrical tonic neck reflex, the symmetrical tonic neck reflex, and associated movements. When these reflexes persist beyond the normal period necessary for their presence, they must be inhibited. They are useful in developing the flexor and extensor tone found in the process of normal development.

A brief description of the reflex, its appearance and integration by the central nervous system, and the sense organ that stimulates the response will be given, after which inhibition of these responses as part of a treatment session will be discussed.

The symmetrical tonic neck reflex is considered to be present during the first month of life and gone by the fourth to sixth month, according to Fiorentino. Barnes et al. said that it is not a true primary response, as it does not appear until 6 months of age, breaking up the total extensor pattern of the child and promoting four-point kneeling. However, they categorized this response with the rest of the primary reflexes because they could find no other place for it.

Extension and flexion of the head cause the stretch receptors in the proprioceptive fibers in the neck to be stimulated. If the symmetrical tonic neck reflex is present, head extension causes the arms to extend and the legs to flex, whereas flexion of the head will promote flexed arms and extended legs. When the response is obligatory, it will interfere with creeping on all fours, kneeling, and the half-kneeling posture needed to get to standing.

The asymmetrical tonic neck reflex is present after 36 weeks of gestation and disappears by the fourth month of life. Fiorentino said that this reflex helps children to first look at their hands and promotes their first experience with eye-hand coordination. As the head is turned, the extremities on the face side will extend, and those on the skull side will flex. Turning the head from one side to the other stimulates the proprioceptive fibers in the neck muscles and joints, and if the reflex is present, the fencer's position will emerge. Persistence of the reflex prevents the infant's hands from coming to the midline and stops the attainment of good visual following. Also, structural changes may take place (e.g., scolioses and hip subluxation).

The tonic labyrinthine reflexes in supine and prone are present from birth until 6 months of age. The labyrinths in the ear are affected by the position of the head and can cause total flexor and extensor postures of the trunk and extremities. The reflex helps to orient the head with the body and extremities and gives needed flexor-extensor tone. In the supine position, extensor tone predominates, and in the prone position the flexor tone will be stronger than extensor tone.

Associated movements are present in the newborn as mass flexor and extensor patterns. The posture of one limb will cause the other to mirror that position, as there are no real individualized movements of head, extremities, and trunk. As the central nervous system is integrated with increasing age, these movements can be inhibited. However, under extreme stress, humans of any age will or can demonstrate the phenomena.

Inhibition and Treatment of Primary Reflexes

Inhibiting the asymmetrical tonic neck reflex (Fig. 1): Position the child with the head in the midline in all positions (Figs. 2–5). Promoting head and extremity flexion in side-lying, supine, or the sitting position often lessens or stops the habitual posture. Positions in which the asymmetrical tonic neck posture is not predominant can be used to get the head and hands to the midline, either passively or actively. Visual following through 180° can also be sought, as the effect of this reflex can keep the eyes turned to the face side.

Inhibiting the tonic labyrinthine reflex in supine (Fig. 6): Position the child correctly (Figs. 2 and 4). A strong extensor posture is present in supine, avoid the position unless the total pattern can be broken by flexing head, trunk, and extremities.

Inhibiting the tonic labyrinthine in prone (Fig. 7): Position the child correctly (Figs. 4, 8, and 9). The prone position encourages flexion, but wedges and pillows in prone can prevent too much flexion. Side-lying (Fig. 4) and, in some instances, supine (Fig. 2) may be better choices for activities. If children can obtain the upright position, they can still be affected by the tonic labyrinthine reflex. For example, if gravity pulls the child forward (Fig. 10), the tonic labyrinthine in prone can be elicited to cause flexion. If gravity pulls the child back (Fig. 11), the tonic labyrinthine in supine can be elicited to cause extension.

Inhibiting the symmetrical tonic neck reflex (Figs. 12 and 13): The reflex is stimulated by neck

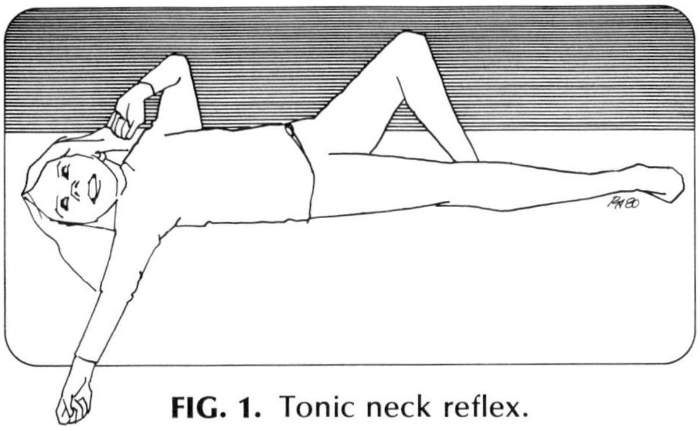

FIG. 1. Tonic neck reflex.

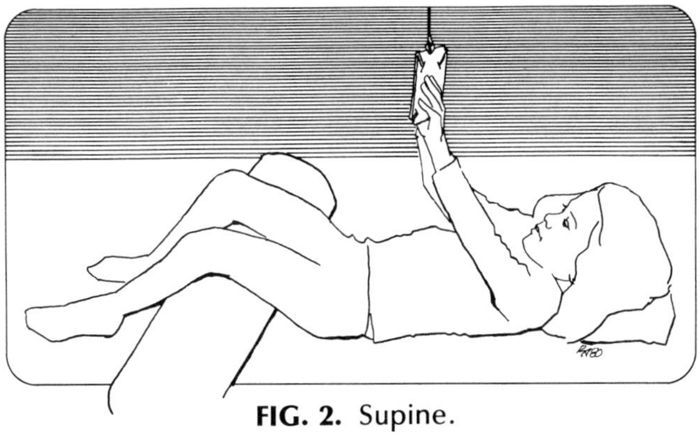

FIG. 2. Supine.

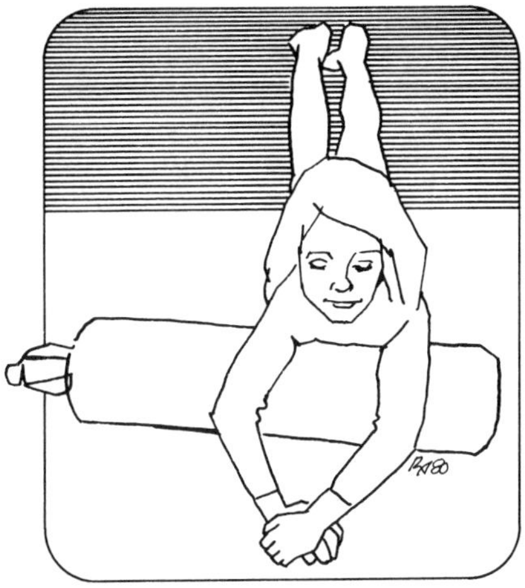

FIG. 3. Prone.

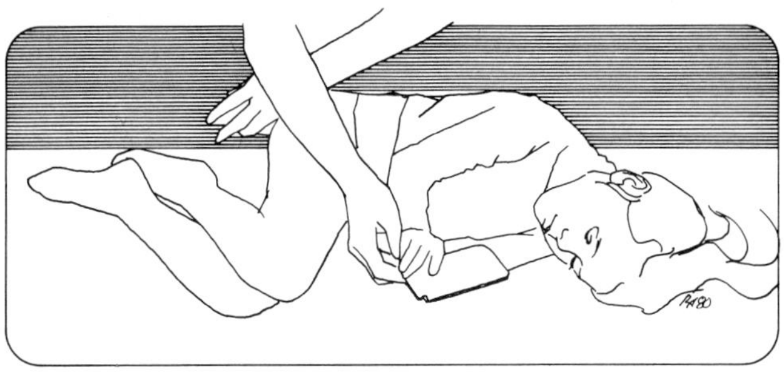

FIG. 4. Sidelying.

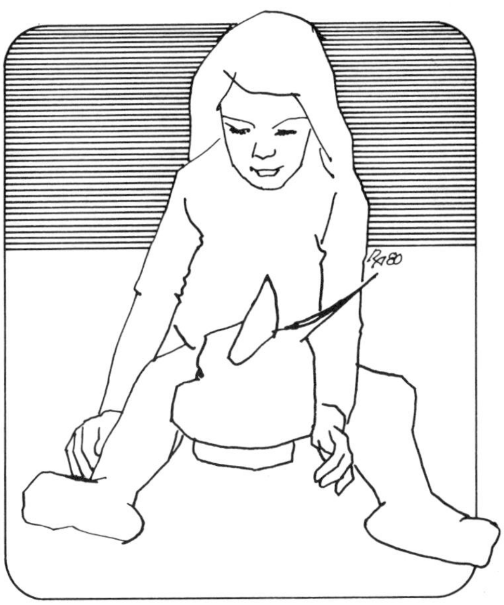

FIG. 5. Sitting.

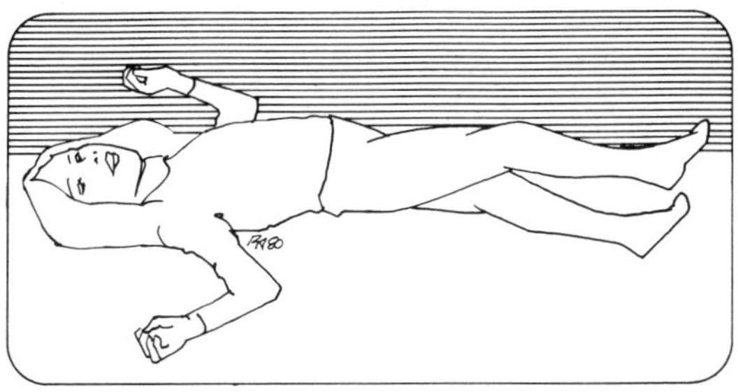

FIG. 6. Tonic labyrinthine reflex supine.

Figs. 1–19: Primary reflexes: Inhibition and treatment positions.

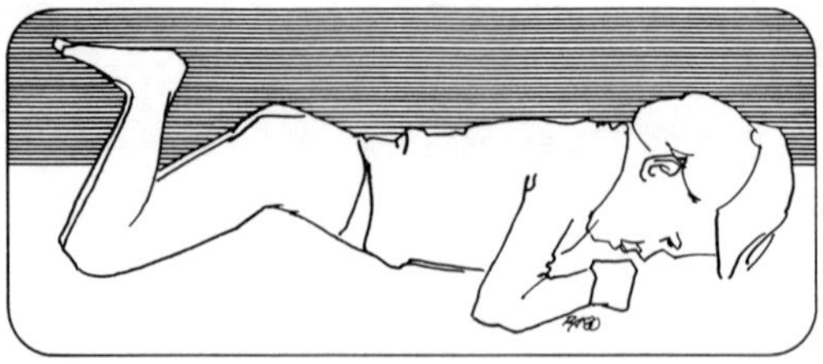

FIG. 7. Tonic labyrinthine reflex prone.

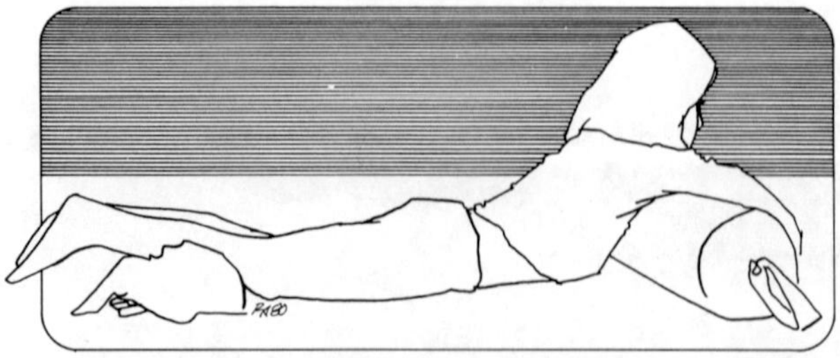

FIG. 8. Prone.

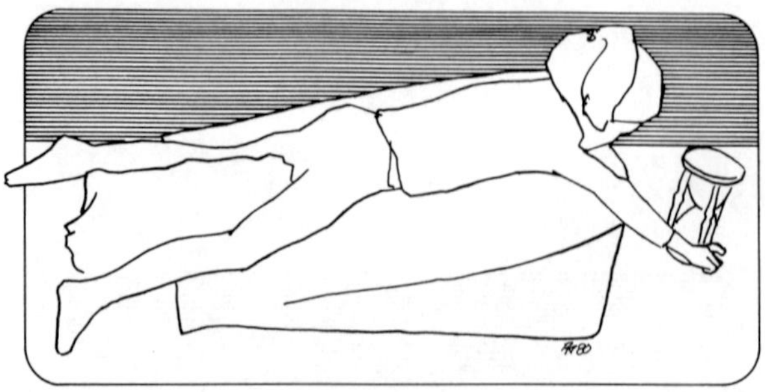

FIG. 9. Prone.

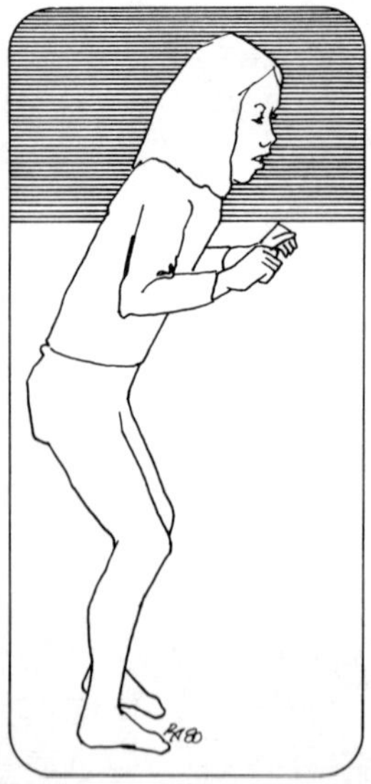

FIG. 10. Standing forward.

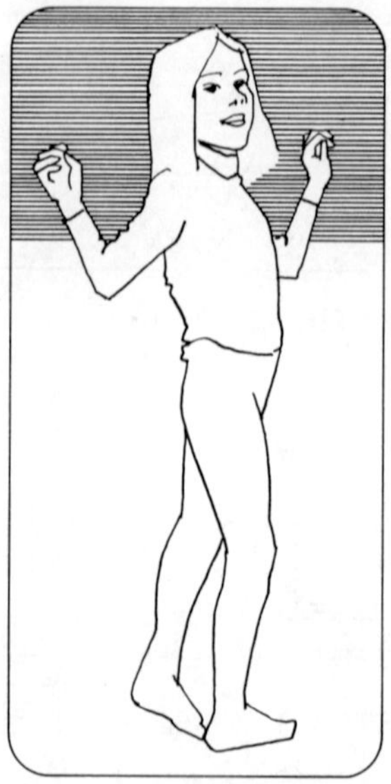

FIG. 11. Standing backward.

flexion or extension; therefore an attempt should be made to keep the head in neutral (Fig. 14). In the higher positions such as kneeling and half-kneeling, the pathological reflex is used to get mass extension of the arms and trunk. This reflex can be prevented by placing the child correctly in these positions and letting the child hold the posture with the head in neutral (Figs. 15–17). This allows the child to sustain a semi-upright posture without using the reflex.

Inhibiting associated movements (Fig. 18): Be aware that associated movements can occur when a child is performing, especially if the motor act requires lots of effort. If the activity causes constant overflow of movements in the nonactive parts, the activity should be modified. Reduction of overflow movements during an activity can be accomplished by recognition of the abnormal posture in the noninvolved active body part and positioning it accordingly (Fig. 19).

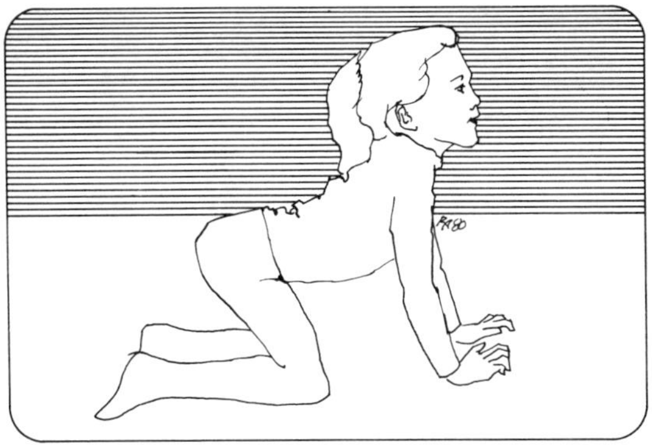

FIG. 12. Symmetrical tonic neck reflex—head extended.

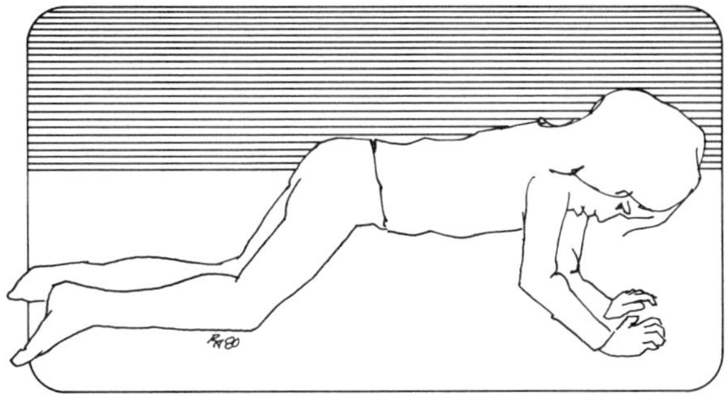

FIG. 13. Symmetrical tonic neck reflex—head flexed.

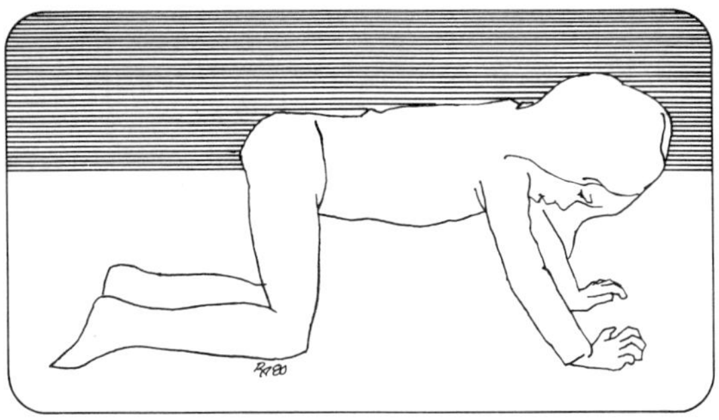

FIG. 14. Head in neutral.

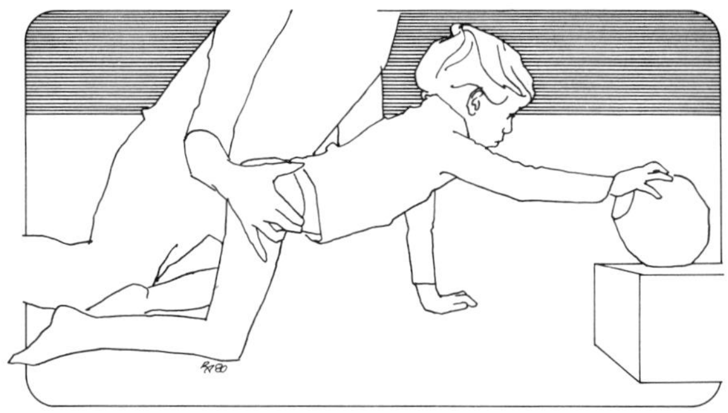

FIG. 15. Quadruped.

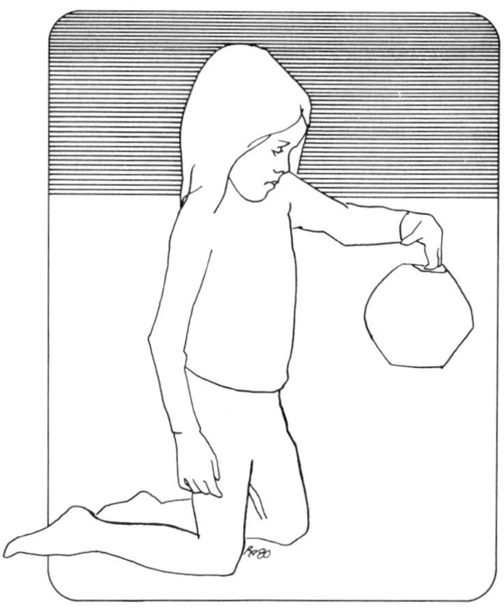

FIG. 16. Kneeling.

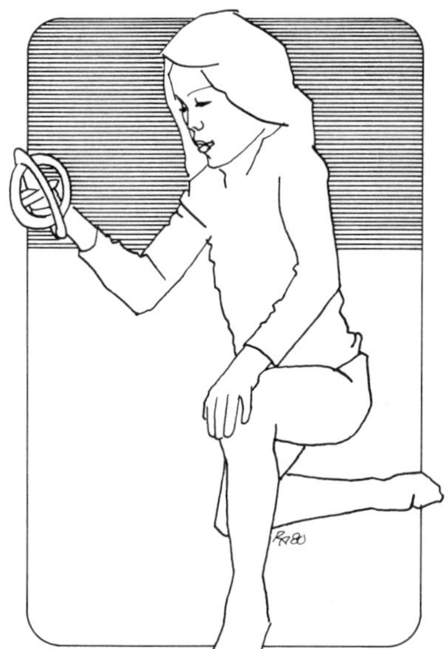

FIG. 17. One-half kneel.

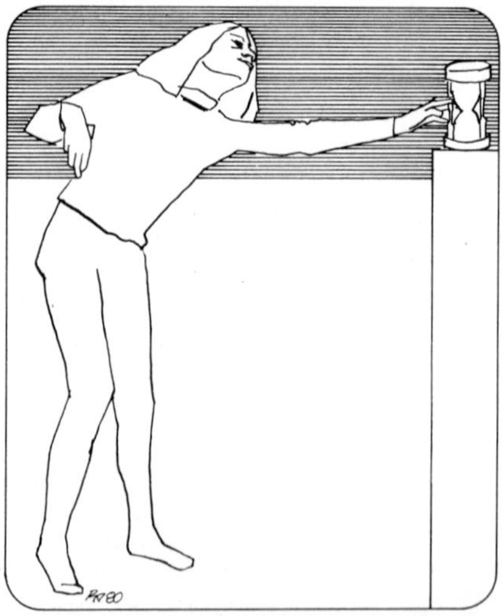

FIG. 18. Associated movements.

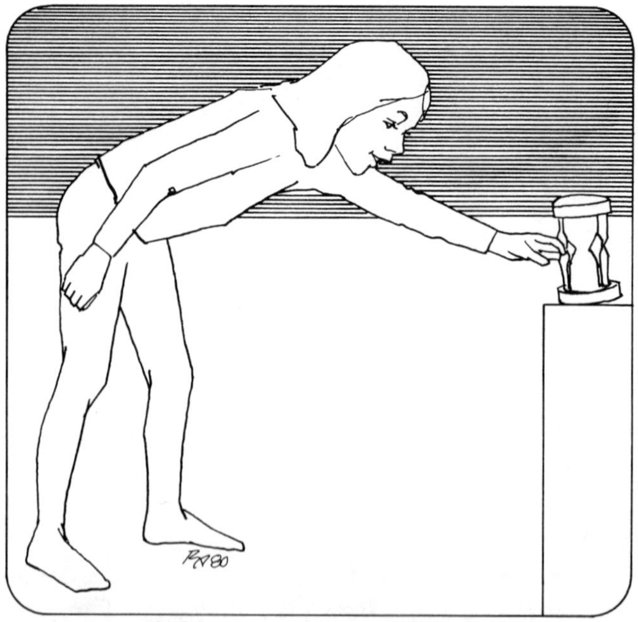

FIG. 19. Inhibition of associated movements.

RIGHTING REACTIONS

Basically, the righting reactions are five different reflexes that serve to keep the head in a normal position, right the body to a normal position, and adjust the body parts in relation to the head and vice versa. These reactions are called the labyrinthine righting reflexes acting on the head, body-righting reflexes acting on the head, neck-righting reflexes, body-righting reflexes acting on the body, and optical righting reflexes. These reflexes enable the child to lift up from prone or supine, sit, get on all fours, kneel, and half-kneel, and finally they put the child in the upright position. They are stimulated by visual and tactile stimuli received from exteroceptors, proprioceptors, and the labyrinths of the inner ear. As cortical control increases, they are generally modified and inhibited, and they disappear by the fifth year; however, in moments of stress they reappear.

In the treatment of developmentally disabled children it is valuable to know how to test for each of these reflexes; such knowledge gives an idea of the child's gross motor functioning. For example, if a child has a head-righting reaction while prone but no other head-righting reaction, it will be expected that on pulling up to sit, the child will have head lag and no ability to sit alone.

Prediction of how far treatment can progress can also be facilitated by such testing. For example, if a child has optical and labyrinthine righting reflexes, the child should be able to roll and should have head control in supine, prone, and support sitting positions. If this is not the case, then the reason must be sought; perhaps there is lack of stimulation in the child's environment, or perhaps there is mental retardation.

In dealing with cerebral palsy, there is the additional problem of muscle tone (e.g., too much, too little, or fluctuating). Abnormal tone does not allow full development and proper working of these reflexes. In the case of older children with severe physical handicaps in whom testing reveals little or no development of these reflexes, one would set very low treatment goals. If a child has failed to achieve at least half of the five righting reactions within the first 2 to 3 years of life, that child's chances of attaining an upright stance are poor. Finally, righting reactions permit a form of treatment that can be very effective: Eliciting righting reactions correctly can at times suppress abnormal and persistent reflexes and facilitate normal development.

A brief description of what the reflex does and what sense organ is being or should be stimulated during treatment will follow, as well as a brief outline of treatment and stimulation of these reflexes.

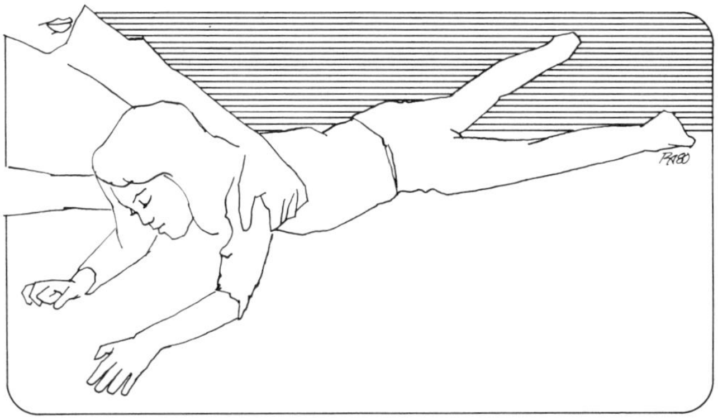

FIG. 20. Prone righting reaction.

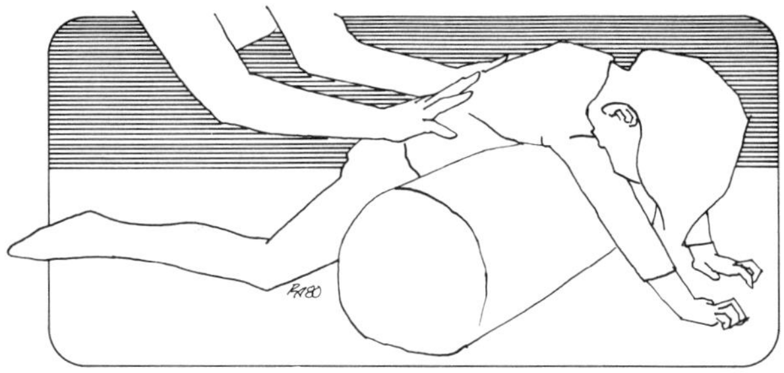

FIG. 21. Roll.

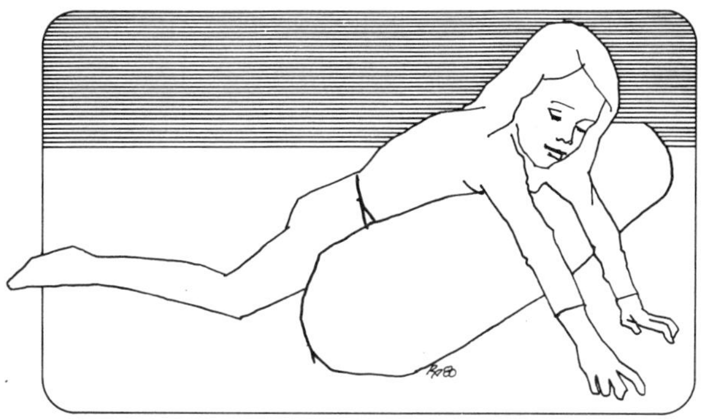

FIG. 22. Roll.

Figs. 20–24: Righting reactions: Facilitatory positions prone.

The labyrinthine head-righting reflex can be stimulated by blocking the child's vision with one's hand and holding the child in various positions in space: prone, supine, and to each side. The head should right itself to the midline. The otoliths of the labyrinths in the middle ear are being stimulated by this action, and the neck muscles will contract and lift the head to the midline. Blindfolding can frighten an infant, and clinicians rarely use blindfolding during testing. Normally, the optical righting reflex is developed

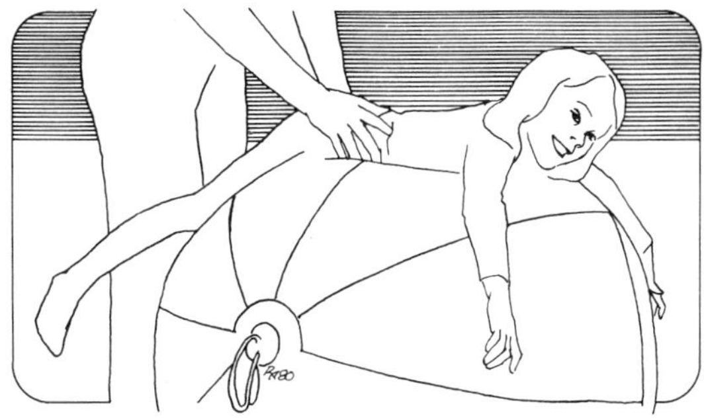

FIG. 23. Ball.

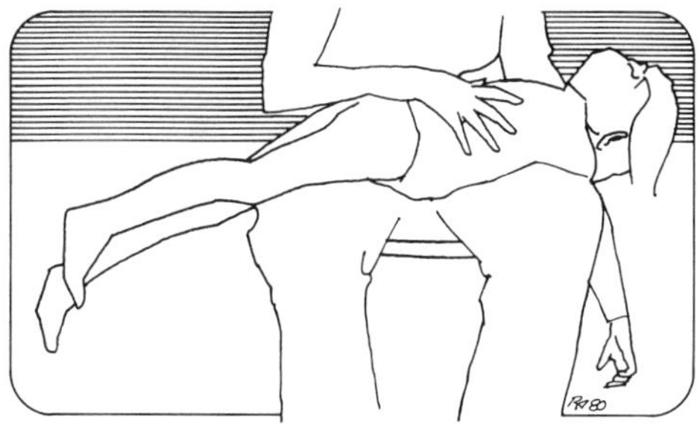

FIG. 24. Lap.

simultaneously with the labyrinthine righting reflex; therefore if one is present, both are present, however the optical righting reaction is often inhibited due to the patient's poor visual control. The optical righting reflex uses vision to right the head. The child is tested as for the labyrinthine head-righting reaction, but without any occlusion of vision.

The body-righting reaction acting on the head, in conjunction with the preceding reflexes, acts to right the head. This is elicited when the child is prone and the chest is in contact with the supporting surface. Tactile contact evokes the pressure sense organs to respond when the child's chest is on a hard surface, stimulating head lifting.

The body-righting reflexes acting on the head contribute with the labyrinthine and optical righting reflexes to righting the head when the child is prone. Contact of the child's chest with the hard surface of a mat will stimulate some exteroceptors-proprioceptors in the chest area, and the head will be lifted. Obviously the child has a few reflexes to ensure prone head righting; this probably is the reason that many severely damaged children have at least this ability, as many reflexes provide this response.

The neck-righting reaction acting on the body

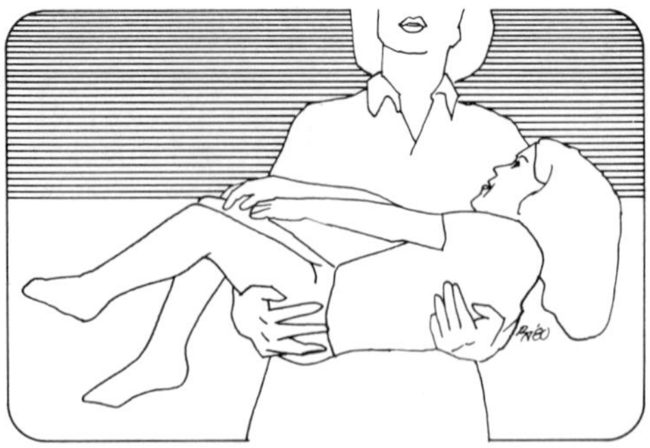

FIG. 25. Supine righting reaction.

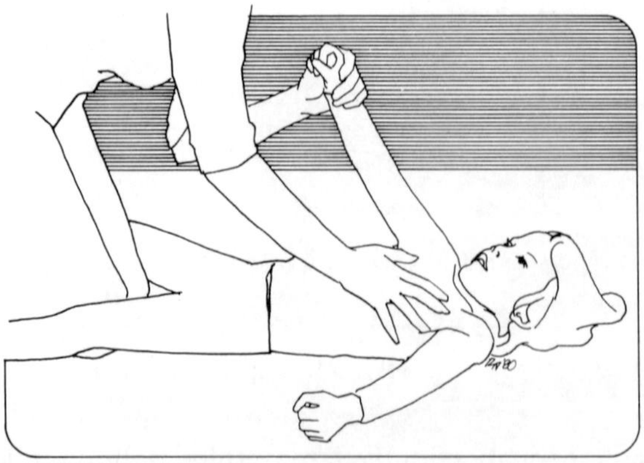

FIG. 27. Pull to sit (a).

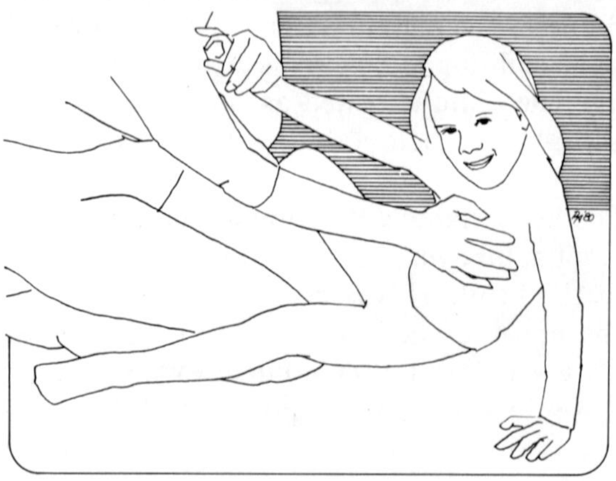

FIG. 29. Pull to sit (c).

assures that if the head is turned to the side, the body will follow. This reflex, which is present at birth, undergoes metamorphosis: from birth to 4 months of age, the body follows the head as one piece; after 4 months, rotation between pelvis and shoulder girdle takes place.

The body-righting reaction acting on the body

Figs. 25–29: Righting reactions: Facilitatory positions supine.

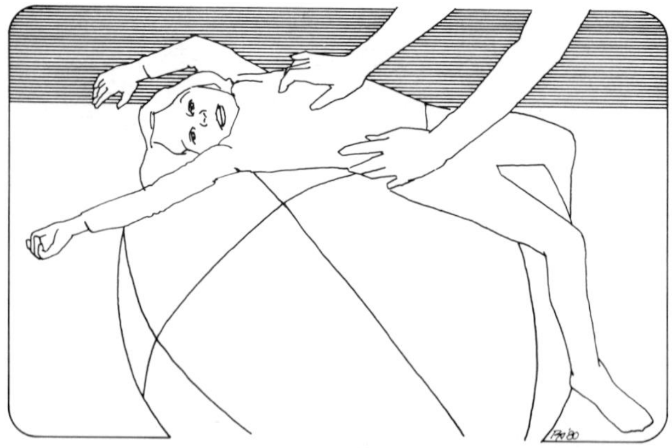

FIG. 26. Large ball.

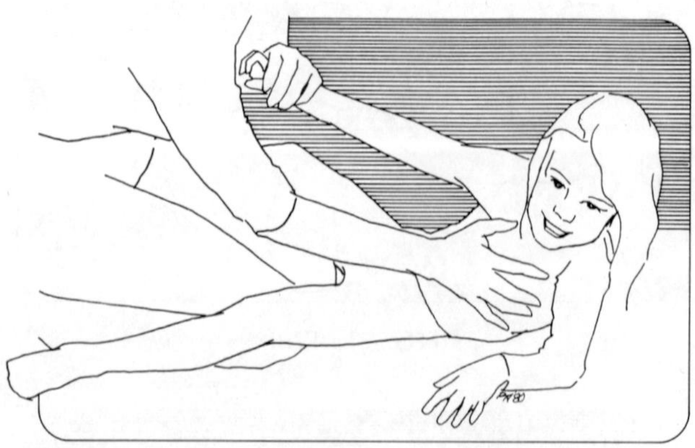

FIG. 28. Pull to sit (b).

keeps the body in the normal position in relation to the supporting surface, even if the head is not in line. It is elicited by exteroceptors, and the body's contact with the ground is the stimulus. There is no special test position for this reflex. One must observe the child and note the rotation between shoulder and pelvis. This reflex comes into play at a later age than the others, usually 10 months of age, and it helps the child obtain the upright position by progressing from prone to all fours, kneeling, half-kneeling, and standing.

Facilitation and Treatment for the Righting Reactions

Facilitating prone righting reactions: Place the child's arms over a pillow or rolled-up blanket so that the head is off the ground and the child is able to freely lift it and turn it. In this position any number of facilitation techniques can be used (e.g., co-contraction or tapping) to get the head up and turning. Visual stimulation by toys or objects together with noise can lure the child into looking up and around in an attempt to visualize

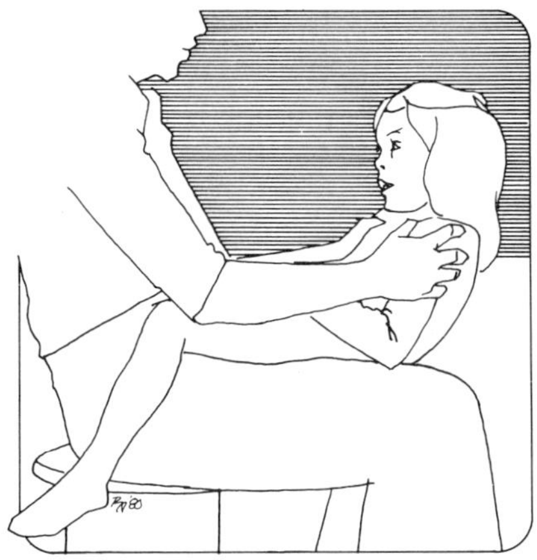

FIG. 30. Sitting on lap (a).

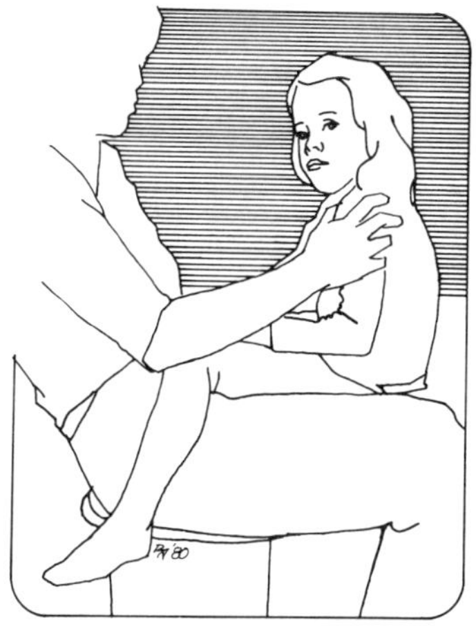

FIG. 31. Sitting on lap (b).

Figs. 30 and 31: Righting positions: Facilitatory positions sitting.

the object (Figs. 20–22). Place the child prone over a large or small ball, and roll the patient back and forth and from side to side with arms up and out to the side. One can do the same stimulation described earlier, only now there is the added movement of the ball, which further stimulates the labyrinths and exteroceptors (Fig. 23). One can place the child lengthwise over one's legs and move the legs up and down and from side to side; the results should be similar to those with the ball activities (Fig. 24).

Facilitating supine righting reactions: Place the child supine on a moving surface such as a large ball or roll, and make sure that the head is supported as the roll is moved back and forth and from side to side. With this activity the flexor musculature, including the neck flexors, will be activated (Fig. 26). To promote functional use of the reaction for sitting, pull the child to sitting on a diagonal with good support and pushing in on the front of the chest. First bring child up onto elbows and then up on extended elbows, or if the child gives no help go back to supine and repeat (Figs. 27–29). One can hold the child upright on one's lap in a sitting position and gently let the head fall back a few degrees. Then aid the child in bringing the head back to the vertical position (Figs. 30 and 31). Sometimes this reflex is difficult to elicit. The prone and vertical responses may develop first, after which the supine righting reflex will finally emerge.

Facilitating vertical lighting reactions (Fig. 32): The child can be straddled on one's lap and tilted slowly from side to side. One can tell if support should be given at chest, midthorax, or hips (Figs 32–34). One should wait a few seconds for the child to respond before assistance is given. Vertical righting to either side can also be done on a roll or small ball (Fig. 36). In some instances the supporting surface can be moved instead of the child (Fig. 35). Stationary supported sitting in an appropriate seating device is important, at least for a few hours a day, so that the child can become oriented to the upright position (Fig. 37). This further strengthens the optical and labyrinthine righting responses, which can help to automatically right the head when suspended.

Facilitating neck-righting reactions acting on the body: On a mat or bed, place child supine, and turn the head or shoulder to either side, assisting in rolling to the side or stomach (Figs. 20, 38, and 39). Note that care must be taken to see that the arms are not unduly stressed by unnatural positions. Some do not like to stimulate rolling in this fashion, as neck righting is usually difficult to elicit, and putting excessive pressure on the head and neck must be avoided. Getting the child to turn can also be done by rotating the shoulders (Fig. 39).

Facilitating body reactions acting on the body: Rotate the pelvis over the shoulder girdle or vice versa, supine and prone (Fig. 40–42). Assist the child after the first few seconds, giving as much opportunity as possible to actively achieve this movement. This activity done on a moving surface, such as a large ball, further stimulates the head and body to right themselves (Figs. 43–45).

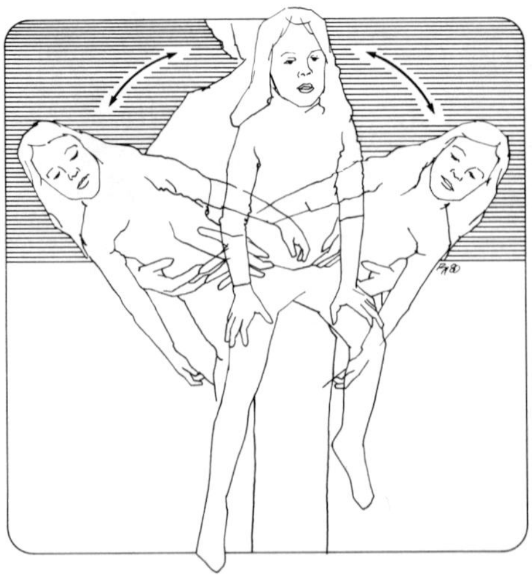

FIG. 32. Vertical righting reactions.

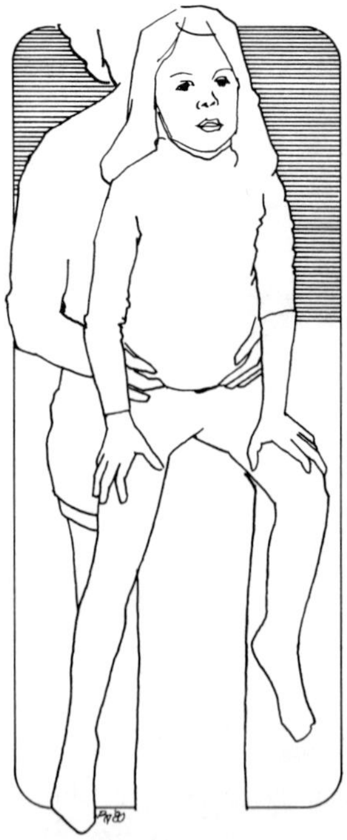

FIG. 33. Lap.

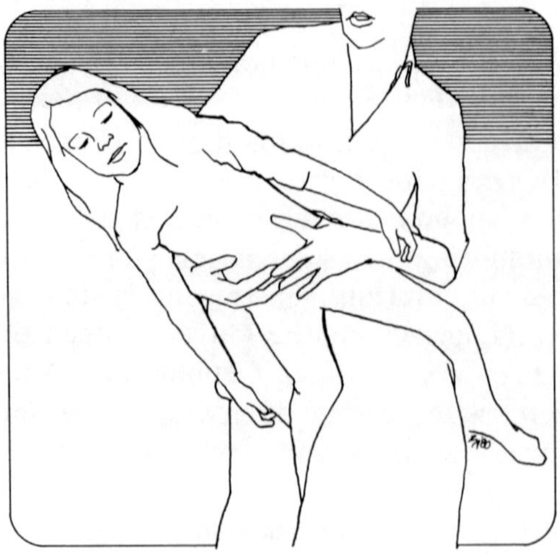

FIG. 34. Lap.

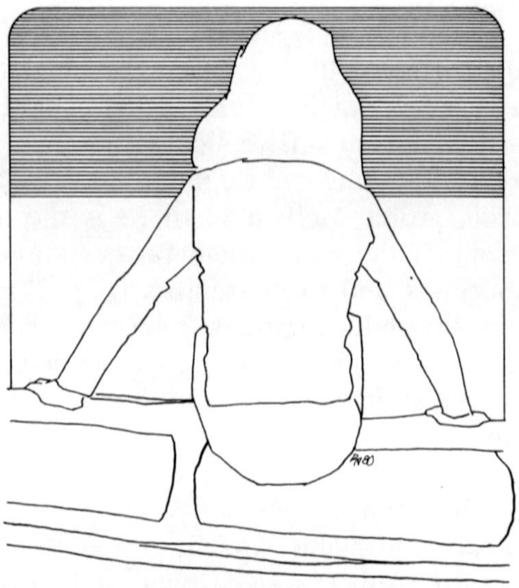

FIG. 35. Roll.

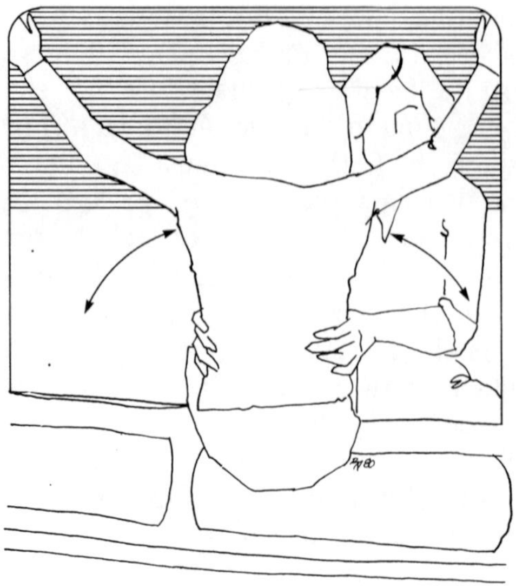

FIG. 36. Roll.

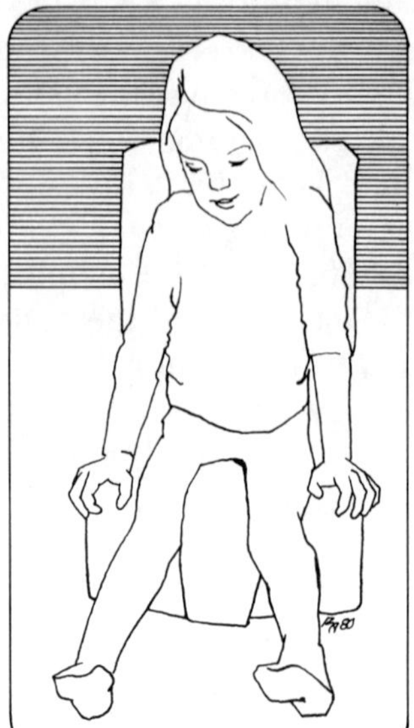

FIG. 37. Sitting.

Figs. 32–37: Righting reactions: Facilitatory positions for vertical righting.

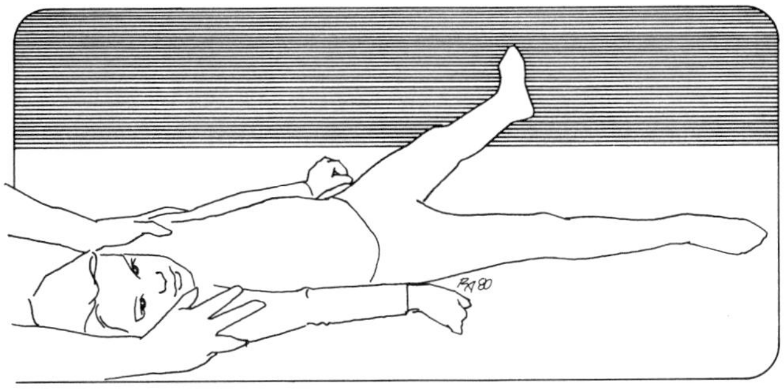

FIG. 38. Rolling initiated at shoulder-neck (a).

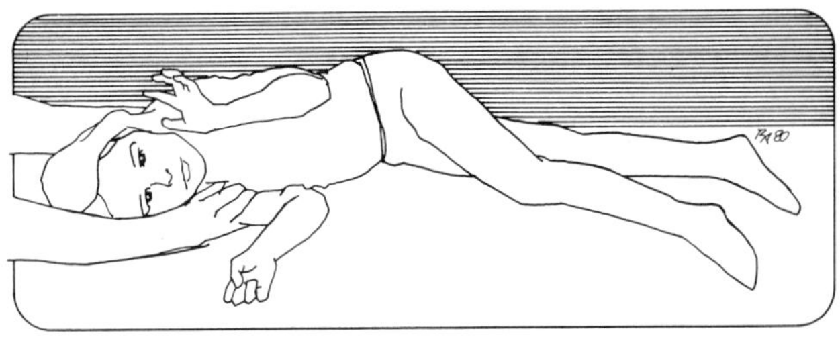

FIG. 39. Rolling (b).

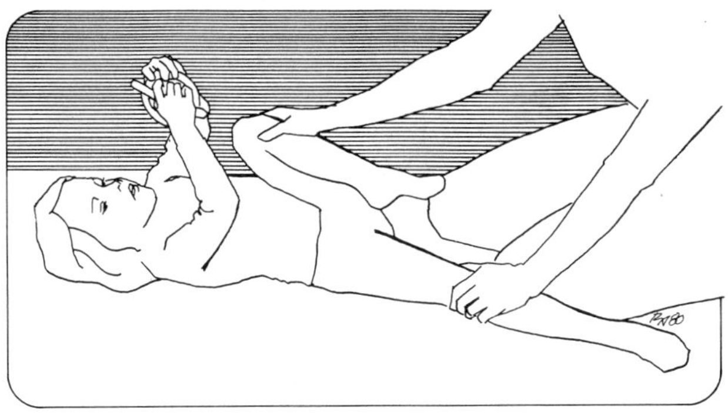

FIG. 40. Rolling initiated at hip (a).

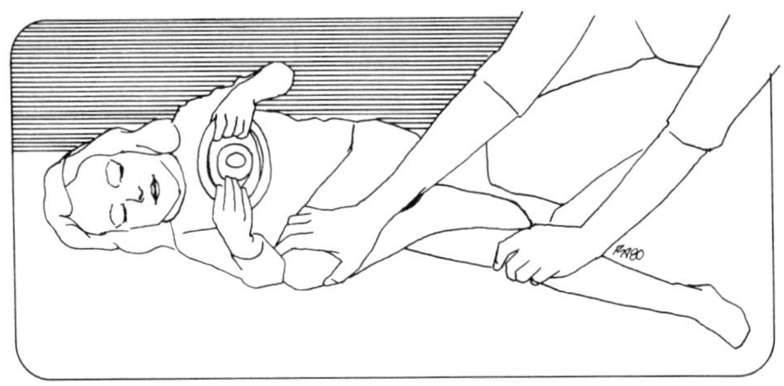

FIG. 41. Rolling (b).

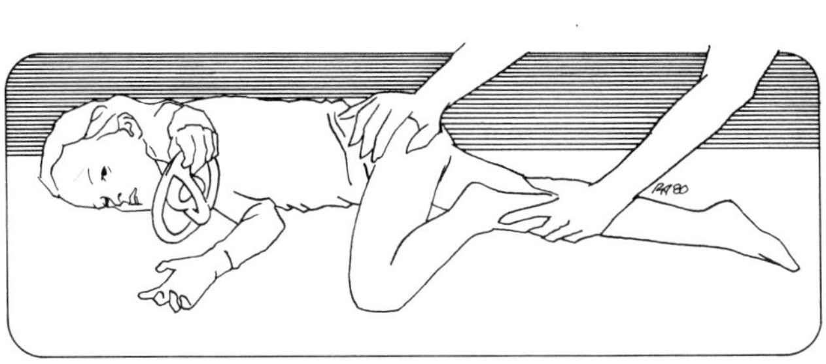

FIG. 42. Rolling (c).

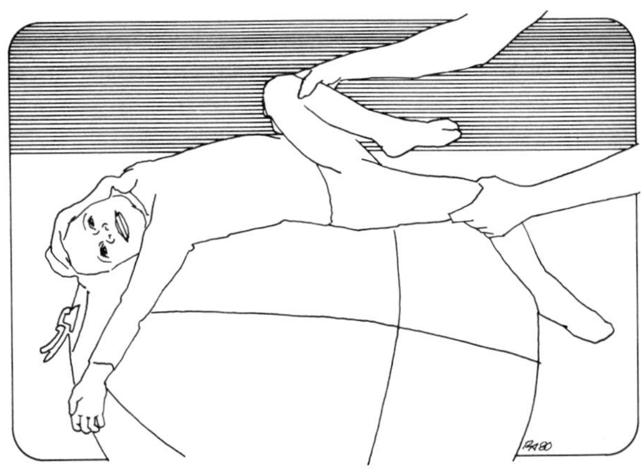

FIG. 43. Rolling on moving surface (a).

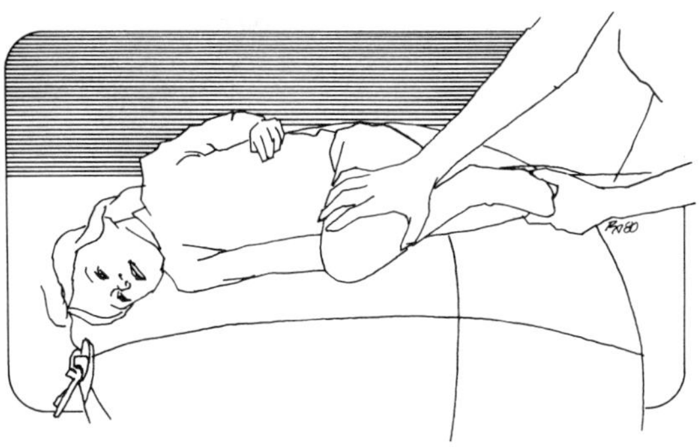

FIG. 44. Rolling (b).

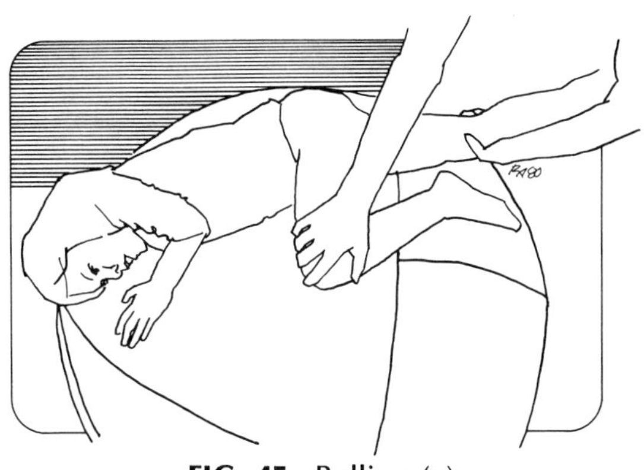

FIG. 45. Rolling (c).

Figs. 38–45: Righting reactions: Facilitatory positions for body righting.

EQUILIBRIUM REACTIONS

Equilibrium reactions are reflexes that provide an automatic balancing mechanism to cope with the upright position. These reactions help to maintain or regain control over the body's center of gravity so that the child will not fall. According to Barnes et al. (1), there are several categories of equilibrium reactions: the protective reactions of the arms and legs, the tilting reactions, and the postural fixating reactions.

The sense organs responsible for the equilibrium reactions are the eyes, body proprioceptors, and the labyrinths, which signal movements of the body's center of gravity. Their information is relayed to the central nervous system, where a coordinated motor response is generated that allows the child to regain or maintain control over the center of gravity.

Protective reactions of the arms include protective extension forward, sideward, and backward. The forward reaction is present at 6 to 7 months of age, the sideward reaction at 7 to 8 months, and the backward reaction at 9 to 10 months. These reactions are present throughout life. When the body's center of gravity is displaced forward, the arms are stimulated into flexion of the shoulders and elbow extension to prevent the child from falling forward. This same catching reaction occurs if one pushes the child to the side or to the back, with shoulder abduction or extensors activated, depending on the direction.

There are protective reactions of the legs that are present from 3 months of age onward. The protective reaction downward is elicited by holding the child suspended vertically, then bringing the child quickly downward toward the floor. The legs will prepare themselves for support standing, with hip extension and abduction, knee extension, and ankle dorsiflexion.

Stepping reactions forward, sideward, and backward are present from approximately 15 months of age and stay throughout life. The legs are required to keep up with the body, no matter what direction the body is projected. The first to develop and the easiest to elicit during a treatment session is the forward stepping reaction. These reactions should be encouraged in preambulatory children by use of assistive devices in preparation for independent standing and ambulation.

The shifting or seesaw reaction comes into play at about the same time as the stepping reactions. If the child is standing on one leg and is pushed toward the non-weight-bearing side, the non-weight-bearing leg will automatically be extended at the hip and knee in order to provide a new base of support.

The sitting reactions, as described by Barnes et al. (1), or the simple equilibrium reactions, as described by Fiorentino and Bobath (2–6), are automatic compensatory movements that occur when the supporting surface is moved or shifted. They can occur in any position, (supine, prone, sitting, all fours, kneeling, half-kneeling, standing). The side of the body that is tilted downward will exhibit abduction and extension downward at the shoulder and hip joints, with extension of the elbow or knee and concavity of the spine upward, whereas the upward side will have a convexity of the spine downward, with the head tilted toward that side and the extremities abducted and usually externally rotated at the large joints and extended at elbow and knee. Tilting reactions occur in the prone and supine positions at approximately 5 to 7 months, in sitting at 7 to 8 months, in quadruped at 9 to 10 months, and in standing at 12 to 24 months.

The postural fixation reactions allow the child to sustain balance while doing any activity in any position. For example, if the child is standing at a blackboard drawing, even though only the arm is moving, the postural fixation reactions are keeping the child balanced in the upright position. If an outside force were to move the child, these reactions would help regain the former state of equilibrium by exactly the same extremity and trunk maneuvers that were seen with the tilting reactions. These reactions are developed by 18 to 24 months of age and remain throughout life.

Facilitation of Protective Arm Reactions

Forward, sideward, and backward propping: In supported long sitting, the arms can be placed in the correct position (forward, sideward, or backward). The child's body weight exerts a downward pressure, which helps elicit a support response of the arms (Figs. 46–51). Manual co-contraction on the extremity musculature can be done before placing the arm. Backward propping is developed last and usually is attempted after

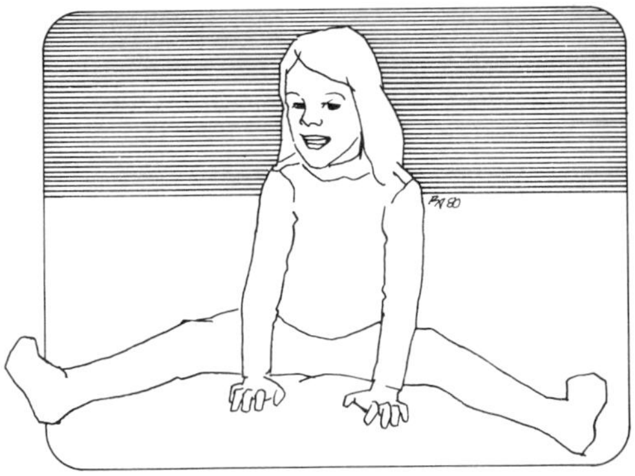

FIG. 46. Forward propping: Long sitting.

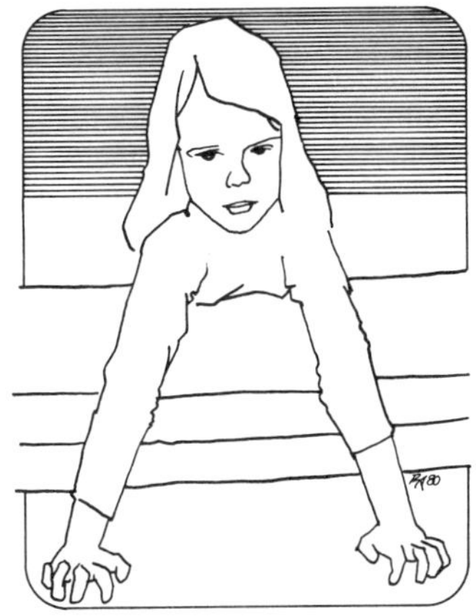

FIG. 47. Forward propping: Over roll.

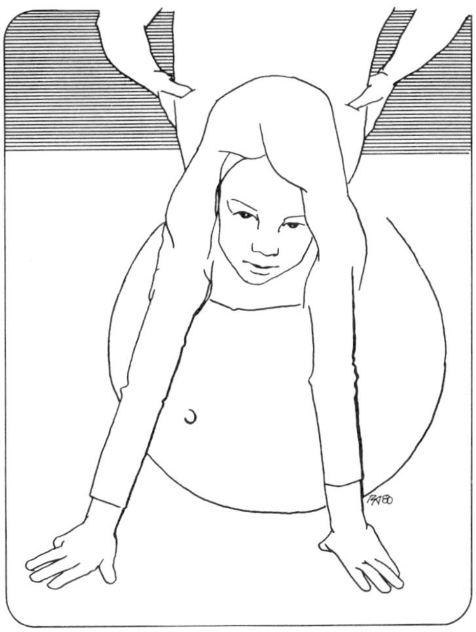

FIG. 48. Forward propping: Over ball.

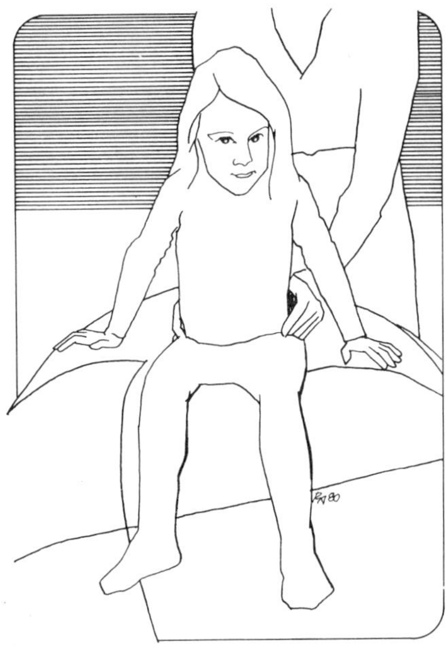

FIG. 49. Sideward propping.

Figs. 46–51: Equilibrium reactions: Facilitatory positions for propping.

forward and sideward propping activities have been practiced. On a moving surface such as a large ball (Figs. 49, 51), with support around the child's chest or waist, gently move the ball in the direction desired. The added stimulation to the labyrinths of the inner ear will help right the head and trunk and make propping less difficult. Rolls (Figs. 47 and 50) are easier to control than the large ball. Place the child supine over a roll, and hold the arms in extension, external rotation and abduction to promote backward propping. Moving the roll back and forth will also aid in supine head righting and stimulate the trunk flexors to contract.

Facilitation of Protective Leg Reactions

Stepping reactions forward, backward, and sideward: Move the child slowly in any direction (Figs. 52–55), holding the child under the arms from the back. A child who needs less assistance can be held by the arms with the therapist in front. As the child becomes more adept in keeping the feet under the body, movement can be more rapid.

Shifting reaction: With the child standing on one leg, hold and flex the non-weight-bearing leg and the arm on the same side. Gently pull the arm on the non-weight-bearing side; the non-weight-bearing extremities will extend in an effort to prevent the body from falling (Fig. 56).

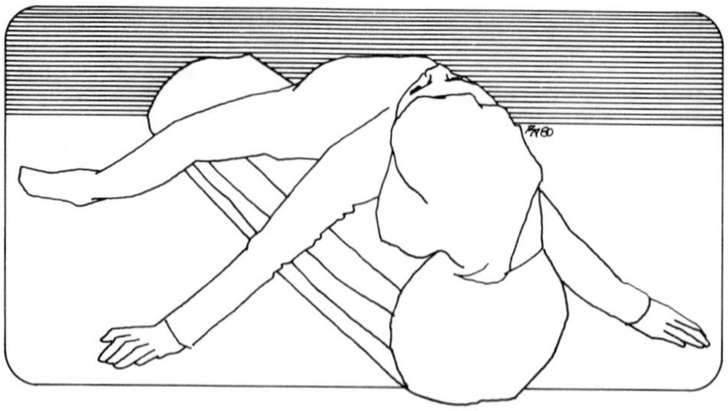

FIG. 50. Backward propping over roll.

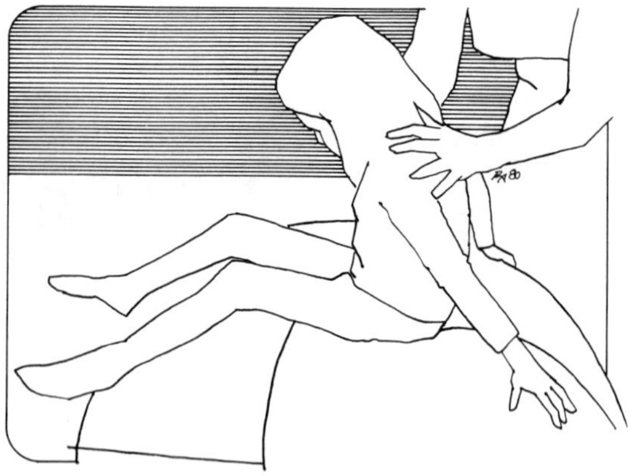

FIG. 51. Backward propping over ball.

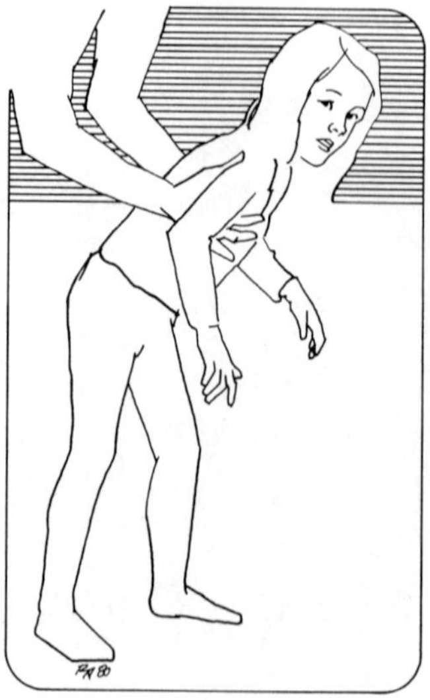

FIG. 52. Stepping reaction forward.

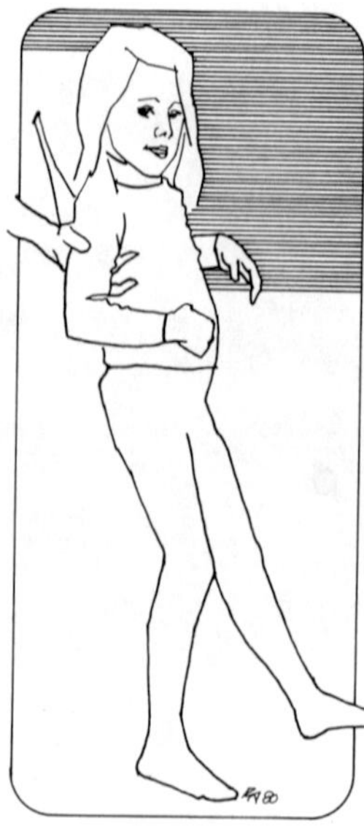

FIG. 53. Stepping reaction backward.

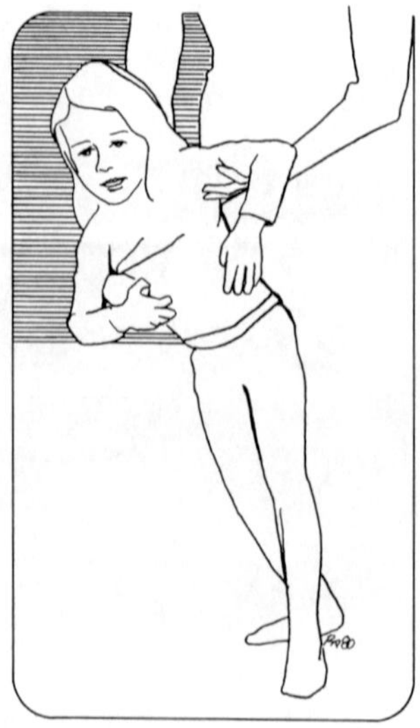

FIG. 54. Stepping reaction sideward.

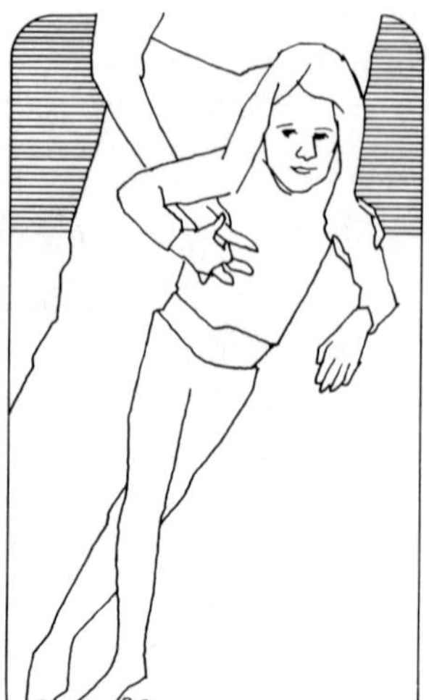

FIG. 55. Stepping reaction sideward.

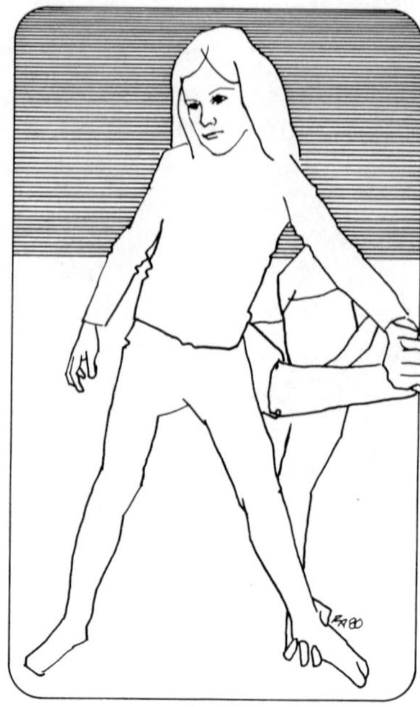

FIG. 56. Shifting reaction.

Figs. 52–56: Stepping reactions: Facilitatory positions for stepping.

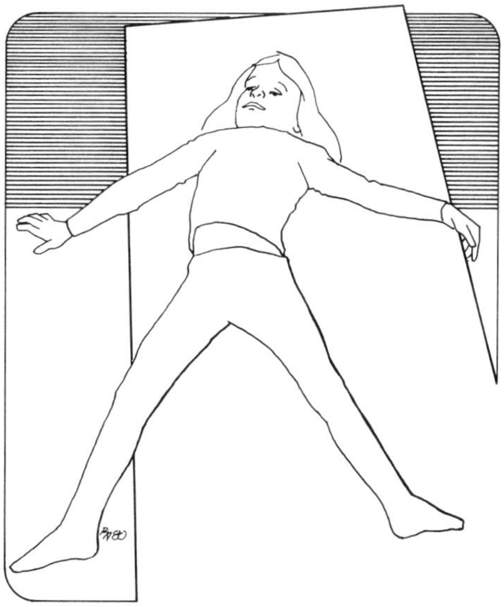

FIG. 57. Supine on vestibular board.

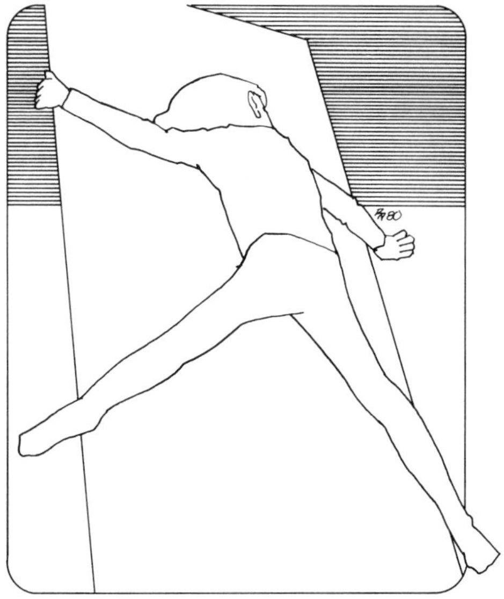

FIG. 58. Prone on vestibular board.

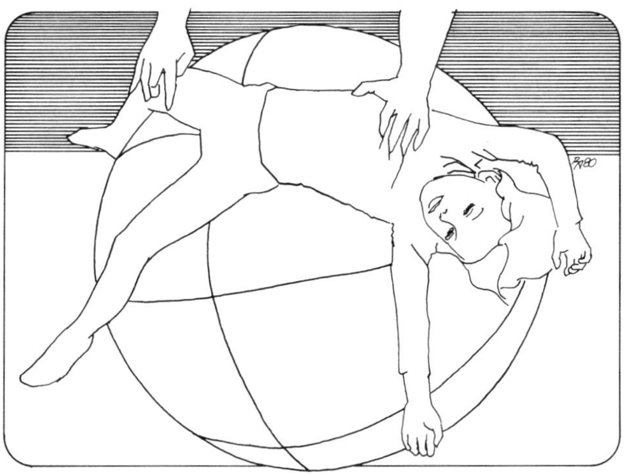

FIG. 59. Supine on large ball.

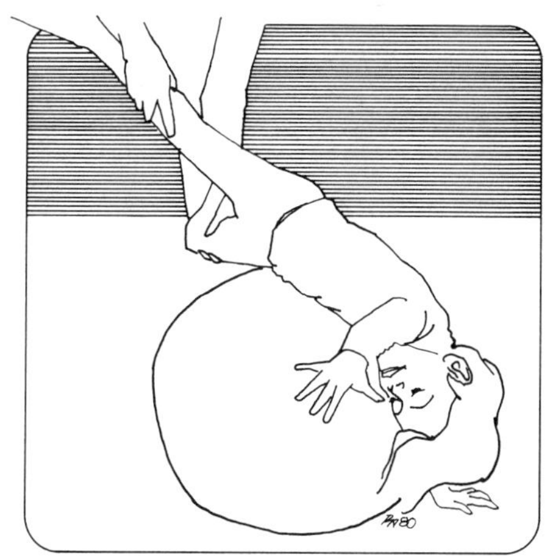

FIG. 60. Prone on ball.

Figs. 57–70: Tilting reactions: Facilitatory positions for tilting.

Facilitation of the Tilting Reactions

Prone and supine: The procedure and equipment are the same as used in eliciting supine and prone righting reactions over the ball or roll (Figs. 57–60). Most children have more control prone; thus a variety of moving surfaces can be used, (barrels, air mattresses, vestibular board (Figs. 59 and 60). Tilting is done by moving either the child or the equipment from side to side or forward and backward.

Sitting: This position (Figs. 61–64) allows for the most varied treatment procedures. Key points for handling the child are at the knees, hips, feet, shoulders, and waist. Find a ball to fit the child's size, so that the hips, knees, and ankles are at 90° and the feet are placed flat on the floor. The child can move or be moved.

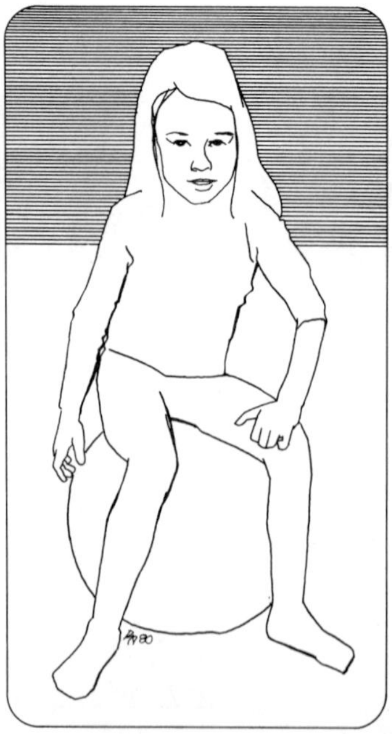

FIG. 61. Sitting.

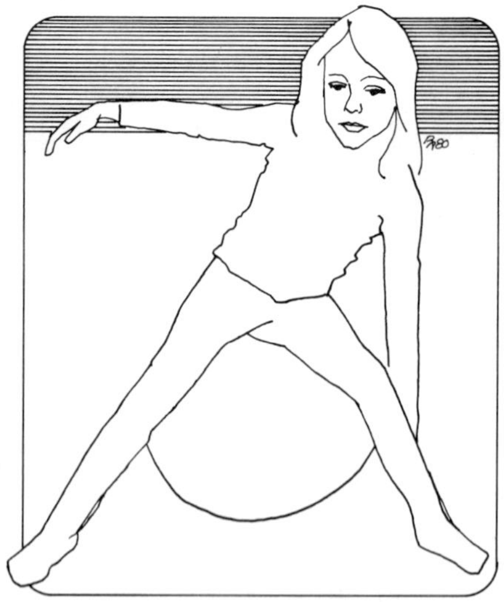

FIG. 62. Sitting.

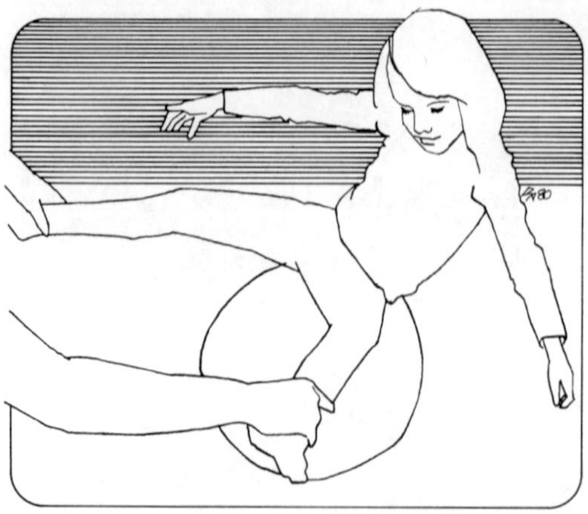

FIG. 63. Sitting.

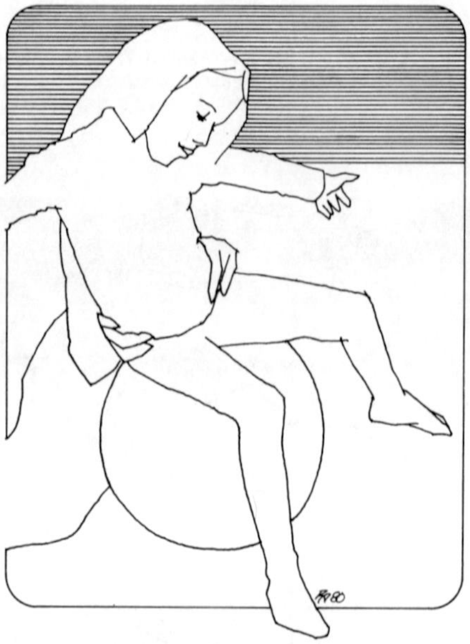

FIG. 64. Sitting.

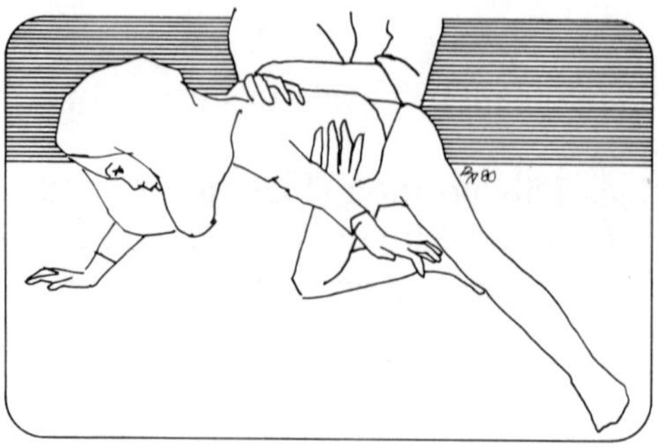

FIG. 65. Quadruped.

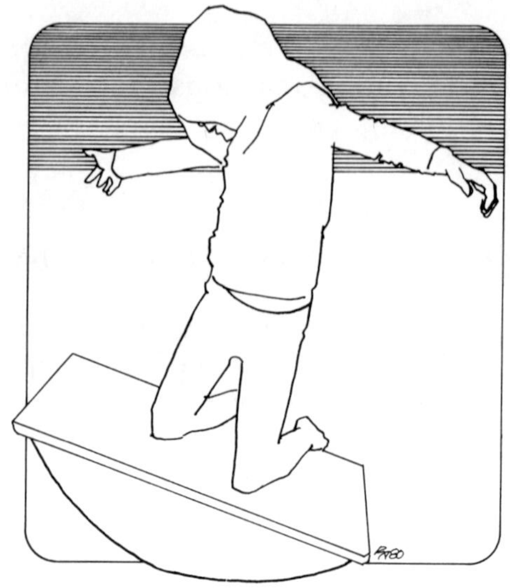

FIG. 66. Kneeling on tilt board.

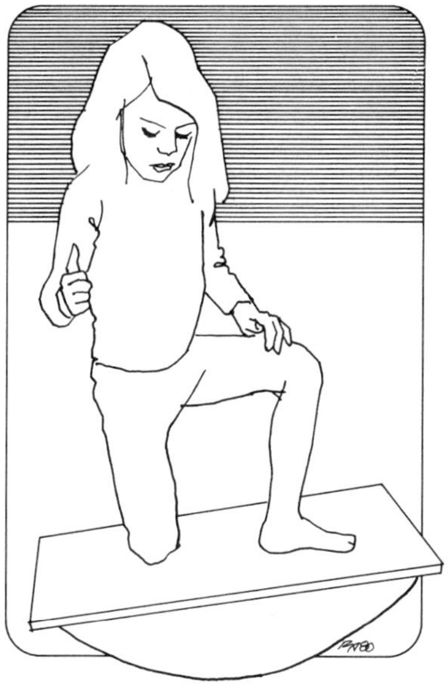

FIG. 67. Half kneeling on tilt board.

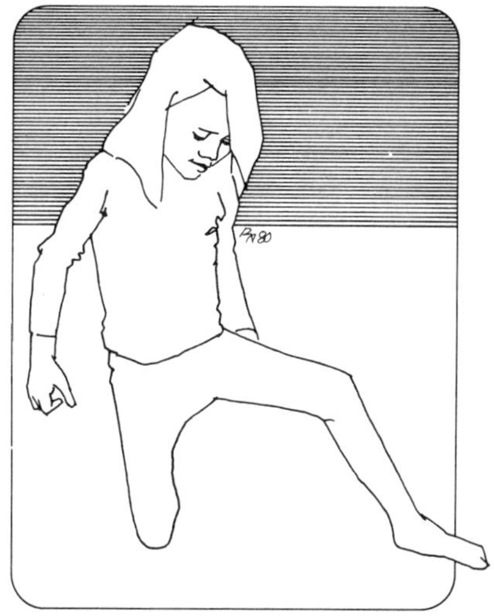

FIG. 68. Half kneel.

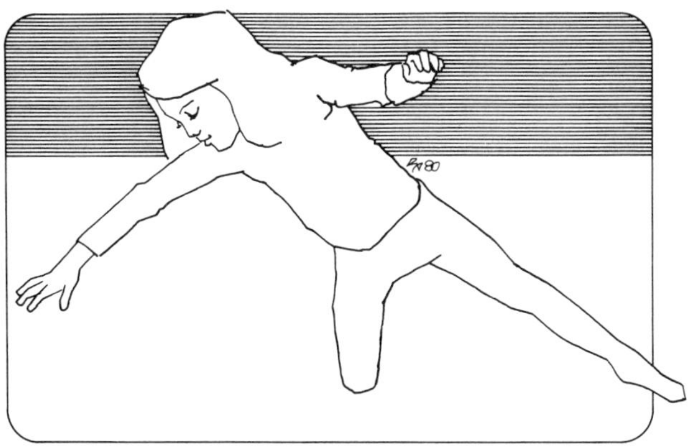

FIG. 69. Half kneel.

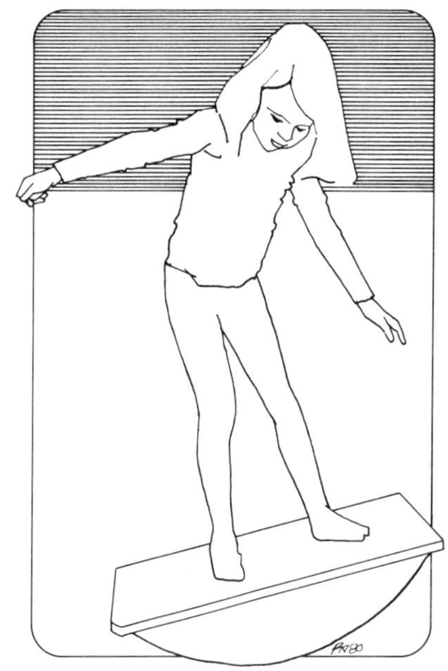

FIG. 70. Standing on tilt board.

Quadruped: To facilitate hand-knee reactions, the child can be placed over a small roll or on a tiltboard, and the apparatus can be pushed by the therapist or child from side to side. The patient can also be held in this position and moved by the therapist (Fig. 65).

Kneeling and half-kneeling: These positions can be done on a large tiltboard, with the child going from side to side or back and forth (Figs. 66 and 67). For some children, just maintaining the position on a level surface is a very difficult task (Figs. 68–69). Rolls and wedges can be used to assist the child in attaining the desired position. Often children use abnormal motor patterns to attain these difficult positions; therefore it is better to assist or place the child in the correct position, and then work on maintaining balance in the correct posture.

Standing: Equilibrium reactions can easily be facilitated on a tiltboard (Fig. 70). However the child should be proficient on the tiltboard in kneeling and one-half kneeling before standing should be attempted.

Facilitation of Postural Fixation Reactions

Postural fixation reactions (Figs. 71–74) can be done in any position, with the child gently pushed from side to side, backward and forward and

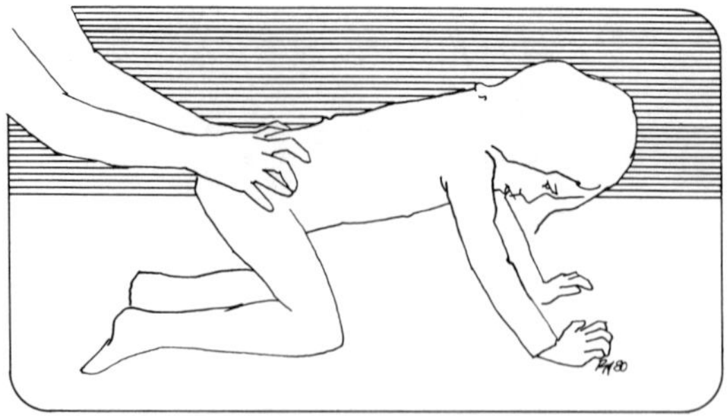

FIG. 71. Quadruped.

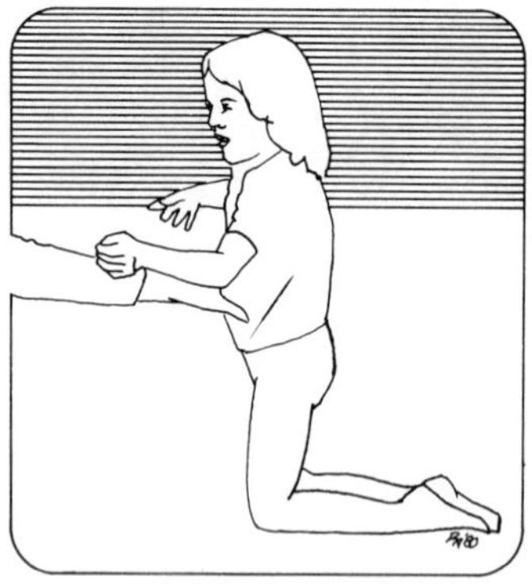

FIG. 72. Kneeling.

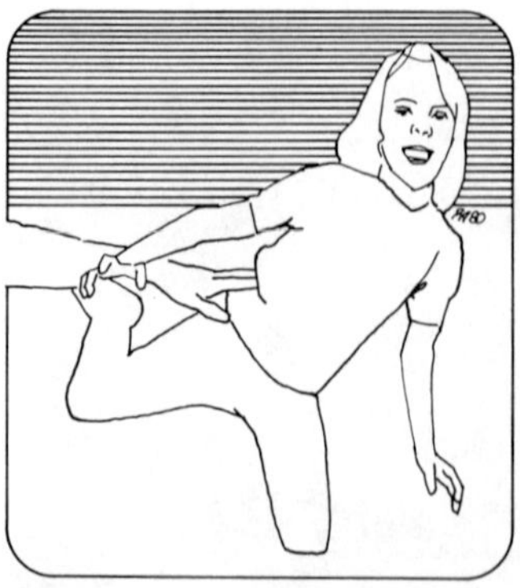

FIG. 73. One-half kneeling.

Figs. 71–74: Postural fixation reactions.

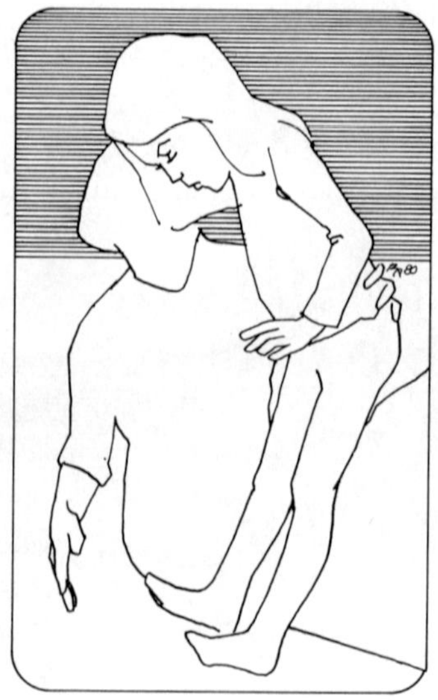

FIG. 74. Standing.

having the patient attempt to maintain his position against the opposing force.

REFERENCES

1. Barnes, M. R., Crutchfield, C. A., and Heriza, C. B. (1978): *The Neurophysiological Basis of Patient Treatment.* Stokesville Publishing, Morgantown, West Virginia.
2. Bleck, E. E. (1975): Locomotion prognosis in cerebral palsy. *Dev. Med. Child Neurol.*, 17:18–25.
3. Bobath, B. (1954): A study of abnormal postural reflex activities in patients with lesions of the central nervous system. *Physiotherapy,* 40:259–280.
4. Bobath, B. (1971): *Abnormal Postural Reflex Activity Caused by Brain Lesions.* William Heinemann, London.
5. Bobath, B. (1967): The very early treatment of cerebral palsy. *Dev. Med. Child Neurol.*, 9:373–390.
6. Fiorentino, M. R. (1972): *Normal and Abnormal Development. The Influences of Primitive Reflexes on Motor Development.* Charles C Thomas, Springfield, Ill.
7. Fiorentino, M. R. (1973): *Reflex Testing Methods for Evaluating CNS Development.* Charles C Thomas, Springfield, Ill.
8. Prechtl, H., and Beintema, D. (1964): *The Neurological Examination of the Full Term Newborn Infant. Clinics in Development Medicine, No. 12.* Spastics International Medical Publications and William Heinemann, London.

Neurobehavioral Evaluation and Management

8

Peggy Strecker Neufeld

Occupational therapy has recently seen considerable growth in the area of treatment approaches for patients with central nervous system (CNS) dysfunction. Brain-damaged patients constitute a complex challenge for the therapist. Various treatment approaches have been developed with specific treatment techniques, but these approaches have a common basis in developmental, neurophysiological, and motor learning theories. The following presentation will be an eclectic view from what we shall term a neurobehavioral frame of reference.

The name neurobehavior is used because the ultimate focus in treatment is on human behavior and not simply on the developmental or physiological processes. Behavior can be defined as the observable actions taken by individuals to manipulate and adapt to their environments. The therapist's goal is to influence patients' behaviors for greater acceptability within their environments. Often this implies qualitative change. Such changes and the ability to learn new behaviors occur through the sensory integrative processes* of the CNS. A motor act is the observable expression of the level of functioning of the sensory integrative process. Therefore, therapy for CNS disorders focuses on effecting changes in the nervous system in order to effect changes in behavior.

Although the sensory-motor, cognitive, psychological, and sociocultural systems are intricately interrelated in providing a background for behavior, this chapter will be concerned only with the functions and dysfunctions of posture and movement. But it must be remembered that meaningful responses produced through sensory integration may take other forms than immediate observable movements. Cognitive planning and social interaction are adaptive behaviors controlled by the CNS. In this light, the concepts presented in this chapter may be applied in the rehabilitation process with the mentally handicapped and the physically handicapped.

This chapter is intended only to highlight the major concepts in the neurobehavioral frame of reference; many excellent resources are available offering detailed illustration of these theoretical and practical concepts, and these resources, plus the numerous continuing education programs offered in this specialty area, should be consulted

* See glossary.

by both beginning and experienced therapists. As new research provides greater understanding of behavioral mechanisms, current treatment programs can be validated or modified for improved effectiveness.

Of particular concern to the occupational therapist is that many of the treatment approaches designed for patients with CNS dysfunction were developed from other disciplines, such as physical therapy. The occupational therapist must accept the challenge of applying these treatment principles within the professional framework by incorporating the use of goal-directed activities. It is important for occupational therapists to realize the significance of correct analysis and choice of treatment.

The following sections will be used to present an overview of the functions and dysfunctions of posture and movement, the significant concepts of normal CNS function and the effects of brain damage, the potential for recovery of function in brain-damaged patients, the evaluation process, and treatment guidelines for brain-damaged patients.

PATIENT POPULATION

CNS dysfunction may be evident in patients with various diagnoses. The criterion for using this approach is that the peripheral pathways and the spinal cord be anatomically intact for transmission of sensory information to the higher cortical centers. It is disorganization within the CNS that accounts for sensory integrative dysfunction and abnormal behavior patterns. Patients with the following conditions are susceptible to loss or impairment of CNS integration: brain damage caused by trauma or cerebral vascular accident, cerebral palsy, congenital psychomotor retardation, multiple sclerosis, Parkinson's disease, minimal brain damage or dysfunction (learning disability), chronic schizophrenia, autism, and emotional disturbances.

This approach has applications in disorders other than those listed. It can also be used to enhance normal movement in patients who have normal CNS function. Often a simple change in sensory input can heighten a desired movement response in the patient with an orthopedic condition or peripheral nervous system disorder.

Finally, it should be emphasized that this approach attempts to promote change through remediation rather than compensation for disorders. This remedial approach may be contraindicated in the presence of certain medical factors. Also, the patient must be willing to work on improvement of qualitative movement while delaying the acquisition of compensatory functions.

NORMAL MOVEMENT AND POSTURE

A thorough understanding of the quality of normal movement and posture will guide the therapist in therapeutic remediation of abnormal movement. Normal posture is important as the foundation from which normal movement occurs. Symmetrical posture in sitting or standing is a comfortable position in which body weight is equally distributed, the head is aligned with the trunk, and the arms are relaxed at the sides of the body. Asymmetrical posture is normal and functional only when normal movement is still easily possible. Normal movement consists of observable changes in total body patterns in which the body parts act dynamically and purposefully in space and time in relation to the environment.

Motor behavior occurs both reflexively and volitionally and can be viewed on a continuum: reflex-volitional-skill (1,2). Both reflex motion and volitional motion should be viewed as patterns of motion. The concept of patterns is demonstrated in the interdependence of movements. Every body part performs relative to its original alignment with the rest of the body and relative to the amount of tension in the rest of the body (3). Reflex motions are observable changes in total body patterns with identifiable causes and effects. As the nervous system develops, the quality of movement improves, and the primitive reflexes provide the foundation for volitional movement. Volitional motions may be defined as observable changes in total body patterns with unidentifiable causes and unpredictable effects. These patterns are refined and are under willed control. Finally, skilled coordinated movement develops as the ultimate performance of volitional motion. Combinations of movement patterns can be observed and categorized in various ways: gross* or fine*, diagonal*, reciprocal, isolated*, symmetrical or asymmetrical.

Qualitatively, normal volitional movement can

be described as efficient, transient, spontaneous, or variable, to meet one's needs. Once a movement pattern is learned, the motor system becomes automatic in following this sensory pattern, called a sensory engram. The quality of movement is also subtly affected by 'personal equations' of movement, i.e., how an individual prefers to move. These influences include personal rhythm, preferred speed, amount of space preferred, and persistence to continue a motor task under varying degrees of comfort (4). The therapist must be aware of the individuality reflected in normal movement.

INTEGRATIVE MECHANISMS

Essential to sound treatment is the therapist's knowledge of how the normal nervous system develops, matures, and functions. This review will highlight a few concepts significant to the rehabilitative process.

Movement depends on information circuits that function both internally and externally (5,6). Sensory input is received through the primary sensory systems (tactile and proprioceptive, visual, auditory, vestibular, gustatory, olfactory) and organized with the CNS. These sensory-motor circuits allow for smooth control of movement and for motor learning (Fig. 1A,B). Effective nervous system function depends on effective integration of environmental experience and somatosensory experience. Therefore, during therapy the sensory input is applied before or during an activity to enhance purposeful movements (7–11).

The CNS needs a balance of facilitory and inhibitory controls. Inhibition (suppression) is as important in functioning as is facilitation (enhancement) of input. Inhibition allows the CNS to focus on only the necessary stimuli. It is accepted that a motor neuron will fire after sensory stimuli accumulate in intensity to the threshold level needed for an action potential. It is the sum of the facilitory and inhibitory impulses that decides if the neuron will fire (12–14). Therefore therapeutic facilitation and inhibition techniques are used selectively to stimulate or increase the probability of muscular contraction (8,15,16).

The nervous system functions as a whole; its parts are interdependent. All levels of the CNS continue to function after maturation, although under the control and influence of the higher cor-

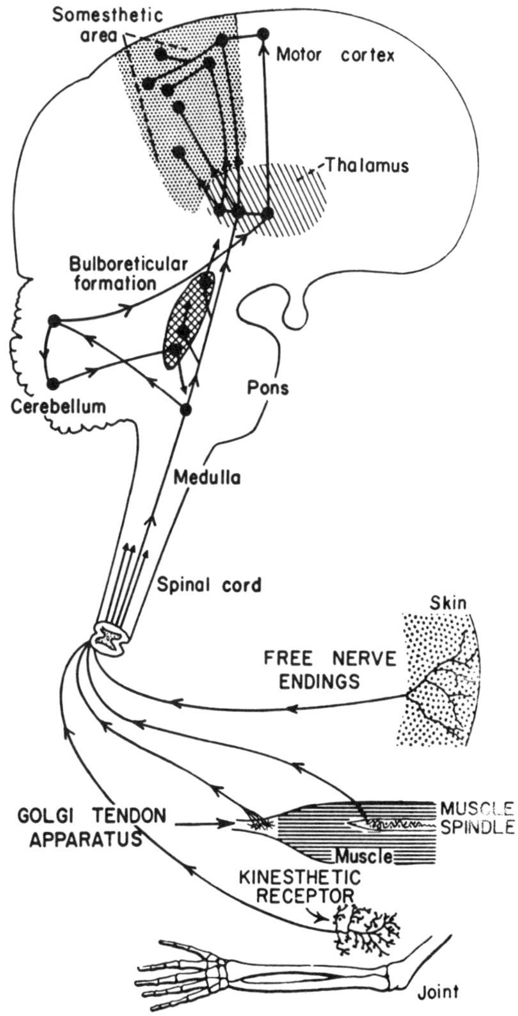

FIG. 1. A. The somatic sensory axis of the nervous system (Courtesy of A. Guyton).

tical centers (1,2,17,18). Even functions such as perception and learning, often thought of as cortical tasks, require effective sensory-motor functioning of the lower brain mechanisms at the brainstem. Therefore therapy aimed at improving the functioning of the lower levels (gross motor coordination) will enhance functioning at higher cortical levels (15).

Movement can be controlled subcortically (through lower brain centers) or cortically (4,14). Subcortically controlled movement is automatic and stereotypic. Most motor learning occurs at this level. Cortically controlled movement is slower and requires more energy, but it is necessary for new learning of highly skilled tasks. Therefore therapy to improve functional movement such as head control or gross motor control is more ef-

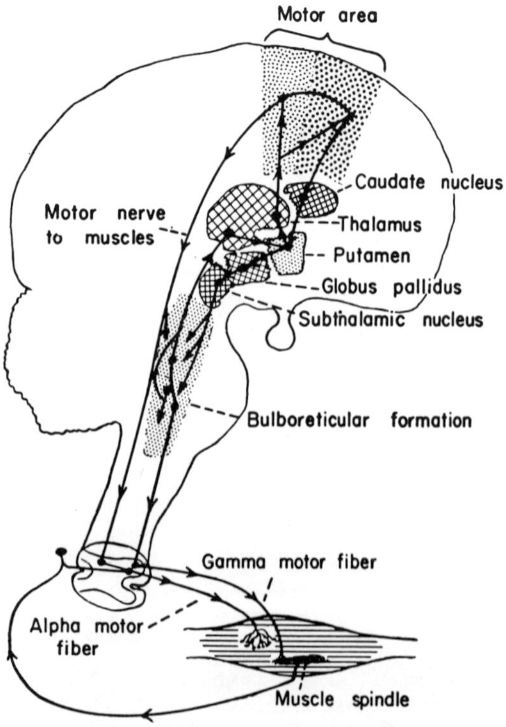

FIG. 1. B. The motor axis of the nervous system (Courtesy of A. Guyton).

fective if the patient is required to learn the task subcortically (1,8,15,16).

Integrative mechanisms are built into the CNS through sensory feedback systems and reverberating circuits allowing comparison and coordination of sensory information. The following neural systems have widespread influences on the brain, since they receive sensory input from many areas of the CNS (6,12–14,19,20). Therapy can help organize the CNS if input is applied that will be integrated in these systems (1,8,15,16). (a) The limbic system functions primarily in driving the organism for survival and integrating emotion with visceral responses. (b) The reticular activating system regulates alertness to allow for more discrete learning. This occurs by focusing on a specific stimulus and inhibiting extraneous stimuli. (c) The autonomic nervous system functions to maintain homeostasis of visceral functions. The sympathetic nervous system functions briefly for alarm reactions (fight or flight). The parasympathetic nervous system operates for normal body function. As the autonomic nervous system and somatic nervous system are interrelated, therapy that affects one will affect the other.

I.	II.
Sympathetic nervous system activated	Parasympathetic nervous system activated
Somatic nervous system active and muscle action	Somatic nervous system inhibited and muscle relaxation
Cortex alerted	Cortex activity decreased

Normal movement requires a base of normal neurophysiology. The alpha-gamma coactivation system maintains a degree of tension (tonus) in the resting muscle (Fig. 2A,B). This system, operating through the muscle spindle, serves to increase or decrease muscle tone in preparing a background for volitional movement (5,13,14,21,22). Therapy can affect movement by biasing* the muscle spindle (1,23,24). Therefore the therapist should know the tonic* and phasic* components of the muscle spindle, the types of sensory stimuli to which the specific sensory receptors will respond, and the nature of their responses (Table 1).

Another neurophysiological phenomenon, reciprocal inhibition, further promotes efficient motion. When a muscle is facilitated, its synergists are also facilitated. Yet inhibitory information is being transmitted to the antagonists. Based on this, facilitation of a weak movement pattern will also aid in inhibiting the stronger movement pattern. Co-contraction of agonists and antagonists occurs when there is rapid fine reciprocation of muscle contraction. This allows co-contraction to provide stability with a dynamic nature (1,24). Posture reflects this, since adjustments are made to meet any change in gravity, as opposed to providing a fixed and stable base.

Motor development occurs sequentially and in predetermined stages (2,17). This demonstrates the principle of ontogeny recapitulating phylogeny. Mass total patterns of movement and posture are developed before fine motions, which are differentiated, selective, and specific. Motor development proceeds cephalad to caudad, from proximal to distal, and from flexion to extension to rotation. Hand function develops from crude ulnar palmar grasp to a radial palmar grasp to a pinch pattern. Thus normal movement can be encouraged by following these same developmental progressions (1,8,25–27).

In normal developmental activities, tonic and

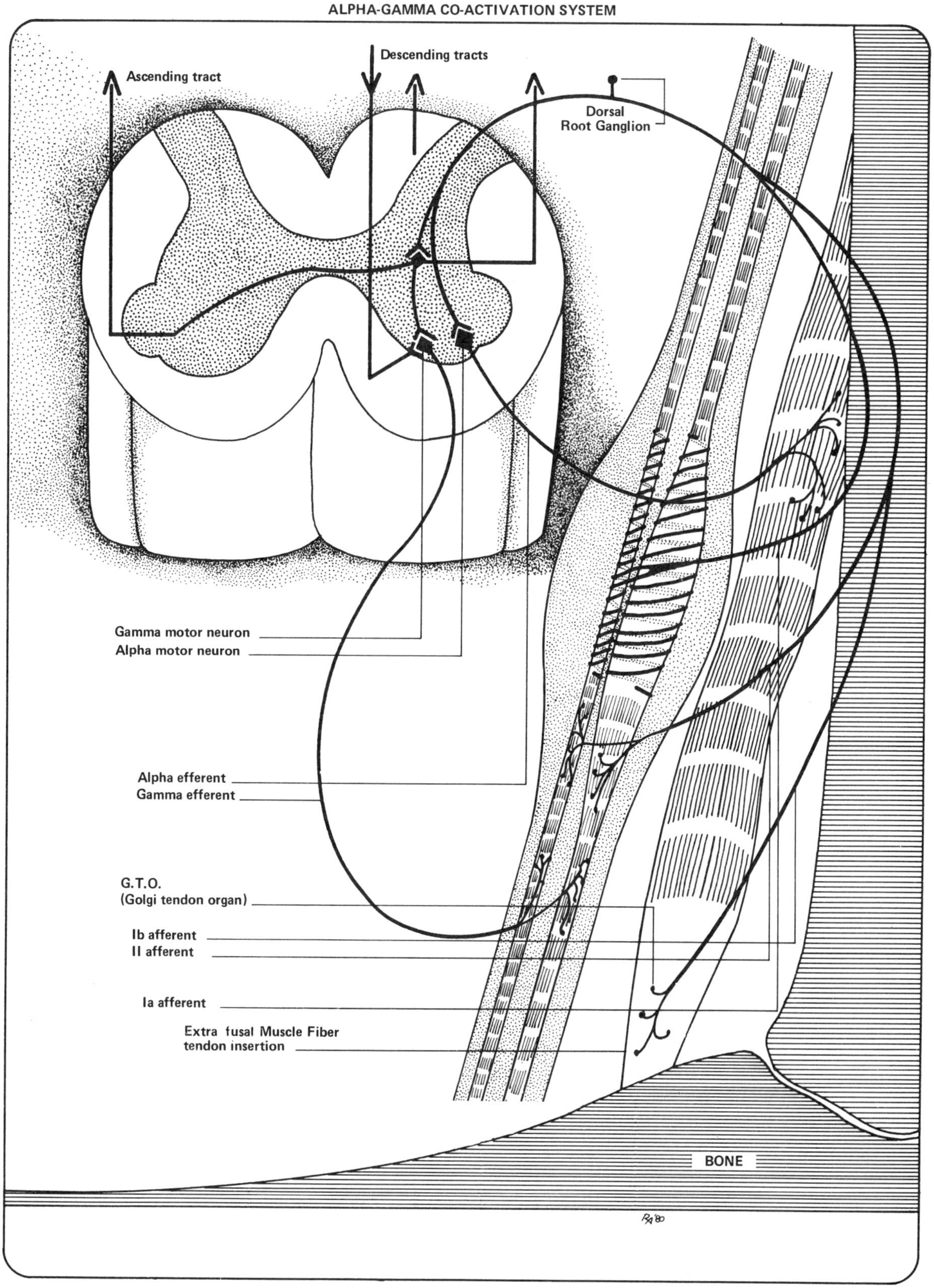

FIG. 2. A. The alpha-gamma coactivation system. This servo-assist phenomenon refers to simultaneous stimulation of the alpha and gamma motor neurons in the control of movement. Direct stimulation through the alpha motor neuron causes rapid contraction. The gamma motor neuron (via gamma loop) regulates the background muscle tone and the amount of muscle shortening needed for an activity. The proportions in this simplified diagram are highly distorted. A typical muscle contains hundreds of muscle spindles. Each muscle spindle contains about twelve or more intrafusal fibers. The diagram shows an enlarged view of the muscle spindle with only two intrafusal fibers.

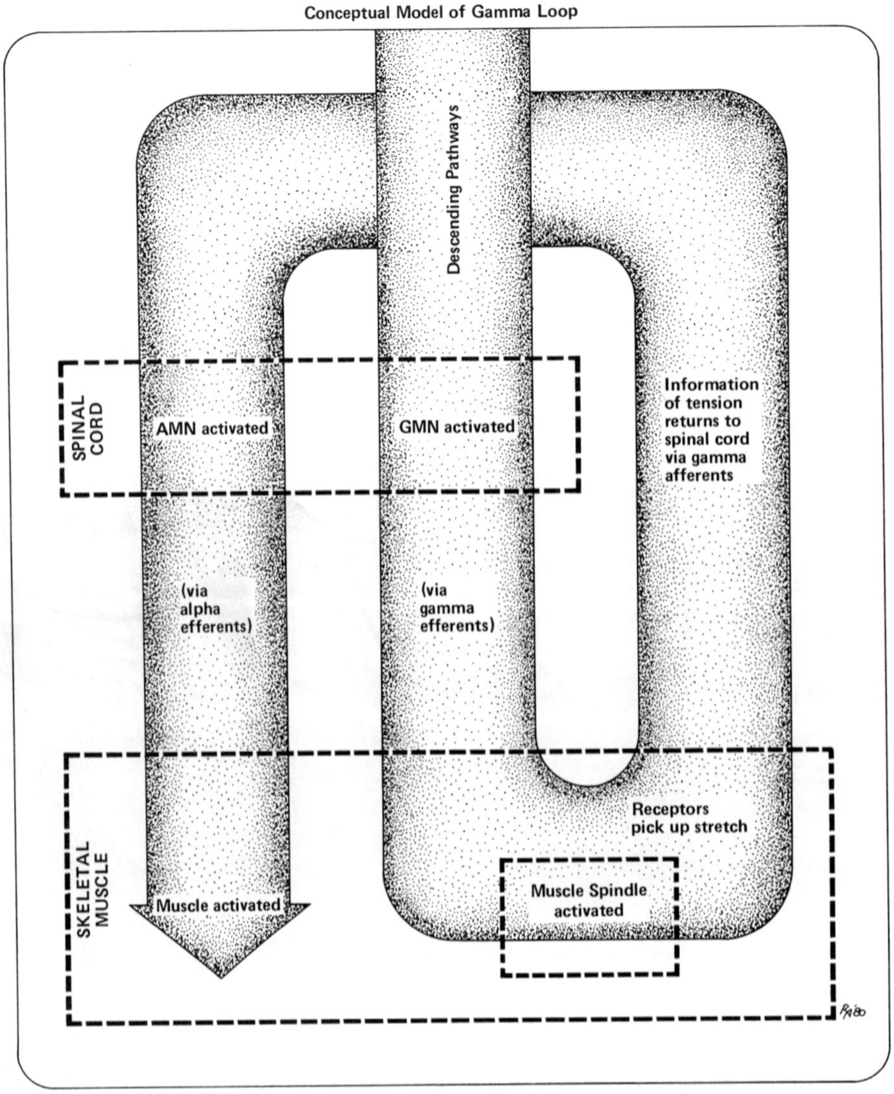

FIG. 2. B. Conceptual model of the gamma loop.

phasic muscles* develop sequentially and reciprocally. The interactions of these muscles in mobilizing and stabilizing actions promote the development of coordinated movement (1,2,10,24). As stability grows out of mobility, it is viewed as a dynamic quality. For example, as a child practices a mobilizing activity such as rocking in quadruped, the phasic hip flexors are used. The muscle spindles of the tonic hip extensors are being biased or put on stretch. This prepares the child to perform the stabilizing activity of hip extension necessary for creeping.

Motor development correlates with the development of cognition, language, social skills and with emotional development (4,15,28,29). Conceptualization occurs as one interacts with tangible objects (earth, gravity, material objects) and as judgments are made on the sensory-motor information and experience. As the neuromuscular system matures, one's ability to explore one's environment improves. Thus learning and growth can occur in all domains of development.

EFFECT OF BRAIN DAMAGE/DYSFUNCTION ON POSTURE AND MOVEMENT

Effects of UMN Lesion on Posture and Movement

The effects of an upper motor neuron (UMN)* lesion on functioning are dependent on the extensiveness of the lesion and its location. Sensory-

TABLE 1. *Components of gamma loop*

Receptor	Afferent	Responds to	Principal response	Basis for treatment technique
Afferent system				
Muscle spindle	Ia tonic fibers	Changes in length of muscle (static component of position)	Facilitates AMN for contraction of muscle from which signals received; quick response; inhibits antagonists	Quick stretch Tapping Vibrating Pressure on muscle belly
	Ia phasic fibers	Speed or velocity of changes (dynamic component) Vibration		Change in muscle length by contraction or mechanically stretching limb
Muscle spindle	II (tonic fibers only)	Changes in length of muscle Responds to static stretch only	Not conclusive Facilitates the muscle stretched Facilitates flexors and inhibits extensors	Maintained stretch of skeletal muscle
Golgi tendon organ	Ib	Changes in tension of skeletal muscle	Inhibits muscle from which signals received (high-threshold fibers) Provides information about tension being generated in muscle (low-threshold fibers)	Stretch Contraction

Receptor	Efferent	Functions
Efferent system		
Gamma motor neuron	Gamma efferent Phasic fibers	Because of small size, requires little excitatory input to discharge Muscle spindle contracts Increases sensitivity of Ia afferent to small stimuli Increases response to large stretches Increases dynamic component of response of Ia endings
	Tonic fibers	Increases static component of responses of Ia and II endings Controls muscle spindle contraction during skeletal muscle contraction
Alpha motor neuron	Alpha efferent	Because of large size, requires much excitatory input to discharge; skeletal muscle contracts

motor deficits are scattered, particularly in the adult. As one focuses on the observable postural and movement disorders, they should be viewed only as symptoms that can be traced to an underlying cause, i.e., the central disorganization of the brain (30–32).

The abnormal neurophysiology of the dysfunctioning alpha-gamma coactivation system can be traced to the UMN lesion. In the presence of a UMN lesion the lower reflex arcs are left intact, no longer regulated by the higher cortical centers. The result is hypertonicity, clinically seen as spasticity or rigidity and sometimes observable as posturing.* A lower motor neuron (LMN)* lesion results in flaccidity. With this lesion, sensory input cannot be received into the CNS; thus reflexes are absent.

An illustration (Table 2) of the subsequent imbalance of facilitory and inhibitory controls may clarify the basis of hypertonicity and hypotonicity. This illustration is an oversimplification since electrical resting levels are not constant. Electrical resting levels of a muscle are influenced by the totality of a situation, including what took place before and during the stimulation and the type and intensity of the stimulation (33).

TABLE 2. *Imbalance of facilitory and inhibitory controls of thresholds of nerve cells*

+10	
0	-----------------------------------
−50	-----------------------------------Threshold potential of anterior horn cell in normal CNS
−60	-----------------------------------Electrical resting level of nerve cell of hypertonic muscle
−70	-----------------------------------Electrical resting level of nerve cell for normal muscle
−80	-----------------------------------Electrical resting level of nerve cell of hypotonic muscle

Note: The normal muscle at rest has a background tension with the threshold resting potential of the nerve cell at approximately −70 mV. In order for a nerve cell to fire and a muscle contraction to occur, this resting potential must be lowered (toward zero). The threshold potential may, in fact, be higher or lower in the normal CNS than the −50 mV suggested here. In the hypertonic muscle (spasticity) the electrical resting level (−60 mV in this case) is closer to threshold (−50 mV), and the excited state causes muscle contraction to occur too quickly and inappropriately. Hypertonic muscles are overly facilitated. In the hypotonic muscle (−80 mV in this case) the electrical resting level is too far from threshold (−50 mV), and the depressed state requires that the muscle receive more excitation for a contraction to occur. Hypotonic muscles are overly inhibited.

Since muscle groups are normally neurophysiologically linked (termed synergistic action), when abnormal tonus occurs it involves muscle groups (25,26,34–36). The result is stereotypic abnormal movement patterns throughout the body. This may be a qualitative impairment involving loss of the variability of motion, or it may be a complete loss of isolated joint motion. Automaticity of movement is reduced. Since one must move in limited patterns, excessive effort is required for even simple motions. A vicious cycle develops as one's increased effort produces even greater spasticity. One becomes locked into abnormal patterns and postures. Functional activities such as self-care and walking become difficult to perform.

The primitive reflexes also reappear, uninhibited by higher cortical centers. With reference to the adult with traumatic brain damage, Hughlings Jackson, in 1884, used the phrase "evolution in reverse" (26). He observed that the nervous system reverted to a lower level of evolution. These reflexes, now pathological, interfere with the quality of movement (8,37). For example, a strong tonic labyrinthine reflex will cause difficulty for the patient in rolling or in assuming a sitting position from the supine. Another example is provided by the patient with a marked symmetrical tonic neck reflex who attempts to stand from sitting. The patient will be unable to extend the head and look up while extending the hips for the stance position.

Clinically, postural and movement disorders are diagnosed when a patient exhibits complexes of behavior. The outline in Appendix A suggests selected disorders indicative of neuropathological processes.

POTENTIAL FOR RECOVERY OF FUNCTION

Therapists have often observed that patients with brain damage do not demonstrate a static condition of primitive functioning. Rather, their motor behavior has a fluctuating quality, changing constantly, during the day and over longer time periods. The plasticity of the CNS is well known, i.e., the ability of the CNS to be influenced and gradually change to increase function.

Although the adult nervous system may not be as plastic or as flexible in recovery as is the child's during normal growth and development, observable behavioral changes can be noted in brain-damaged adults as they learn, adapt, and compensate for lost functions (38).

In the past the neurophysiological basis for this compensation was believed to be reorganization of the existing neural pathways. It was postulated that in brain-damaged patients therapy could promote the use of different or less frequently used neural circuits (latent, dormant pathways). This is classified as a functional neurophysiological change in the CNS. Redundancy in brain function accounts for this ability to reroute impulses around damaged areas to the intact parts of the brain.

But the neurophysiological basis of plasticity is yet to be fully understood. It is hoped that research relating to the regenerative and growth capabilities of the CNS will clarify the theoretical basis for the neurobehavioral frame of reference. It is known that when damage occurs no new neurons can develop, but maturation during normal growth and development through increased myelination of neural processes implies that structural changes in the CNS are possible.

The structural basis of neurophysiological plasticity has been postulated to lie in synaptic changes brought about by hypertrophy, regression, or budding of additional synapses (23,39,40). Regression of dendritic spine synapses in pyramidal cells secondary to disuse has been well demonstrated in laboratory animals. Also, experiments with brain-injured animals have demonstrated that increased sensation brought about by exercise and handling results in recovery of function and a histological increase in dendritic growth (1,41). Goldberger (39) has shown that damaged axons in the midbrain in cats grow sprouts and regenerate new synapses. He postulated that axonal sprouting accounts for the return of reflex activity during the first two weeks after lesioning, since reflexes disappear again once axonal sprouting is destroyed. He reported that healthy motor axons will also develop collateral sprouts to form new synapses. These new pathways, possibly accounting for the return of function, have been seen in the autonomic nervous system, spinal cord, and parts of the brain. But, in summary, it must be recognized that it is still only theory that these structural changes are indeed the basis for relearning movement. Also, since research cannot be easily carried out on humans, postulates about recovery of brain function in humans require a major jump from their basis in animal research.

EVALUATION

As the neurobehavioral frame of reference is eclectic, evaluation procedures are available from each theorist. All theorists agree that treatment should be initiated only after thorough analysis of the patient's needs. The evaluation must assess the normal movement patterns that are present or absent and the abnormal movement patterns that are interfering. Areas to be evaluated include sensation, muscle tone, control of mobilizing and stabilizing actions, joint mobility, integration of primitive reflexes, the presence of righting and equilibrium reactions, coordination, control and speed of normal movement patterns, and sensory-motor development.

Skill in clinical observation is essential. Qualitative observation of posture and movement is used to analyze the disorder, as opposed to a quantitative assessment. As the patient performs a task, the therapist must ask, "How is the patient moving?" For example, is the patient exhibiting stereotypic patterns or demonstrating adequate proximal stability or mobility? At this stage of the evaluation, the therapist should attempt to clearly describe the patient's motor performance. Next the therapist must ask, "Why does the patient move in this manner?" The answer to this will uncover the underlying problems (e.g., flexor spasticity predominance, interference from the tonic labyrinthine reflex).

Consider this evaluative process with a patient who initially exhibits poor sitting posture. The answer to the question "How does the patient sit?" may reveal the following: posturing of the arms and trunk; asymmetry of the trunk, with unequal weight-bearing of the hips; head and trunk misalignment with regard to the midline; the patient holding tightly onto the chair; the legs rotated so that the feet are not positioned flat on the floor. Next, the question "Why is the patient sitting this way?" may reveal one of these possibilities: spastic abdominals that are laterally flexing the trunk; spastic hamstrings with lower extremity extensor hypertonus causing difficulty in maintaining hip flexion; unstable trunk caused by hypotonicity and inability to maintain spinal extension; absence of righting reactions; presence of a primitive reflex; impaired body scheme; contractures of extremities; depressed state of mind.

Evaluation should be done initially and throughout the treatment session for continual reappraisal of the patient's status. During a treatment session, quick reassessment of tone will indicate if changes are needed in treatment. Often evaluation and treatment activities will be quite similar.

The following sequence of evaluation procedures is suggested as a general guide; it assumes familiarity with commonly used occupational therapy assessments:

All patients should be interviewed initially, specifically concerning medical history, chief complaints, and goals for therapy. This information can be used to confirm how and why the patients move as they do.

Each patient's posture in sitting and standing should be observed, checking for equal weight-bearing and ability to assume and maintain alignment of head, trunk, arms and legs.

Next, the patient's performance of functional movement patterns should be observed, with emphasis on movement patterns that will elicit behaviors indicative of dysfunction. The patient should be observed for total body patterns such as posturing and compensatory movements of "uninvolved" muscle groups. The following activities should be sequenced generally from gross to fine motions for a smooth flow of movement during the evaluation: (a) Self-care activities: bed mobility (rolling, sitting up, etc.), hygiene, feeding, dressing, homemaking. (b) Gross body motions: transfer from wheelchair to chair, rise to standing, move from standing to sitting, performing the developmental positions on a mat or on a bed (roll; prone on elbows, then on extended arms; quadruped on elbows and knees, then on hands and knees; kneel standing, half-kneel standing, standing, and walking). (c) Arm and trunk motions in sitting and standing: assess quality of motion during unilateral movements, bilateral symmetrical motion, and bilateral asymmetrical motion. Active isolated trunk motion is requested: trunk forward and backward, diagonal to both sides, rotation. Trunk motions may also be elicited when arm motions are requested. (d) Hand function: perform buttoning, pegboard placements of various shapes and sizes requiring progressively finer hand coordination, tasks requiring various prehension patterns.

As the patient's muscle tone normalizes during recovery, movement can then be assessed as to strength and endurance by means of resistive tests such as the manual muscle test and pinch meters.

Then the patient should be moved passively, allowing the therapist to feel tonal changes as well as observe the patient's responses to various movements. Before manipulation, and if indicated (as in stroke victims), the shoulder joint should be palpated to determine if subluxation is present. The patient will already have been interviewed in regard to pain. Edema should also be noted as a possible limiting factor to motion. The passive range-of-motion assessment can determine both joint mobility and degree of spasticity or flaccidity. To determine actual joint range, the effect of excess muscle tone should be minimized by first moving the limbs in gross diagonal patterns, as opposed to movement in the cardinal planes. Then mobility should be tested in different positions (sitting, supine, prone) to check the influences of reflex control.

On the basis of the active and passive movement tests described, muscle tone may be defined. Strong spasticity is identified when the patient cannot perform the motion and marked resistance is felt. Moderate spasticity is identified when the patient can perform some or all of a motion, but only with much effort and abnormal patterning. Minimal spasticity is identified when the patient can perform motion in a fairly normal manner, but only slowly and with effort. Flaccidity is identified when the patient cannot perform the motion and the stretch reflex cannot be elicited by quick stretch to the limb. Hypotonicity is distinguished from flaccidity when the patient cannot perform motion but a stretch reflex can be elicited.

Reflex testing for adults should involve modifications of the methods of Fiorentino (43) to account for the larger size of the patient or the medical condition. Some positions may even be contraindicated. In adults, changes in muscle tone are more often noted during palpation than actual observation of joint motion.

Other evaluation forms and procedures available include the following: (a) Bobath (25) has provided assessment for adults using three groups of tests: tests for postural reactions in response to being moved; tests for voluntary movement on request; tests for balance and other automatic protective reactions. (b) Brunnstrom (26) has assessed hemiplegic patients according to the presence of limb synergies and the recovery stage at which the patient is functioning. Brunnstrom's six stages of recovery are well illustrated in her text. Timed tests of rapid successions of movements or tasks are suggested. (c) Rood (1,8,42) evaluated four levels of motor control (mobility, stability, proximal mobility on distal stability, proximal stability on distal mobility) while putting patients through the ontogenetic motor patterns (supine withdrawal, roll over, pivot prone, neck co-contraction, on elbows, quadruped, standing, walking). (d) The proprioceptive neuromuscular facilitation (PNF) approach developed by Kabot (51,52) and expanded by Knott and Voss (44) is used to evaluate the quality of motor performance during assumption of positions, followed by progression in all directions from those positions, by means of a developmental sequence. Performance of the diagonal patterns is assessed as to flexor/extensor dominance, rate of movement, mobility/stability, and types of muscle contraction possible. No form is available, but suggestions for the process are provided in their text (44).

POSTULATES FOR CHANGE AND TREATMENT

In applying the neurobehavioral approach, specific treatment techniques have been suggested by Brunnstrom, Bobath, Rood, Knott, and Voss, as well as others. Although there are differences in terminology, the treatment principles are common to all.

Consistent with developmental frames of reference, therapy follows a graded sequential progression, beginning at the level of the patient's current function. Obviously, bed mobility and positioning are facilitated before sitting posture; this is followed by head, neck, and trunk control, then coordinated limb movements. Treatment priorities are established in accordance with the underlying causes of the movement and postural disorders, as identified by the answer to the question why the patient moves in a particular way. Short-term goals are the responses the therapist expects during treatment. Answering the question "What type of behavior needs to be facilitated?" can help the therapist select an appropriate activity or handling techniques for the goal. This selection is based on an activity analysis, especially focusing on developmental and neurophysiological components. Since developmental activities occur in an overlapping manner, not step by step, treatment should allow attempts at new activities while current activities are being perfected.

"Normalization" of abnormal muscle tone is an immediate goal in treatment. Reestablishing normal tone will provide a balance of agonists and antagonists and facilitate skilled motion. Control of postural reflexes is another prerequisite. All theorists agree that abnormal movement patterns are to be avoided. Brunnstrom allowed an exception to this when she encouraged primitive reflexes in patients with minimal spasticity to facilitate volitional synergistic motion; but even she agreed that once volitional movement appears, the primitive reflex movement should be avoided.

Facilitory or inhibitory sensory stimuli are used to enhance normal movement. Sensory stimuli are selected to help organize the nervous system, avoiding overstressing of an already disorganized CNS. The primary sensory systems are selectively stimulated. Parasympathetic nervous system control is encouraged initially in treatment. Since the autonomic nervous system determines which sensory input will be received, it is important that any physical or emotional fight-or-flight reactions be reduced and the normal parasympathetic nervous system be in control.

Control of developmental components of motion and establishment of normal patterns of movement are common treatment goals. The head and trunk are emphasized as the postural foundation for distal movement. Normal posture will prepare tonus and alignment for normal movement. Patterns of mobility and stability are emphasized according to the patient's needs. Spinal diagonal patterns are emphasized, as opposed to isolated joint motion in the cardinal planes (e.g., forward shoulder flexion).

Another point of agreement is the necessity of therapeutic activity for the acquisition of skill. Activities provide appropriate sensory stimuli that further encourage normal movement, giving accurate sensory feedback concerning improved performance. Also, a challenging goal-directed activity requires the cortex to focus attention on the end act and allows subcortical control of the performance. This subcortical control requires the integration of sensory-motor processes in the CNS. In addition, the repetitive nature of activities encourages development of skills. Finally, as Moore (33) said, "one needs stimuli that are meaningful, for a system to respond purposefully." There is a direct correlation between the amounts of learning and growth and development and the nature of the environment. In occupational therapy, environment and activity are the keys to prevention and remediation of dysfunction.

The following suggestions are offered as guidelines in selecting treatment activities useful for patients with movement and postural disorders. Other dysfunctions such as ataxia and rigidity may also be treated within this frame of reference. Treatment examples are given in the parentheses.

Hypertonicity is inhibited by the following: (a) activities that require or provide slow, repetitive, reciprocal movement (cephalad to caudad, proximal to distal) and diagonal reciprocal motions (the patient can be slowly rolled from side-lying to prone repeatedly until muscle tension reduces; activities in which the patient picks up objects from the floor on one side and places them high on the opposite side); (b) activities that prevent abnormally linked postural and movement patterns from occurring (the therapist controls the patient at key points proximally, such as head, neck, shoulders, and pelvic girdle; limbs are placed or moved into positions directly opposite to abnormal patterns; flexor spasticity of trunk and arm can be counteracted by extension of neck and spine, external rotation at shoulder, extension at elbow, and thumb abduction); (c) activities that require or maintain a balance between agonist and antagonist muscles and motions (sensory input of tapping, icing, brushing to muscles antagonistic to spastic musculature; activities requiring tonic contraction of extensors will reciprocally inhibit flexor spasticity); (d) activities that avoid strong volitional effort on the patient's part (do not use weights or heavy equipment on spastic muscles, e.g., weighted sanders, printing press).

Hypotonicity is facilitated by the following: (a) activities that provide an increase in fast, irregular tactile and proprioceptive stimuli (brushing, tapping, vibration, quick icing over muscle belly; joint compression applied with more than body weight increases proprioceptive input); (b) activities that encourage tonic muscle action (patient performs activities while positioned in all fours or prone on elbows, a position that increases co-contraction proximally); (c) activities that encourage movement, reflexive at first, then voluntary (resistance through gravity, manually, or equipment will increase muscle tension; asymmetrical tonic neck reflex, (ATNR) will produce increased tonus changes in extremities).

Inability to regulate postural reflexes is decreased by the following: (a) activities that require automatic voluntary gross movement (throwing and catching ball, ring toss from sitting or standing); (b) activities that avoid or prevent specific stimulus positions for abnormal primitive reflexes (do not use ATNR to facilitate volitional motion; decrease control of tonic labyrinthine reflex supine when patient is supine in bed by flexing head and knee with small pillow).

Symmetrical and normal postural and movement patterns are facilitated by the following: (a) activities that require the use of all available musculature in gross and fine motion (increase weight-bearing on both feet or buttocks; activities producing swaying motions of total body, e.g., sanding large board); (b) activities that require interaction of both sides of the body (large objects, bilateral handles, etc.).

Learning of normal motor behavior is enhanced by the following: (a) activities that require repetition of specified motions with increased sensory feedback from successful movements (allow normal movements only during repetitive activities, e.g., sanding, weaving, leather lacing, sewing); (b) activities that incorporate specific learned motor components into a functional goal-directed activity (vibration and tapping over elbow extensors applied during checkers game, in which positioning requires extension of elbow; slow rolling in bed is followed up with activity of sitting up in bed from supine).

OVERVIEW OF SOME SPECIFIC TREATMENT TECHNIQUES

Since many good resources for the following therapies are available, only key concepts will be highlighted here (see Bibliography). Appendix B presents an outline of possible facilitation and inhibition techniques. There are many other theorists and therapists in this area whose work should be considered.

Brunnstrom (1,8,9,26,42,45,55) promoted movement therapy for hemiplegic patients based on extensive study and clinical work. The core of this approach is recognition that recovery of the hemiplegic patient proceeds through six stages of increasing control over posture and movement. Treatment follows and encourages this progression. The primitive patterns of concern are the associated reactions, flexion and extension synergies of the extremities, and attitudinal and postural reflexes. Combinations of patterns deviating from the stereotypic synergies are facilitated once volitional synergistic motion is initiated. Synergies are not facilitated until they are strongly developed.

In occupational therapy, Brunnstrom's technique can be used in preparation for goal-directed activities, especially since many techniques are carried out while sitting. If a synergy is being facilitated, the following activity should be positioned to encourage the same synergy pattern. If the patient is recovering from synergy control, functional activities should be used to encourage the movement pattern (e.g., instead of having the patient move a hand to the opposite arm, the patient can use a washcloth to wash the arm). If the patient reaches a plateau at any stage, it is time to teach functional use of the available pattern of motion for self-care activities.

Bobath developed the neurodevelopmental treatment (NDT) approach for patients with cerebral palsy (1,8,9,25,34,42,45–48). Bobath's text (25) on adult hemiplegic patients provides excellent illustrated resources. Bobath's method teaches patients to determine when their muscle tone increases and how to modify or inhibit spasticity. Handling activities performed by the therapist are used before, during, and after an activity. The therapist guides the patient using proximal points of control without applying resistance to promote mobility or stability. Spasticity is inhibited by moving the patient in reflex-inhibiting patterns. All abnormal movement patterns are avoided. Rotation movements are especially important in unlocking spasticity. Once normal tone is established, therapy facilitates more selective complex movements and the righting and equilibrium reactions.

Rood (1,8,9,11,42,45) constantly changes and validates her techniques by applying the latest results of neurophysiological research. Although a recent workshop demonstrated the growth of this approach, there is little in the literature on her evolving treatment methods. Rood is particularly known for her use of proprioceptive and tactile stimulation procedures to influence tone. Another important aspect is the developmental sequences of motor control through phases of mobility and stability and the ontogenetic motor patterns. Appendix C shows her suggested outline for treatment.

Interest in the proprioceptive neuromuscular facilitation (PNF) approach developed by Knott and Voss (1,8,9,42,44,45,49–54) has recently increased, although no recent literature is available. PNF uses total body patterns, with emphasis on spiral and diagonal patterns. Resistance is used to reinforce and define a direction of motion for the patient. Treatment is directed toward a balance of muscle power and the ability to perform smooth rhythmic motions. Well-defined patterns are elicited through specific manual contacts and by using a sequence of developmental positions.

In the PNF treatment planning process the therapist asks questions: "Which diagonal pattern is needed to promote a balance of muscle tone?" "Should resistance be applied or not?" "Would isotonic or isometric muscle contraction be more effective at the weakened body part?" "Where is joint range within the diagonal patterns limited?" "Would unilateral or bilateral motion

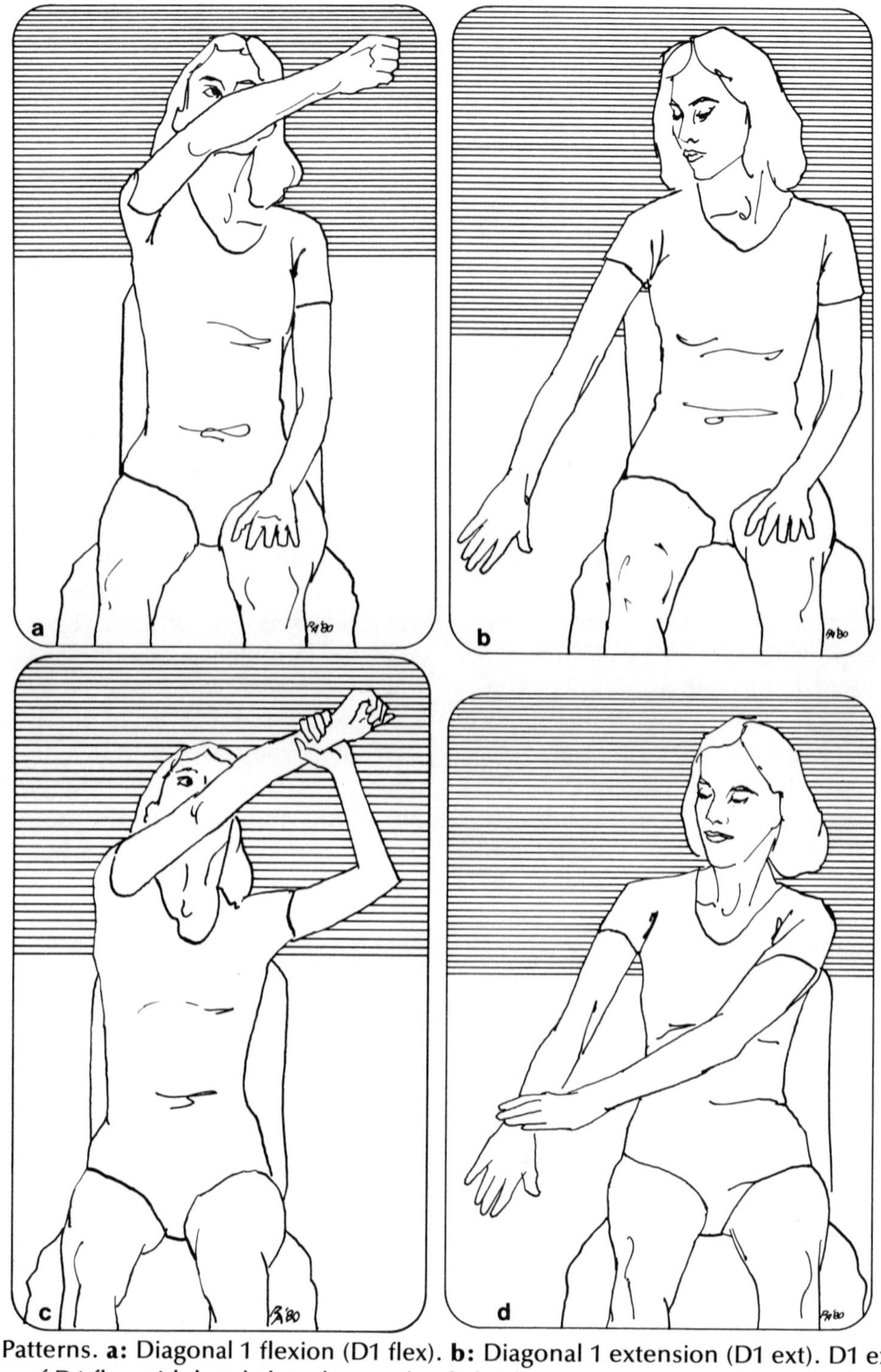

FIG. 3. A. PNF Patterns. **a:** Diagonal 1 flexion (D1 flex). **b:** Diagonal 1 extension (D1 ext). D1 ext begins in the shortened range of D1 flex with hand closed toward radial side. Movement into D1 ext leads with hand opening toward ulnar side. Eyes follow hand so head and hand cross midline. **c** and **d:** Bilateral Asymmetrical "Chopping." Leading arm goes from D1 flex to D1 ext. Opposite extremity moves in D2 patterns. The assist hand grips the volar wrist of the leading arm (Right in this illustration). Eyes follow hand of leading arm. Reversing from extension (D1 and D2) to flexion (D1 and D2) is "reversal of chop." Elbows may remain in extension or flexion (Courtesy of Dorothy Voss).

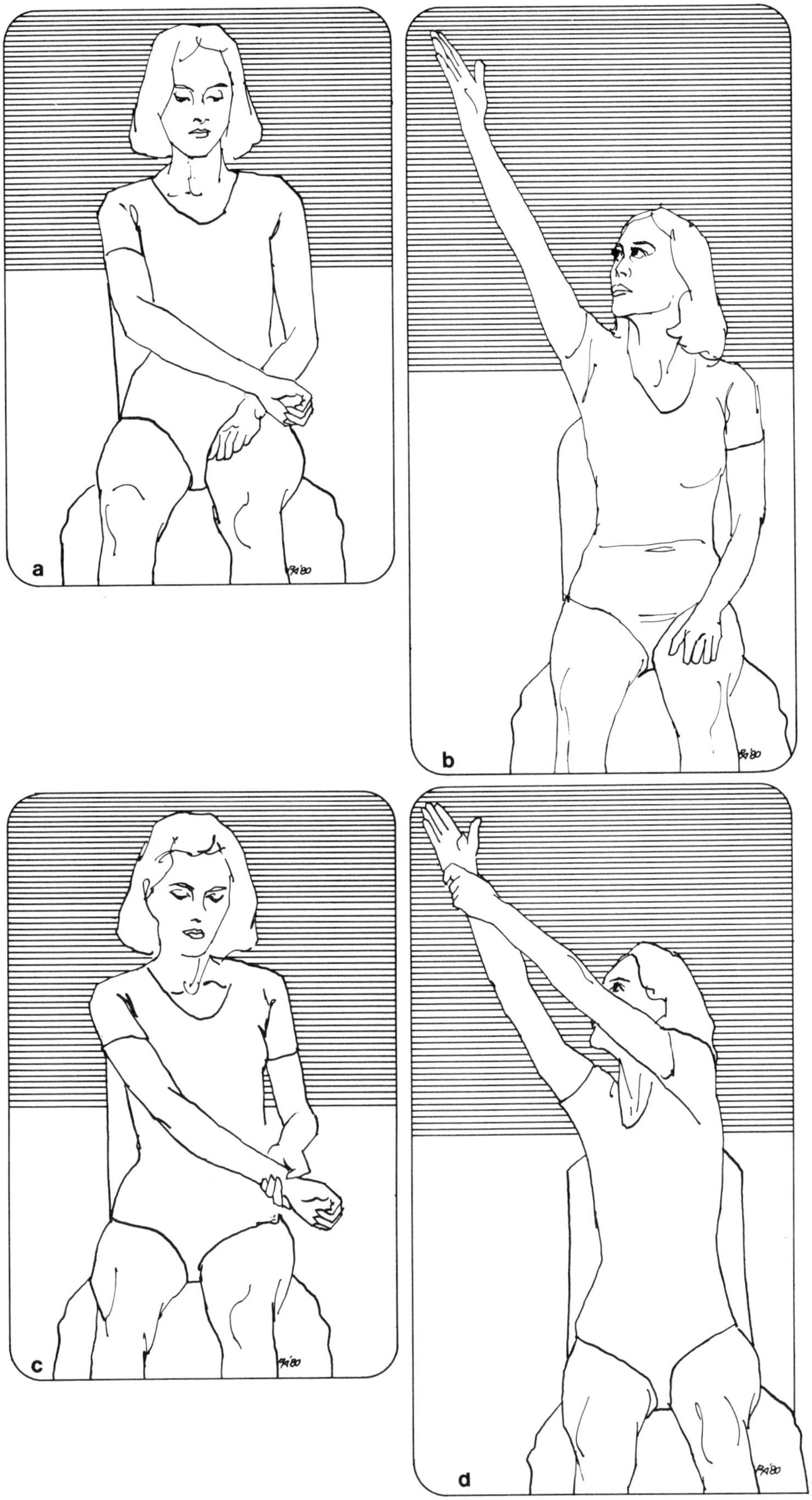

FIG. 3. B. PNF Patterns. **a:** Diagonal 2 extension (D2 ext). **b:** Diagonal 2 flexion (D2 flex). D2 flex begins in the shortened range of D2 ext with hand closed toward the ulnar side. Movement into D2 flex leads with hand opening toward radial side. All diagonal patterns, head to foot, cross midline when performed through full range. **c** and **d:** Bilateral Asymmetrical "Lifting." Leading arm goes through D2 ext to D2 flex. The opposite extremity moves in D1 patterns. The leading hand (Right in this illustration) opens with shoulder abduction and closes with shoulder adduction. Hand grips volar wrist of leading arm. Contact with an opposite extremity, self-touching, promotes stability and perception (Courtesy of Dorothy Voss).

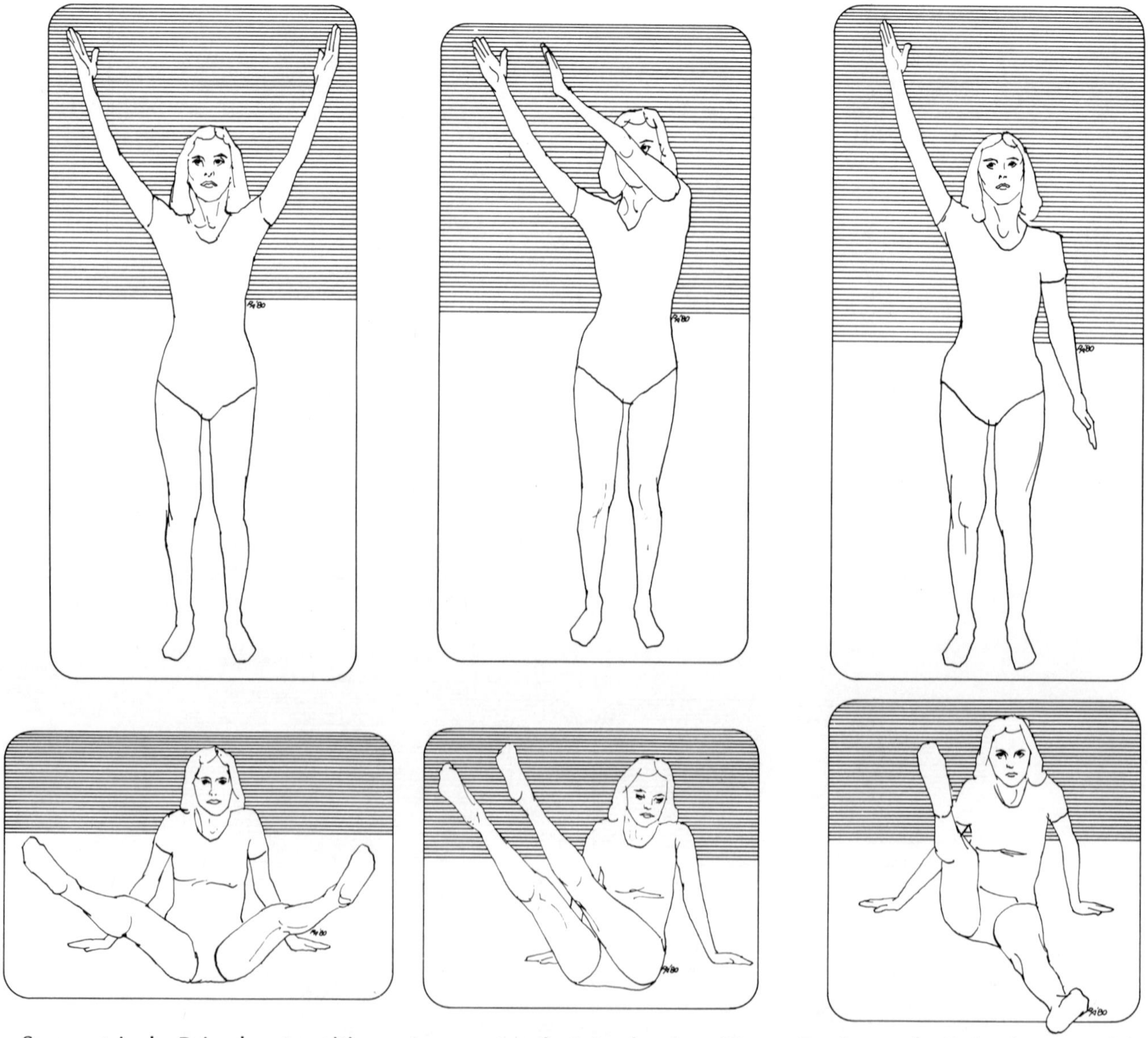

Symmetrical: Paired extremities perform like movements at the same time

Asymmetrical: Paired extremities perform movements toward one side at the same time

Reciprocal: Paired extremities perform movements in opposite direction at the same time.

FIG. 4. A. Total body patterns: interactions of body segments producing combined movements of upper or lower extremities.
(Courtesy of Dorothy E. Voss.)

be more effective for the patient?" The PNF diagonal patterns can be done using passive, active, active assisted, and resisted motions.

In occupational therapy, numerous craft, recreational, and self-care activities have therapeutic potential, since diagonal patterns are inherent or can be elicited with simple adaptations of the position of the patient or craft media and equipment. The two basic diagonal patterns of the upper extremities and the bilateral patterns of chopping and lifting are shown in Figs. 3A and 3B. Again, these are used before and during goal-directed activity. Different total body patterns and interactions of body parts may be used in treatment as in Fig. 4. For treatment suggestions refer to Appendix D.

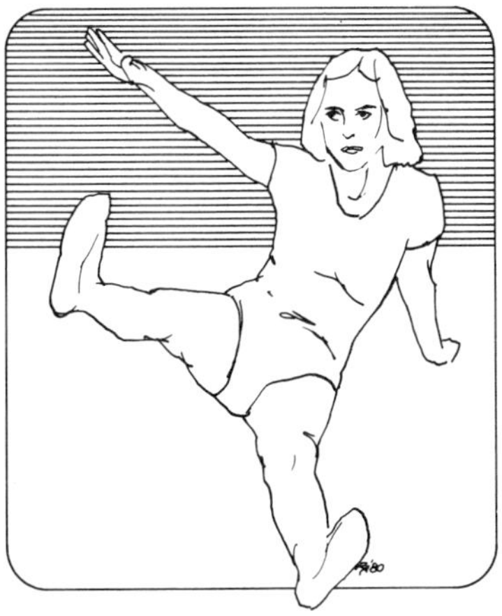

Ipsilateral: extremities of same side move in same direction at same time

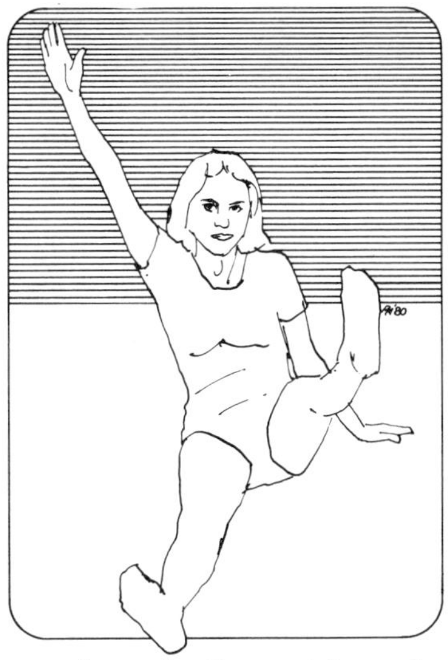

Contralateral: Extremities of opposite sides move in same direction at the same time

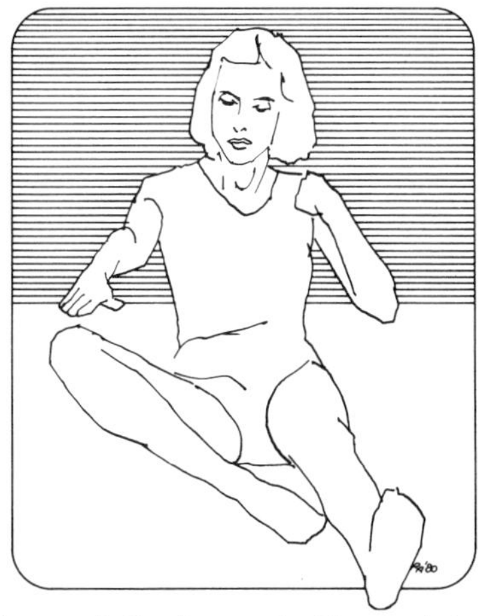

Diagonal Reciprocal: Contralateral extremities move in same direction at the same time while opposite contralateral extremities move in the opposite direction

FIG. 4. B. Total body patterns: interaction of body segments combined movements of upper and lower extremities.
(Courtesy of Dorothy E. Voss.)

REFERENCES

1. Northwestern University Special Therapeutic Exercise Project (NUSTEP) (1967): An exploratory and analytical survey of therapeutic exercise. *Am. J. Phys. Med.,* 46.
2. Payton, O., Hirt, S., and Newton, R. (1977): *Scientific Bases for Neurophysiologic Approaches to Therapeutic Exercises, An Anthology.* F. A. Davis, Philadelphia.
3. O'Connell, A., and Gardner, E. (1972): *Understanding the Scientific Bases of Human Movement.* Williams & Wilkins, Baltimore.
4. Cratty, B. (1973): *Movement Behavior and Motor Learning,* ed. 3. Lea & Febiger, Philadelphia.
5. Vander, A., Sherman, J., and Luciano, D. (1975): *Human Physiology: The Mechanisms of Body Function,* ed. 2. McGraw-Hill, New York.
6. Eccles, J. (1977): *The Understanding of the Brain,* McGraw-Hill, New York.
7. Bishop, B. (1975): Vibratory stimulation: Possible applications of in treatment of motor dysfunctions. *Phys. Ther.,* 55:139–143.
8. Trombly, C., and Scott, A. (1977): *Occupational Therapy for Physical Dysfunction.* Williams & Wilkins, Baltimore.
9. Harris, F. A. (1978): Facilitation exercises in therapeutic exercise. In: *Therapeutic Exercise,* ed. 3, edited by J. Basmajian, pp. 93–139. Williams & Wilkins, Baltimore.
10. Goff, B. (1972): The application of recent advances in neurophysiology to Miss M. Rood's concept of neuromuscular facilitation. *Physiotherapy,* 58:405–415.
11. Rood, M. (1956): Neurophysiological mechanisms utilized in the treatment of neuromuscular dysfunction. *Am. J. Occup. Ther.,* 10:220–224.
12. Schmidt, R. (editor) (1978): *Fundamentals of Sensory Physiology.* Springer-Verlag, New York.
13. Schmidt, R. (editor) (1978): *Fundamentals of Neurophysiology.* Springer-Verlag, New York.
14. Guyton, A. (1972): *Structure and Function of the Nervous System.* W. B. Saunders, Philadelphia.
15. Ayres, A. J. (1973): *Sensory Integration and Learning Disorders.* Western Psychological Services, Los Angeles.
16. Farber, S., and Huss, A. J. (1974): *Sensorimotor Evaluation and Treatment Procedures for Allied Health Personnel.* Indiana University Foundation, Indianapolis.
17. McGraw, N. (1945): *The Neuromuscular Maturation of the Human Infant.* Hafner, New York.
18. Fiorentino, M. (1972): *Normal and Abnormal Development.* Charles C Thomas, Springfield, Ill.
19. Moore, J. (1976): Behavior, bias, limbic system. *Am. J. Occup. Ther.,* 30:11–19.
20. Gellhorn, E. (1967): *Principles of Autonomic*

Somatic Integration. University of Minnesota Press, Minneapolis.

21. Moore, J. (1974): The Golgi tendon organ and the muscle spindle. *Am. J. Occup. Ther.*, 28:415–520.
22. Moore, J. (1973): Terminology today. *Am. J. Occup. Ther.*, 27:149–155.
23. Bishop, B. (1977): Spasticity, part I–IV. *Phys. Ther.*, 57:371–401.
24. Crutchfield, C., and Barnes, M. (1975): *Neurophysiological Basis of Patient Treatment. Vol. I: The Muscle Spindle*, ed. 2. Stokesville Publishing, Morgantown, W. Va.
25. Bobath, B. (1978): *Adult Hemiplegia: Evaluation and Treatment*. William Heinemann, New York.
26. Brunnstrom, S. (1970): *Movement Therapy in Hemiplegia*. Harper & Row, New York.
27. Ayres, A. J. (1954): Ontogenetic principles in the development of arm and hand function. *Am. J. Occup. Ther.*, 8:95–99.
28. Tiffany, E. (1978): The developmental treatment approach: Cognitive, social, and emotional aspects. In: *Willard and Spackman's Occupational Therapy*, ed. 5, edited by H. Hopkins and H. Smith. pp. 123–125. J. B. Lippincott, Philadelphia.
29. Silberyahn, N. (1978): Sensory integrative theory. In: *Willard and Spackman's Occupational Therapy*, ed. 5, edited by H. Hopkins and H. Smith. pp. 134–140. J. B. Lippincott, Philadelphia.
30. Cash, J. (1974): *Neurophysiology for Physiotherapists*. Faker & Faker, London.
31. Marmo, N. (1974): A new look at the brain damaged adult. *Am. J. Occup. Ther.*, 28:199–206.
32. Chusid, J. (1979): *Correlative Neuroanatomy and Functional Neurology*, ed. 17. Lange Medical, Los Altos.
33. Moore, J. (1969): *Neuroanatomy Simplified, Some Basic Concepts for Understanding Rehabilitation Techniques*. Kendall/Hunt, Dubuque, Iowa.
34. Bobath, B. The effect of spasticity on adult hemiplegia and its treatment. From a manual in Workshop.
35. Brunnstrom, S. (1961): Motor behavior of adult hemiplegic patients: Hints for training. *Am. J. Occup. Ther.*, 25:6–12.
36. Twitchell, T. (1951): The restoration of motor function following hemiplegia in man. *Brain*, 74:443–480.
37. Bobath, B. (1971): *Abnormal Reflex Activity Caused by Brain Lesions*. ed. 2. William Heinemann, New York.
38. Moore, J. (1973): *Concepts from the Neurobehavioral Sciences*. Kendall/Hunt, Dubuque, Iowa.
39. Goldberger, M. (1974): Recovery of movement after central nervous system lesions in monkeys. In: *Plasticity and Recovery of Function in the Central Nervous System*, edited by J. Stein, D. Rosen, N. Butters. pp. 365–387. Academic Press, New York.
40. Buerger, A., and Tobis, J. (editors) (1976): *Neurophysiologic Aspects of Rehabilitation Medicine*. Charles C Thomas, Springfield.
41. Noback, C. R. (1977): *The Human Nervous System*. McGraw-Hill, New York.
42. Chartered Society of Physiotherapy (1974): *Facilitation of Movement*, ed. 4 (reprint of six articles from *Physiotherapy*). CSP, London.
43. Fiorentino, N. (1963): *Reflex Testing Methods for Evaluating Central Nervous System Development*, Charles C Thomas, Springfield.
44. Knott, M., and Voss, D. (1968): *Proprioceptive Neuromuscular Facilitation*. Harper & Row, New York.
45. Huss, J. (1978): Sensorimotor approaches. In: *Willard and Spackman's Occupational Therapy*, ed. 5, edited by H. Hopkins and H. Smith, pp. 125–134. J. B. Lippincott, Philadelphia.
46. Bobath, B. (1969): The treatment of neuromuscular disorders by improving patterns of coordination. *Physiotherapy*, 55:18–22.
47. Bobath, B. (1960): Observations on adult hemiplegia and suggestions for treatment. *Physiotherapy Journal*, 47:31.
48. Bobath, B. (1954): A study of abnormal postural reflex activity in patients with lesions of the central nervous system. *Physiotherapy Journal*, 40:259, 295, 326, 369.
49. Surburg, P. (1977): The effect of proprioceptive facilitation patterning upon reaction, response, and movement times. *Phys. Ther.*, 57:513–517.
50. Wynn Parry, C. B. (1973): *Rehabilitation of the Hand*, ed. 3. Butterworth, London.
51. Kabot, H. (1958): Proprioceptive facilitation in therapeutic exercise. In: *Therapeutic Exercise*, edited by S. Licht, pp. 301–318. Elizabeth Licht, New Haven.
52. Kabot, H. (1950): Concepts and techniques of occupational therapy for neuro-muscular disorders. *Am. J. Occup. Ther.*, 4:6–11.
53. Ayres, A. J. (1955): Proprioceptive facilitation elicited through the upper extremities. Part I. Background. Part II. Application. Part III. Specific application. *Am. J. Occup. Ther.* 9:1–9, 57–58, 76–77, 121–126.
54. Voss, D. (1959): PNF: Applications of patterns and techniques in occupational therapy. *Am. J. Occup. Ther.*, 13:191–194.

BIBLIOGRAPHY

Ayres, A. J. (1975): Sensorimotor foundations of academic ability. In: *Perceptual and Learning Abilities in Children, Vol. 2,* edited by W. Cruickshank and D. Hallohan. Syracuse University Press, New York.

Ball, T., and Mumpei, G. (1978): Brushing and physiological arousal. *Am. J. Phys. Med.,* 57:295–299.

Banus, B. S., Kent, C. A., Norton, Y. deS., Sukiennicki, D. R., and Becker, M. L. (1979): *The Developmental Therapist.* Charles B. Slack, Thorofare, New Jersey.

Barnes, M., Crutchfield, C., and Heriza, C. (1978): Reflexes in motor development. In: *The Neurophysiological Basis of Patient Treatment,* Vol. 2, edited by Stokesville Publishing Company, Morgantown, West Virginia.

Cooke, D. (1958): The effects of resistance on multiple sclerosis patients with intention tremor. *Am. J. Occup. Ther.,* Vol. XII, No. 2, Part II, pps. 89–92.

Downey, J., and Darling, R. (1971): *Physiological Basis of Rehabilitation Medicine.* W. B. Saunders, Philadelphia.

Eyzagvirre, C., and Fidone, S. (1975): *Physiology of the Nervous System,* ed. 2. Year Book, Chicago.

Fay, T. (1958): Neuromuscular reflex therapy for spastic disorders. *J. Fla. Med. Assoc.,* 44:1234–1240.

Gowitzke, B., and Milner, M. (1980): *Understanding the Scientific Bases of Human Movement,* ed. 2. Williams and Wilkins, Baltimore.

Granit, R. (1970): *The Basis of Motor Control.* John Wiley, New York.

Harris, F. (1969): Control of gamma efferents through the reticular activating system. *Am. J. Occup. Ther.,* 23:397–409.

Harris, F. (1971): Multiple loop input control of efferent activity: A physiological basis for facilitation techniques. *Phys. Ther.,* 51:391–397.

Huss, J. (1977): Touch with care or a caring touch? *Am. J. Occup. Ther.,* 31:11–18.

Johnstone, M. (1978): *Restoration of Motor Function in the Stroke Patient.* Churchhill Livingston, New York.

Ketty, S. (1979): Disorders of the human brain. *Sci. Am.* 241:202–214.

King, L. J. (1974): A sensory integrative approach to schizophrenia. *Am. J. Occup. Ther.,* 28:529–536.

King, L. J. (1978): Occupational therapy research in psychiatry: A perspective. *Am. J. Occup. Ther.,* 32:15–18.

Lance, J., and Burke, D. (1974): Mechanisms of spasticity. *Arch. Phys. Med. Rehabil.,* 55:332–337.

Langworthy, O. R. (1970): *The Sensory Control of Posture and Movement.* Williams & Wilkins, Baltimore.

Luria, A. R. (1963): *Restoration of Function after Brain Injury.* Macmillan, New York.

Mathews, P. B. C. (1972): *Mammalian Muscle Receptors and Their Central Actions.* Williams & Wilkins, Baltimore.

Montagu, A. (1971): *Touching, The Hyman Significance of the Skin.* Harper & Row, New York.

Raisman, G., and Field, P. M. (1973): A quantitative investigation of the development of collateral reinnervation of the septal nuclei. *Brain Res.,* 50:241–264.

Retzlaff, E., and Fontaine, T. (1965): Functional and structural changes in motor neurons with age. In: *Behavior, Aging, and the Nervous System,* edited by A. T. Welford and J. Birren. Charles C Thomas, Springfield, Ill.

Roberts, T. (1967): *Neurophysiology of Postural Mechanism.* Butterworth and Company, New York.

Rushworth, G. (1960): Spasticity and rigidity: An experimental study and review. *J. Neurol. Neurosurg. Psychiatry,* 23:99.

Stejskal, L. (1979): Postural reflexes in man. *Am. J. Phys. Med.,* 58:1–25.

Treanor, W. (1973): Restitution of movement following brain injury. *Phys. Ther. Rev.,* 34:606–610.

Voss, D. (1972): Proprioceptive neuromuscular facilitation: The PNF method. In: *Physical Therapy Services in the Developmental Disabilities,* edited by P. H. Pearson and C. A. Williams, pp. 223–282. Charles C Thomas, Springfield, Ill.

Wickstrom, R. (1977): *Fundamental Motor Patterns,* ed. 2. Lea & Febiger, Philadelphia.

APPENDIX A: OUTLINE OF SELECTED DISORDERS INDICATIVE OF NEUROPATHOLOGY

1. Hypertonicity
   a. Hyperactive deep tendon reflexes.
   b. Sudden resistance felt on passive motion or quick stretch of a joint when motion is against the involved muscle's action.
   c. Motions are linked into total body patterns that prevent isolated joint motion, reduce the variability of active joint motion, and decrease relative consistency of strength and joint range.
   d. Isolated joint motions are slow, weak, in-

efficient, and incoordinated, especially in reciprocal movements.
   e. Inability to produce stabilizing and mobilizing components for skilled motor performance.
   f. Patient's conscious effort reinforces hypertonus and abnormal movement patterns.
2. Hypotonicity
   a. Diminished or lost deep tendon reflexes.
   b. Less than normal resilience or resistance felt on passive joint range, i.e., limb feels heavy when moved.
   c. Involved muscles atrophy and feel flabby and soft when palpated.
   d. Instability or laxity of joints observed or palpated on active or passive motion.
   e. Weakened or lost reflexive and/or voluntary motion.
3. Inability to regulate postural reflexes
   a. Specific head and neck positions or motions produce predictable changes in tonus (when muscle is palpated) or stereotypic observable movement.
   b. Presence of primitive reflexes (i.e., ATNR, TLR) interferes with or prevents the performance of normal movement.
   c. Absence of normal righting reflexes prevents realignment of total body in space during movement, i.e., posture against gravity is difficult to maintain or achieve, and postural adjustments to active or passive motions are delayed, slow, or absent.
4. Asymmetrical postures and motions
   a. Uninvolved muscles overcompensate for deficits by exaggeration of normal motion.
   b. Difficulty in using or coordinating the two sides of the body, i.e., avoidance of using or bearing weight on involved body segments and avoidance of moving in diagonal patterns.

APPENDIX B: FACILITATION AND INHIBITION TECHNIQUES[1]

The treatment modalities for facilitation are applied to the weaker muscles or those muscle groups needed for the proper development sequence. The therapist must be familiar with all of the modalities and must have properly evaluated the patient so that techniques that will most benefit the patient can be used.

Inhibition or Relaxation Techniques

1. *General rule of inhibition.* Activity that is slow and repetitive is usually inhibitory. Slow repetitive activity sends inhibitory impulses to the bulbar section of the brain (in the reticular area), which in turn causes total body inhibition.

2. *Slow stroking.* Slow stroking is alternate stroking of the posterior primary rami with a firm but light pressure, done in such a manner that one hand starts at the occiput and progresses down to the coccyx. Before lifting the first hand, the therapist should place the other hand at the occiput. Thus there is continuous contact. This is repeated for 3 min. Do not use this technique if the hair growth on the back is in sworls or irregular in pattern (this will stimulate instead of inhibit the patient). Slow stroking is more effective if done directly on the skin.

3. *Neutral warmth.* Extremes of temperature may produce relaxation initially; however, rebound may result. Neutral warmth is helpful in cases of spasticity, rigidity, extreme tension, or painful joint and/or muscles. If the total body is to be treated, the patient is wrapped in a cotton blanket for 10–20 min at the beginning of treatment. If water is used, it should be tepid or at body temperature, not hot. If kept within the neutral range (body temperature), there will be no rebound affect in 2–3 hr. However, if the temperature is too high, the patient will tighten up in 2–3 hr and may find pain associated with this rebound.

4. *Slow rolling.* The therapist places one hand on the patient's pelvis and the other hand on a shoulder. The patient is rolled from supine to side and returned to supine. Slow rolling should be repeated for several minutes until the patient shows signs of relaxing (reduced tension).

5. *Rocking in a rocking chair or over a beach ball.* A rocking chair can be therapeutic for both the patient and the therapist. When rocking a child over a beach ball, the therapist should stabilize the patient at the pelvis. The patient is generally in the prone position and rocked only in a forward and backward direction.

6. *Pressure on the insertion of a muscle.* For specific inhibition of a tight muscle group, apply pressure on the insertion of the muscle (i.e., for wrist flexors, place a hand cone in the hand).

[1] Compiled from Huss (45) and other sources.

7. *Reflex-inhibiting patterns.* Movement patterns that inhibit abnormal postural reactions and facilitate active voluntary movements. Proximal key points of control are used: neck, shoulder, and pelvic girdle. (e.g., a reflex-inhibiting pattern to counteract flexor spasticity of the trunk and arm is to extend the neck and spine, externally rotate the shoulder, extend elbow, followed by supination and thumb abduction).

8. *Auditory stimuli.* Soft regular rhythms are inhibitory. The therapist should be aware of the speaking voice when attempting to inhibit a patient.

9. *Taste and smell.* Warm fluids are inhibitory to hyperactive oral pathology. Perfume or other pleasant odors will have a calming effect.

10. *Reciprocal inhibition.* This is a normal neurophysiological process. As motor neurons transmit impulses to agonist muscles, causing them to contract, the motor neurons that supply their antagonists are simultaneously and reciprocally inhibited. In treatment of spastic biceps, facilitation to the triceps reciprocally inhibits the biceps.

11. *Rotary joint compression.* For frozen shoulder, start with the patient's arm next to the body. The therapist stabilizes the shoulder with one hand, with the other hand on the elbow to apply force up the humerus into the shoulder joint. Then the therapist gently rotates the arm, increasing the amount of flexion and abduction. It may take as long as 20 min to get up to 90°. Joint compression of less than patient's body weight will be inhibitory to all the muscles around that joint.

Facilitation Techniques

1. *General rule.* Fast irregular rhythms in an activity have a stimulatory effect. Rolling, rocking, and shaking can be done rapidly for a stimulatory effect. Emotions also can activate the gamma-alpha coactivation system, i.e., increased spasticity when crying.

2. *Brushing.* Brushing is done with a battery-operated rotary mixer into which has been inserted a soft camel hair quill brush. The stimulus is applied over the dermatomal representation of the muscle to be facilitated, which, in most cases, corresponds with the area over the muscle belly. It is applied for approximately 10–15 sec per area. The fast repetitive stimulation is specifically received by exteroceptors and probably C fibers, with resultant effects on the gamma system. It is also beneficial in increasing circulation and thus aiding in skin care. This fast brushing can be used in cases of athetosis as well as spasticity and flaccidity. Since there is a latency period in the strongest effect of the brushing (10–30 min), this should be done first in the treatment period. Brush for either a flexor pattern or extensor pattern, but not both at the same time. Do not brush on children under 6 years of age or on seizure-prone patients. Do not brush across the midline above the forehead.

3. *Icing.* This is also facilitory to exteroceptors and probably C fibers. An ice cube that has been wrapped on one end for ease of handling is rubbed with pressure over the muscle belly that is to be facilitated for approximately 5 sec. The water is then wiped off. Three quick swipes on both sides of the abdomen following the curve of and just below the last rib are facilitory to the diaphragm. Remember that the temperature receptors respond to a critical change in temperature; so the response to the icing will be more effective if the part to be iced is warm or at least normal body temperature. Apply ice distal to proximal, since distal areas have greater cortical representation. Chewing ice is good for facilitating the tongue and swallowing. Don't flavor the ice. Anything with sugar, citric acid, or a dairy product will thicken the mucus and make swallowing difficult. Knott and Voss (PNF) use prolonged icing for 20 min as inhibitory to hypertonus. Precautions: Do not ice the head; do not ice anterior midline of trunk; do not ice posterior trunk. This gives a sympathetic nervous system reaction and could increase high blood pressure, etc. (caution for patients with cardiovascular problems). One can ice sternocleidomastoid, under chin, or around lips for lip closure.

Brushing and icing have bilateral effects. Therefore, in cases of hemiplegia, the noninvolved extremities should be brushed and iced before applying stimulation to the involved extremities.

4. *Vibrations.* Vibration is carried out with a battery-operated cosmetic vibrator. Vibration is a fast repetitive stimulus that yields immediate response but wears off in 3 min. It causes maintained arousal of the reticular system, which in turn activates the cortex. It is much safer than brushing because there is no afterdischarge. It

stimulates proprioceptors; therefore muscles and tendons are vibrated. Apply gentle pressure for more facilitory input when vibrating. Caution: Do not use with seizure-prone patients or children under 6 years of age.

5. *Vestibular stimulation.* In cases of hypotonia, the patient will benefit from fast rolling, spinning, tilting, and swinging in all planes. The patient must be watched for emotional reactions and sympathetic nervous system reaction! If fear is evident, stop and begin with a more gentle modified stimulus. This stimulation will increase tone generally. Use caution! Do not spin seizure-prone patients!

6. *Pressure.* Pressure acts through the muscle spindles and other proprioceptors and is effective as long as the stimulation is applied. Pressure to the muscle belly can be applied by tapping, rubbing, or hacking to facilitate that specific muscle. A quick stretch is facilitory for movement to the muscle stretched (through the stretch reflex). Joint compression applied with more than body weight will facilitate an extensor pattern and a co-contraction pattern. Joint traction, basically a form of stretch, will facilitate a pattern of flexion. Precaution: Do not use in the presence of fractures or for patients with poor skin condition.

7. *Resistance.* Resistance is a major tool in muscle stimulation and strengthening in the normal as well as in the neurologically damaged individual. It is a form of stretch in which the proprioceptors are stimulated and more motor units are called on to fire. When applying resistance, avoid patterns of incoordination. The amount of resistance must be graded for the particular patient, particular pattern, and position. If the resistance is strong, steady, and static, then a co-contraction will result. If movement is desired, downgrade the amount of resistance. In most cases it has been found beneficial when applying resistance to do so in a pattern of apply, hold, release, apply, hold, release, rather than applying a steady pull. The first procedure allows the muscle fibers to adjust, whereas the second procedure fatigues the muscle faster. Using resistance against a total pattern of movement increases sensory input because of the principle of irradiation (PNF).

8. *Taste and smell.* Taste reactions are especially important in patients with swallowing problems. Warm fluids will inhibit hyperactive swallowing, and salty and oily fluids (meat juices) will thin the mucus. These foods will make swallowing less difficult. Noxious oders have a stimulatory effect.

9. *Successive induction.* Successive induction is based on Sherrington's law that a muscle will contract more strongly if preceded by contraction of the antagonist. Clinically, apply alternating agonist and antagonist patterns of resistance (e.g., for weak wrist flexors, first give maximum resistance to wrist extensors, then without relaxing, give resistance to wrist flexors).

10. *Visual and auditory stimuli.* Bright colors are stimulatory. Fast, loud, irregular rhythms are stimulatory.

APPENDIX C: TREATMENT TECHNIQUES DEVELOPED BY ROOD[1]

Treatment Techniques Suggested for Hypotonic Patients: Floppy Baby Syndrome

Overall general stimulation: swinging, rolling, spinning, fast rocking in all planes for labyrinthine stimulation. Specific exteroceptive and proprioceptive stimulation for specific developmental patterns in proper sequence.

Treatment Techniques Suggested for Hypertonic Patients: Maintained Tone in Flexors or Extensors: Spastic CVA, CP, MS, MD

1. Neutral warmth for relaxation may be helpful (also slow rolling, slow stroking).
2. Exteroceptive and proprioceptive stimulation of antagonists of spastic (tight) musculature in appropriate developmental sequence.
3. Do not stretch the spastic musculature.

Treatment Techniques Suggested for Rigidity: Co-contraction of Both Flexors and Extensors: Parkinson's Disease

1. Neutral warmth and slow rolling for relaxation.
2. Stimulation for reciprocal movement patterns.

Treatment Techniques Suggested for Hyperkinetic patients where There Is Uncontrolled

[1] Compiled from Miss Joy Huss, O.T.R., R.P.T.; Mrs. S. Randolph, R.P.T.; and Mrs. S. Farber, O.T.R.

Movement: Athetosis, Chorea, Ataxia, Hyperactive Behavior

1. Slow stroking down the posterior primary rami for relaxation.
2. Stimulate for maintained holding patterns, keeping the distal segment stabilized until proximal control is obtained (prone on elbows, all-fours).
3. Progress to movement patterns of crawling, creeping, etc.

Follow-up Activities

It is very important that once the stimulation has been applied, it be followed with activity that will use the input on a cortical level. The patient's attention should be directed toward the activity itself, not the movements or performance per se. Activities should be selected that spontaneously elicit the automatic motor responses that have been facilitated through the previously described techniques. Once the patient is able to use the motor responses facilitated during therapy in meaningful activities, further mastery of motor skills occurs, and the level of functioning is enhanced. With a young child, activities will include toys and games of proper level. An older child or adult may engage in a craft, activity, game, gardening, or even household chores. These activities will be performed in the developmental position or pattern currently being stressed. For instance, checkers may be played in the prone-on-elbows position, or a craft activity such as block printing may be done in the all-fours position.

APPENDIX D: INTRODUCTION TO PNF AND APPLICATION TO OCCUPATIONAL THERAPY ACTIVITIES

Assisting to Positions

Side-lying to Side-sitting

Manual contacts: shoulders.

Techniques: quick stretch.

Verbal command: On the count of three, I want you to look back at me. One, two, three. Look (quick stretch with "look") at me.

Variation: may go from side-lying to side-lying on elbows before progressing to side-sitting. Side-lying on elbows is a position often used by paraplegic and quadriplegic patients on carts for eating and hygiene.

Side-sitting position is good for increasing trunk balance and enhancing facilitation and/or movement of upper arm, with stability, co-contraction, and joint compression of lower arm. Activities to do in this position: rhythmic stabilization, vibration of triceps (lower arm) for contraction, table buffer exercises, stacking cones (reaching behind body to pick them up), turning pages of newspaper or magazine, playing chess, watching TV, eating a snack, doing a rug punch stabilized in a vise.

Side-sitting to Long-sitting

Manual contacts: scapula and shoulder.

Procedure: Turn patient so that weight is distributed on both hips. Have patient look in direction of turn and reach over to support self with free arm. Position legs in extension, if necessary.

Long-sitting helps to increase sitting balance and provide stability for dressing legs in bed. It is easily applied to a variety of one-handed or two-handed activities. Some activities are the following: One-handed: stacking cones in a diagonal pattern, playing checkers, throwing bean bags, hitting ball with stick, sanding project positioned on slant board, painting. Two-handed: pulling putty, throwing and catching ball, rolling ball around body, macrame, leather stamping, throwing and molding clay, mixing ingredients in a bowl, preparing vegetables. Variation: small lapboard with legs placed over patient's legs provides hard working surface and expands type of activities that can be done in this position.

Prone to Prone on Elbows

Manual contact: shoulders.

Techniques: quick stretch (QS).

Verbal command: On the count of three, I want you to look up. One, two, three, Look (QS) up! (shift weight from one side to the other in order to get optimal position of forearm).

Prone on elbows increases head and neck control and stability of scapula. Applied activities vary according to strength and endurance in the position. Initially may just shift weight and practice lifting head or press down on elbows. Then progress to mildly resistive activities confined to

[1] Reprinted by the courtesy of Beverly Ritt, O.T.R., Supervisor, Rehabilitation Institute, Chicago, from Manual at Workshop on PNF for O.T., 1978.

small area within easy reach of hands, i.e., tile project, bringing crackers or pretzel to mouth, crocheting or drawing. Later perform an activity that requires balance on one arm only, i.e., typing one-handed, playing checkers, stacking cones, combing hair, and other grasp and release tasks.

Prone to Hands and Knees

Manual contacts: hips, then shoulders (stand with one foot at waist and other foot at knees).

Sequence: Tell the patient what you are going to do, and tell the patient to relax. Slide hips back over knees and hold firmly with your legs. Hold shoulders, and quick stretch to full extension of arms.

Verbal command: On count of three, I want you to look up. One, two, three, Look up!

Position provides opportunity to increase balance and stability in hips and shoulders. May begin activity by rhythmic stabilization and/or rocking in different directions: forward, backward, sideways, diagonally. Follow stabilizing tasks with simultaneous static/dynamic activity, i.e., stacking cones, sanding, hammering, placing tiles in trivet.

Application of all-fours position in daily activities would be washing and waxing floor, cleaning under bed, picking up item on floor, cleaning low shelves or oven, or working in garden.

Modified Plantigrade Position

This position is easily applied to most occupational therapy activities. A few are the following: washing dishes, wiping table, making bed, painting, grasp and release tasks, playing cards with card holder, throwing beanbags in a game of "toss across," getting out of bathtub.

GLOSSARY

Sensory-integrative process: As defined by Dr. Jean Ayres, this is the process of receiving sensory information or stimule, organizing it, and interpreting it, in order to produce a meaningful response.

Gross movement: performance of total body, especially postural activities, or of a number of body segments interacting.

Fine movement: performance of smaller units of body segments interacting in the motion, such as hand motion.

Isolated movement: performance of a specific body segment, in a separate and uncombined action.

Diagonal movement: motion obliquely across body midline.

Bias: a normal constant discharge of stimulation through the gamma motor neuron maintains muscle spindle tension and allows receptors to be highly sensitive to changes in skeletal length. This "gamma bias" provides background tension in the skeletal muscle. Therapy attempts to influence muscle tone in the abnormal CNS by biasing the muscle spindle through the use of sensory input.

Tonic: refers to a long lasting or maintained response, or a long-lasting input.

Phasic: refers to a short-lasting response or a short-lasting input.

Tonic muscles: also called stabilizers, these muscles function in a maintained continuous response for endurance activities or for weight-bearing.

Phasic muscles: also called mobilizers, these muscles function to provide a rapid response for flexibility and speed.

Upper Motor Neuron (UMN): "consists of a nerve cell in the motor cortex with its processes which pass through the internal capsule, brain stem, and spinal cord by way of corticobulbar or corticospinal tract to the lower motor neuron." (Ref. 32)

Lower Motor Neuron (LMN): "also called the final common pathway, this consists of a cell body in the anterior gray column of the spinal cord and an axon passing by way of peripheral nerves to the motor end plates of muscles" (Ref. 32)

Posturing: the body assumes and maintains an abnormal static postural attitude due to an imbalance of muscle tone.

Functional Effects of Sensory Input in Neurobiological Disorders

9

Arthur J. Nelson

The central nervous system (CNS) has been termed a pattern generator that has inherent movement sequences that are subsequently guided by sensory messages from the periphery. When there are disorders of the CNS, at least three general problems can arise: (a) dyskinesia or akinesia, (b) loss of appropriateness of control, (c) imbalance between tone and motor control. An explanation of the effects of sensory input on functioning when there is disordered functioning requires exploration of the role of sensory input in movement control in the intact individual.

CONCEPTS OF MOTOR CONTROL

The idea that movement is a sensory-motor phenomenon is attributed to Mott and Sherrington (1). This concept was expanded by Sherrington (2) to form a basis for a hierarchical organization of the nervous system whereby discrete stereotyped reflexes are linked together with sensory feedback involved at each level added. These early investigators formed this concept on the basis of findings that an animal became paralyzed when the muscular and cutaneous afferents were sectioned. Lassek (3) and Twitchell (4) replicated these studies and found that afferent impulses from the skin, muscles, and joints were essential for the production of "higher-level" movement.

A diametrically opposite view was offered by Lashley and Ball (5), who reported that severance of the proprioceptive afferents in rats resulted in no loss in running proficiency. Taub and Berman (6) found that unilateral deafferentation resulted in greater deficiencies in functioning than if both limbs were deafferented. Taub et al. (7) went on to claim that sensory feedback is not even necessary in the early stages of learning movements. Bossom (8) criticized the latter on the basis that vision was preserved and was found to be an important source of recovery of motor function in deafferented limbs. Granit (9) suggested that deafferentation may not result in profound disability because the CNS may press alternate circuits into action.

Studies by Coggeshall et al. (10) also suggested that some unmyelinated afferents may enter the ventral root and that therefore deafferentation of dorsal roots may not interrupt all sensory feedback. Shik and Orlovsky (11) demonstrated that mesencephalic cats can ambulate (once the pattern is established) when electrical stimulation is applied to the midbrain, despite deafferentation. Apparently there are centrally generated motor programs that can be executed when the movement has been practiced and is somewhat automatic. Significantly, these investigators found that unexpected changes in the environment required the presence of afferents for appropriate response. Evarts (12) and Thach (13) have also discovered that there are internal afferent feedback mechanisms, as evidenced by the finding that the precentral gyrus motor cortical cells discharge prior to movement in rhesus monkeys. Eccles (14) has shown the existence of cerebral-cerebellar loops in humans as well as animals that provide for a check on motor accuracy considerably prior to the influence of peripheral feedback. Peripheral feedback is thereby placed on a background of a centrally generated motor program that is checked internally by cerebellar-cerebral loops that are reinforced by peripheral feedback that arrives in a pattern that serves to predict the next sequence in the motor plan. Sensory feedback from the periphery, then, is involved not only in providing knowledge of results but also in formulating predictors of future actions. Evarts (12) demonstrated in primates that there are predictor discharges within cortical circuits 18 to 40 msec prior to initiation of motor cortical cellular action. He also found in another study (15) that the stretch reflex response could be enhanced through anticipation of a movement in that same muscle group, whereas the stretch response became diminished when the anticipation was to the opposite muscle group.

MOTOR UNIT PATTERNS OF ACTIVITY

Skeletal muscle action or inaction is ultimately determined by the state of depolarization of the anterior horn cell membrane. In the resting state the cell is negatively charged to 70 mV or more. Two opposite-acting nerve endings on the anterior horn cell influence the cell either toward depolarization or toward hyperpolarization. Small motor neurons will fire an all-or-none spike potential when 30 mV of depolarization is reached, whereas the larger motor neurons require 50 mV to fire them. It is believed that physiological flexor muscles have a higher percentage of motor neurons that require greater levels of depolarization or a higher threshold (Fig. 1).

Burke and Edgerton (16) have indicated that human muscle is a checkerboard of at least three muscle fiber types. On one extreme there is the phasic, pale, type II muscle fiber that is rich in glycolytic enzymes; when activated, it responds with a fast-twitch short-lived response. On the other extreme there is the tonic, dark, type I muscle fiber that is also quite endurant. In between these extremes is type III fiber, which has a relatively fast twitch and is moderately endurant, with oxidative glycolytic enzymes. This is the fiber type that can perhaps be modified most (Fig. 2).

Kugelberg and Engels (17) identified the human soleus muscle as having 65% type I fibers, with the major balance being of type III. Conversely, they identified the extensor digitorum longus as being composed of 60% type II, with an admixture of types I and III. Obviously a muscle with increased density of type I will be a slower-acting muscle and will be more endurant, but also will not produce high levels of force. Endurance training of this muscle will result in an enhanced capillary bed, improved mitochondrial density, and an improved oxidative enzyme state, according to Burke and Edgerton (16). They also indicated that high power production by a muscle results in hypertrophy of the type II fibers. Thorstensson et al. (18) found in healthy young males that high-velocity training was correlated with increased density of type II fibers in the vastus lateralis (biopsy histological survey).

The muscle spindle afferents also have a much more significant influence on the smaller type I fibers than on type III and even more than on type II. Thus reflex influences from the spindle have the greatest impact on muscles with greater quantities of type I, such as the soleus muscle. Conversely, a muscle like the extensor digitorum longus will have less reflex influence. The more phasic the muscle, the more direct the control from higher centers. In CNS disorders there is a common observation that patients can engage in low-level motor output but cannot develop tension rapidly. Tokizane and Shimazu (19), using frequency analysis, demonstrated preservation of tonic motor unit discharge and generally an ab-

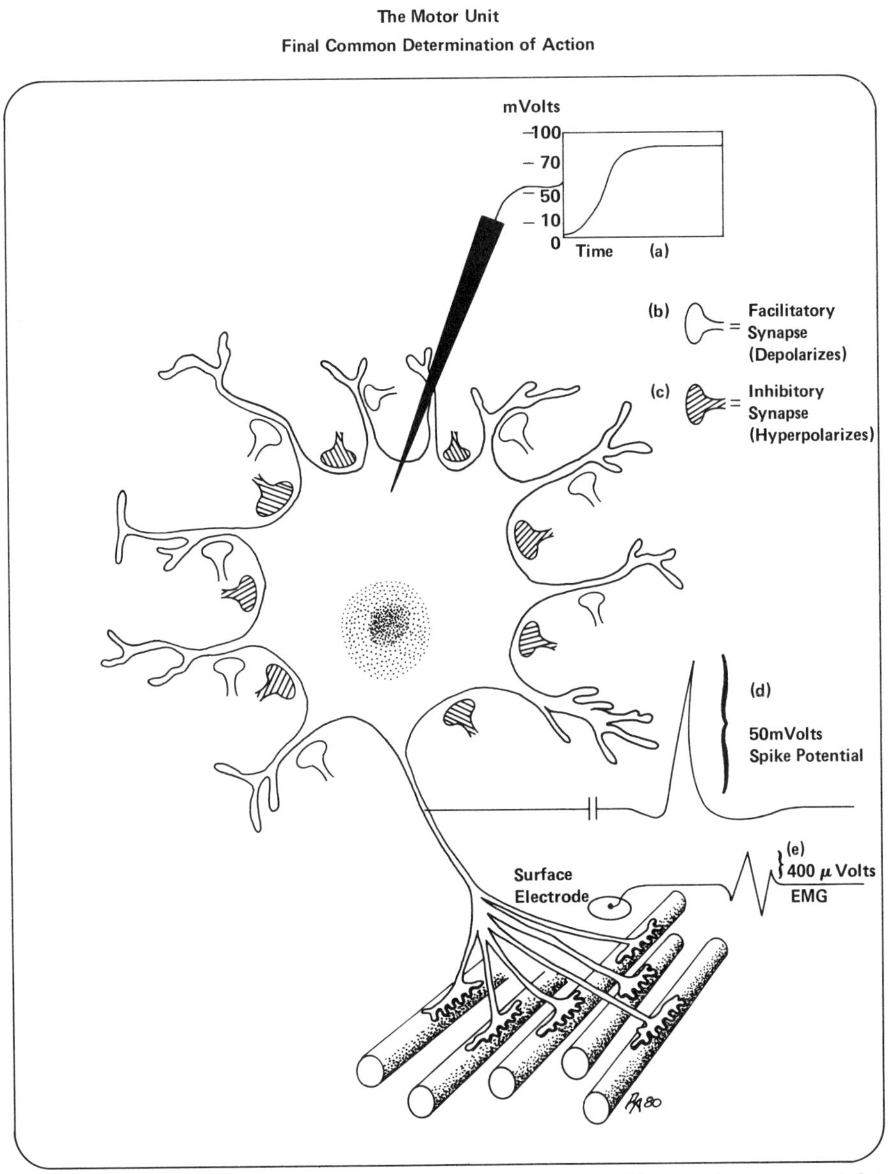

FIG. 1. The motor unit is the final determinant of action or inaction. The resting potential **(a)** is generally −70 to −90 mV. The synapses are either facilitory **(b)** or inhibitory **(c)**. Should the depolarization **(b)** achieve threshold, a spike potential occurs **(d)**.

sence of phasic motor unit activity. Electromyographic (EMG) feedback techniques may then be employed to terminate motor unit activity abruptly, because the low-level tonic activity is also quite endurant and therefore will persist for protracted periods of time.

Another general problem for the CNS-lesioned patient is execution of the appropriate amount of tension. For example, during locomotion it is essential that the quadriceps muscle contract rapidly to decelerate the forward momentum from heel strike to mid-stance. If the power produced is inadequate, the knee will collapse; if the tension developed is excessive, the knee will remain in extension instead of flexing slightly during mid-stance. Another challenge to the patient is to develop not only sufficient tension but also rapid application of the tension; otherwise the knee will not decelerate the knee rapidly enough, and when the tension finally achieves the proper level, the knee will snap back because the sustained calf muscle action will assist the late quad-

Motor-Unit Composition of Human Skeletal Muscle

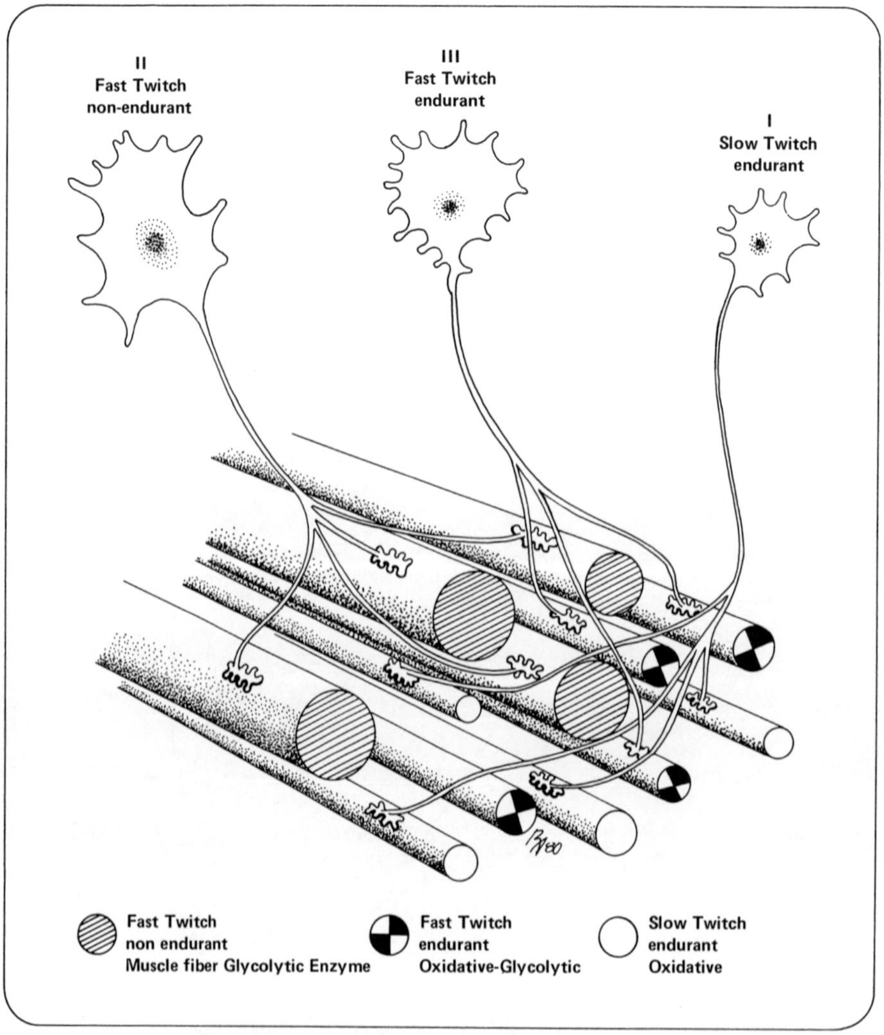

FIG. 2. Motor unit composition of human skeletal muscle. Symbolic representation of the extremes possible within skeletal muscle. The fast-twitch fibers provide high-amplitude short-duration responses, and the slow-twitch fibers provide responses of lower amplitude and longer duration.

riceps to extend the knee. This mechanism may predispose the knee to recurvation.

INTEGRATIVE PROPERTIES OF NEURONS

The neurons in the spinal cord (and elsewhere) are covered with synapses, with the excitatory ones tending to synapse on dendrites and the inhibitory ones on the cell body. The algebraic and temporal summation of these excitatory and inhibitory inputs ultimately determines action or inaction in the system (Fig. 1). The neuron is thereby able to respond to input from many sources and provide a coding by modulating the frequency of firing. For instance, a large number of excitatory postsynaptic potentials (EPSP) in a brief period of time will depolarize the cell with a series of spike potentials. If excitation is very intense, the cell will remain depolarized above its threshold and tend to fire at a higher frequency of firing, proportional to the input intensity, which is referred to as frequency coding by modulation.

Following repeated discharge of a synaptic pathway, the transmitters are readily released. This phenomenon has been called the first physiological evidence of simple learning.

RECEPTORS AS ERROR DETECTORS

Mosaic patterns of proprioceptive (muscle stretch, tension, and joint movement), exteroceptive (touch, heat, and pressure), and distance (sight, smell, and sound) messages incessantly bombard the nervous system. All receptors are specialized endings of nerves that transform some physical or mechanical stimuli into an electrical code. When a nerve ending is distorted, its membrane creates a graded depolarization known as a generator potential. When this generator potential reaches the axon's threshold, it results in a spike potential. Increased strength of stimulus increases the frequency of firing, thereby creating a code for the CNS to formulate patterns of response appropriate to the input.

The anatomic structure of the receptor determines to a major extent the nature of the events it will respond to. When a receptor is encapsulated, there is a tendency for it to adapt mechanically to the stimulus more rapidly. Most exteroceptors tend to have a rapid rate of adaptation. This adaptation prevents overstimulation of the system and also provides distinct frequency modulation, eventually formulating distinct patterns of responses to specific stimuli.

During movement, the adaptation property of receptors assures continual updating of information to the motor neurons. If the cutaneous receptors have a steady contact, they will adapt, and there will be no continual change of input, thereby supporting a response of static posture. The structures of the exteroceptors then give messages that increasingly discharge with wider or more rapid contact. The action brought about continues the change in contact, thereby keeping the motion maintained. Constant contact will signal error should movement be taking place simultaneously.

A review of the properties of receptors found within muscles, tendons, and joints supports the previous notion that sensory input detects departure of the motor program from the initial plan of action. They can generally be classified as error detectors that provide feedback in increasing amounts when the movement does not meet with the expected interactional environmental requirements.

The joint receptors are responsive to joint position and movement in the extremes of motion, but not in the mid-region, according to Eyzaquire and Fidone (20) and Somjen (21). Ralston (22) demonstrated in cineplastic arm amputees that extreme positions of the elbow joint resulted in a significant decrease in isometric tension in the biceps brachii (detached distal tendon). Apparently the mid-position of the joint provides minimal biomechanical advantage in this mid-range. It is evident that this area becomes an optimal site for action and is a type of target. As the movement goes farther from this target area, the nerve endings fire with increasing frequency.

Monitoring of tension in muscles as signaled by the neurotendinous organs (Golgi tendon organs) has revealed that they are more sensitive to active tension, according to Eldred (23).

These series-connected tension recorders result in inhibition of the motor neurons supplying the originating muscle, thereby autogenetically limiting the rate of tension development, keeping the movement within a given range. The tendon receptors are increasingly active when tension moves above 20% of the maximum capacity of the muscle, which suggests that higher levels of tension fall outside most routine motor patterns. Should a movement require more than this moderate to low-level output, the higher centers must overcome the inhibition of the tendon organs. This would imply that these receptors detect error and guide tension toward specific levels.

Length change in a muscle is monitored by the muscle spindle. Because muscles are predominantly arranged mechanically to enhance speed and range of movement, a small amount of length change in the muscle will be enhanced markedly by the time it is manifested distally. Small oscillations of the muscle will result in a tremor peripherally of greater magnitude. Obviously, the spindles will fire if the gross muscle tension is being overcome, thereby increasing the firing of the motor units to bring the muscle to the appropriate length. The spindles within the shortening muscle are capable of responding to changes in load (and therefore length change) because of dual independent motor control of the spindles that makes them tighten in proportion to the gross muscle shortening. Their role then is to provide increasing afferent discharge when the length of the muscle deviates from the planned amount (Fig. 3).

When a muscle is contracted, given numbers of smaller motor units are recruited initially, and as the contraction increases, larger motor units are brought in. Vallbo (24) has demonstrated that in addition to these alpha motor neurons discharg-

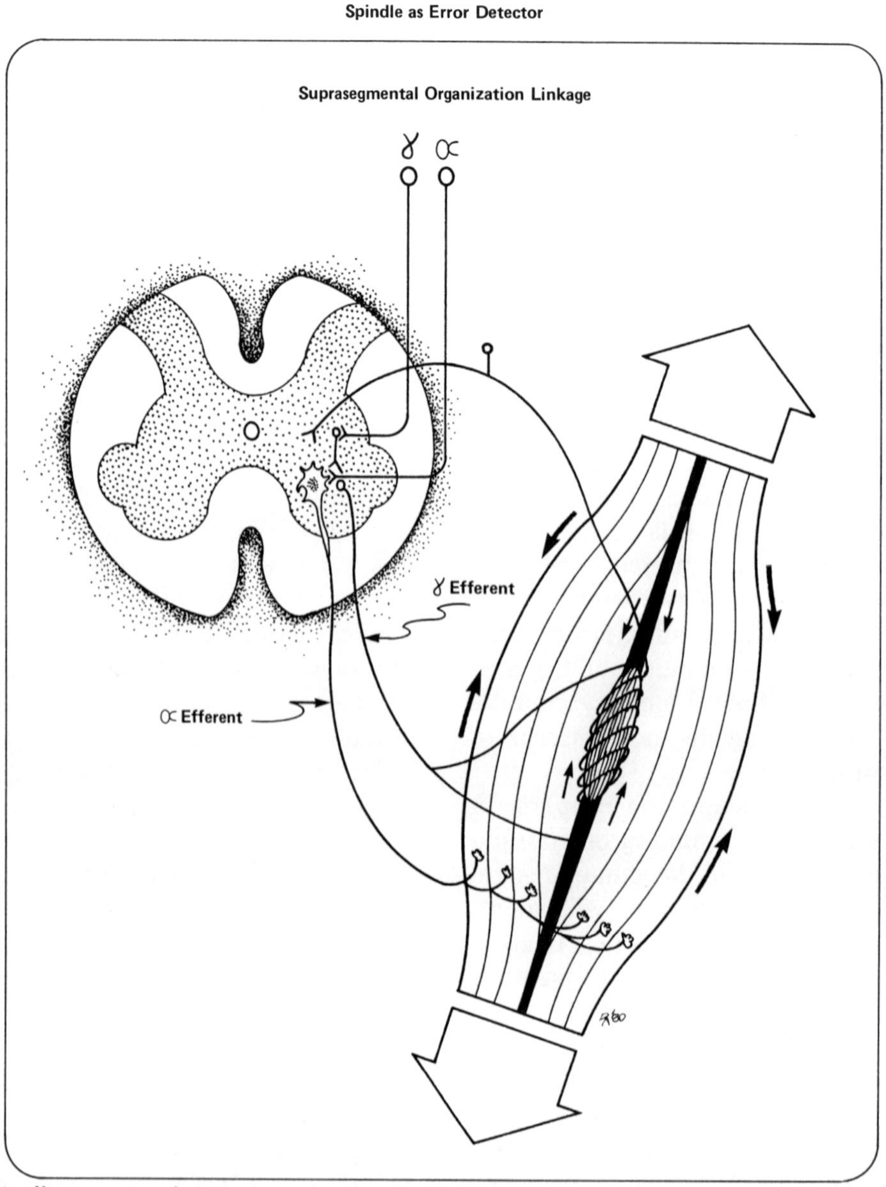

FIG. 3. Muscle spindle as error detector: suprasegmental organization. Alpha efferent discharge is paired with fusimotor discharge, and if the skeletal muscle is insufficiently contracted, this will result in stretch. The spindle is activated, and increased alpha efferent discharge provides the correction.

ing, there is a parallel discharge of the muscle spindle's efferent neurons (gamma efferents) during activation of the muscle. This matching of alpha and gamma discharges, as proposed by Granit (25), has been altered in tests of normal subjects by Smith (26) and Nelson (27) through fusimotor deafferentation. Both investigators found that fusimotor blockade resulted in no change in the maximum force developed; however, there was decreased accuracy when attempting to attain specific target levels of power. This would suggest that the spindle is involved in the process of attaining accurate motor control. Because loss of motor control is a major problem in CNS-lesioned patients, control of the fusimotor system is essential for retraining (Fig. 4).

In CNS disorders there is a release of these primitive tuning reflexes resulting in increased muscle stretch responses that Hughlings Jackson referred to as a release phenomenon. This release is manifested as spasticity or as dystonia. Absence of fusimotor input has resulted in improved movement in tests by some investigators (28), but no improvement for others (29). Brudny et al. (30)

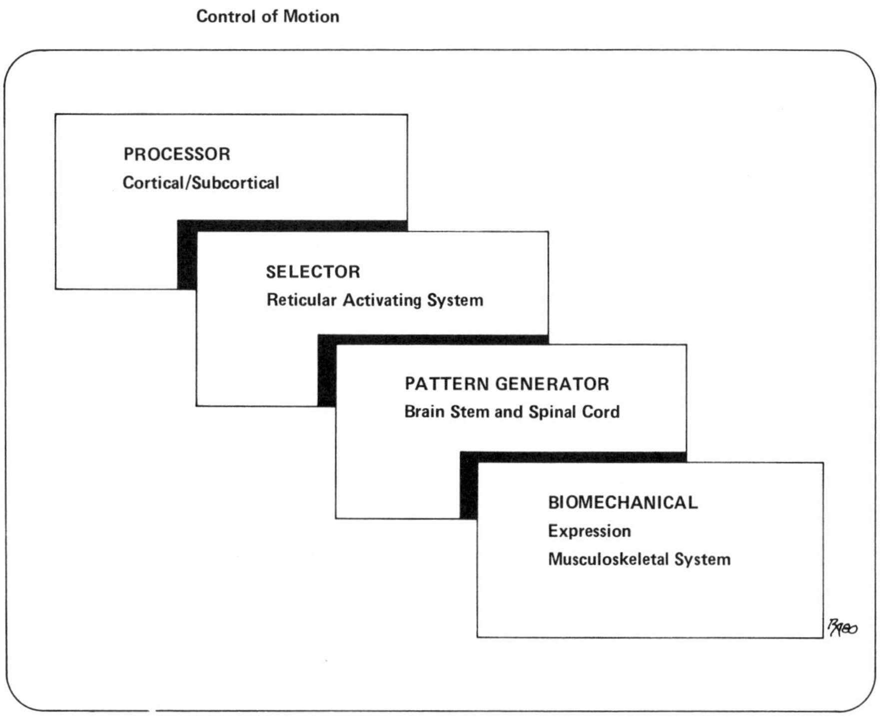

FIG. 4. Control of motion.

found that skeletal muscle EMG feedback was most effective in rectifying dystonic imbalance in torticollis patients. This implies that dystonia results from prolonged low-level motor neuron discharge, not from excessive fusimotor discharge, as noted by Wiesendanger (31). The latter investigator suggested that some forms of increased muscle stretch responses result from loss of presynaptic spindle afferent (Ia) inhibition, which is a corollary function of corticospinal tracts. Improved activation of motor neurons through improved feedback should then be simultaneously involved in presynaptic inhibition of proprioceptive afferents (Fig. 5).

Another prominent feature of CNS motor system lesions is loss of distal, highly developed, learned motor behavior. The need for feedback in this type of movement control is demonstrated by the direct studies of Goldring and Ratcheson (32) involving motor cortex units in conscious human subjects. They found that these units responded vigorously to passive joint movement with bilateral sensory and motor correlation. Superficial somatic and auditory inputs were ineffective in producing motor cortex neuronal activity. They implied that multisensory integration probably occurs to a greater extent at lower levels in humans than in animals.

The corticospinal tracts, in view of Lawrence and Kuyper (33), superimpose speed and agility on the subcortical spinal pathways that provide for total body activity.

The contention that motor control can be improved in spastic patients with fusimotor blockade has been refuted by recent investigations by Sahrman and Norton (34). They suggested emphasis on the appropriate quantity and quality of discharges of alpha as well as fusimotor neurons to effect controlled movement. This suggests that strategies that give the patient accurate information about the motor neuron discharge, either directly or through function, will be most effective in improving subsequent control of those motor neuron pools. Furthermore, the timing of the pairing of alpha and gamma discharges will be closer to the normal relationship if the movements are executed with appropriate force production in a specified period of time. It has been suggested by Landau (35) that tactile and visual feedback dominates distal precise motor control in the intact subject. Conversely, in the CNS-lesioned patient, mass movement responses are

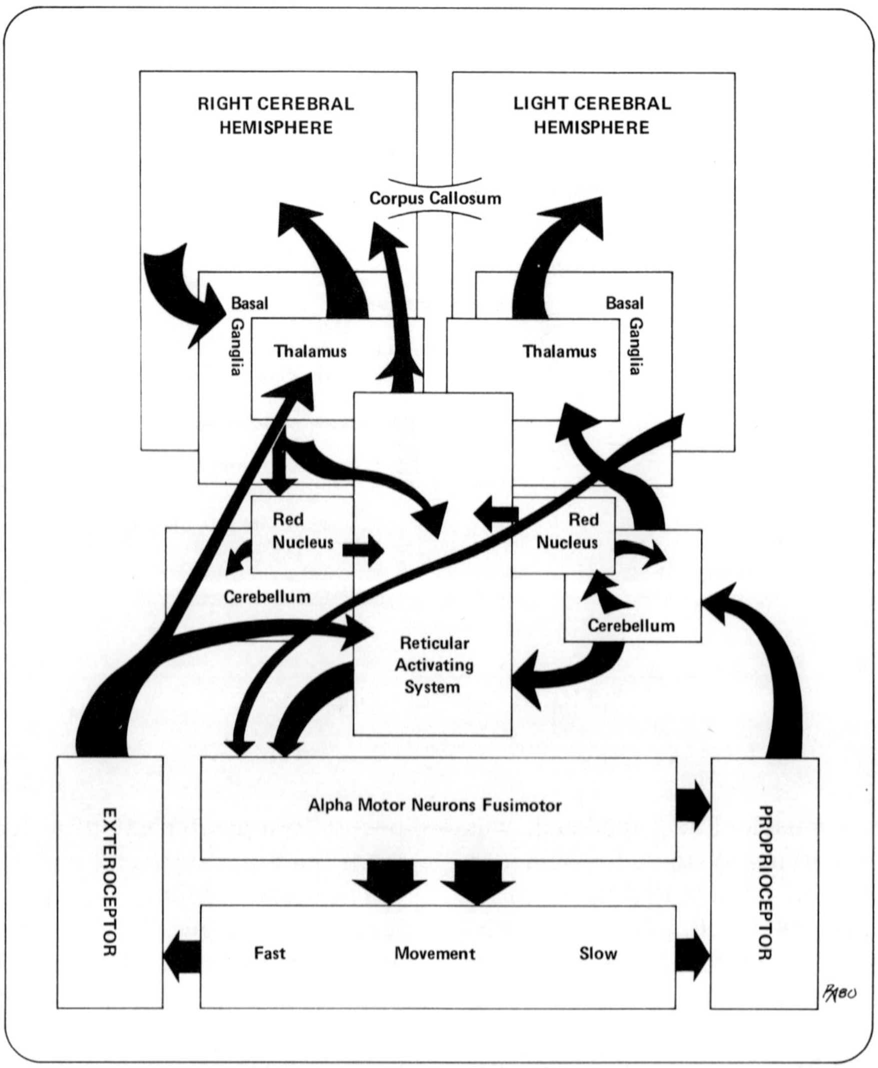

FIG. 5. Neural substrate of motion.

produced by even superficial tactile stimuli. Therefore, the more the sensory stimuli are involved with movement actively produced, the less mass response may be elicited. Activation of corticospinal pathways is reportedly (36) a source of inhibition to the nuclei cuneatus and gracilis, thereby diminishing generalized hypersensitivity and providing for more selective sensory-motor integration.

SUMMARY

The CNS can be considered a pattern generator that ultimately discharges motor units in muscles that respond in a range of actions extending from rapid and short-lived to slow and sustained. Sensory input appears to have a major role in error detection in the execution of the motor patterns. Augmentation of these patterns with EMG feedback should stress rate of motor unit production, appropriateness of output level, and abrupt termination. The roles of selected receptors have been outlined, with implications for the improvement of motor control in neurobiological disorders. Neurobiological disorders generally manifest (a) loss of rate of tension development, (b) loss of appropriate level of motor power, and (c) inability to rapidly inhibit motor output. Providing knowledge of results, from patient-initiated actions, through internal sensory pathways or through augmented external sensory mechanisms is essential in reformulating a central, outgoing program of motor control. Sensory response is most effective when it is occasioned by activity patterns that approximate those usually encountered by the individual.

REFERENCES

1. Mott, F. W., and Sherrington, C. S. (1895): *Proc. R. Soc.*, 57:481–488.
2. Sherrington, C. S. (1906): *The Integrative Action of the Nervous System*. Yale University Press, New Haven.
3. Lassek, A. M. (1953): Inactivation of voluntary motor function following rhizotomy. *J. Neuropathol. Exp. Neurol.*, 12:83–87.
4. Twitchell, T. E. (1954): Sensory factors in purposive movement. *J. Neurophysiol.*, 17:239–252.
5. Lashley, K. S., and Ball, J. (1929): *J. Comp. Physiol.*, 9:71–106.
6. Taub, E., and Berman, A. J. (1968): Movement and learning in absence of sensory feedback. In: *The Neurophysiology of Spatially Oriented Behavior*, edited by S. J. Freedman, pp. 173–192. Dorsey, Homewood, Ill.
7. Taub, E., Perrella, P., and Barro, G. (1973): Alertness, level of activity, and purposive movement following somato-sensory deafferation in monkeys. *Annals N.Y. Acad. Science*, 290:959–960.
8. Bossom, J. (1974): Visual responses in deafferented recovery. *Brain Res.*, 21:285–296.
9. Granit, R. (1970): *The Basis of Motor Control*. Academic Press, New York.
10. Coggeshall, R. E., Coulter, J. D., and Willis, W. D. (1973): *Abst. Proc. Neurosci. Soc.*, p. 387.
11. Shik, M. L., Orlovski, G. N. (1976): Neurophysiology of locomotor automatism. *Physiol. Rev.*, 56:465–501.
12. Evarts, E. V. (1973): Motor cortex reflexes associated with learned movement. *Science*, 179:501–503.
13. Thach, W. T. (1970): Discharge of cerebellar neurons related to two maintained postures and two prompt movements and nuclear cell output. *J. Neurophysiol.*, 33:527–547.
14. Eccles, J. C. (1973): *The Understanding of the Brain*. McGraw-Hill, New York.
15. Evarts, E. V. (1968): Relation of pyramidal tract activity to force exerted during voluntary movement. *J. Neurophysiol.*, 31:14.
16. Burke, R. E., and Edgerton, V. R. (1975): Motor unit properties and selective involvement in movement. In: *Exercise and Sport Sciences Reviews, Vol. 3*, edited by J. H. Wilmore and J. F. Keough, pp. 31–81. Academic Press, New York.
17. Kugelberg, E., and Engels, K. (1973): The motor unit. In: *New Developments in EMG and Clinical Neurophysiology, Vol. 1*, edited by J. E. Desmedt, pp. 2–13, Karger Publishing, Belgium.
18. Thorstensson, A., Grimby, G., and Karlsson, J. (1976): Force-velocity relations and fiber composition in human knee extensor muscles. *J. Appl. Physiol.*, 40:12–16.
19. Tokizane, T., and Shimazu, H. (1964): *Functional Differentiation of Human Skeletal Muscle*. Charles C Thomas, Springfield, Ill.
20. Eyzaquire, C., and Fidone, S. N. (1975): *Physiology of the Nervous System*, ed. 2. Year Book, Chicago.
21. Somjen, G. (1972): *Sensory Coding in the Mammalian Nervous System*. Appleton-Century-Crofts, New York.
22. Ralston, J. (1958): *Recent Advances in Neurophysiology*. Institute for Rehabilitation, New York University, New York.
23. Eldred, E. (1976): Recent advances in physiology of muscle receptors. In: *Neurophysiological Aspects of Rehabilitation Medicine*, edited by E. Buerger and J. Tobis, pp. 2–15. Charles C Thomas, Springfield, Ill.
24. Vallbo, A. B. Muscle spindle afferent discharge from resting and contrasting muscles in normal human subjects. In: *Neurophysiological Aspects* of Rehabilitation Medicine, edited by E. Buerger and J. Tobis, pp. 251–262. Charles C Thomas, Springfield, Ill.
25. Granit, R., and Burke, R. E. (1973): The control of movement and posture. *Brain Res.*, 53:1–28.
26. Smith, J. L. (1972): Fusimotor neuron block and voluntary arm movement in man. *Am. J. Phys. Med.*, 51:225–239.
27. Nelson, A. J. (1976): Fusimotor influence on performance of ankle dorsiflexion in young adults. *Physiotherapy*, 62:117–124.
28. Khalili, A. A., and Betts, H. B. (1970): *Management of Spasticity with Phenol Nerve Block*. Report RD-2529M, Social and Rehabilitation Service, U.S. Public Health Service, Washington, D.C.
29. Landau, W. M. (1969): Spasticity and rigidity. In: *Recent Advances in Neurology, Vol. 6*, edited by F. Plum, pp. 1–32. F. A. Davis Co., Philadelphia.
30. Brudny, J., Korein, J., Grynbaum, B., and Sachs-Frankel, G. (1977): Sensory feedback therapy in patients with brain insult. *Scand. J. Rehabil. Med.*, 9:155–163.
31. Wiesendanger, M. (1972): *Pathophysiology of Muscle Tone*. Springer-Verlag, New York.

32. Goldring, S., and Ratcheson, R. (1972): Human motor cortex: Sensory input data from single neuron recordings. *Science,* 175:1493–1495.
33. Lawrence, D. G., and Kuypers, H. G. J. M. (1965): Pyramidal and nonpyramidal pathways in monkeys: Anatomical and functional correlates. *Science,* 148:973–975.
34. Sahrman, S. A., and Norton, B. J. (1977): The relation of voluntary movement to spasticity in the upper motor neuron syndrome. *Ann. Neurol.,* 2:460–465.
35. Landau, W. M. (1974): Movement disorders. In: *Neurological Pathophysiology,* edited by S. G. Eliassen, A. L. Prensky, and W. B. Hardin, pp. 132–140. Oxford University Press, London.
36. Eliassen, S. G., Prensky, A. L., and Hardin, W. B. (editors) (1974): *Neurological Pathophysiology.* Oxford University Press, London.

Interdisciplinary Approach to the Adult Visual Perceptual Function-Dysfunction Continuum

10

Beatriz Colon Abreu

This chapter presents a review of interdisciplinary concepts in the areas of neurophysiology, neuroanatomy, cognitive psychology, psychophysics and rehabilitation as they relate to perception. It proposes an eclectic and interdisciplinary approach for the adult visual perception function-dysfunction continuum. The evaluation and intervention strategies are based on extensive clinical experience with acquired brain injured adults. The concepts of environmental enrichment and structural reorganization are postulated as efficient treatment techniques to ameliorate perceptual motor deficits in these patients.

The character of the cortical relationship will differ at different stages of functional development. The factor of age is often neglected in the Occupational Therapy educational experience relative to visual perception function-dysfunction continuum. The theoretical background provided in basic professional education, then, fails to prepare the student or the clinician for the responsibility of dealing with the "matured" patient that acquired visual perceptual dysfunctions. Many clinicians in an attempt to design evaluation and treatment techniques tend to generalize directly from the pediatrics visual-perceptual frames of reference. This is unfortunate and many times leads to incomplete and or incorrect interpretation of this patient population's functions and dysfunctions. The theories established for children with visual perceptual problems were not designed for the adolescent, adult or aged.

More detailed examination of the adult visual perceptual process is needed at the college level as well as the postgraduate and continuing education levels. Such programs should help to improve the quality of care for brain-injured adults.

PERCEPTION

Perception is a personal, subjective, and sometimes puzzling process by which each individual actively searches and judges the external environment. Thus far, the process of perception can be formulated only in vague terms. It is not known how light reflected from an object creates an optic stimulus that leads to visual perception.

Humans are more than just information-processing devices that gather and transform information through sensory and motor systems. Expectations, motivations, and past experiences, as well as genetic factors inherent in the sensory-motor system, can change the processing of incoming stimuli and their interpretation. This ability to change programs that have been established by genetics or experience separates humans from machines and other processing devices; these devices inevitably respond to stimuli in a preprogrammed manner (1–5).

Luria (6) pointed out that human perception is a complex process of coding perceived material that takes place in close conjunction with speech. Human perceptual activity never takes place without the direct participation of language. Language involves systematic communication of ideas or feelings by the use of conventionalized signs, gestures, marks, and articulate vocal sounds. Language has a productive aspect and a receptive aspect. Perception, language, and memory must be combined into one picture in order to understand the information-processing mechanism.

NEURONS AND SYNAPSES

All levels of the nervous system are involved in perception. The nervous system is an organized constellation of nerve cells and associated nonneural cells (Figs. 1 and 2). Specialized functions of this system are reception, integration, and transmission of neuronal impulses, by means of which the individual perceives. The nerve cell or neuron is the system's communicating device. Nerve cells do not communicate with one another by direct contact; they must bridge the tiny gaps between them. These gaps between nerve cells are called synapses. They can be bridged by chemical or electrical means and thus are classified as chemical or electric synapses (7–9) (Fig. 3).

In the case of chemical synapses, the nerve cells communicate by secreting neurotransmitter substances that traverse the tiny gap. In the case of electrical synapses, communication between cells is accomplished by flow of electrical current not involving chemical action (Fig. 3). The synapses seem to be the most likely structural elements whose changes could underlie changes in behavior (7–10).

Both types of synapses carry information by means of electrical signals. The electrical or electrophysiological potentials between neurons have various characteristics. They are classified into two kinds of potentials: action potentials, or spikes, and graded potentials.

The action potentials involve active voltage; they are excitatory and self-propagating, producing an all-or-none response. They cannot sum; therefore they are nondecremental. They are considered to be of digital frequency and seem to be created for traveling long distances.

The graded potentials involve passive voltage. They can be excitatory or inhibitory; they can add temporally and spatially and can algebraically cancel each other out. They can also decay. They are considered to be of analog frequency and seem to be created for integration, lasting longer and for shorter distances.

Regardless of shape, size, location, and function, most nerve cells can be described in terms of a neuron containing signaling potentials: resting, excitatory, and inhibitory synaptic potentials (7,11,12). Examples of macroneurons are the pyramidal neurons, Purkinje neurons, and spinal motor neurons (Fig. 4). They develop early in life; they are relatively inflexible, rigidly structured, forming true circuits; they appear to be for fast speeds and long distances. Their resting potential is −70 or −90 mu. They involve chemical synapses, and they conduct in both graded and spike potentials. They are also classic in the manner they communicate, going from cell axon to dendrite.

Examples of microneurons are the stellate cells and granule cells; others are called local neuronal circuits (LNCs) (Fig. 4). These cells become both more complex and more numerous with progression up the phylogenetic scale. They develop late in life and seem to be slower, for shorter distances, such as in integration. They appear to be relatively flexible in their synaptic communication patterns, connecting, for example, axon-dendrite, axon-axon, and dendrite-dendrite. They involve both chemical and electrical synapses, and their resting potential is −20 mu (Fig. 5).

VISUAL PATHWAY AND RECEPTIVE FIELD

Experiments in subhuman primates have contributed to perception theory. Kuffler, working with cats at Johns Hopkins Hospital, discovered that some analysis of visual patterns takes place outside the brain in the retina. Hubel and Weisel

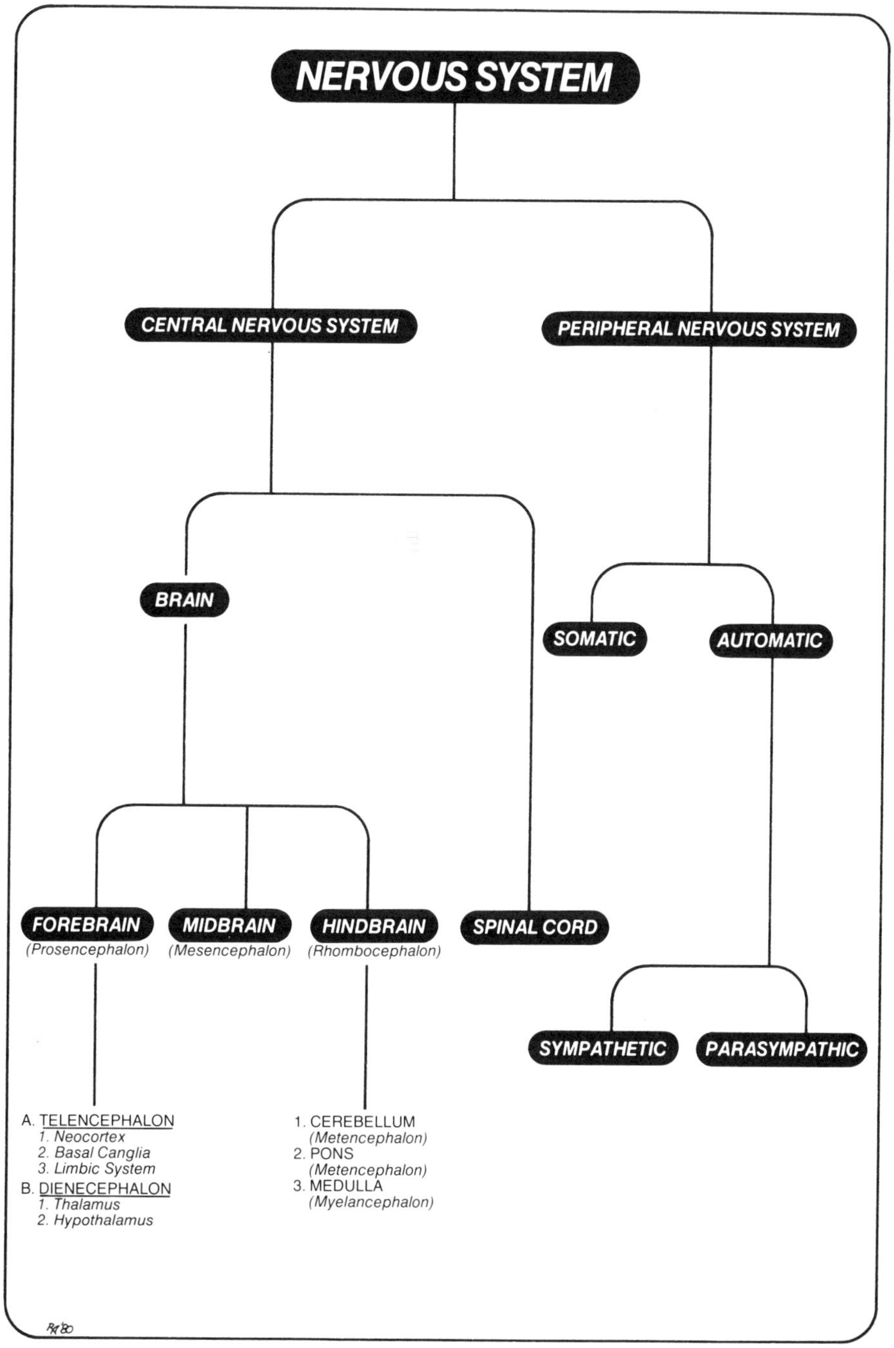

FIG. 1. Adapted from Dr. Ausma Rabe.

at Harvard Medical School continued to elaborate this concept and mapped the visual pathway a little farther, establishing six steps from the retina to the cortex. This information provided some idea of the mechanisms and circuitry of the visual system. Extrapolation of data from the visual system of the cat to the human model has influenced the theory of perception. Information about feature-processing cells has been used by psychologists to explain letter recognition, visual illusion, visual acuity, line orientation, and motion aftereffect. These experiments were landmarks in the development of an understanding of how the visual neurons respond to visual stimuli. Figures 5 and 6 show the theoretical representation of the visual pathway and the characteristics

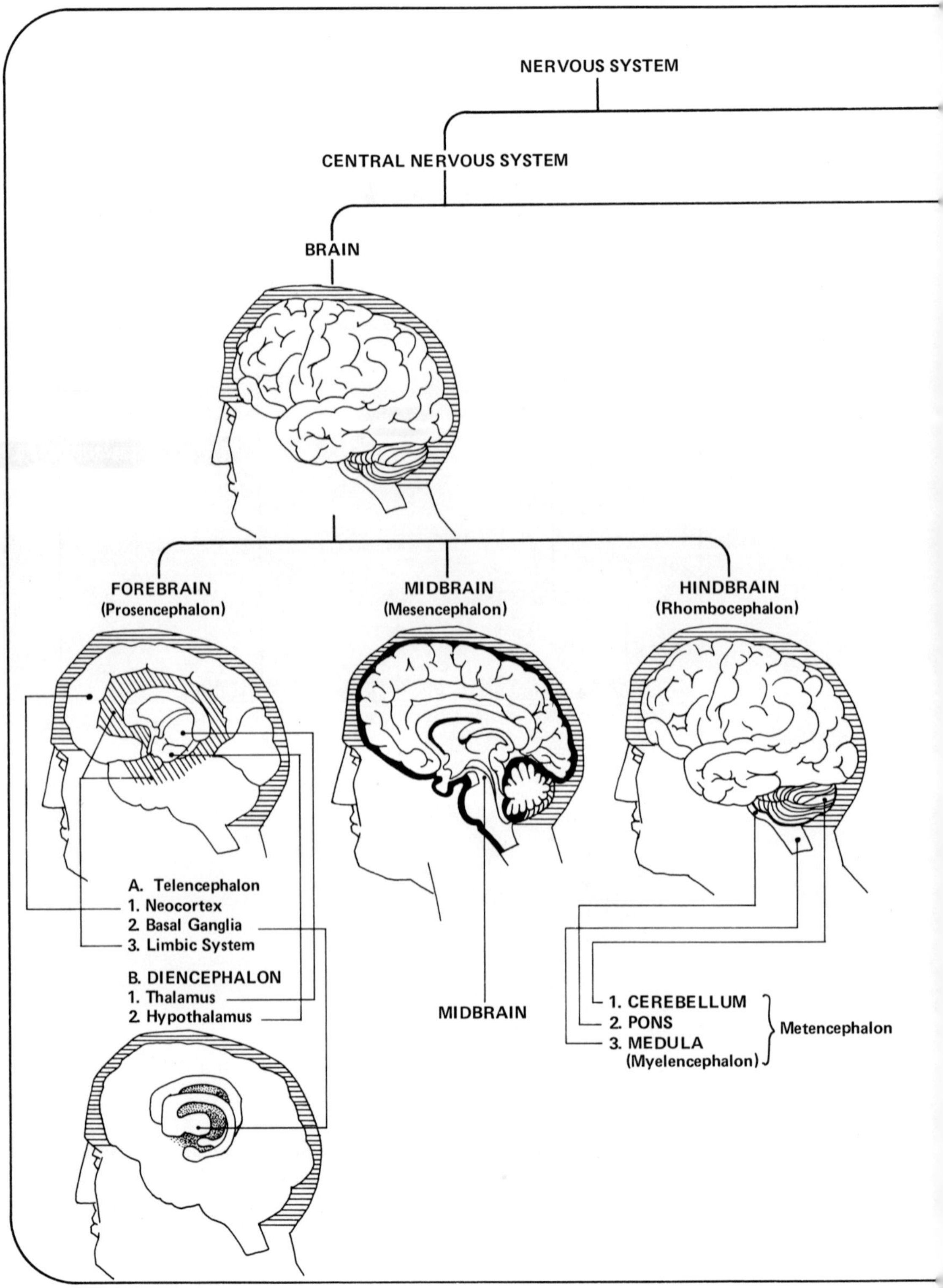
NERVOUS SYSTEM
CENTRAL NERVOUS SYSTEM
BRAIN
FOREBRAIN
(Prosencephalon)
MIDBRAIN
(Mesencephalon)
HINDBRAIN
(Rhombocephalon)
A. Telencephalon
1. Neocortex
2. Basal Ganglia
3. Limbic System
B. DIENCEPHALON
1. Thalamus
2. Hypothalamus
MIDBRAIN
1. CEREBELLUM
2. PONS
3. MEDULA
(Myelencephalon)
Metencephalon

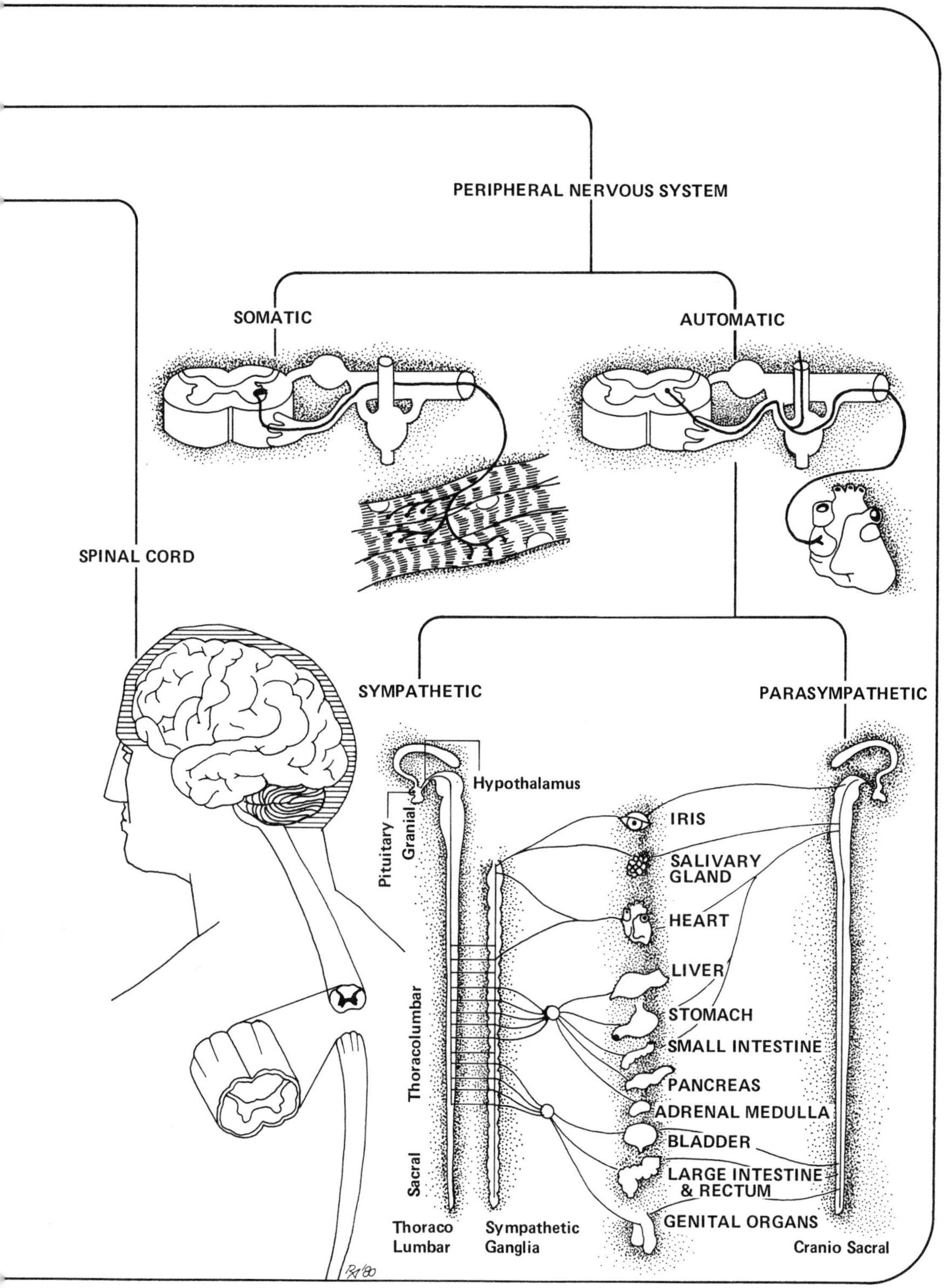
PERIPHERAL NERVOUS SYSTEM
SOMATIC
AUTOMATIC
SPINAL CORD
SYMPATHETIC
PARASYMPATHETIC
Hypothalamus
Pituitary
Granial
Thoracolumbar
Sacral
IRIS
SALIVARY GLAND
HEART
LIVER
STOMACH
SMALL INTESTINE
PANCREAS
ADRENAL MEDULLA
BLADDER
LARGE INTESTINE & RECTUM
GENITAL ORGANS
Thoraco Lumbar
Sympathetic Ganglia
Cranio Sacral

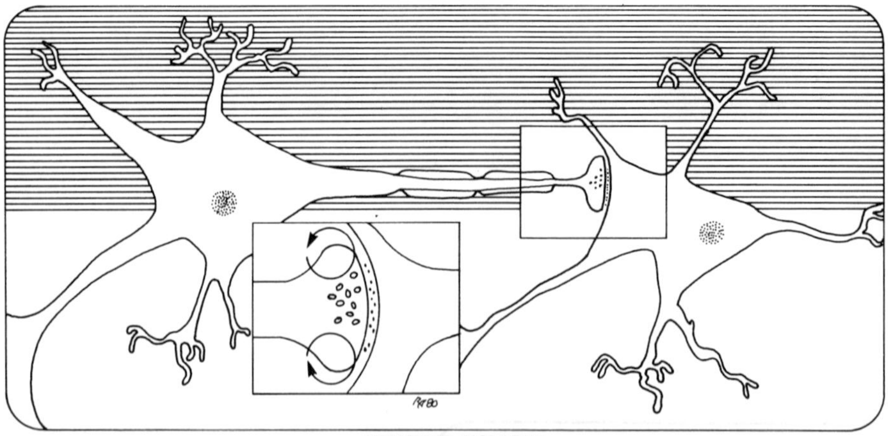

a. CHEMICAL SYNAPSE

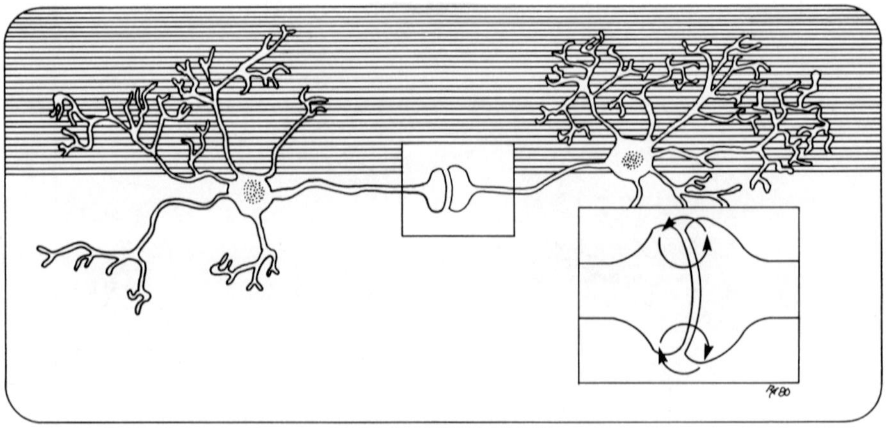

b. ELECTRICAL SYNAPSE

FIG. 3.

of receptive fields at successive levels of the visual system (1,8–10,12–14).

Figure 5 shows the human visual pathway from retina to cortex. At the retinal level there is some analysis; then, through the optic nerve, some fibers cross over to the other side of the brain, and others remain. They all lead to the lateral geniculate bodies in each side of the brain and from there to the visual area of the cerebral cortex, areas 17, 18, and 19.

Figure 6 shows the characteristics of the visual system concerning the cells' receptive fields. A receptive field is that region of the retina where illumination changes the firing rate of a cell. It can be excitatory or inhibitory. This theory has received criticism from Bishop and Stone in Australia. In their experiments they measured the latency of response of a complex cell and compared it with the latency of a simple cell. They found that the complex cell responded before the simple cell. Therefore there is doubt that this hierarchy of projections is stable; there is the possibility that there may be different types of projections to the cortex. Experimental analysis in primates has been informative, but limited. The central aim in studying visual perception is to find the relationship between the retinal image as the input and the perceived world of objects as the output. There still are no cues to how the electrical signals are reconstituted into images. Another limitation is that human processing involves cognitive and conscious elements that are lacking in subhuman primates (12,15).

NERVOUS SYSTEM

Perception involves intersensory and interhemispheric integration. Although the cortex is important in perception, other levels of the central nervous system (CNS) are also involved. This can be appreciated from studies in lower animals, who exhibit relatively fine perceptual motor skills.

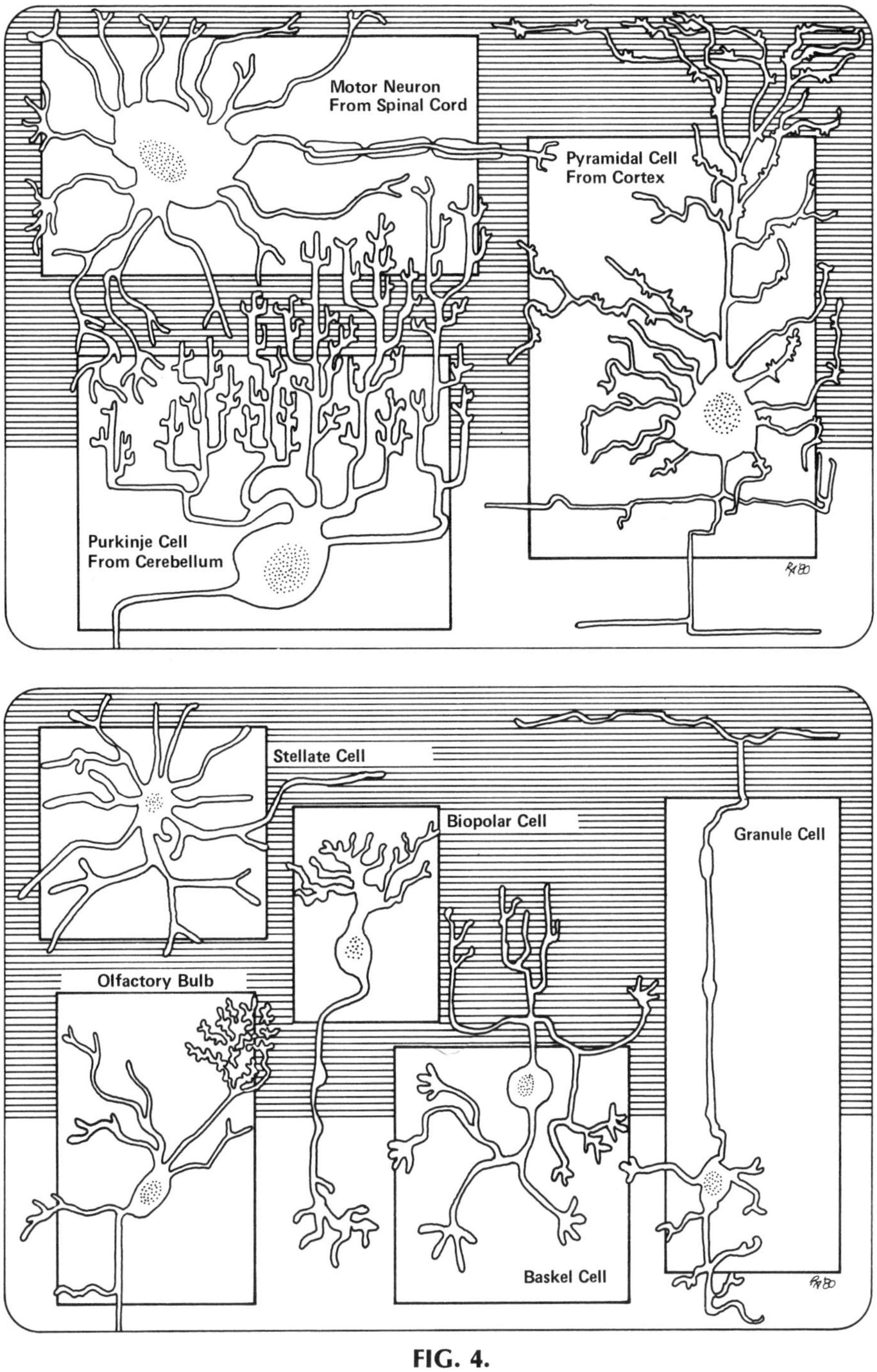

FIG. 4.

The association areas of the cerebral cortex are the regions that seem most specialized for mediation of complex processes like thought and language (8–10,14). Brain correlates of human language, such as cortical-cortical connections, appear to be of crucial importance in the human brain. Behavioral tests that have been used extensively in evaluating the effects of cortical damage include discrimination learning, particularly visual discrimination, learning sets, delayed responses, and delayed alternation.

One most impressive aspect of the human brain is the relatively large size of the frontal lobe, particularly the prefrontal areas, those that lie anterior to the motor region. Nauta (16) stated that this lobe appears not to contain a single subfield

VISUAL PATHWAYS

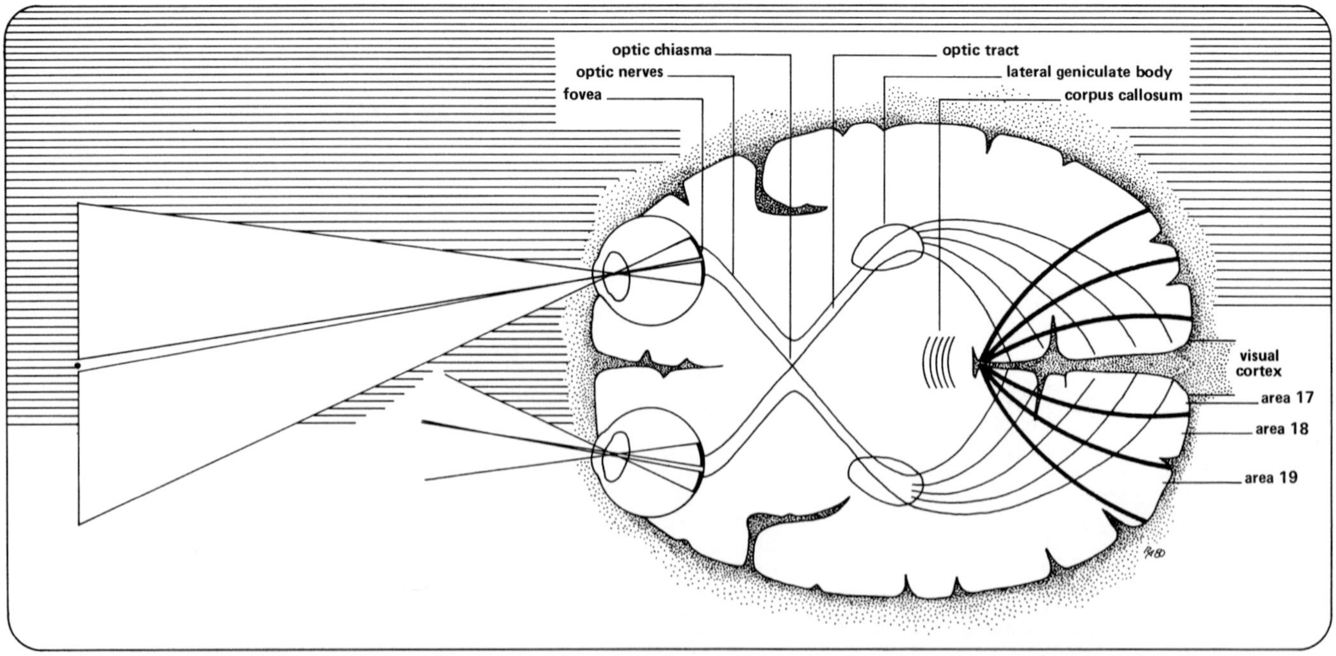

FIG. 5.

that can be identified with any particular sensory modality, and its entire expansion must accordingly be considered association cortex.

The neural circuitry places this lobe in a reciprocal relationship with the parietal and temporal regions involved in the processing of visual, auditory, and somatic information. The reciprocity in the anatomic relationship with the limbic system suggests that the frontal cortex both monitors and modulates limbic mechanisms. It appears certain that their functional states manifest themselves subjectively in the form of affects and motivations. Perhaps the phenomenon of behavioral anticipation and the loss of foresight in patients with frontal lobe lesions are associated to this frontolimbic relationship. Luria (6) stated that this disturbance affects the preliminary synthesis underlying the regulation of complex forms of motor operations and also affects the evaluation of the effect of the patient's own actions, without which goal-directed and selected behavior is impossible. He stated that the frontal lobes synthesize information about the outside world and information about the internal states of the body and that they are the means whereby the behavior of the organism is regulated in conformity with the effect produced by its actions.

The intellectual changes that are part of the frontal lobe syndrome are not specific: emotional "incontinence," crying and laughing alternating rapidly, often not related to sadness or mirth. Patients seen in the clinical setting may be in a state of apathy, not responding to spoken commands. These patients appear to be awake, and therefore they are not considered to be in coma; yet there is little more cognitive functioning than in a comatose patient.

The posterior association cortex studies have emphasized the temporal lobe. The temporal region is complex in structure and in functional organization. The temporal lobe and the angular gyrus (lying at the posterior tip of the lateral fissure where the temporal, parietal, and occipital lobes all come together) are especially important for many of the intellectual functions of the cerebral cortex, particularly for interpretation of the different sensory experiences, whether they be visual, auditory, or somatic. Following severe damage in these regions, patients may hear perfectly well, even recognize different words, but still be unable to arrange these words into coherent thought. Likewise, they may be able to read words from a printed page, but again be unable to recognize the thought the words should convey. Electrical stimulation elicits visual and auditory hallucinations, and for this reason it is believed

Type of cell	Shape of field	What is best stimulus?	How good is diffuse light as a stimulus?	Is orien-tation of stimulus important?	Is position of stimulus important?	Are there distinct "on" and "off" areas within recep-tor fields?	Are cells driven by both eyes?	Can cells respond selectively to movement in one direction?
Receptor	⊗	Light	Good	No	Yes	No	No	No
Ganglion	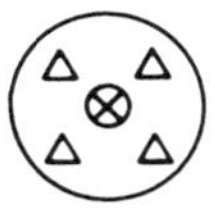	Small spot or narrow bar over center	Moderate	No	Yes	Yes	No	No
Geniculate	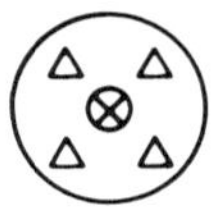	Small spot or narrow bar over center	Poor	No	Yes	Yes	No	No
Simple	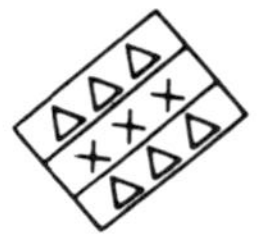	Narrow bar or edge	Ineffective	Yes	Yes	Yes	Yes (except in monkey layer IV)	Some can
Complex	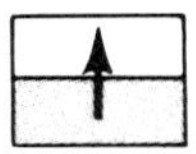	Bar or edge	Ineffective	Yes	No	No	Yes	Some can
Hypercomplex	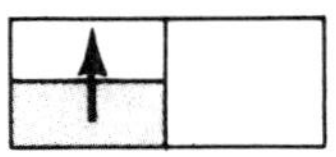	Line or edge that stops; corner or angle	Ineffective	Yes	Yes	Yes	Yes	Some can

FIG. 6. Characteristics of receptive fields at successive levels of the visual system. Courtesy of Sinauer Associates, Inc., from: From Neuron to Brain, Stephen W. Kuffler and John G. Nicholls.

that the lobe stores memory patterns. The interpretive functions of the temporal lobe and angular gyrus are usually highly developed in only one cerebral hemisphere, which is called the dominant hemisphere. The speech area (premotor) is almost always located on the dominant lobe. Thus it can be seen that temporal lobe or angular gyrus dysfunction or destruction will lead to speech and language deficits. On the average, left-handed patients show milder disorders when speech regions are damaged. Damage to Broca's area results in slow and labored speech, but comprehension remains intact. When Wernicke's area is damaged, speech is fluent, but it lacks content and comprehensibility (8–10,14).

It is not possible to designate a region as being responsible for perception. Speech plays a decisive role in the mediation of mental processes. It not only gives names to the objects of the outside world but also distinguishes among their essential properties and includes them in a system of relationships to other objects. But the material basis of higher nervous processes is the brain as a whole, and even though the brain is highly differentiated, its parts constitute a unified whole.

SENSATION AND PERCEPTION

Perception is a dynamic process in which sensory messages play an integral part but are not the sole basis for perception. The individual is not a passive complex, made up of receptor systems; there are also active programmed systems in the form of motor actions that besides passively perceiving also actively search for information (4,5). This interrelationship of sensation impulses passively imposed and actively obtained results in exploration and performance as responses to stimuli. In other words, motor activity changes as a result of sensory input; also, sensory input changes as the direction of the individual changes. There are feedforward mechanisms as well as feedback mechanisms inherent in the process of perception (17,18). The most widely accepted notion of the importance of sensation implies absolute dependence of individual performance on sensation, as represented by stimulus response. This notion of Gibson (4,5) has been modified as shown in Fig. 7.

This process of perception begins at birth and continues throughout the life-span. The individual searches for and receives from internal and external environments sensation stimuli that are organized and interpreted, involving constant interaction between the individual and the environment.

Swiss psychologist Jean Piaget proposed a model in which the individual plays a very active role in this cognitive interchange with the environment, but he also took into account intelligence, which he called the knowledge that subsists after perception takes place (15).

Many psychologists have described the distinction between sensation and perception, presenting sensation as a simpler concept involving the responses of sensory receptors to stimuli, and perception as a more complex process involving the encoding of sensory messages by the higher centers of the brain (1,19,20). Current understanding of the brain is so incomplete that it would be fruitless if not impossible to attempt to establish boundary lines between sensory organization and perceptual organization.

EYE STRUCTURES

The eye structures and muscles are described in Figs. 8 and 11 (8,10,11,21–28). The thick outside layer that gives the eye its shape is called the sclera. The conjunctiva is the infiltrating white connective tissue. It does not cover the cornea, which is where light enters and is completely

(S→R)
↓
PASSIVE SENSORY INPUT → INDIVIDUAL PERCEPTUAL PROCESS → MOTOR RESPONSE TO STIMULUS
↓
ACTIVE SENSORY INPUT ← MOTOR RESPONSE AS AN ACTIVE SEARCH FOR SENSORY INPUT

Adapted with permission.

FIG. 7. James J. Gibson: The Senses Considered as Perceptual Systems, 1966, adapted with permission from Houghton Mifflin Company.

transparent. The light that enters the eye through the cornea passes to the anterior chamber, which is the space between the cornea and pupil. This chamber is filled with an aqueous solution called the aqueous humor; it bends the light rays so that an image can form. Behind the cornea is the iris, a circular muscle that determines the size of the pupil; it is the colored portion of the eye, its color being genetically determined depending on the quantity and manner of distribution of the pigment cells. The amount of light that reaches the retina depends on the iris and pupil. The pupil is the central perforation in the iris; this circular opening contracts and dilates in a manner similar to the aperture of a camera. The pupil varies in size; if it is constricted, there is a reduction in the amount of light entering the eye; if it is dilated, there is an increase in the amount of light entering the eye. The occupational therapist can assess the three basic pupillary functions (pupillary constriction, consensuality, and convergence constriction) by the following procedures. To test for pupillary constriction, one should first determine the patient's pupil size. Then the light from a flashlight is directed into the right pupil, and the speed of dilation (fast or slow) is compared with that in the left eye and recorded. Then, with two flashlights at the same time, light is directed to both eyes simultaneously, and responses are recorded. The two pupils should dilate and constrict together. To test for the second pupillary function, consensuality, is to test for the reflex that enables the pupil of the nonstimulated eye to constrict and dilate at the same time as that of the stimulated eye. This phenomenon occurs because stimulation of the pupil with light stimulates the optic nerve that carries the light stimulus to the brain. Bilateral oculomotor stimulation results in constriction of the pupils. The therapist must remember to darken the room before assessment and cover one eye. The third function, reflex convergence, is tested with an object, a ruler or pencil held in front of the patient about 18 inches away from the eyes. The patient is told to keep looking at the object as it is moved closer. The therapist records any constriction of the pupils and records the distance at which convergence was broken. Since the pupil of the eye constricts when the eye accommodates for near vision, this association is used by physicians as a tool to diagnose parasympathetic nerve damage (28). Other conditions, such as Horner's syndrome, which is caused by sympathetic nerve interruption, also cause pupillary constriction. In these

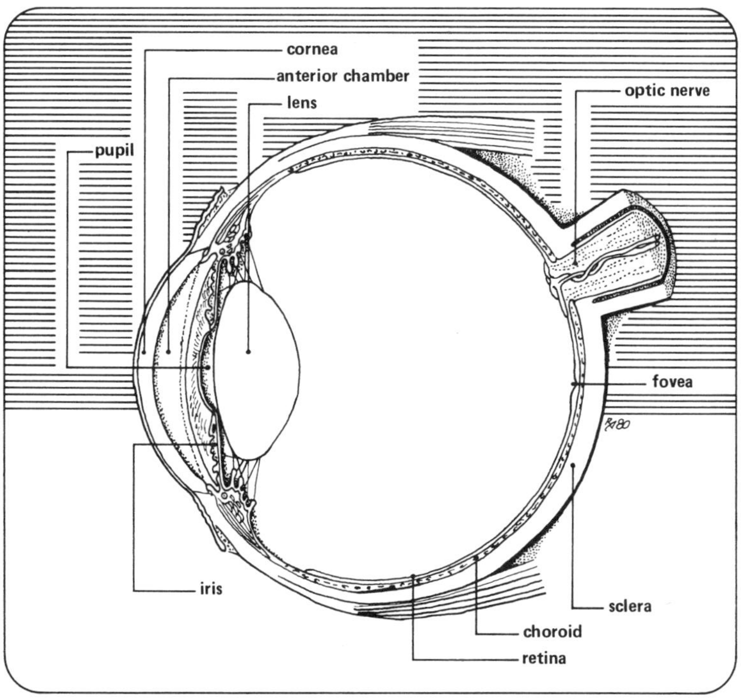

FIG. 8. The eye structures.

TABLE 1. *The perceptual systems*

Name	Mode of Attention	Receptive Units	Anatomy of the Organ	Activity of the Organ	Stimuli Available	External Information Obtained
The Basic Orienting System	General orientation	Mechano-receptors	Vestibular organs	Body equilibrium	Forces of gravity and acceleration	Direction of gravity, being pushed
The Auditory System	Listening	Mechano-receptors	Cochlear organs with middle ear and auricle	Orienting to sounds	Vibration in the air	Nature and location of vibratory events
The Haptic System	Touching	Mechano-receptors and possibly Thermo-receptors	Skin (including attachments and openings) Joints (including ligaments) Muscles (including tendons	Exploration of many kinds	Deformations of tissues Configuration of joints Stretching of muscle fibers	Contact with the earth Mechanical encounters Object shapes Solidity or viscosity
The Taste-Smell System	Smelling	Chemo-receptors	Nasal cavity (nose)	Sniffing	Composition of the medium	Nature of volatile sources
	Tasting	Chemo- and mechano-receptors	Oral cavity (mouth)	Savoring	Composition of ingested objects	Nutritive and biochemical values
The Visual System	Looking	Photo-receptors	Ocular mechanism (eyes, with intrinsic and extrinsic eye muscles, as related to the vestibular organs, the head and the whole body)	Accommodation, Pupillary adjustment, Fixation, convergence Exploration	The variables of structure in ambient light	Everything that can be specified by the variables of optical structure (information about objects, animals, motions, events, and places)

James J. Gibson: The Senses Considered as Perceptual Systems, 1966, Reprinted with permission from Houghton Mifflin Company.

cases, patients also show ptosis (drooping of the upper lid) and no sweating on the same side of the face. Other diseases such as syphilis, occasionally alcoholism, encephalitis, and central nervous system damage may cause dysfunction of pupillary constriction.

The retina is the layer that lines the posterior part of the inside of the eyeball; it has light-sensitive cells (receptors), pigment cells, and other nerve cells. The receptor layer of rods and cones has a ratio of 18 rods to 1 cone, and there are about 13 million rods. The rods mediate perception of luminosity or brightness, and the cones mediate perception of color. The rods are considerably more sensitive to changes of light and darkness than the cones, but they are less well equipped for reception of clear-cut images. The function of the cones is to secure sharp reception of a well-focused image; they are responsible for pattern discrimination and are very well packed in the fovea. The fovea is the central portion of the retina, a small indentation located in its posterior surface, where only cones exist. It is the region of greatest acuity. It is tinted yellow, thus producing the yellow spot called the macula lutea.

The optic disk or papilla nervi optici represents the point of makeup of the optic nerve; it converges cells from all regions of the retina on the point of exit. It is a roundish white area at the posterior surface of the retina. At the point of exit, the optic nerve of the retina, a blind spot, scotoma, or circular hole can be detected in the corresponding temporal part of the visual field. The data required for assessment of the optic nerve include the results of a visual acuity test, the results of a visual field test, and the results of a funduscopic examination. This information is part of the data reported from examination by the physician or neurologist; if it is not available in the patient's chart, it should be obtained before visual perceptual tests are administered in occupational therapy.

The retina obtains its blood supply and nourishment from the choroid layer, which is the membrane on which the entire retina lies. It is heavily pigmented and therefore prevents light from leaking back to the retina or to the inside.

The lens changes the focus of the eye. It is held in place by the suspensory ligaments. It bends the light rays. It has refractive power of 18 diopters. The ability of the lens to accommodate, or its power to focus, varies with nearsightedness (myopia), farsightedness (hyperopia), and presbyopia (a condition of old age in which the lens loses its elasticity and becomes almost nonaccommodating, unable to focus for near vision). Thus it is important that the patient's history prior to brain injury be obtained from the chart or from family members.

LIGHT, ENERGY, AND PSYCHOPHYSICS

The clinician or student studying perception should understand at least in an elementary fashion the physical principles of the light energy that stimulates the retina. This light energy is complex vibratory energy that forms part of the electromagnetic radiation spectrum. Only light of certain wavelengths stimulates the retina. Wavelength is measured in millimicrons or nanometers (1 mμ = 1 nm). The wavelengths of the visible spectrum range between 400 and 750 nm; electromagnetic radiation of other wavelengths is not visible to the human eye (1,19,20,24) (Fig. 9).

The individual can apprehend only a small portion of the outer world; this limited capacity is determined by the sensitivity of the individual's sensory receptors (15). The analytical properties of the sensory receptors permit assessment of the quality, intensity, location, and duration of stimuli.

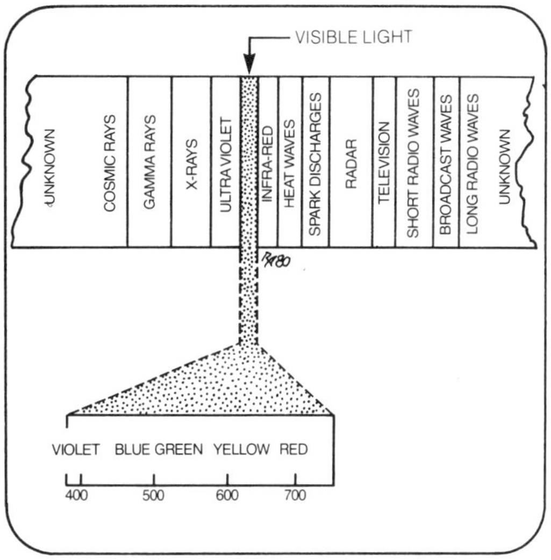

FIG. 9.

The sensations from physical stimuli in the environment are processed as different perceptions. The objects or physical stimuli in the environment may transmit, reflect, absorb, refract, or radiate light. This means that the light reaching the eye is varied. These variations in light will be perceived in different ways, depending on the wavelength. For example, light of wavelengths between 440 and 490 nm is perceived as blue (between 490 and 570 nm, green; between 570 and 600 nm, yellow; between 600 and 660 nm, red) (1,14).

If a light wave varies in amplitude or intensity, this can be perceived as changes in brightness; if the mixture of wavelengths changes, this can be perceived as changes in color.

If a beam of sunlight, which is a heterogeneous mixture of visible and invisible wavelengths, is passed through a prism, the various wavelengths will refract or bend, some more than others, resulting in a spectrum of color. The longer the wavelength, the less the ray bends while going through the prism. The shorter wavelengths bend more, and thus there is created an orderly array of wavelengths producing different colors: violet, indigo, blue, green, yellow, orange, and red. An individual can genetically inherit defective color vision or even color blindness. This defect can be detected by using the Ishihara test plates. These plates are composed of dotted figures in one color against a dotted background in a different color. A patient with defective color vision will not see the dotted figure seen by those with normal color vision. Bevan (27) reported that 10% of all men and less than 1% of women have inherited color vision deficits. The most common deficit involves perception of red and green, and the rarest involves blue. Some occupational therapists erroneously consider the ability to match colors a test for color perception.

Psychophysics is the science dealing with the relationship between stimulation and perception of sensation. Occupational therapists can benefit from the principles and laws of psychophysics when trying to interpret findings and analyze patients' responses to perceptual tests. As mentioned earlier, the physical properties of stimuli along with individual judgments contribute to perception of phenomena. Inability to respond to stimuli may result if the stimuli are subthreshold or subliminal. A threshold or limen is a boundary value for stimuli, separating a stimulus that elicits a response from a stimulus that elicits a different response or no response. An absolute threshold, stimulus threshold, or R.L. (after Reis Limen, German psychologist) is the value that can be detected 60% of the time (14,29,30).

In 1860 Gustav Fechner first approached the study of thresholds (1). A pioneer in experimental psychology, he studied the relationships between mind and body, between the psychic world and physical world. His philosophical notion was that mind and body are one, merely different sides of the coin. Fechner's law states that sensation intensity is proportional to the logarithm of stimulus intensity. In other words, perception of a sensation tends to increase linearly with an increase in stimulus intensity. The stronger the stimulus, the stronger the response, the better the perception of the sensation. This psychophysical relationship postulated by Fechner was based on Weber's law, which related the sensation's physical magnitude to perception. In 1930 Weber studied the differences required to perceive different sensations (15,29). For example, it is easier for a poor man to detect a dollar missing from his wallet than for a millionaire to detect a dollar missing from his wallet. Another example: It is easier to detect a spot of light of given intensity in the dark than in a well-illuminated room. All these psychophysiological laws have been tested in laboratory experiments and found almost never to hold true. The relationship between sensation and perception is not linear; there are many other factors that affect perception. Another name relevant to the study of psychophysics is that of Stevens. He also postulated a relationship between perception and the intensity of the stimulus, but his relationship was more general than that of Fechner. He presented systematized mathematical equations that transferred one set of intensity values to perceptual values. This transformation of value in psychophysics is called scaling. Scaling the intensity of the stimulus to the magnitude of perception depends on many variables. For example, in brightness perception, the observation depends on (a) the intensity or quality of the stimulus, (b) the spatial context or location of the stimulus, (c) the temporal context or time dimension, and (d) the subjective context of individual inherent and learned factors (14,29).

All these scientific concepts are typical of the classic approach to perception. All methods and concepts reviewed were attempts to answer the classic question about the boundary value of the physical stimulus. Another psychophysical concept concerns detection or discrimination as it relates to judgment. The detection theory emphasizes the relationship between two kind of responses: correct responses or "hits" and false responses or "false alarms." Therefore this theory is addressed to judgmental aspects of the individual rather than to the relationship between stimulus and response or to the sensory aspects of perception (29,31,32).

Detection theory takes into account the expectation or anticipation of error, habituation, and other biases related to the individual's reward and punishment. These concepts are very important for occupational therapists evaluating perceptual motor skills in their patients. The student as well as the clinician must carefully examine the evaluation tools and tasks and account for a nonlinear relationship between stimulus and response and also account for the variable judgmental errors of the patient. That a patient fails or succeeds in detecting or discriminating a task or stimulus does not correlate with whether or not the patient has perceptual problems. The judgmental aspects influence the discriminatory skills; the therapist needs to distinguish to what extent motivation, fatigue, previous practice, expectations, and indirect losses or gains from the response account for the judgment error or correctness. Thus a test in perception must be correlated with self-care performance, with cognitive performance, with function. We cannot test in isolation for 1 or 2 hr and arrive at definite conclusions without further observation of the patient interacting with the environment. Many patients evaluated at different times and in different situations display not only different but conflicting detection and discriminatory skills. Others seem to have visual perceptual problems but show a great deal of adaptation with minimal effort.

MEMORY AND PERCEPTION

Memory is a mental process that allows the individual to store experiences and perceptions for recall at a later date (33). Perception occurs rapidly and automatically, and although there are some innate perceptual skills (34), there are also those that depend on previous experiences. We believe that the nature-nurture elements in perception are compatible. The roles of experience, learning, and perception are unclear. Perception, learning, and memory fit into one picture when we are analyzing information processing. By information processing we mean the storage of information in memory, the retrieval of information from memory, and the movement in response to information (3).

We cannot make definitive statements regarding the capacity limits of memory, but we can state that there are limitations to human memory in terms of time and space. The rather low numbers of new unrelated items that we can recall after a single exposure are among the puzzles of memory. At the other end of the spectrum are echoic memory and iconic memory, which enable some individuals to record incredible amounts of information after visual presentation (iconic) or auditory presentation (echoic) in an almost nonassociative manner. These gifted individuals possess almost photographic memory.

There are various memory theories. The most popular postulates a distinction between short-term memory and long-term memory. Some psychologists propose a memory model with three stages of processing information: sensory memory (echoic and iconic memory), short-term memory (span of 5+ − 2, 30–60 sec), and long-term memory (high capacity, unlimited, where organization and categories are critical) (35–37). Later studies have presented arguments against this theory. Reed (31) presented evidence that the strength dynamics of short-term memory and long-term memory follow the same equation. He wrote of the one-trace theory and stated that memory can be explained more elegantly by assuming that there are passive and active memory systems.

Surprisingly little is clear when one considers the anatomic structures and pathways concerned in memory processing and storage. The suggested relationship between memory disorders and hippocampal damage has received its most detailed support from Milner (38) and Scoville (36), who carried out extensive studies on a patient called

H.M. This patient, who had a long history of uncontrollable seizures, underwent temporal lobe resection in the hope of lessening his seizures. The seizures lessened in frequency and severity, but the patient showed a profound postoperative memory disturbance. This led to the suggestion that amnesia is caused by hippocampal lesions. The so-called short-term memory of H.M. seemed normal, but his ability to form new long-term traces was virtually completely lost. This case was also used to support the two-trace theory of memory. The majority of experiments have failed to find general impairments of learning and memory with hippocampal lesions. The apparent lack of correspondence between the results with human and animal hippocampal lesions creates a major barrier to our study of memory (39). Horel's argument (40) is that we simply have not used tests with animals that are comparable to the ones by which we recognize these memory functions in humans.

The possibility that certain parts of the brain play especially important roles in processes related to learning and memory has been extensively pursued by authors (41–44) who have supported the idea that there are neural changes related exclusively to learning and memory and perception. Recent data from lesion studies, recording studies, and chemical studies all give a picture of plasticity of the nervous system. They also suggest the need for more subtle anatomic and functional analysis in order to understand the role of memory. Memory studies by these scientists focus on individual neurons and their interconnections, detecting changes in connections among neurons in the brain. These changes, whether chemical (related to transmitter substance) or anatomic (related to form, shape, and structure of the synapse) or both, produce electrophysiological changes that affect behavior, perception, learning, and memory (Fig. 9). The presence of these changes in synaptic contact or synaptic effectiveness has been supported by studies that correlate maturation, growth, deprivation, enrichment, malnutrition, and senility with neural connectivity (45–56).

Synapses still appear to be the most likely structural elements whose changes could underlie changes in behavior, but this hypothesis has yet to be tested. We know that the conditions of sensory stimulation during development appear to influence the numbers and sizes of synapses in cortical layers. This suggests that synaptic numbers are influenced by environmental factors, which may provide occupational therapists a neurophysiological rationale for the efficacy of intervention techniques in perceptual motor training. It also appears that reduction in learning capacity tends to be dependent on the extent rather than the site of lesions. However, it has also been documented that destruction of even large amounts of cortical tissue in many patients may result in only minor demonstrable changes in behavior and competence. The problem of the neural basis for perception, learning, and memory continues.

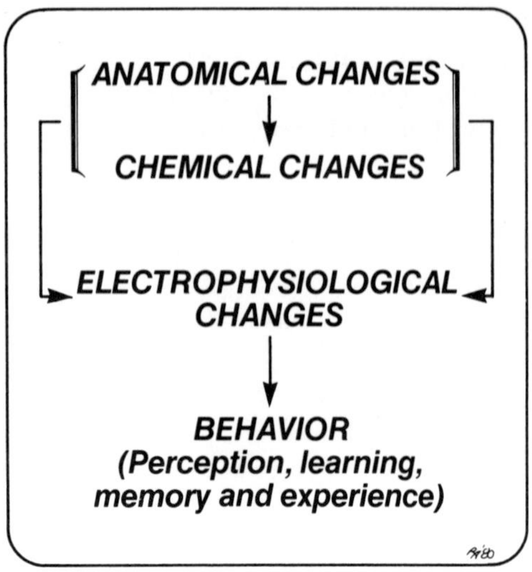

FIG. 10.
Courtesy of Dr. Ausma Rabe

VISUAL PERCEPTIVE EVALUATION AND INTERVENTION STRATEGIES

Adult patients with local brain lesions like the classic lesion studied by Luria display abnormal behaviors and disorganized performances, but hardly ever do they display total loss of function. Luria suggested that the brain is a highly differentiated system whose parts are responsible for different aspects of the unified whole. According to Luria, recovery of function can be attributed to structural reorganization into a new dynamic system widely dispersed in the cerebral cortex and lower formations. This concept regards the individual cortical areas as junctions or complex functional centers with dynamic levels of localization, rather than a matter of fixed functional assignment to particular areas of the brain.

The clinician and the student will benefit from the methods of investigation used by Luria in studying this patient population. The difference in approaches to investigation is that Luria used his logical method for functional identification of the primary defect, whereas the therapist will use these investigations or evaluation methods to plan intervention programs for rehabilitation. The student and clinician, like Luria, will find that patients with brain injury resulting from cerebrovascular accidents, head trauma, tumors, and postoperative lesions do not display isolated symptoms but display groups of disturbances or behaviors indicative of dysfunction. Grouping and identification of these behaviors, symptoms, and syndromes are essential in order to effectively plan and execute intervention procedures. Clinicians will differ in their interpretations of these symptoms, depending on their frames of reference. A first attempt to organize the observed symptoms has led to the following tentative classification:

1. Speech and language comprehension dysfunction
2. Attentional dysfunction
3. Sensory reception dysfunction
4. Motor dysfunction: (a) total paralysis, (b) incomplete or partial paralysis, (c) paresis, (d) apraxia, (e) motor perseveration, (f) incoordination

Speech and Language Comprehension

Luria (6) said that speech not only gives names to the objects in the outside world but also distinguishes among their essential properties and includes them in a system of relationships to other objects. Because of language, man can evoke an image of a particular object and use it in the absence of the object. In this category of symptoms the occupational therapist may group all the patients diagnosed as aphasics by the speech pathologist. The term aphasia is used here to denote language disorder following brain injury in patients who had previously been normal speakers and hearers. No developmental aphasias are considered (57). It is strongly recommended that speech pathologists and occupational therapists work together; their work will be complementary, and ultimately the patient will benefit from a more integrated program. A list of techniques for use in aphasia is provided by Halpern, with permission from Bobbs-Merrill (58); many of these are used by occupational therapists for different behaviors indicative of visual perceptual dysfunction. The Institute of Rehabilitation Medicine, N.Y.U. Medical Center, uses the following list of the various forms of aphasia therapy:

1. Exposing the patient to language stimulation, such as watching television, reading aloud, and participating as much as possible in speaking situations. Improvement is seen as the result of the combined effects of spontaneous recovery and verbal stimulation, and they are substituted for a formal program of treatment.
2. Interaction between the therapist and the patient, with emphasis on technique rather than content.
3. Permitting the patient to make all speech attempts without inhibition or control from a therapist.
4. Activities that simulate real-life situations acted out by the patient.
5. Role playing, pantomime, impersonation.
6. Conventional remedial reading, writing, and articulatory exercise materials adapted to adult interest.
7. Multisensory approach, rather than an attempt to isolate modalities.
8. For phonemic impairment, phonetic placement techniques taken from traditional articulation therapy.
9. Imitation practice.
10. Reading words aloud.
11. Speaking practice in a crowded room.
12. Playing commercially available word games.
13. Grammar drills.
14. Selection of a vocabulary based on its potential usefulness in daily life.
15. Use of teaching materials selected according to patient's premorbid interests.
16. Conversational practice.
17. Rhythm practice.

18. Training in lip reading to increase patient's understanding.
19. Teasing, playing pranks, telling jokes.
20. Attempts to shift dominance.
21. Singing.
22. A highly structured approach to language therapy based on modern linguistic theory.
23. Building vocabularies around a common theme such as parts of the body or house furnishings.
24. Teaching associated words, e.g., when teaching the word "shoe," the word "shine" is also introduced.
25. Using the patient's spontaneous responses as the material for treatment.
26. Singing greetings, questions, and answers.
27. Using card index plan where the patient is trained to write down on separate cards fragments of the theme he has to relate. He is then to arrange the cards in their proper order and speak from them.
28. Teaching phonemes according to the order of acquisition observed in children.
29. Group therapy (a) exclusively, (b) combined with individual therapy (c), to manipulate treatment conditions, (d) as social medium, (e) to provide natural milieu, (f) for psychotherapeutic gains.
30. Short frequent sessions rather than occasional and lengthy ones.
31. Daily sessions are more fruitful than sessions on alternate days.
32. Full-time intensive schedule, where patients attend language training classes for several hours daily.
33. Language training for 2 hr daily.
34. Treatment at home to supplement or substitute for formal speech therapy.
35. Patients teaching themselves by following a self-prescribed treatment regime.
36. Use of the patient's intact modalities to teach those skills for which he has the greatest loss.
37. Use of incidental learning more than goal-directed learning.
38. Direct psychotherapy for concomitant emotional problems.
39. Group psychotherapy to reduce anxiety in order to help verbal functioning.
40. Drug therapy to cut down on anxiety to help verbal functioning.
41. Reading aloud with and without the binaural introduction of pure tones.
42. Stimulation therapy, where the content of therapy is not as important as the manner in which it is conducted.
43. Primary use of auditory stimulation.

Aphasic patients are varied. They display different degrees and mixtures of expressive and receptive dysfunctions. They also display spontaneous and uncontrolled emotional responses. At times these responses are very disturbing to the patients, to family, and to friends, depending on their levels of understanding and comprehension. The occupational therapist and the speech pathologist will find themselves holding council over this behavior involving loss of inhibition of emotions in brain-injured patients.

The clinician and student working with this patient population will soon discover that alternative communication channels are needed in order to evaluate dysfunctions: signs, gestures, and tactile and kinesthetic cues. Because aphasic patients may or may not have attentional or other visual perceptual problems, this must be investigated and documented when awareness status allows it.

Attentional Dysfunction Syndrome

Aphasic patients display various degrees of dysfunction in their ability to selectively sustain function or interest in stimuli from the environment. Voluntary and reflexive eye movements, cancellation tasks, and figure group tasks, auditory or visual, may be used to detect behaviors indicative of attentional dysfunction. A review of the evaluation of eye movements is in order.

The eyeball approximates a globe 1 inch in diameter, with six muscles that control its movement (Fig. 10). The occupational therapist should check for pursuit movements, eye fixation, and saccade movements before attempting any other task in visual motor perceptual evaluation of brain-injured adults.

Eye fixation movements include all the ocular rotations and movements that allow the individual to hold or align the fovea on a particular portion of the visual field. Fixation movements involve both voluntary and involuntary control. It will be remembered that fixation movements

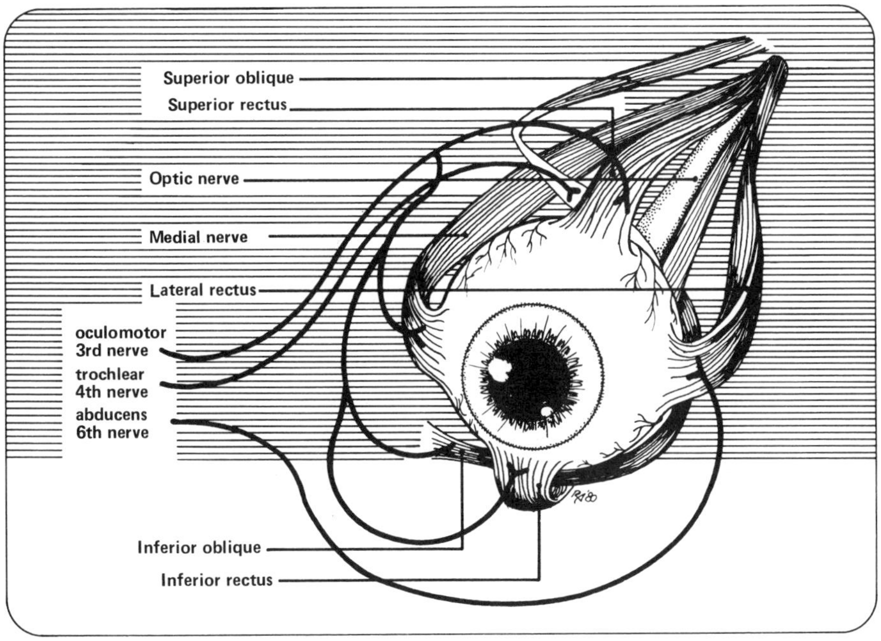

FIG. 11.

were tested while testing for pupillary vergence. They are the disjunctive movements of the eyes such as convergence and divergence. Patients converge and constrict the pupils when tested for ability to maintain fixation. The oculomotor system adducts the patient's eyes simultaneously and synchronously when the object of focus is brought nearer.

The eyes also fix in pursuit movements. They are slow conjugate (simultaneously and in the same direction) movements of the two eyes following a moving object.

The clinician testing the patient will stand in front of the patient and will move a pencil, finger, or bright small object along the directions that correspond to the eye muscle movements up, down, in, and out. Wavelike pursuit movement may also be used. When testing for eye movement, the clinician is also testing for integrity of the cranial nerves that innervate these six muscles: trochlear, oculomotor, and abducens. These three visual nerves have interrelated functions and usually are examined together. In addition to innervating the muscles of the eye, the oculomotor nerve also controls pupillary constriction and dilatation as well as the muscle of the upper lid (21–23).

The six muscles of the eyes can be divided in two sets: oblique and rectus. The obliques consist of superior oblique and inferior oblique. The rectus set has four muscles: superior rectus, inferior rectus, medial rectus, and lateral rectus.

The superior oblique muscle rotates the eye downward and outward. The trochlear (fourth cranial) nerve innervates this muscle; the trochlear originates in the midbrain just inferior to the third cranial nerve. The assistance of the inferior rectus is also needed in making the eye look down; this muscle receives its innervation from the oculomotor nerve, which also originates in the midbrain. The third muscle assisting in this motion is the lateral rectus, which rotates the eyeball outward; it receives its motor supply from the sixth cranial nerve, the abducens, which originates from the pons. The three muscles that participate in this movement are supplied by three nerves (11,21–23,26,27).

The inferior oblique muscle rotates the eye upward and outward. The superior rectus muscle assists in this movement to pull the eye back and to look up, along with the medial rectus. These three muscles are innervated by the oculomotor nerve.

The rapid eye movements involved in looking from one target to another are called saccadic eye movements. Research has shown that infants have greater corrective saccadic ability than adults (1). The saccades vary in amplitude, and the larger ones often occur along with supplementary head movements. Between the saccades there are brief periods of fixation (11).

Determination of visual perception requires thorough investigation of eye movements and direction of gaze (6). Eye movements, according to Luria, are used for detecting, identifying, integrating, and deriving meaning from objects and visual signs in the environment. The eye movement mechanism facilitates orienting and exploratory activity (6).

Saccadic reflexive movements are associated with redirection of attention to a new object (11). An individual engaged in observing an object alternates between saccade and fixation movements. Eye movements are determined by the contour of the object.

Luria (6) suggested two methods for evaluating these reflex movements. The first tests what he called elementary reflex eye movements. The clinician stands in front of the patient and uses a flashlight; no verbal instructions are needed. The clinician turns the flashlight on and moves it to the right visual field and then to the left visual field. The patient's responses, eye movements, and attention are noted. Luria stated that this movement is the responsibility of the brainstem. The other method tests what he called complex movement. It calls for suppression of the saccade reflexive tendency to look at the flashlight by giving the patient verbal instructions to look to the right or look to the left while shining the flashlight to the opposite side. He believed that the frontal lobe areas of the anterior oculomotor centers are involved in this response. If both eye movements tested appear the same in range, smoothness, and speed, the response is considered to be normal.

Clinical experience indicates that almost all brain-injured patients who have visual perceptual problems also have problems with eye movements, as well as attentional problems.

Another clinical observation is that in many cases a patient will not follow a moving object visually, but will be aware of its presence and displacement in the visual field. If asked, the patient will verbally account for the finger or object displacement, but the patient appears to be visually hypoactive.

The presence of spontaneous nystagmus should also be investigated. When the head is rotating in one direction, the eyes must rotate in the opposite direction if they are to remain fixed long enough to gain a clear image. After they have rotated far to one side, they jump suddenly in the direction of rotation of the head to fix on a new object and then rotates slowly backward again. This is known as nystagmus. The jumping motion is called the fast component of nystagmus, and the slow movement is called the slow component. Nystagmus always occurs automatically when the semicircular canals are stimulated. There are various kinds of nystagmus: rotational, compensating eye reflexes caused by rapid rotational acceleration; positional, related to a particular position of the head and canals; optokinetic, evoked by a succession of moving objects passing before the eyes.

The precise pathways that transmit nystagmus information from the vestibular apparatus to the ocular nuclei are not known. A probable pathway is through the medial longitudinal fasciculus, which connects the vestibular nuclei directly with this nuclei. However, complete transection of this fasciculus does not prevent vestibular nystagmus, which indicates that other pathways are undoubtedly involved (15,28). Nystagmus is probably the most thoroughly studied integration process in the whole of neurology, and it is widely accepted as an index for vestibular integration. The hypothesis that vestibular integration may account for learning disabilities and CNS and psychiatric conditions requires further examination (59–63). The greatest accuracy in measuring and analyzing nystagmic eye movements is achieved through electronystagmographic techniques (64).

Eye movements are of paramount importance as behavior modes indicative of perceptual dysfunction, and they are strongly linked to attention. Arousal precedes attention, and alertness is a property of arousal. If a patient is awake but is in a low state of arousal, such as lethargy, any attempt at testing will reveal poor attention. It is not lack of attention but rather lack of arousal that is the cause of inability to respond in such a situation. Clinical experience indicates the greatest arousal deficits in patients who have sustained traumatic head injury or undergone operation for brain tumors, as compared with pa-

SENSORY RECEPTORS

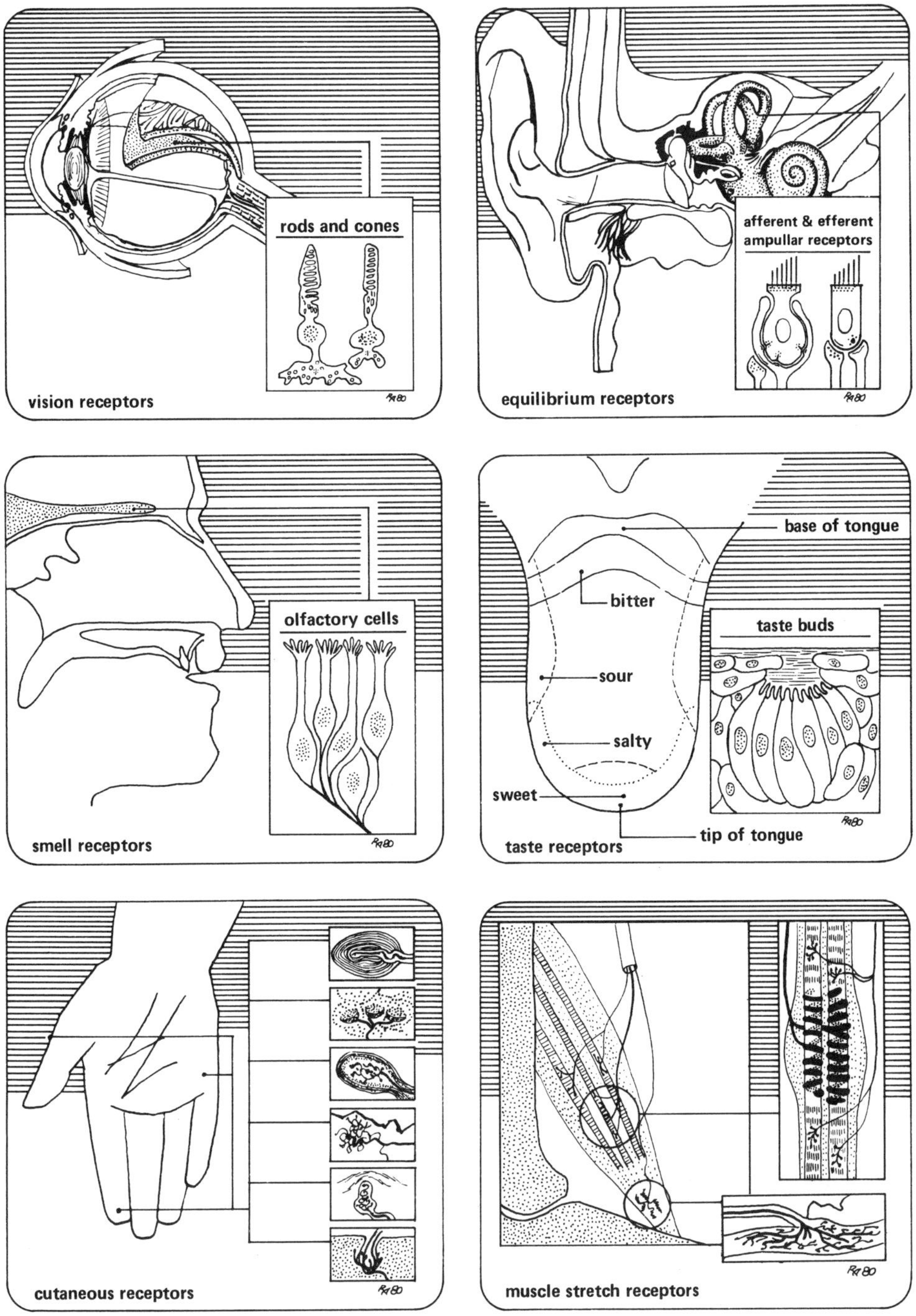

FIG. 12.

tients who have sustained acute cerebrovascular accidents. Such cases have been managed by means of intensive sensory environmental enrichment techniques administered by rehabilitation therapists, nurses, and visitors. Some examples are olfactory stimulation, tactile stimulation, tapping, brushing, icing, passive movement, auditory stimulation using an earplug and alternating it between ears, vestibular stimulation, pressure splints for deep pressure and positioning. Such stimulations are given at different frequencies and patterns to avoid adaptation. Such programs appear to be effective, but further investigations are needed. Basically, the therapy is stimulating the reticular activating system, and as a result it may be increasing the level of arousal.

Other patients will manifest a better state of arousal but will have attentional problems requiring extra cueing and structuring. Other patients may have both attentional and perceptual problems. The beginning therapist should not think that because there is an attentional problem there will automatically be other visual perceptual problems. Still other patients will have motivational problems. The therapist will develop the ability to recognize some of the motivational patterns. These are purely subjective behavior judgments that cannot be objectively documented, but with prolonged observation and documentation of fluctuations in performance they may become salient not only to the therapist but also to other rehabilitation personnel and to the family of the patient. The tool is as good as the practitioner.

Other tools that have been found effective include the following: environmental structuring; setting goals, time limits, and speed limits; amplification of stimuli; techniques to make the stimuli more salient to the patient. This approach has been used not only with attentional problems but also with all the perceptual motor dysfunctions in adults who have suffered brain injury. Facility in task analysis and activity analysis, along with good imagination, will ensure that the clinician working with these patients has a surplus of techniques involving the concepts of environmental enrichment and structuring.

Sensory-Reception Dysfunction

In this category the therapist may group all patients who show perceptual dysfunction not resulting from severe arousal or attentional problems but resulting from integrational or functional derangement in sensory detection secondary to brain injury or a premorbid condition (Figs. 11 and 12). These patients cannot see well and hear well and do not feel well because their receptor cells are not functioning properly, for whatever reason of structural or functional integration. Their impairments of sense reception slow them down and diminish their ability to detect and respond quickly to environmental changes and demands. A report of visual and auditory acuity should be obtained along with a detailed cutaneous evaluation, including pain, temperature, static and dynamic touch, position sense, stereognosis, and vibration. The same procedures of environmental structuring and enrichment can be applied for this patient population. The patient must be reeducated in the proper appreciation of the senses. Sunderland (65) stated that sensory reeducation can greatly improve sensory acuity after nerve damage if the patient is well motivated. The same should be true for brain-injured patients who do not have peripheral but rather central readjustment problems that prohibit them from discriminating or appreciating sensory phenomena. It seems that the sensory cortex in these patients fails to detect, and therefore the signal does not reach consciousness. With training and practice, the patient can convert a less efficient system into a more efficient one, with accuracy and refinement being increased by demanding the patient's full capacity and by providing new situations and novel stimuli.

Since 1940, clinicians using neurophysiological techniques, such as Bobath, Brunnstrom, Fay, and Kabat, had emphasized the relationship between human brain and movement patterns. It is only since Basmajian's studies on the training of single motor units that rehabilitation emphasis included individual muscle training. Electromyographic (EMG) biofeedback grew out of his work (Fig. 13).

Biofeedback has been called electronic yoga, the yoga of the West, electronic proprioception, sensory feedback therapy, and placebo. These names imply various frames of reference with physical and psychiatric implications. An increasing body of clinical and research evidence suggests that biofeedback represents a relatively effective technique for the shaping of self-control over certain physiologic events (66–74). These events are usually autonomous in that they tend to occur automatically and below the level of awareness. Patients who have done poorly with traditional rehabilitation techniques and patients who have had poor motivation have shown effective results in motor control with EMG biofeedback. Speculation about how it works has produced some suggestions: (a) information feedback, (b) shaping responses, (c) motivation, (d) placebo effect. Only those things that the organism pays attention to are preserved in the record (engram) or added to the automatic mecha-

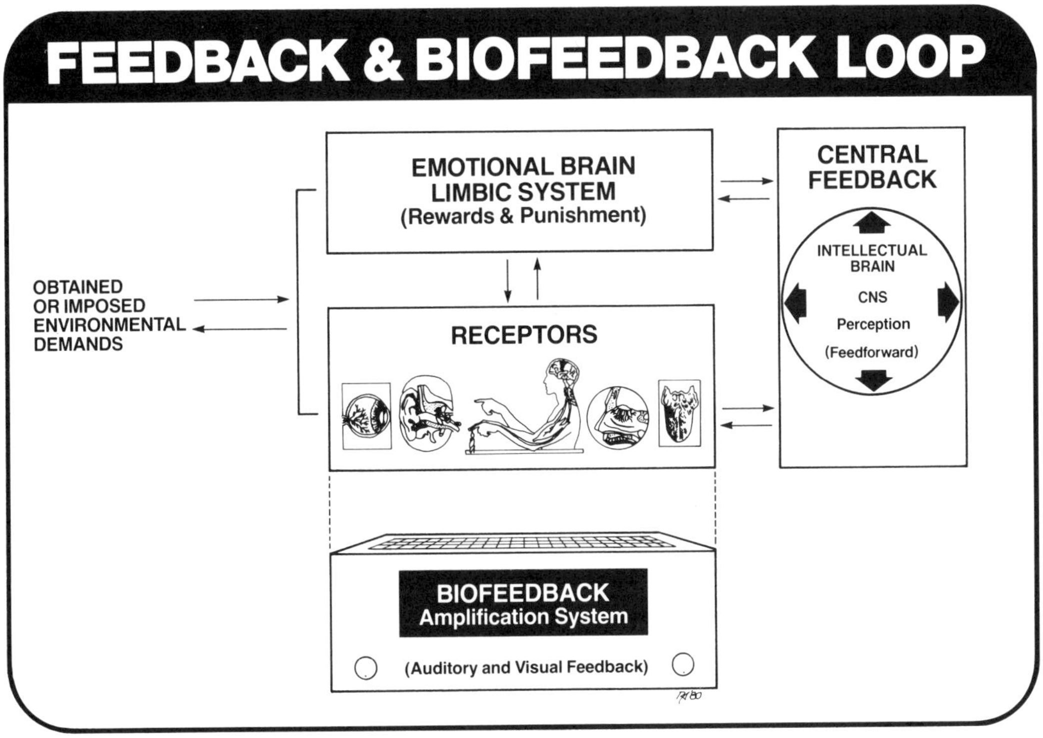

FIG. 13.

nism (75). With biofeedback, attention is greatly increased by feedback from the surface electrodes that pick up the patient's motor responses; they provide immediate and continuing qualitative and quantitative information. This electronic proprioceptive feedback depends on visual and auditory monitoring of the patient's muscular contractions.

Clinicians are using behavior modification through operant conditioning, as Skinner and Miller did in guiding and shaping behavior through reinforcement. The patient's cognitive aspect seems to accept feedback (visual/auditory) as a reward.

Biofeedback provides an element of motivation, an impulsion to action, and an element of alertness and hyperawareness of mental processes. It reinforces the patient's favorable expectations of treatment. The symbolism of the EMG instrumentation and the symbolic implications of clinician enthusiasm in using a new technique create a placebo effect. The research thus far marks the merest beginning of a new attempt to apply modern technology to inner processes.

No sensory education technique will be tolerated if the patient is experiencing severe pain. Pain is a complicated and puzzling phenomenon that impedes rehabilitation. Brain-injured patients on occasion develop pain-hand syndromes, and a close working relationship between physical therapists and occupational therapists is necessary for a more integrated approach. A brief review of pain theory seems indicated. Pain changes or alters behavior in various ways, and the reaction to pain may not be proportional to the degree of pain.

Pain is an individual perception. Tolerance and perception vary significantly from patient to patient. Figure 14 shows the anatomic structures believed to be related to pain perception, the proposed chemical neurotransmitters, the integration centers, and the multidisciplinary frame of reference applicable to pain perception (76–88).

Peptides are the combinations of amino acids formed by linkage of the amino groups of some of the acids with the carboxyl groups of others. Enkephalins are low-molecular-weight peptides or endogenous substances in the brain that act as agonists at the opiate receptor site. Endorphins are all the endogenous peptides with morphinelike agents.

Erlanger and Gasser divided the action poten-

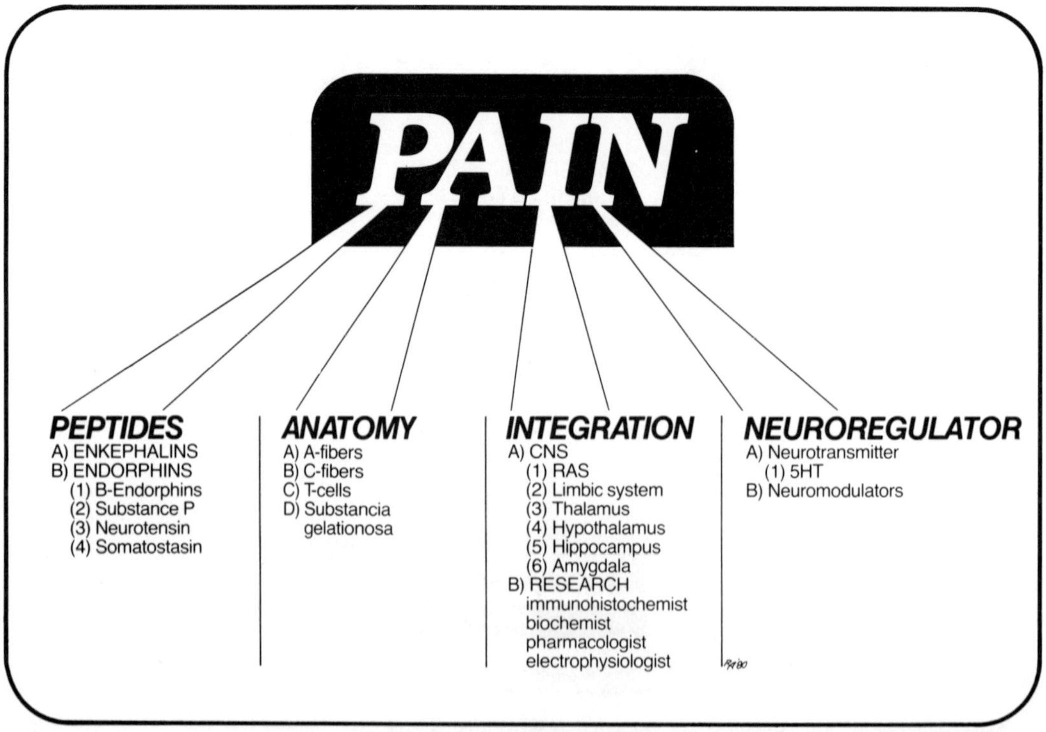

FIG. 14.

tials of a mixed nerve, according to their speeds of conduction, into three groups of potentials (A, B, and C), each group corresponding to a specific fiber. The A fibers are large, richly myelinated fast-conducting fibers of the motor and sensory systems. These A fibers can be subdivided into four groups, alpha, beta, gamma, and delta, progressing in size and conduction capacity. The delta fiber has been proposed to mediate well-localized primary sensations of pain corresponding to epicritical sensibility through the dorsal column gracile and cuneate ascending tracts. C fibers are often considered as specific pain receptors or nociceptors. They are small unmyelinated fibers sensitive to noxious stimuli. They discharge at a slow rate during stimulation and even after cessation of stimulation. They mediate secondary diffuse pain through the spinothalamic tract.

T cells (postulated and named by Melzak and Wall in 1965) have been described as injury-detecting cells in the spinal cord. The axons of T cells supposedly are contained in lamina V. They are believed to play a critical role in perception and response. If they are activated, pain results. But there is no experimental evidence that a particular cell or axon is crucial in response to injury.

The cells of the substantia gelatinosa are in the dorsal horn of the spinal cord. Melzak and Wall also proposed that the substantia gelatinosa functions as a gate control system that modulates transmission from the peripheral fibers to the T cells, but the role of the substantia gelatinosa in any function is unknown.

The structures shown in Fig. 14 are functionally connected with the neural basis of pain perception. The reticular activating system (RAS) is responsible for awareness, alertness, and behavior. The limbic system is concerned with emotional behavior and inhibition of the RAS. The thalamus is the relay station for sensory information. The hypothalamus is the linkage of the nervous system, monitoring and regulating the autonomic nervous system. The hippocampus is related to learning and memory, as is the amygdala.

The neuroregulators are chemical substances that can change behavior. They include the neurotransmitters and neuromodulators. Their presence can be detected in the cerebrospinal fluid, blood, and urine. Neurotransmitters are chemical substances that are released from nerve terminals and cross the synaptic spaces to influence other nerve cells. They mediate functions ranging from muscle contractions to behavioral responses. Neuromodulators are the chemicals that enhance or inhibit the actions of neurotransmitters. They are also called the second messengers of the brain. Unlike the neurotransmitter, the neuromodulator must have a specific receptor; examples are cyclic AMP and endorphins. 5-Hydroxytryptamine (5-HT), also known as serotonin, is a synaptic transmitter found in the raphe nuclei in the midbrain. The raphe nuclei have been implicated in psychosis and in pain control, and brain levels of serotonin have been implicated in psychosis and in pain control. Brain levels of serotonin are dramatically altered by tranquilizers like reserpine, and application of electrical transcutaneous stimulation as treatment for pain seems to increase blood and urine levels of serotonin.

The mechanisms by which pain is controlled remain completely unknown (87). The general clinical considerations are the following: (a) location, superficial or deep; (b) quality; (c) intensity; (d) time relationships; (e) modifying factors; (f) physiological factors, e.g., nausea and vomiting; (g) mental changes, e.g., irritability, lack of concentration and anticipation (65). The physical modalities for pain control are many. Most of them are administered by physical therapists: ultraviolet, cold, biofeedback, electrotherapy, heat, ultrasound, hydrotherapy, manual therapy, mechanical therapy, splints, assistive devices, therapeutic activity (88).

Motor Dysfunction

Various treatment approaches have been developed with specific treatment techniques. Refer to the chapters on neurobehavioral evaluation and management and apraxia.

Ability to function in self-care activities and social activities, motivation, and ability to learn and adapt are judged not so much in the therapeutic environment as when the patient is alone on the ward or at home. Other members of the rehabilitation team, nurses, family members, and visitors should be recruited for this investigation. The method of investigation proposed here to assess function in brain-injured patients will not be completed in 1 or 2 days. Therapeutic sessions must be designed to elicit functions and dysfunctions. These findings must be documented and then compared with more realistic functional adaptation and performance. A report on the patient's performance of skills is incomplete, as the only reported behaviors indicative of dysfunctions are those skills displayed by the patient in the experimental situation created by the clinician.

SUMMARY

This chapter has presented a review of visual perceptual function concepts. It is hoped that this information assists the therapist in understanding the complexity and importance of this area in occupational therapy. For without concepts one cannot build theories and without theoretical framework one cannot design adequate evaluation tools and treatment strategies. Appendix A and the occupational therapy outline are presented as tentative outlines to guide the occupational therapist in dealing with visual perceptual evaluation and treatment strategies. These are open to questions and modifications and although it is the result of extensive clinical experience with brain injured adults, it is considered but the first step toward the goal of improving our theoretical framework in visual perceptual testing and management for adults.

APPENDIX A: SCIENCES RELATED IN A MULTIDISCIPLINARY APPROACH TO VISUAL PERCEPTUAL EVALUATION AND TREATMENT STRATEGIES IN OCCUPATIONAL THERAPY

Neuroanatomy: (a) medical records; reports and history on pathology of specific structures in the nervous system; (b) medical records, reports and history on pathology of the oculomotor structures.

Physiology: (a) medical records; reports and history on dysfunction of the nervous system; (b) medical records, reports and history of visual dysfunction.

Psychology: medical records; reports and history of psychosocial dysfunction, emotional status, and cognition.

Psychophysics: awareness and accountability

of perceptual judgments (correctness and errors) for the relationship of physical and psychic stimulus or between the magnitude of the stimulus and the perception of the stimulus.

Rehabilitation: Occupational therapy assessment and training of functional performance; reports from other rehabilitation specialists and other personnel are also included when they are relevant to the following areas: (a) speech and language skills (receptive, expressive, and function); (b) visual motor skills (receptive, expressive and function); (c) self-care independence skills (motivation, learning, and motor skills); (d) school-home-work patterns (motivation, efficiency, and independence); (e) leisure and play patterns (personality, socioeconomic, age status).

Common postulates used in rehabilitation

1. Reflexively dominated versus integrated reflex relationships
2. Proximal-distal relationship
3. Cephalocaudal relationship
4. Gross-fine relationship
5. Imposed–self-initiated relationship
6. Sensory-motor relationship
7. Motosensory relationship
8. Active-passive relationship
9. Sensory-function–sensory-integration relationship
10. Hemispheric function–interhemispheric integration
11. Agonist-antagonist relationship
12. Emotional-physical relationship
13. Conscious-unconscious relationship
14. Part-total relationship
15. Motivation-learning relationship
16. Nature-nurture relationship
17. Noise–single-detection relationship
18. Practice-performance relationship
19. Structuring-performance relationship
20. Increased stimulus-performance relationship
21. Decreased stimulus-performance relationship
22. Sensation-magnitude–nonlinear-perception relationship
23. Memory-perception relationship
24. Abnormal-movement-patterns–normal-movement-patterns relationship
25. Individual muscle movement pattern

OCCUPATIONAL THERAPY OUTLINE

Rehabilitation Assessment for Nature and Definition or Problem

Normal	Mild	Mod.	Sev.
N	1	2	3

- I. Speech and language skills
  - A. Receptive ability
    1. Responds to gross noise
    2. Responds to name
    3. Recognizes family names
    4. Follows gestural instructions
    5. Follows verbal instructions
    6. Follows written instructions
    7. Follows spatial or directionality instructions
  - B. Expressive ability
    1. Attempts to communicate
    2. Able to indicate yes and no
    3. Says own name
    4. Uses expressions voluntarily
    5. Gives messages
  - C. Visual retention and/or memory
    1. Recalling a name
    2. Recalling a telephone number
    3. Recalling a postural pattern; imitation of posture
- II. Motor behaviors
  - A. Asymmetrical postures (head, shoulders, trunk, hips, & limbs)
  - B. Deep tendon reflexes status
  - C. Passive resistance to stretch
  - D. Stereotypic observable movement
  - E. Postural, righting and equilibrium
  - F. Active motion
  - G. Motor planning

Left		Right
	Hand to mouth (elbow flexion)	

Hand to opposite wrist (elbow flexion with adduction)
Hand to opposite elbow (elbow flexion with adduction)
Hand to opposite shoulder (elbow with adduction & sh. flexion.)
Hand to same shoulder (elbow flexion with supination)
Middle of waist (shoulder abduction)
Side reach (shoulder abduction with elbow extension)
Nape of neck (external rotation)
Behind back (internal rotation)
Forward reach (shoulder flexion with elbow extension)
Overhead (shoulder flexion with external rotation)
Palm up (supination)
Palm down (pronation)
Wrist extension
Wrist flexion

III. Hand function
  A. Grasp type: Gross ☐ Lateral ☐ Oppose ☐ 4-Fingertip preh. ☐ None ☐
  B. Release: Dropping ☐ Placement ☐ Nonfunctional ☐
  C. Finger manipulation ______________
  D. Spontaneous use ☐

IV. Limitations
  A. Contractures ______________
  B. Deformities ______________
  C. Subluxation ______________
  D. Pain ______________
  E. Edema ______________

V. Sensation or cutaneous senses
  A. Superficial: Temperature ☐ Pain ☐ Touch ☐ 2-Point discrimination ☐
  B. Combined: Stereognosis ☐ Topognosis ☐
  C. Deep: Myo. & joint position sense: Gross ☐ Fine ☐ Vibration ☐

VI. Nature and definition of the problem and its relationship to function
  A. Statement on attention skills: ability to selectively sustain function or interest in stimuli from the environment
    1. Report visual acuity and eye glasses need and usage
    2. Report eye movement quality and range
      a. Vergence:convergence
      b. Pursuit movement:
        1) Upward gaze
        2) Downward gaze
        3) Side to side
        4) Sinusoidal
        5) Nystagmus
        6) Visual attention to flashlight without verbal instructions
        7) Visual inhibition to flashlight stimuli over verbal instructions to look at the opposite side
        8) Sustaining fixed gaze for 20 sec (in two different directions)
        9) Cancellation tasks
        10) Visual hemianopsia or field test
        11) Visual neglect
        12) Figure-ground
  B. Ability to discriminate essential stimulus features and establish relationships
    1. Shape discrimination
      a. Form boards: simple shapes
      b. Form boards: abstract shapes
      c. Form boards: numbers
      d. Form boards: letters
      e. Flashcard language signs: #, $, %, ¢, &, *, ?, +, =, −, etc.

2. Size discrimination
   a. Form boards: sizes
   b. Flashcards: sizes, signs
   c. Budgets: graph comparisons
   d. Coins: size comparison and value
   e. Shopping: cost and value comparison
   f. Size: figure-ground discrimination tasks
3. Spatial variance discrimination
   a. Spatial variance form boards such as Ayres's
   b. Dot-to-dot design
   c. Spatial test such as Mertens's
   d. Directionality map test

C. Ability to integrate the parts into a total whole
   1. Hand puzzle
   2. Man puzzle
   3. Closure tests
   4. Hooper test

D. Organizational skills, categorization, sequence, judgment, and flexibility
   1. Categorize card stack on large groups, i.e., animals vs. objects
   2. Categorize card stack on subcategories, i.e., dogs vs. birds
   3. Card sequence: story telling
   4. Picture caption telling
   5. Picture caption writing
   6. Time telling
   7. Read paragraph: answer a question
   8. Mathematics problem solving: carry numbers

VII. Functional performance: speech and language; ADL; school, work, and home or institution patterns; leisure and play patterns
   A. Reads newspaper, magazine, or books
   B. Watches television, understands it
   C. Uses telephone
   D. Signs checks and official forms
   E. Uses writing as a substitute for speech
   F. Uses gesturing as a substitute for speech
   G. Sits
   H. Stands
   I. Ambulates
   J. Wheelchair mobility
   K. Transfers
   L. Dresses
   M. Grooms
   N. Feeds
   O. Awareness of limitations
   P. Self-corrects
   Q. Problem-solve
   R. Motivation
   S. Hobbies and interest

VIII. Strategy, tactics, goals, and datelines to attain goals

REFERENCES

1. Murch, G. M. (1973): *Visual and Auditory Perception*. Bobbs-Merrill, Indianapolis.
2. Norman, D. A. (1976): *Memory and Attention*. John Wiley & Sons, New York.
3. Keele, S. W. (1973): *Attention and Human Performance*. Goodyear Publishing, Pacific Palisades, Ca.
4. Gibson, E. J. (1969): *Principles of Perceptual Learning and Development*. Appleton-Century-Crofts, New York.
5. Gibson, J. J. (1966): *The Senses Considered as Perceptual Systems*. Houghton Mifflin, Boston.
6. Luria, A. R. (1966): *Higher Cortical Functions in Man*. Basic Books, New York.
7. Bullock, T. H. (1977): *Introduction to Nervous Systems*. W. H. Freeman, San Francisco.
8. Thompson, R. (1975): *Progress in Psychobiology: Readings from Scientific American*. W. H. Freeman, San Francisco.
9. Thompson, R. F. (1971): *Physiological Psychology: Readings from Scientific American*. W. H. Freeman, San Francisco.
10. Thompson, R. (1975): *Introduction to Physiological Psychology*. Harper & Row, New York.
11. Schmidt, R. F. (1978): *Fundamentals of Sensory Physiology*. Springer-Verlag, New York.
12. Kuffler, S., and Nicholls, J. (1977): *From Neuron to Brain*. Sinauer Associates, Sunderland, Mass.
13. Hubel, D. H., and Wiesel, T. N. (1962): Receptive fields, binocular interaction and functional architecture in cat's visual cortex. *J. Physiol.*, 160:106–154.
14. Thompson, R. F. (1967): *Foundations of Physiological Psychology*. Harper & Row, New York.
15. Monnier, M. (1975): *Functions of the Nervous*

System, Vol. 3: Sensory Functions and Perception. Elsevier, Amsterdam.
16. Nauta, W. J. H. (1971): The problem of the frontal lobe: A reinterpretation. *J. Psychiatr. Res.*, 3:167–187.
17. Evarts, E. V. (1979): Brain mechanisms in movement. *Sci. Am.*, 241:3.
18. Jones, B. (1974): Is proprioception important for skilled performance? *Journal of Motor Behavior*, 6:33–45.
19. Rock, I. (1975): *An Introduction to Perception*. Macmillan, New York.
20. Kaufman, L. (1974): *Sight and Mind: An Introduction to Visual Perception*. Oxford University Press, London.
21. Mechner, F. (1975): Patient assessment: Neurological examination. Part I. *Am. J. Nurs.*, 75:1–22.
22. Mechner, F. (1975): Patient assessment: Neurological examination. Part II. *Am. J. Nurs.*, 75:1–22.
23. Mechner, F. (1974): Patient assessment: Examination of the eye. Part I. *Am. J. Nurs.*, 74:1–22.
24. Held, R., and Whitman, R. (1976): *Recent Progress in Perception: Scientific American Readings*. W. H. Freeman, San Francisco.
25. Brown, L. J. (1973): *Sensory Systems*. Williams & Wilkins, Baltimore.
26. Chusid, J. (1970): *Correlative Neuroanatomy and Functional Neurology*. Lange Medical, Los Altos.
27. Bevan, J. (1978): *The Simon & Schuster Handbook of Anatomy and Physiology*. Mitchell Beazly, London.
28. Guyton, C. A. (1971): *Textbook of Medical Physiology*, ed. 4, edited by A. C. Guyton. W. B. Saunders, Philadelphia.
29. Stevens, S. S. (1951): Measurement and psychophysics. In: *Handbook of Experimental Psychology*, pp. 1–49. John Wiley & Sons, New York.
30. Kling, J. W., and Riggs, A. (1971): *Experimental Psychology*. Holt, Rinehart, & Winston, New York.
31. Reed, V. A. (1973): Speed accuracy trade-off in recognition memory. *Science*, 181:574–576.
32. Wickelgren, W. (1977): *Learning and Memory*. Prentice-Hall, Englewood Cliffs, N.J.
33. Strub, R. L., and Black, W. F. (1977): *The Mental Status Examination in Neurology*. F. A. Davis, Philadelphia.
34. Bower, T. G. R. (1974): Development of infant behavior. *Br. Med. Bull.*, 30:175–178.
35. Milner, B., Corkin, S., and Teuber, H. L. (1968): Further analysis of the hippocampal amnesic syndrome: 14-year follow-up study of H.M. *Neuropsychologia*, 6:215–234.
36. Scoville, W. B. (1968): Amnesia after bilateral mesial temporal lobe excision: Introduction to case H.M. *Neuropsychologia*, 6:211–213.
37. Wickelgren, W. (1968): Sparing of short-term memory in an amnesic patient: Implications for strength theory of memory. *Neuropsychologia*, 6:235–244.
38. Milner, B. (1954): Intellectual function of the temporal lobes: *Psychol. Bull.*, 51:42–62.
39. Weiskrantz, L. (1977): Trying to bridge some neuropsychological gaps between monkey and man. *Br. J. Psychol.*, 68:431–445.
40. Horel J. A. (1978): The neuroanatomy of amnesia. *Brain*, 101:403–445.
41. Miskin, M., and Manning, F. J. (1978): Nonspatial memory after selective prefrontal lesions in monkeys. *Brain Res.*, 143:313–323.
42. Miskin, M. (1978): Memory in monkeys severely impaired by combined but not separate removal of amygdala and hippocampus. *Nature*, 273: 297–299.
43. Sahgal, A., and Iversen, S. D. (1978): Categorization and retrieval after selective inferotemporal lesions in monkeys. *Brain Res.* 146:341–350.
44. Izquierdo, I., and Elizabetsky, E. (1978): Four memory channels in the rat brain. *Psychopharmacology*, 67:215–222.
45. Popper, K. R., and Eccles, J. C. (1977): *The Self and Its Brain: An Argument for Interactionism*. Springer-Verlag, New York.
46. Diamond, M. C. (1978): The aging brain: Some enlightening and optimistic results. *Am. Sci.*, 66:71.
47. Dyson, S. E., and Jones, D. G. (1976): Undernutrition and the developing nervous system. *Prog. Neurobiol.* 7:171–196.
48. Winick, M. (1976): *Malnutrition and Brain Development*. Oxford University Press, London.
49. Jacobson, M. (1978): *Developmental Neurobiology*. Plenum Press, New York.
50. Cummins, R. A., Livesey, P. J., and Evan, J. G. M. (1977): A developmental theory of environmental enrichment. *Science*, 197:692–695.
51. Bondy, S., and Harrington, M. (1978): Brain blood flow: Alteration by exposure to a learned task. *Science*, 20:318–319.
52. Tizard, J. (1974): Early malnutrition, growth and mental development in man. *Br. Med. Bull.*, 30:169–174.
53. Dobbing, J., and Smart, L. (1974): Vulnerability of developing brain and behavior. *Br. Med. Bull.*, 5:129–135.

54. Walsh, R. N., and Greenough, W. T. (editors) (1976): *Environments as Therapy for Brain Dysfunction*. Plenum Press, New York.
55. Cragg, B. G. (1974): Plasticity of synapses. *Br. Med. Bull.*, 30:141–144.
56. Cottlieb, A. A. (editor) (1978): *The Development of Behavior and the Nervous System, Vol. 4: Early Influences*. Academic Press, New York.
57. Lesser, R. (1978): *Linguistic Investigations of Aphasia*. Elsevier, New York.
58. Halpern, H. (1977): *Adult Aphasia*. Bobbs-Merrill, Indianapolis.
59. Ornitz, E., Brown, M. B., Mason, A., and Putman, M. (1974): Effect of visual input on vestibular nystagmus in autistic children. *Arch. Gen. Psychiatry*, 31:369–375.
60. Ritvo, E., Ornitz, E., Eviatar, A., Abraham, A., Markham, C., Brown, M. B., and Mason, A. (1969): Decreased postrotary nystagmus in early infantile autism. *Neurology*, 19:653–658.
61. Eviatar, L. A., Eviatar, A., and Naray, I. (1974): Maturation of neurovestibular responses in infants. *Dev. Med. Child Neurol.*, 16:435–466.
62. Angyal, A., and Blackman, N. (1974): Vestibular reactivity in schizophrenia. *Arch. Neurol. Psychiatry*, 611–620.
63. Rachman, O. O., and Berger, M. (1963): Whirling and postural control in schizophrenic children. *J. Child Psychol. Psychiatry*, 4:137–155.
64. Wallace, R. (1975): Electronystagmography. A review of 17 years experience. *Ann. Otol. Rhinol. Laryngol.*, 84:541–543.
65. Sunderland, S. (1978): *Nerves and Nerve Injuries*. Churchill Livingstone, London.
66. Basmajian, J. V. (1972): EMG comes of age. *Science*, 176:603–609.
67. Basmajian, J. V. (1974): *Muscles Alive: Their Functions Revealed by Electromyography*, ed. 3. Williams & Wilkins, Baltimore.
68. Basmajian, J. V., Kukulka, C. G., Narayan, M. G., and Takebe, K. (1975): Biofeedback treatment of foot-drop after stroke compared with standard rehabilitation techniques: Effects on voluntary control and strength. *Arch. Phys. Med. Rehabil.*, 56:231–236.
69. Benson, H. (1975): *The Relaxation Response*. William Morrow, New York.
70. Brudny, J., Korein, J., and Levidow, L. (1974): Sensory feedback therapy as a modality of treatment in central nervous system disorders of voluntary movement. *Neurology*, 24:925–932.
71. Engel, B. T. (1972): Operant conditioning of cardiac function: A status report. *Psychophysiology*, 9:161–177.
72. Kukulka, C. G., and Basmajian, J. V. (1975): Assessment of an audiovisual feedback device used in motor training. *Am. J. Phys. Med.*, 54:194–208.
73. Kukulka, C. G., Brown, D. M., and Basmajian, J. V. (1975): A preliminary report: Biofeedback training for early finger joint mobilization. *Am. J. Occup. Ther.*, 29:469–470.
74. Shapiro, A. K. (1960): A contribution to a history of the placebo effect. *Behav. Sci.*, 5:109–135.
75. Penfield W. R. (1968): Engrams in the human brain. *Proc. R. Soc. Med.*, 61:831–840.
76. Almay, B. L. G., Johansson, F., Knorring, L. V., Terenius, L., and Wahlstrom, A. (1978): Endorphins in chronic pain. Differences in CSF endorphins level between organic and psychogenic pain syndromes. *Pain*, 5:153–162.
77. Augustinsson, L. E., Bohlin, P., Bundsen, P., Carlsson, C. A., Forssman, L., Sjoberg, P., and Tyreman, N. O. (1977): Pain relief during delivery by transcutaneous electrical nerve stimulation. *Pain*, 4:59–65.
78. Hughes, J., Kosterlitz, H., and Leslie, F. M. (1975): Effect of morphine on adrenergic transmission in the mouse vas deferens. Assessment of agonist and antagonist potencies of narcotic analgesis. *Br. J. Pharmacol.* 53:371–381.
79. Marx, J. L. (1979): Brain peptides: Is substance Pa transmitter of pain signals? *Science*, 205:886–889.
80. Messing, R. B., and Lytle, L. D. (1977): Serotonin containing neurons: Their role in pain and analgesia. *Pain*, 4:1–21.
81. Nathan, P. W. (1977): Pain. *Br. Med. Bull.*, 33: 149–151.
82. Procacci, P., Zoppi, M., and Maresca, M. (1979): Experimental pain in man. *Pain*, 6:123–140.
83. Ray, C. D. (1977): On opiates, pain and the nervous system. *Neurosurgery*, 1(2):188–189.
84. Snyder, S. (1978): The opiate receptor and morphine-like peptides in the brain. *Am. J. Psychiatry*, 135:645–652.
85. Suda, T., Liotta, A. S., and Krieger, D. J. (1978): B-endorphin is not detectable in plasma from normal human subjects. *Science*, 202:221–223.
86. Sweet, W. H. (1977): The neuropeptides. *Neurosurgery*, (3) Nov-Dec.
87. Wall, P. D. (1978): The gate control theory of pain mechanisms—a re-examination and re-statement. *Brain*, 101:1–18.

88. Zohn, A. D., and Mennel, J. (1976): *Musculoskeletal Pain: Diagnosis and Physical Treatment.* Little, Brown, Boston.

BIBLIOGRAPHY

Ayres, J. (1976): Southern California Postrotary Nystagmus Test Manual. Western Psychological Services, Los Angeles.

Barchas, J. D., Berger, P. A., Ciaranello, R. D., and Elliott, G. R. Behavioral neurochemistry, neuroregulators and behavioral states. *Sciences,* 200:964–972.

Clark, L., Kreutzberg, J., and Chee, F. (1977): Vestibular stimulation influence on motor development in infants. *Science,* 196:1228–1229.

Luria, A. R. *The Working Brain: An Introduction to Neuropsychology.* Basic Books, New York.

Mechner, F. (1976): Patient assessment: Neurological examination. Part III. *Am. J. Nurs.,* 76:1–22.

Rossier, J., et al. (1979): Stimulation of human peraqueductal gray for pain relief increases immunoreactive B-endorphin in ventricular fluid. *Science,* 203:279–281.

Snyder, S. H. (1977): Opiate receptors and internal opiates. *Sci. Am.* 236(3):44–56.

Warrington, E. K., and Weiskrantz, L. (1968): A study of learning and retention in amnesia patients. *Neuropsychologia,* 6:283–291.

Weiskrantz, L., and Warrington, E. K. (1976). The problem of the amnesic syndrome in man and animals. In: *The Hippocampus, Vol. 2,* edited by R. L. Isaacson and K. Pribram, pp. 434–439. Plenum Press, New York.

Occupational Therapy and Cardiac Rehabilitation

11

Cecilia Sattely Seiser

Cardiac rehabilitation programs have flourished in the 1970s, and many more are currently in the design stage. Most of the programs now in effect began as pioneer programs developed around research that occurred over the last 20 to 25 years.

HISTORICAL REVIEW

Traditionally, patients were put on strict bed rest following myocardial infarction. In the 1940s and 1950s patients were kept in bed for 6 to 8 weeks following uncomplicated coronary attack. The belief was that rest was important to allow the damaged heart muscles to heal. Patients were cautioned to lie as still as possible and to use as little energy as possible, for fear that arrhythmia or myocardial aneurysm would occur. However, as early as 1944 there were individual physicians who questioned the wisdom of complete bed rest. Harrison (1) spoke of the "abuse" of bed rest for patients with cardiovascular disease and suggested that the excessive caution would result in cardiac neurosis in postinfarction patients. Levine (2) stated that long-continued bed rest "saps morale, provokes desperation, unleashes anxiety and ushers in hopelessness of the capacity of resuming a normal life." Dock (3), in the same year, favored the use of a bedside commode rather than a bedpan as a means of avoiding the Valsalva maneuver.

Many working in the cardiac field at that time believed that the traditional attitudes of both physicians and lay people seemed to be emotional responses to their own fears of death. Perhaps the reluctance to change from the traditional bed rest was the result of interpretation of the Hippocratic oath, which counseled that it was wiser to do the patient "no harm" when in doubt of the efficacy of a specific treatment.

Progress continued, however, and in 1951 Levine (4) published an article in which he recommended the "chair treatment of acute coronary thrombosis." He suggested that the patient be allowed to sit in a chair for 1 to 2 hours beginning the first day after myocardial infarction. He believed that this sitting position would be beneficial because it resulted in increased peripheral venous pooling, decreased venous return, and therefore resulted in reduction of cardiac work. Many studies in the 1950s and 1960s indicated that hospitals were making cardiac "cripples" out of patients who had suffered simple myocardial infarctions. Ignorance and fear among medical personnel were important factors in preventing adoption of the new information that had become available (5).

As physicians began to realize that long periods of bed rest were in fact deleterious to patients, the care of cardiac patients gradually changed. It was in 1950 that the famous Bellevue study (6) showed that more oxygen was consumed in using a bedpan than in using a bedside commode. This study was the first of many that measured oxygen consumption or energy expenditure in various activities. This concept has proved extremely useful in determining graded activity programs and exercise prescriptions in current rehabilitation programs.

The work of Kottke, Danz, and Kubicek and their associates (7–10) at the University of Minnesota during the 1950s and 1960s contributed considerably to the documentation of the energy costs of various activities. Their reports were of special interest to occupational therapists because they documented the energy costs of occupational therapy crafts activities as well as activities of daily living. The energy requirements in these early studies were reported in calories per square meter per minute or liters of oxygen per kilogram of body weight per minute. Since that time, the American Heart Association has established a standard measure for reporting energy requirements, the metabolic equivalent (MET). One MET is the energy expenditure at rest, equivalent to approximately 3.5 ml O_2 per kilogram of body weight per minute (11). In other words, the MET is the unit of energy consumption equivalent to the basal oxygen consumption of the patient in a rested, fasting, relaxed, fully supported state, sitting or lying supine. One MET is equal to the patient's basal metabolic rate (BMR). METs express how many times higher the energy requirements of any activity are than the BMR; METs describe a ratio between the energy requirement for a given activity and the individual's BMR. Thus, 2 METs indicate energy expenditure twice the BMR; 3 METs are three times the BMR. BMR depends on body weight, sex, age, muscle tonus, glandular activity, etc.

However, it should be noted that in almost all of the studies of energy consumption done in the 1940s, 1950s, and early 1960s, the subjects were "normal" college students, athletes, and physical education majors; this was to obtain normal standards for the energy required for various activities. Kottke's subjects, observed during a site visit in the middle 1950s, were college student volunteers and hospital personnel.

The question remained: Does the cardiac patient respond in a manner similar to that of the "normal" person? Studies conducted in the 1960s and 1970s have addressed this issue and found that the responses are indeed similar. Zohman (12), of Montefiore Hospital in New York City, has been one of the pioneers in evaluating the effects of activity on the cardiac patient.

In the late 1960s and 1970s there has been increasing emphasis on early ambulation and early mobilization programs. This approach is designed to offset the deleterious effects of prolonged immobilization in bed. An interesting article by Saltin and associates (13) in 1968 reported a study of the effects of extended bed rest on a group of healthy college students. They were placed on bed rest for 21 days, with physical fitness being measured before and after the period of bed rest. Following the period of bed rest, all subjects showed a decrease in cardiac output, a decrease in stroke volume, and an increase in heart rate during exercise. This study also indicated that the higher the level of physical fitness prior to bed rest, the longer the training period required to return to the prior functional level. Rehabilitation personnel began to wonder if perhaps the weakness and fatigue experienced by cardiac patients beginning an exercise program were the result of extended bed rest, rather than the result of the disease process of myocardial infarction. A study conducted by Bonner (14) in 1969 demonstrated that there are decreases in skeletal muscle mass, contractile strength, and efficiency after 1 week of bed rest. Therefore, because of inefficiently contracting muscles, a greater demand for oxygen is imposed on an already impaired circulatory system. Early ambulation efforts in the cardiac rehabilitation programs are designed to lessen the deleterious effects of bed rest and the resultant deconditioning of the cardiovascular system.

Occupational therapists have been in the forefront in applying the information reported in the studies previously mentioned. As early as 1952 the Veterans Administration Hospital, Bronx,

New York, had a cardiac program that involved three basic elements: (a) a graded program to increase exercise tolerance through activities, based on the concepts promulgated by Kottke and others; (b) teaching conservation of energy for long-term, chronic cardiac patients, based on time-motion studies performed in industry; (c) patient education regarding the need for activity and the benefits of activity for developing a healthy cardiovascular system. The program has since developed into a full team program that incorporates the contributions of many health professionals.

DEFINITION OF CARDIAC REHABILITATION

"Cardiac Rehabilitation is the process concerned with the full development of each cardiac patient's physical, mental, social and vocational potential. It is designed to restore the patient to an optimally productive, active and satisfying life as soon as possible after the recognition of heart disease.

"Rehabilitation should include diagnosis, medical and surgical treatment, assessment of physical, social, emotional, educational and vocational resources of the patient and the provision of any services or training needed to provide optimal restoration. It should include measures to prevent progression of disease. In short it is inseparable from the philosophy and programming of comprehensive continuing health care" (5).

Most of the work in cardiac rehabilitation programs has been done with patients who have suffered uncomplicated myocardial infarction (without arrhythmias). Despite their infarctions, these patients have good left ventricular function and do not have congestive heart failure. Although high-risk cardiac patients who have suffered complications can also benefit from cardiac rehabilitation programs (15), additional caution must be observed with these patients, and greater amounts of time and effort must be devoted to monitoring their therapy sessions.

GOALS OF CARDIAC REHABILITATION PROGRAMS

Most of the rehabilitation programs throughout the United States are based on the model created by Wenger (16) at Grady Memorial Hospital in Atlanta, Georgia, and the program developed by Zohman and Tobis (12) of Montefiore Hospital in New York City. Cardiac rehabilitation programs are essentially mobilization programs, beginning the first to third day after admission to the hospital. These programs are based on increasing the activity of patients by means of a sequence of graded exercises designed to develop capacity and to demonstrate to the patients that they are capable of such activity without deleterious effects.

Occupational therapists, with their emphasis on "function" and "independent living," have much to contribute to these programs. They have developed many outstanding programs in cooperation with other health professionals on cardiac rehabilitation teams.

The goals of various cardiac rehabilitation programs may vary slightly. Most will follow a general outline such as the program at the Bronx VA Medical Center:

Preventive

1. To prevent further myocardial infarctions by instituting a program of reconditioning early.

Psychological

2. To assist patients to be optimistic regarding the future so that they become interested in reconditioning.
3. To control the anxiety and depression that result from suddenly decreased activity and inadequate knowledge of the disease process.
4. To prevent psychological as well as physical problems arising from inactivity.
5. To assess neurotic traits that may interfere with a program and to teach patients to cope with them. For example: (a) Passive dependent types. Patients want to sit back and be treated, and therefore there is a poor rehabilitation prognosis. (b) Obsessive-compulsive types. Patients are overactive and want to do things; these patients may overdo. (c) Maladaptive types. Patients are overly concerned with their careers or their health. They tend to be anxious and irritable, which interferes with their ability to cooperate in the rehabilitation program.
6. To provide psychological counseling when problems exist (problems relating to reaction

to disability, family relations, sexual activity, etc.).

Functional

7. To increase functional capacity by gradually increasing activity or exercise level based on the results of exercise tolerance testing.
8. To limit energy consumption to safe levels within patients' functional capacities.

Educational

9. To provide education regarding risk factors (diet, smoking, physical activity, life-style) in order to reduce these risks.
10. To encourage changes in life-styles to include leisure activities that can help to reduce tension and pressure.

Vocational

11. To assist patients in returning to their previous jobs or to new vocations through vocational rehabilitation or vocational counseling, as necessary.

Thus the cardiac rehabilitation program is concerned with prevention of further myocardial infarction, as well as with the functional, psychological, educational, and vocational rehabilitation of the patient. A major activity in a cardiac rehabilitation program is testing to determine the level of function, together with the teaching of energy conservation. However, the initial thrust of the program is to motivate patients and get them involved. This helps to alleviate their fears and anxieties, which are common occurrences following hospitalization for myocardial infarction. Unfortunately, at the present time the health care system does little to reduce the fear and anxiety aroused by hospitalization. Perhaps another aspect of the cardiac rehabilitation program should be to educate hospital personnel, including cardiologists and other members of the rehabilitation staff, regarding the value of the rehabilitation program.

THE CARDIAC TEAM

The cardiac team may be small, but if a particular institution has adequate support funds, the team can be much larger. The cardiac team should be led by a combination cardiologist-physiatrist and may include a number of members, depending on the availability of suitable personnel. The following are suggested:

1. The cardiologist assigns the patient as soon as possible to the treatment team, gives the cardiac history and diagnosis, including a functional diagnosis, and may supervise the program, if desired.
2. The physiatrist assesses the patient's clinical status and issues the exercise prescription based on exercise tolerance testing. A complete prescription includes the intensity, frequency, and type of exercise and the rate of progression. It indicates the stage of the program to which the patient should be assigned and the need for additional exercise testing, monitoring, and precautions. The physiatrist is available during exercise training for immediate management of complications.
3. The coordinator of the program may be an exercise physiologist at the Ph.D. level or one of the physicians listed previously or any other competent member of the team. This person organizes the program and the professionals involved in the program, interviews and counsels patients, and oversees the testing and monitoring. The coordinator of the program obtains the medical history, including risk factors, social factors, symptoms, etc., communicates this information to other team members, and assists in planning a program for the patient.
4. Depending on the availability of personnel, team members may represent a few specialties or as broad a diversity of health professions as a particular facility can support. The occupational therapist and physical therapist are essential. The physical therapist plans the exercise program, beginning with the acute stage in the coronary care unit and progressing to active exercise with the patient in more advanced stages. The physical therapist may also work with the physiologist or physical educator in the exercise tolerance testing program.
5. The occupational therapist's contribution is threefold: (a) to determine activity guidelines for the cardiac patient using monitored task evaluation in the areas of ADL, leisure ac-

tivities, and work; (b) to modify activities in order to reduce the cardiac workload by means of energy conservation, as indicated in severe or chronic cardiac conditions; (c) to provide education for patients, family, and other interested individuals regarding the concepts discussed here, as well as the risk factors contributing to coronary disease.

6. The team may also include a physical educator. The physical educator should be well trained in exercise physiology and the physiology of activity and thus should be able to contribute considerably to the stress testing and exercise programs. In our team we have both a physical therapist and a physical educator who is a corrective therapist. We find that both make valuable contributions to the program.
7. The recreation therapist helps patients adjust to those leisure activities that are within the prescribed MET level and assists patients in changing their life-styles through participation in a number of leisure activities.
8. There are other individuals who can make valuable contributions to the cardiac team: the cardiac nurse, dietitian, psychologist, social worker, sex therapist, vocational counselor, educational therapist, manual arts therapist, and other concerned individuals who may represent the strengths of any given institution.

CONTRAINDICATIONS TO AN EXERCISE PROGRAM

The following contraindications provided by the American Heart Association are important, for there are some patients who should not exercise. Patients who have any of the following conditions are not candidates for an exercise program (5):

1. Severe decompensated heart failure; dyspnea at rest
2. Active myocarditis
3. Severe uncontrollable arrhythmia
4. Thrombophlebitis
5. Ventricular aneurysm
6. Heart block
7. Anemia
8. Cyanotic heart disease
9. Recent history of embolism, either systemic or pulmonary
10. Acute infectious disease
11. Severe aortic stenosis

Although not candidates for an exercise program, these patients can benefit greatly from an energy conservation program. This rehabilitation goal should not be overlooked.

PRECAUTIONS

Team members must be knowledgeable of the MET requirements of various activities, or at least have the list available as essential reference material, so that MET requirements will not be exceeded. Team members must be aware of the precautions necessary in cardiac treatment and must be familiar with symptoms that necessitate at least temporary cessation of the program.

1. Symptoms: (a) anginal pain or pressure or discomfort, (b) dyspnea, (c) fatigue, (d) faintness or dizziness (decreased blood supply to brain), (e) palpitations, (f) claudication pain in legs.
2. Signs: (a) pallor, localized or general; (b) excessive sweating, particularly cold sweating; (c) ataxic gait and/or glassy stare with mental deterioration; (d) irregular pulse (120 upper limit; one of the indications for EKG monitoring); (e) extreme elevation of systolic or diastolic blood pressure; (f) lowered blood pressure on exercise; (g) EKG changes (arrhythmias, ischemic changes, second- or third-degree heart block).

Special care must be taken in situations involving insufficient flow of blood to the brain. Ischemia of the brain can be caused by insufficient cardiac output or decreased vasomotor tone (syncope). Faintness, dizziness, ataxic gait, and a glassy stare are indications of ischemia of the brain. Other symptoms of failure of the heart as a pumping mechanism are pallor, which indicates cutaneous vasoconstriction, and lowered blood pressure on exercise. Therefore it is important that all members of the cardiac rehabilitation team, whether they are concerned with the evaluation of functioning, grading exercise, or conducting the activities program, be aware of the meaning and seriousness of such symptoms.

EMERGENCY MANAGEMENT

Medical personnel as well as patients should be acquainted with the steps in emergency management of any symptoms observed. For example:

1. Paleness, low blood pressure, dizziness, ataxic gait: Put the patient in a supine position; lower the head; elevate the legs.
2. Anginal pain: Stop activity. Have the patient take nitroglycerin.
3. Claudication: Stop exercise. Have the patient rest.
4. Dyspnea, fatigue: Stop activity. Have the patient rest.

MONITORING THE PROGRAM

In setting up a cardiac rehabilitation program, it is important to decide with the medical staff how the patients will be monitored and who will be in charge of making decisions regarding monitoring. Depending on the available equipment, various methods of monitoring may be used at different stages of the rehabilitation program. For instance, most programs monitor blood pressure and heart rate on all patients during ADL, exercise, and ambulation testing. The heart rate is probably more meaningful than any other single test. Therefore, although a program can function without EKG monitoring, a cardiac program should minimally monitor the blood pressure and heart rate (pulse).

Most programs use EKG monitoring at least at the beginning of a new activity. It may be desirable to monitor some patients continuously. In other words, at each session the blood pressure, heart rate, and EKG should be monitored in those patients who are unstable or who have had day-to-day changes in their capacities. A therapist may recommend continuous monitoring based on clinical observation; the prescribing physician must order this.

Thus the occupational therapist must know how to read and interpret EKGs for signs of ischemia of the heart and for danger signals in order to determine when to diminish or discontinue an activity. This might be accomplished with a portable EKG unit with oscilloscope or with more sophisticated equipment for 24-hr long-term monitoring (e.g., Holter Monitor). Telemetry can be used for monitoring as well.

The general procedure followed during monitoring is as follows: (a) Record the blood pressure, the heart rate, and/or the EKG readings at rest. (b) Have an activity period with 2 or 3 min of exercise initially, and increase the time and intensity of exercise periods as the program proceeds. (c) Record the blood pressure, heart rate, and EKG readings following the exercise. (d) Have a rest period for a minimum of 2 min. (e) Measure the time required for the blood pressure, heart rate, and EKG readings to return to pretest levels. This procedure will be repeated for each session, gradually increasing the time of the exercise or activity period, and gradually checking less often after the patient is past the acute stage. Following each level of activity, blood pressure, heart rate, and EKG readings should return to resting levels within 5 to 10 min. If these measurements do not return to normal in that time, activity should be reduced to the next lower level, with the time being increased to build endurance at that level of activity. After the patient builds endurance at the lower level, the level of intensity of the activity may be increased again to determine if the patient can accommodate the higher level. The highest level of achievement will indicate the maximum level of activity at which the patient can perform. This level should be considered a peak level, rather than a routine level of performance.

EQUIPMENT

For evaluation of the cardiac patient, there are some standard pieces of equipment that should be available to the occupational therapist:

1. A sphygmomanometer (blood pressure cuff) for monitoring blood pressure. There are two types generally available: a mercury type and an aneroid type. The aneroid type is more portable and less expensive, but it requires calibration approximately once a year. The mercury type is usually a desk or wall type; it is generally more stable and is more commonly used. However, there is no essential difference in accuracy between the two types. The aneroid type is probably easier for ward work. Either type is good for clinic use.
2. A stethoscope for listening to the K sounds during monitoring of blood pressure. If a

stethoscope must be shared with other members of the team, it is wise to have alcohol wipes available to clean the earpieces after each use.

3. A watch or stopwatch with a sweep second hand for counting the pulse rate. Although a regular wristwatch is most often used, a digital watch or a pocket stopwatch is more accurate.
4. Single-channel EKG unit with oscilloscope for continuous monitoring. Although multichannel EKG units are available in clinics, the paper is quite expensive, and a multichannel EKG unit usually is not portable. Therefore, a single-channel unit with oscilloscope is best. A single-channel unit enables the therapist to monitor a patient during bedside and clinic activities.

The preceding devices are essential for a cardiac rehabilitation program in occupational therapy. There are additional pieces of equipment that are desirable and quite helpful:

5. A telemetry unit. Telemetry enables the therapist to monitor the patient during exercise or activity anywhere within 200 feet of the unit. It allows the therapist to see the effects of exercise or activity as it is being performed. Although the ST segment cannot be read qualitatively, the rate and rhythm can be accurately monitored.
6. Holter Monitor. The cardiac division of the hospital may already have a Holter Monitor. It may not be necessary, and it is probably cost inefficient, to have the entire unit in the occupational therapy department. In using the Holter Monitor, the therapist places EKG leads on the patient. These leads are connected to a compact recording unit that is worn by the patient and stores the EKG information. The patient is sent home for a period of 12 to 24 hr, and the EKG is recorded during ADL. The patient is directed to follow the usual routine at home and carry out normal activities: household chores, mowing the lawn, shopping, golfing, sexual activity, etc. The patient is directed to keep a chronological record of activities on an hour-to-hour or minute-to-minute basis so that it can be correlated with the recorded information. Also, the patient is directed to record any cardiac symptoms experienced and the times of their occurrences. Also, any other significant facts are recorded, e.g., the times of meals, times of medication, occasions of emotional stress. When the patient returns to the clinic, the recorded information is put through the Holter Scanner, and the EKG is analyzed to determine any changes indicative of ischemia, arrhythmia, or heart block. This information, when correlated with the information the patient has recorded, pinpoints the effects of specific activities on the patient.
7. A stress test system. An elaborate program may include a treadmill, a bicycle ergometer, and an arm ergometer. The factors entering into the choice between a treadmill and a bicycle ergometer are discussed in the stress test literature. A stress test system must also include a defibrillator and medications for emergency use. Generally, the physiologist, physical therapist, or physical educator will use this equipment for testing. In a true team approach the occupational therapist should also be able to use this equipment and administer the stress test or exercise tolerance test if necessary. (Stress test and exercise tolerance test are used interchangeably.) When an exercise tolerance test is administered, a physician must be available in case cardiac emergencies arise.

There is an additional piece of equipment that is nice to have, but it may be a luxury for some programs; it is necessary in programs involving research and when building an intensely active cardiac rehabilitation program:

8. Metabolic Measurement Cart. This highly sophisticated piece of equipment calculates the actual MET requirement for a patient during activity. The equipment is expensive and is usually used by the occupational therapist who works closely with an exercise physiologist, cardiologist, or physiatrist. The advantage of the metabolic measurement cart is that it provides direct measurements of the patient's responses to specific activities, in contrast to the former method of using predicted values. There is considerable individual variation in cardiac work, especially in the

TABLE 1. *Cardiac Rehabilitation Program**

Stage	Self-care (OT)	Exercise and ambulation (PT, CT)	Leisure (MAT, ET, OT, RT)[b]	METs
Stage 1[a]	Positioning: Same as PT ADL: Begin self-feeding liquids; progress to complete feeding; bed raised to 45°, with trunk & arms supported by pillow & tray; progress to a.m. care, including washing hands and face, brushing teeth in bed.	PT: Positioning: Check correct position of patient in bed: legs in neutral (prevent external rotation), footboard in bed to prevent drop; bed to 45°; trunk & arms supported by pillow and tray. TED: Stocking application to enhance deep saphenous circulation & reduce likelihood of thromboembolic complications. Passive range of motion to arms and legs 5 repetitions (once daily); shoulder flex; elbow flex, ext, pron, supin; hip flex, ext, abd, add; knee flex & ext; ankle dorsi & plantar flex, inversion & eversion; toe flex & ext. Active range of motion: Flex feet against footboard for 3–5 min every hour; progress to active ROM on same planes as above.	Activity: OT: Light handcrafts involving finger and wrist motion: patient supported at 45° in bed.	1–1.5
Stage 2	ADL: Continue feeding & a.m. care; begin dressing self; progress to sitting at bedside, self-feeding three times per day, shaving, combing hair; begin ambulation in room; progress to walking toward bathroom; bathe in tub (2.5); MET requirements for walking: mph km/hr METs Strolling 1 1.6 1.5–2 Level walk 2 3.2 2–3	PT: Active exercises: (1) Warmup with active ROM as in stage 1; (2) add as indicated[c] (a) resistance in same movements (including from minimal to moderate as feasible); (b) hands on shoulder, elbow circling, 5 × BID; (c) breathing exercises at bedside (deep inhale & exhale) 5 × BID; (d) trunk movement at bedside, 5 × each (lateral, flex.) BID; (3) cooldown period, decreasing ROM, as in (1) above.	Education: ET: Viewing of audiovisual program on risk reduction. Activities (according to patient interest): MAT (art, wood, radio) or OT activity (using minimal resistance, and finger, wrist, & elbow motion) ½ to 1 hr total time.	1.5–2.5

Stage 3	Complete dressing, bathing (3.0 METs), including legs, and progress to entire body (4.0 METs); Comb hair.	PT: (1) Warmup stage 2 exercises; (2) add (a) alternating straight leg exercises BID; (b) breathing exercises in standing position 5 × BID; (c) standing exercises; trunk movement as stage 2, add rotation, BID (2.5 METs); (3) cool-down period with stage 2 exercises. CT: Begin ambulation for endurance; begin 15 meters (50 ft), increasing to 90 meters; progress to stair descending; orient to CT clinic: (elevator for return to ward) (4.0 METs); MET requirements for walking: (walking table below)	Education: ET: expansion of previous program; progress to group discussion and individual planning; coordinate with nurse, vocational counselor, psychologist, dietitian, sex therapist, etc. Activities: According to patient interest; use resisted arm motions; bedside and/or on-ward activity room. ET, MAT, or OT and REC ½–1 hr each	2.5–4
Stage 4	Continue previous program; add Showering (4 METs); washing hair; add household activities if required; make home visit if required to teach energy conservation; instructions re continuation of program at home.	CT: (1) Warmup (continue PT warmup); continue stair descending; (2) add (a) monitored treadmill exercise (5–7 METs); (b) stair climbing (5–6 METs); (c) monitored progressive resistive exercises with weights; PT and/or CT make home visit, as required; instructions re continuation of program at home.	Education: ET: Continue group program and reading. Recreation: Walk to recreation hall; billiards, shuffleboard, Ping-Pong to tolerance Activities: ET, MAT, OT in clinics 1–1.5 hr; instructions re continuation of activities at home.	4–7

MET requirements for walking (Stage 3, CT):

	mph	km/hr	METs
Strolling	1	1.6	1.5–2
Level walk	2	3.2	2–3
	3	4.8	3–4
	3.5	5.2	4–5
	4.0	6.4	5–6
	5	8.0	6–7

[a] Stage 1: initial interview by coordinator to obtain history, to introduce the patient to the program, including the theory of graded activity, and to answer questions. Aim: to improve or maintain function, to minimize psychological stress, to educate for modification of life-style as necessary.

[b] OT: occupational therapy; PT: physical therapy; MAT: manual arts therapy; ET: educational therapy; RT: recreation therapy; CT: corrective therapy.

[c] Indications for increased exercise tolerance; no cardiac ischemia indication, no dyspnea, no acute change in EKG.

* VA Medical Center, Bronx, New York.

TABLE 2. *Energy expenditures (stage 1, 1–1.5 METs)*

Activity	METs	Activity	METs
General		Leisure	
Bed exercise, arm movement		Chip carving	1.3
(supine or sitting)	1.2–1.5	Copper tooling	1.3
Conversation	1.0	Leather carving, sitting	1.4
Resting, supine	1.0	Leather (light) punch & lace	1.1
Sitting in bed	1.2	Leather tooling, reclined	1.1
Sitting in chair	1.2	Leather stamping, at table	1.3
		Leather, link belt, reclined	1.1
		Rug hooking, sitting	1.04
		Weaving, table loom	1.2–1.4
ADL		Vocational	
Eating	1.2–2	Box maker	1.3–1.7
Washing hands, face	1.3	Inspector	1.2
		Maintenance electrician	1.3–2.2
		Plant guard	1.4–3.5
		Printer	1.6
		Watch repair	1.2–1.5
Household			
Knitting, hand sewing	1.2–2		

early subacute stage and in high-risk cardiac patients.

MANAGEMENT METHODS

A cardiac program is graded according to the numbers of METs required to carry out specific activities (12). There have been many studies on the requirements of activities for normal individuals, and the therapist can be guided by the general comparative energy expenditures of the various activities.

Although there is a strong correlation between energy expenditure and cardiac work, the MET requirement is not the only consideration. Astrand and associates (17,18) have concluded that given a constant level of oxygen consumption, the heart rate is significantly higher when the activity is performed (a) in a hot environment, (b) under emotional stress, (c) with the arms as opposed to the trunk and legs, or (d) using isometric rather than isotonic muscular effort. These factors were found to have greater influence at low levels of 2 to 3 METs, and therefore they are especially meaningful for the treatment of hospitalized patients. Ogden (19), reporting on the cardiac work load of self-care activities, stated that maximum heart rates do not appear to be related to the MET level of the task, indicating that cardiac work load is not predictable on the basis of energy expenditure alone. Thus the other previously mentioned influences must be considered.

A usual rule of thumb is that the use of larger and more massive muscles requires more energy than the use of smaller and more delicate muscles. When possible, the patient should be taught to perform activities with the larger muscles of the body. Strenuous activity involving the smaller muscles should be avoided. A given amount of work requires the same amount of energy whether performed by the smaller or larger muscles. However, when this work is performed by the larger muscles, it represents a lesser percentage of the larger muscles' maximal capacity. In effect, the work is "spread out," resulting in reduced cardiac work, lower heart rate, and lower blood pressure.

In addition to the physical requirements of any given activity, an excess metabolic increase may also be caused by excitement, anxiety, or impatience. The therapist must assess the emotional qualities of any given activity for the individual patient.

TABLE 3. *Energy expenditures (stage 2, 1.5–2.5 METs)*

Activity	METs
General	
Driving a car	2.2–3
Standing, quietly	1.5
Walking, level, 1.5 km/hr or 1 mph	1.5–2
Walking, level, 3.2 km/hr or 2 mph	2–3
Wheelchair propulsion	1.9
Cycling, level, 8.0 km/hr or 5 mph	2–3
ADL	
Dressing, undressing	1.8–3
Shaving	2.0
Washing face, combing hair	2.0
Household	
Baking	2
Cooking	2.5
Lawn mower, riding	2–3
Light housework, sweeping, polishing, ironing	2–4
Peeling potatoes	2.0
Power saw	2–4
Washing small clothes	2.4
Woodwork, light	2–3
Leisure	
Bookbinding	2.5
Bowling	2–4
Chisel carving with mallet, standing	1.5–2
Chisel carving without mallet, sitting	1.76
Drawing	2.0
Fishing, from bank or boat or ice	2–4
Flying[a]	1.5–2
Golf, power cart	2–3
Horseshoe pitching	2–3
Motorcycling[a]	1.5–2
Music playing[a]	
Accordion	1.8–3
Cello, sitting	1.8–3
Flute, sitting	2.0
Horn, sitting	1.68
Piano	2.0
Trumpet, standing	1.8
Violin, sitting	2.6
Woodwinds, sitting	1.8
Playing cards[a]	1.5–2
Shuffleboard	2–3
Sailing	2–5
Woodwork, light	2–3
Vocational	
Armature winding	1.7
Assembler	2–3
Auto repair	2–3
Bartending	2–3
Calculating, electric	1.5–2
Desk work	1.5–2
Drill press operator	2.4
Farming, driving harvester	2.4
Driving tractor	2.0
Janitorial	2–3
Judge	2.5
Radio, TV repair	2–3
Sewing, machine	2–3
Typing, electric	1.5–2
Typing, manual	2–3
Writing, sitting	1.6–2

[a] A major excess metabolic increase may occur in some of these activities because of excitement, anxiety, or impatience, and a physician must assess the patient's psychological reactivity.

Our program is divided into four energy stages graded according to MET requirements. For instance, in stage 1 patients are usually in the coronary care unit. They are allowed to exert 1 to 1.5 METs to perform very light activities of self-care and to participate in minimal activity. When patients are transferred from the acute coronary care unit to an intermediate ward where they are

TABLE 4. *Energy expenditures (stage 3, 2.5–4 METs)*

Activity	METs	Activity	METs
General		Leisure	
Cycling, 5.5 mph, uneven ground	3.5–5	Archery	3–4
		Badminton, social doubles	3–4
		Canoeing, rowing, kayaking	3–8
		Conditioning exercises (calisthenics)	3–8
		Croquet	3–4
		Dancing[a]	3–7
		Hiking, cross-country	3–6
ADL		Horseback riding, sit to trot	3–4
Showering	3.5	Softball	3–6
Using bedpan	3.8	Table tennis[a]	3–5
		Volleyball[a]	3–6
Household		Vocational	
Carpet sweeping	2.7	Carpentry	2–7
Cleaning windows	3–4	Farming, feeding hens & dogs	3.5–4.5
Food shopping	3–4	Farming, milking by hand	3–4
Gardening	3–6	Electrical work	3–4
Hanging wash	3.6	Janitor	3–4
		Matron	3–4
Heavy housework, scrubbing floors, making beds	3–7	Paper hanging	3–8
Ironing	3.6	Plastering	3–5
Kneading dough	2.6	Plumbing	3–8
Mopping	3.6	Pulling on wires, twisting cables, e.g., rewiring house	2–7
Raking	3–6	Sanding floors, power sander	2.5–5
Weeding	3–6	Standing, light assembly	2.5–5
Wringing wash by hand	3.5	Stocking shelves	2.5–5
		Tractor plowing	3–4
		Trailer truck in traffic	3–4
		Welding	3–4

[a] See note to Table 3.

still monitored, they can advance to stage 2. They are allowed to do 1.5 to 2.5 METs, which allows a gradual increase in the number of activities. Our program is described in Table 1. Patients are increased from level to level with approval of the physician. An increase in activity level may also be recommended by the therapist. When patients can perform activities at a given level without abnormal or excessive changes in blood pressure, heart rate, and EKG readings, they are then advanced to the next level.

At each stage patients are begun on an activity for a short period of time. Gradually the time is increased for endurance within that MET range.

Progress notes are written daily during the acute stages and once a week or once every 2 weeks during the more stable stages. Progress notes state the activity, the time, the pulse and pressure changes, and the EKG changes. EKG readings are reported as follows: (a) heart rate as beats per minute, (b) rhythm, (c) ST segment and T wave, (d) PR interval, indicating whether abnormal or prolonged, (e) observation of the QRS complex.

The EKG results should be studied by the therapist prior to implementing a cardiac rehabilitation program. There is a self-study program for understanding EKGs that is used as a standard reference in most departments (20).

TABLE 5. *Energy expenditures (stage 4, 4–7 METs)*

Activity	METs
General	
Ambulation, braces & crutches	6.4
Climbing stairs	
17-lb load 27 ft/min	7.0
Cycling, 12.9 km/hr or 8 mph	4–5
16.1 km/hr or 10 mph	5–6
17.7 km/hr or 11 mph	6–7
20.9 km/hr or 13 mph	8–9
Deep knee bends, 16/min	5.4
Push-ups	6.0
Running in place	6–7
Running 8.9 km/hr or 5.5 mph	8–9
Walking, fields & hillside	4.64
Walking, plowed field	4.4
Walking, steep grade	6–8
Walking, upstairs	4–8
Walking, downstairs	4–5
Household	
Beating carpets	4
Digging	4–8
Hoeing	4–8
Mowing lawn, power	4–5
Hand mower	4–7
Planing hardwood	7.0
Planting seedling	4.0
Sawing hardwood	6.0
Shoveling, light earth	5–6
Snow shoveling, wet	8–15
Snow shoveling, powder	6–9
Splitting logs, cutting trees by hand	5–10
Wheelbarrow	4–10
Vocational	
Coal mining, drilling	5.36
Erecting roof supports	4.86–6.2
Carpentry, hammering, planing	6.0
Carpentry, light	4–5
Chopping wood, hand axe or saw	5–5.5
Farming, feeding cattle	4.8
Shoveling grain	4.8
Fireman (boiler)	5.3–7
Forestry, barking trees	7.0
Chopping	5–6
Hoeing	5.2
Planting by hand	6.2
Sawing by hand	7.0
Leisure	
Back-packing	5–11
Badminton, singles	4–9
Badminton, competition	6–7
Basketball, non-game	3–9
Basektball, game play	7–12
Canoeing, 6.4 km/hr or 4 mph	5–6
Canoeing, 8.0 km/hr or 5 mph	7–8
Cricket, batting	4–7
Cricket, bowling	5.1
Dancing, twist & wiggle	5.8
Fencing	6–10
Fishing, stream (wading)	5–6
Folk (square) dancing	6–7
Football, touch	6–10
Golf, walking	4–7
Handball	8–12
Horseback riding	3–8
"Posting" to trot	5–7
Gallop	7–8
Hunting, bow or gun, small game, carry light load	3–7
Hunting, big game, dragging carcass	3–14
Jogging	7–15
Mountain climbing	5–10
Paddleball	7–12
Scuba diving	5–10
Skating, ice & roller	5–8
Skiing, snow, downhill,	5–8
Skiing, cross-country	6–12
Skiing, water	5–7
Sledding & Tobogganing	4–8
Snowshoeing	7–14
Squash	8–13
Soccer	5–12
Swimming	4–8
Swimming, side stroke	6.9
Tennis	4–9

TABLE 5. *Energy expenditures (stage 4, 4–7 METs)*

Vocational	
Sawing by power	4.24
Stacking fire wood	4.96
Weeding	4.72
Furriery	4.72
Heavy tools	
Pneumatic tools (jack-hammers, drills, spades)	6.0
Shovel, pick, tunnel bar	8.0
Shovel, 10/minute, 16 lb	10+
Heavy construction	5.2
Laborer	4.8–6
Laying railroad track	7.0
Lifting & carrying objects	
20–44 lb	4.5
45–64 lb	6.0
65–84 lb	7.5
85–100 lb	8.5
Machine tooling, operating punch press	5.0
Moving, pushing heavy object, 75 lb or more (moving van work)	8.0+
Painting outside	4.4
Postman	8.0
Sawing hardwood, hand	7–8
Shoveling coal	6.16
Steel mill, fettling	5.04
Forging	5.6
Tipping molds	5.2
Surveyor	4–5

Other helpful books are listed in the Bibliography. If possible, therapists should take a course in cardiac rehabilitation.

We have found that a listing of MET requirements for various activities has been most helpful in acquainting new therapists, patients, physicians, nurses, and others with the concept of MET requirements (Tables 2–6). This listing has been made as broad as possible from as many resources as possible to suit the needs of various groups. The list has been used to initiate discussion during group meetings and has been used to teach MET levels to other hospital personnel. It is useful when used in conjunction with the metabolic measurement cart to compare a patient's MET requirement for a given activity with the average.

The concept of "equicaloric matching" is used to help patients transfer their knowledge regarding monitored activities to other activities of similar MET levels. For instance, if a patient can walk on level ground at 1 mile per hour (strolling), which requires 1.5 to 2 METs, without significant cardiac signs or symptoms, then it should be possible to perform any other activity that requires 1.5 to 2 METs (e.g., typing on an electric typewriter or performing clerical desk work). Similarly, if the patient can walk at a moderate pace of 3 miles per hour (3–4 METs) without distress, then it should be possible to perform any other activity using the same amount of METs.

SUMMARY

Occupational therapists have contributed to the early studies in the field of cardiac rehabilitation,

TABLE 6. *Energy expenditure (stage 4, 7+ METs)*

General		Leisure	
Climbing hills, 7-kg load	7.4	Boxing in a ring	7.84
10-kg load	7.9	Boxing, sparring	12.6
20-kg load	8.3	Dancing, choreographer, vigorous	9.52
Cycling, racing	9.6	Field hockey	7.6
Running in place	6–7	Football	7.5
Running 8.9 km/hr or 5.5 mph	8–9	Judo	11.04
Walking upstairs fast	11.2	Marching, rapid	8.08
		Skiing hard snow, level walking	8.16
		Uphill, max. speed	15.6
		Swimming, back stroke	9.6
		Breast stroke	9.2
		Crawl, fast	8.9
		Crawl, slow	7.28
		Treading fast	9.68
		Vocational	
		Digging trenches	8.24
		Farming	
		Cleaning animal stalls	7.68
		Forking straw bales	7.8
		Forestry, axe chopping, fast	16.88
		Carrying logs	10.56
		Felling trees	7.52
		Trimming trees	7.36
		Horse grooming	7.28
		Skin diving, maximum motion	15.68
		Moderate motion	11.68
		Steel mill, merchant mill rolling	8.24
		Hand rolling	7.76
		Removing slag	10.08
		Tending furnace	7.72

and they are active in the design and formulation of new programs. The role of the occupational therapist is threefold:

1. To determine activity guidelines for cardiac patients using monitored task evaluation in the areas of ADL, leisure activities, and work. The amount of activity permitted is determined by the monitoring of the activity as it is performed by the individual patient. It is guided by general charts of MET requirements of activity, supplemented by knowledge of environmental and psychological factors influencing cardiac output.
2. To modify activity for high-risk cardiac patients by reducing cardiac work and teaching the principles of energy conservation.
3. To provide education for patients, family, and other interested individuals regarding the concepts discussed here, as well as risk factors contributing to coronary disease.

Thus the purpose of cardiac rehabilitation is to create and reinforce a pattern of activities that will permit the patient to return to as active a life as possible within the limits of cardiac function.

ACKNOWLEDGMENTS

Sincere appreciation is extended to Andrew A. Fischer, M.D., Ph.D., and Kerry Stewart, Ed.D., for their professional suggestions and editing and to Mrs. Patricia Harris for her skill and patience in preparing the manuscript.

REFERENCES

1. Harrison, T. R. (1944): Abuse of rest as a therapeutic measure for patients with cardiovascular disease. *J.A.M.A.*, 125:1075.
2. Levine, S. A. (1944): Some harmful effects of recumbency in the treatment of heart disease. *J.A.M.A.*, 125:80.
3. Dock, W. (1944): The evil sequelae of complete bedrest. *J.A.M.A.*, 125:1083.
4. Levine, S. A., and Lown, B. (1951): The "chair" treatment of acute coronary thrombosis. *Trans. Assoc. Am. Physicians,* 64:316.
5. American Heart Association Sub-Committee on Rehabilitation (1977): *Cardiac Rehabilitation Unit Program Guide.* American Heart Association, Dallas.
6. Benton, J. G., Brown, H., and Rusk, H. A. (1950): Energy expended by patients on the bedpan and bedside commode. *J.A.M.A.*, 144:1443.
7. Kottke, F. J., Kubicek, W. G., Danz, J. N., and Olsen, M. E. (1978): Studies of cardiac output during the early phase of rehabilitation. *Postgrad. Med.*, 23:533.
8. Kottke, F. J., Danz, J. N., and Kubicek, W. G. (1957): Study of cardiac output during rehabilitation activities. *Arch. Phys. Med.*, 38:75.
9. Kottke, F. J., Kubicek, W. G., Olsen, M. E., Hastings, R. H., and Quast, K. (1962): Five stage test of cardiac performance during occupational therapy. *Arch. Phys. Med.*, 43:228.
10. Quiggle, A. B., Kottke, F. J., and Magney, J. (1954): Metabolic requirements of occupational therapy activities. *Arch. Phys. Med.*, 35:567.
11. American Heart Association Committee on Exercise (1975): *Exercise Testing and Training of Individuals with Heart Disease or at High Risk for Its Development: A Handbook for Physicians.* American Heart Association, Dallas.
12. Zohman, L. R., and Tobis, J. S. (1970): *Cardiac Rehabilitation.* Grune & Stratton, New York.
13. Saltin, B., Blomqvist, G., Mitchell, J. H., Johnson, R. L., Wildenthal, K., and Chapman, C. B. (1968): Response to exercise after bedrest and training. *Circulation* [*Suppl. 7*], 37–38:1.
14. Bonner, C. D. (1969): Rehabilitation instead of bed rest? *Geriatrics,* 24:109.
15. Abraham, A. S., Yitzhak, S., Wienstein, M., Dollderg, M., and Menczel, J. (1975): Value of early ambulation in patients with and without complications after acute myocardial infarction. *N. Engl. J. Med.*, 292:719.
16. Wenger, N. C., and Hellerstein, H. K. (1978): *Rehabilitation of the Coronary Patient.* John Wiley & Sons, New York.
17. Astrand, P. O., and Rodahl, K. (1970): *Textbook of Work Physiology.* McGraw-Hill, New York.
18. Astrand, I. (1972): ST depression, heart rate and blood pressure during arm and leg work. *Scand. J. Lab. Invest.*, 30:411.
19. Ogden, L. D. (1979): Activity guidelines for early subacute and high risk cardiac patients. *Am. J. Occup. Ther.*, 33:291.
20. Dubin, D. (1974): *Rapid Interpretation of EKGs.* Cover Publishing, Tampa.

BIBLIOGRAPHY

Background

American Heart Association (1973): *Coronary Risk Handbook: Estimating Risk of Coronary Heart Disease in Daily Practice.* American Heart Association, New York.

Katz, A. M. (1977): *Physiology of the Heart.* Raven Press, New York.

Kirkendall, W. M., Burton, A. C., Epstein, F. H., and Freis, E. D. (1967): *Recommendations for Human Blood Pressure Determination by Sphygmomanometers.* American Heart Association, New York.

Lancour, J. (1976): How to avoid pitfalls in measuring blood pressure. *Am. J. Nurs.*, 72:1242–1246.

Cardiac Rehabilitation, General

Grace, W. H. (1973): *Pre-hospital Care of Acute Myocardial Infarction.* American Heart Association, New York.

Johnston, B. L., Cantwell, J. D., and Fletcher, G. F. (1976): Eight steps to inpatient cardiac rehabilitation: The team effort. *Heart and Lung,* 58:97–111.

Matheson, L. N., Selvester, R. H., and Rice, H. E. (1975): The interdisciplinary team in cardiac rehabilitation. *Rehabil. Lit.*, 36:366–375.

Huntley, N., and Mullvain, M. A. (editors) (1978): *Basics of Cardiac Rehabilitation.* Minnesota Occupational Therapy Association, Minneapolis (available from Mary Sue Davitt, P.O. Box 822, Minneapolis Minn. 55440).

Pollock, M. L., Wilmore, J. H., and Fox, S. M.

(1978): *Health and Fitness through Physical Activity*. John Wiley & Sons, New York.
Trombly, C. A., and Scott, A. D. (1977): *Occupational Therapy for Physical Dysfunction*. Williams & Wilkins, Baltimore.
Wenger, N. K. (1973): *Rehabilitation after Myocardial Infarction*. American Heart Association, New York.
Wilson, P. K. (1975): *Adult Fitness and Cardiac Rehabilitation*. University Park Press, Baltimore.

Energy Costs of Activity

Passamore, R., and Durnin, J. V. G. A. (1955): Human energy expenditure. *Physiol. Rev.*, 35:801–840.
Katch, F. I., and McArdle, W. D. (1977): *Nutrition, Weight Control and Exercise*. Houghton Mifflin, Boston.

Exercise

American College of Sports Medicine (1976): *Guidelines for Graded Exercise Testing and Exercise Prescription*. Lea & Febiger, Philadelphia.
American Heart Association (1972): *Exercise Testing and Training of Apparently Healthy Individuals: A Handbook for Physicians*. American Heart Association, New York.
Amsterdam, E., Wilmore, J. H., and DeMaria, A. N. (1977): *Exercise in Cardio-vascular Health and Disease*. Yorke Medical Books, New York.
Morse, R. L. (1972): *Exercise and the Heart—Guidelines for Exercise Programs*. Charles C Thomas, Springfield, Ill.
Naughton, J. (1977): Exercise programs for patients with acute myocardial infarction. *Practical Cardiology*.
Silvarajan, E., Lerman, J., Mansfield, L. W., and Bruce, R. A. (1977): Progressive ambulation and treadmill testing of patients with acute myocardial infarction during hospitalization: A feasibility study. *Arch. Phys. Med. Rehabil.*, Vol. 58.

EKG Study and Interpretation

Alexander, S. (1965): Arrhythmias associated with acute myocardial infarction. *Med. Clin. North Am*.
Butler, H. H. (1973): How to read an ECG. *R.N.*, January, February, March.
Chernoff, H. M. (1972): *Workbook in Clinical Electro-cardiography*. Medcom Learning Systems, New York.
Hoffman, B. F. (1966): The genesis of cardiac arrhythmias. *Prog. Cardiovasc. Dis.*, 8:319–329.
Margolis, J. R., and Wagner, G. (1976): *Arrhythmias in Acute Myocardial Infarction*. American Heart Association, New York.
Meltzer, L., Pinneo, R., and Kitchell, J. R. (1970): *Intensive Coronary Care, A Manual for Nurses*. Charles Press, Philadelphia.
Menard, R. (1968): *Introduction to Arrhythmia Recognition*. California Heart Association, Los Angeles.

Psychological and Social Effects

Friedman, M., and Rosenman, R. H. (1975): *Type A Behavior and Your Heart*. Fawcett Publications, Greenwich, Conn.
Hackett, T. P., and Cassem, N. H. (1975): *Patient Psychology*. American Heart Association, New York.
Stern, M. J., Pascale, L., and McLoone, J. B. (1976): Psycho-social adaptation following an acute myocardial infarction. *J. Chronic Dis.*, 29:513–526.
Wheatley, D. (1977): *Stress and the Heart: Interactions of the Cardio-vascular System, Behavioral State, and Psychotropic Drugs*. Raven Press, New York.

Patient Education

American Heart Association (1973): *The Heart and Blood Vessels*. American Heart Association, New York.
Blakeslee, A., and Stamler, J. (1963): *Your Heart Has Nine Lives*. Prentice-Hall, Englewood Cliffs, N.J.
Bracken, M. B., Bracken, M., and Landry, A. B. (1977): Patient education by videotape after myocardial infarction: An empirical evaluation. *Arch. Phys. Med. Rehabil.*, 58:213–219.
Hollander, L. L. (1977): *Hypertension: Manual for Patients*. Massachusetts Rehabilitation Hospital, Boston.
Hollander, L. L. (1976): *Take Heart!* Massachusetts Rehabilitation Hospital, Boston.
Jenkins, D.: *Coronary Artery Disease*. North Carolina Heart Association, Chapel Hill.
Massachusetts General Hospital (1977): *Smoke Gets in Your Eyes!* Massachusetts Rehabilitation Hospital, Boston.
North Carolina Heart Association: *Back in Circulation*. North Carolina Heart Association, Chapel Hill.

A Psychoneurophysiologically Based Activity Analysis 12

Elsi Dicmonas

This chapter presents a guide for determining the cognitive-sensory-perceptual-motor functions necessary for learning and using a skill, defining its subskills and their components, and understanding the neurophysiological requirements for mastering the components of subskill processes. This model of activity analysis is designed to assist the therapist in (a) appraising the complexity of subskills of which an activity is composed, (b) determining which behavioral constructs and physiological mechanisms of skills acquisition the disabled person retains and which have been lost, (c) integrating the remedies for identified impairments into the natural sequence of a purposeful task performance, and (d) defining and implementing the function of occupational therapy, which is "the art and science of directing man's participation in selected tasks to restore, reinforce and enhance performance, facilitate learning of those skills and functions essential for adaptation and productivity, diminish and correct pathology, and to promote and maintain health. Its fundamental concern is the development and maintenance of the capacity, throughout the life span, to perform with satisfaction to self and others those tasks and roles essential to productive living and to the mastery of self and the environment" (1).

The organization and procedures of this activity analysis are applicable primarily to skills involving the use of one or both arms. The structure of this analysis arises from the conviction that all movements result from a conscious decision and subsequent events revolving around the wish to achieve a specific purpose. The analysis proceeds to the hierarchical sequences through which goal-oriented movements are learned and integrated.

The preceding definition of occupational therapy describes the therapist's basic concern for the patient's capacity to master selected life tasks. The therapist assists the patient in learning new skills and adapting old skills that are necessary for achieving the patient's goals, which have been altered because of changes in cognitive, psychosocial, or physical capacities.

Most of our life tasks involve problems that must be solved by planned motor actions (2). We orient ourselves in the environment through movements, and we respond to human and nonhuman objects through movements. Beginning at birth, we learn to interact with the environment by means of sequential progressive tuning of our sensory-motor mechanisms in response to events that occur in the environment. As infants, our first movements were random. Then, inadvertently, we began to cause events to happen, and thereby we came to recognize the interaction between our movements and the environment. Our motions became deliberate. A motion fulfilled a specific purpose, and through that motion we achieved a goal. At the same time, we started to accumulate numerous environmental-interaction experiences; later, in modified form, these were recruited for learning and performing additional skills. It was at an early stage of life that our cognitive processes began to lead movement planning and execution.

There is a tendency to equate skills acquisition with physical activity, specifically the execution of motion. The occupational therapist knows that the principal goal of the profession is to restore function, not isolated movement. The ability to move one's joints does not assure acquisition of skills or restoration of function, since a functional movement is an adaptive response (3) to a decision-making process, to environmental and internal stimuli, involving analysis and synthesis of incoming sensory information. This adaptive response or motor output represents the sum total of sequentially interrelated cognitive, sensory, and perceptual events that preceded and predetermined the movement composition. The term "adaptive response" also connotes that memory or recall plays an important part in the problem-solving function of task achievement. A goal-specific response is built on previously learned cognitive-sensory-perceptual-motor matches, but it is modified to the sensory-motor requirements of the task at hand. Therefore an individual must have the ability to integrate and adapt existing interaction matches to the receptor-effector processing of concurrent ongoing movement sequences necessary to achieve a predefined goal.

Movement, we conclude, is the final process that derives from desire to achieve a purpose, recognition of the pertinent environmental factors, and recall and use of similar past experiences. It is not just a conglomeration of motor outputs involving various joints.

By means of such activity analysis we can follow, step by step, the development of those sequentially interrelated factors that produce movement. The author used this model as a device for teaching the skill of activity analysis to occupational therapy students prior to becoming acquainted with Gentile's parameters of motor learning (3). Gentile's concepts of motor learning correlate very closely with the theories and principles of occupational therapy. Through her publications and teaching Gentile has reinforced the author's belief that rehabilitation must be oriented toward the patient's life-style. Her writings, in conjunction with the theories of the dynamics of movement developed by behaviorists and psychologists such as Piaget, Miller, Galanter, and Pribram, neurophysiologists such as Bernstein, Guyton, Luria, and Teuber, and many others, have provided the theoretical background for this description of the underlying behavioral and neurophysiological processes through which a meaningful activity is learned and performed.

VALUE OF LIFE-STYLE-ORIENTED ACTIVITIES

To the able individual, as well as to the disabled, skills acquisition is a never-ending endeavor as life proceeds from its evolutionary phases to its involutionary phases. Therefore the goals and tasks pursued during these progressing and regressing life stages vary. In addition, some learned skills lose their usefulness and applicability after various periods of time, and then they begin to compete with the requirement for new achievements.

The first step toward engaging in an activity is to define its goal, so that its relevance to current life-style and future plans and expectations can be determined and appraised by the individual.

From a behavioral point of view, task-oriented activities can be grouped into three types: those common to all people, such as the activities of daily living; those that are specific to the successive phases of life, such as play, work, and leisure activities; those that meet an individual's personal needs and reflect individual personality traits, such as vocational and recreational pursuits. It might be suggested that the activities in all these categories are meaningful to most individuals. Nevertheless, contact with many people who have had to reorganize their life goals, tasks, and modes of operation makes it apparent that even such generalized activities as those of daily living have gradations and are modified by the individual's life-style, needs, and cultural-ethnic influences. Success in assisting an individual to adapt existing skills or acquire new skills requires consideration of the following factors.

An individual who experiences a physical trauma of catastrophic disease does not easily realize that previous life-style, tasks, and related activities can no longer be pursued, that there must be redefinition of goals, adaptation of skills, and learning of new activities. Without such realization, any attempt at retraining and adapting activities will be fruitless because of lack of goal orientation and hence lack of incentive and intrinsic motivation.

Adults who come to occupational therapy had at some time in the past organized and structured their life-styles and had accordingly learned those activities by which they pursued their life tasks. Before they experienced physical catastrophe, their selections of activities and plans for implementation reflected the priorities they attached to role actualization, meeting vital and nonvital needs, and social-interaction objectives. Individuals often categorize their activities according to relevance; at various times a given activity might be perceived as necessary but not enjoyable, enjoyable because of a special interest but not necessary, or interesting and personally challenging and therefore meaningful. Activities can become personalized for a variety of reasons: because of past experiences, needs and interests, hopes and fears, personality traits, anticipation of goal achievement.

There is great variation in the number and diversity of skills individuals acquire during their life phases. Miller, Galanter, and Pribram (4) and Welford (5) have discussed numerous strategies by which individuals select their activities: (a) Some activities are pursued as ends in themselves because they are perceived as enjoyable and self-fulfilling. A given job-related activity may provide gratification because an individual simply finds it interesting; for another individual the same activity may serve as a means to an end, providing an opportunity to enhance one's life-style, pursue interests that are not job-related, or work toward other goals. (b) There are individuals who recognize various possible applications of a skill and have the resourcefulness to apply a few learned skills in many different situations. (c) Other individuals make an effort to learn additional skills in a search for alternatives to job boredom or in preparation for future life tasks. (d) Some individuals engage in a multitude of activities without ever mastering specific skills because they feel compelled to keep busy in order to counteract restlessness or feelings that their lives are empty. (e) There are others who feel no need to add to their repertoire of learned activities because most of their interests revolve around a single focus. Their vocational activities differ little from the activities with which they relax or interact socially. (f) Some individuals organize their activities into neat self-contained packages of role-related activities, activities for self-gratification, activities tailored to their specific social needs. These self-centered individuals often find themselves stripped of these protective activity shields when health, vocational, financial, or social mishaps occur. Unexpectedly, a life-style that is encapsulated in a rigid and narrow structure disintegrates, and for many of these individuals self-pity prevents adaptation to the new life situation. (g) Some individuals find it difficult to develop skills because they have too many activities competing for their time. (h) Some individuals are inner-directed; that is, they choose to remain independent of others as they plan their lives, set their goals, and make their choices in the area of skills acquisition and implementation. If the self-image of such an individual is shattered by catastrophe, it will be difficult to accept the fact that once-familiar skills must be relearned with the assistance of another person and that physical dysfunction will limit the choice of goal achievement (6). To these individuals, inability to achieve their goals independently is a source of frustration that can prevent them from adapting their existing skills and learning new ones. Tasks that are seen as foreign do not provide great incentive for learning, and hence no progress can be made in skills acquisition.

A therapist should not use an activity as a therapeutic medium unless the individual being treated understands the purpose of the activity and recognizes and accepts its value as a goal-directed activity that contributes to the individual's own plan of achievement, role actualization, and fulfillment of personal and social needs. "When activities match or are related to the developmental needs and interests of the individual, these activities not only afford the necessary learning for development or restoration, but provide an intrinsic gratification which promotes and sustains health and evokes a strong investment in the restorative process" (7). Also, we must realize that during the process of adjusting to temporary or permanent impairment of cognitive-sensory-perceptual-motor functions, an individual may have little interest in acquring skills if this involves making adaptations. The patient's vision of the goal may be obscured by physical and emotional stress (8) and by the hope of full restoration of capacity within a short time. Why, in the patient's view, waste time learning adaptations and substitute skills?

In concluding this discussion of the importance of individual life-styles and life-task-oriented activity used as a therapeutic medium, it should be emphasized that the therapist must be fully aware of the value the patient places on the skill that is to be learned or adapted. Cooperation is assured if the patient finds meaning in the activity, not only because it has therapeutic value but also because the patient sees personal-interest value or specific goal value, either temporary or permanent.

The patient who takes a significant interest in an activity mobilizes and integrates in a much more natural way the cognitive functions involved in the following processes: (a) decisions regarding goals and choices of activities; (b) judgments regarding the pertinence of a task to personal needs, medical and physical status, and current and future personal and economic priorities; (c) acquisition and use of academic skills, as demonstrated by comprehending and following written and verbal instructions; (d) recall of information from recent sensory input (immediate memory), environmental events, and past experiences related to the activity (long-term memory); (e) anticipation of events and sequences involved in handling materials and performing tasks; (f) demonstration of creativity based on synthesis of past experiences and production of new thought.

Such cognitive processes can be sucessfully nurtured through life-style-oriented activities to promote self-value and self-respect.

IMPORTANCE OF ENVIRONMENTAL EVENTS IN PLANNING AND PERFORMANCE

Activity, as already indicated, involves some kind of direct or indirect interaction with the environment. Before engaging in activity, one would prefer to know as much as possible about characteristics of events in the environment. How does one acquire such knowledge?

As social beings who must interact with our own kind as well as with the rest of our environment, we frequently find ourselves in surroundings that are neither of our choosing nor of our making. By recognizing and assessing the environmental elements, we learn to adapt ourselves to the uncontrollable factors, and we learn to change and use those aspects of the environment that can be modified or controlled. This dual process of partial subordination to the environment and partial control over the environment is called by Piaget (9) a process of assimilation and accommodation. It is an ongoing process throughout life, and it is fundamental to motor learning and skills acquisition.

As we mature we develop percepts and later concepts regarding the various characteristics of the elements we encounter in the environment, e.g., shape, size, weight, color, texture, and usefulness. We learn to label them with symbols, and we attach these symbolic properties to human and nonhuman objects. This enables us to think of environmental elements as having tangible qualities. Furthermore, during our exploration of the environment, external stimuli are being monitored (with proprioceptive-kinesthetic feedback) by means of orienting movements of head, eyes, trunk, and limbs. This information contributes to the development of space and time perception, which in turn produces in the individual a specific movement image of interaction with an object (10). Piaget described this development of environment-movement constructs in a similar way when he discussed the development of spatial-temporal concepts. He considered spatial concepts to be "internalized actions, not merely mental images of external things or events, or even images of the results of actions"

(11). Miller, Galanter, and Pribram discussed the same development of environment-movement constructs. They characterized these environment-oriented actions as "internal representation of the universe" (12). Konorski's concept of tactile, visual, and auditory kinesthetic gnostic units is most descriptive for understanding the complex integration of neurophysiological processes involved in skills acquisition. Bernstein used the term "engram" for describing movement images and their formulas existing in the central nervous system "containing in some form of brain trace the whole process of the movement in its entire course in time" (13). During each environmental interaction, specific compositions of cognitive-sensory-perceptual-motor processes form concurrent and successive signal-impulse chains (14) with their unique synapse-transmission imprint patterns that carry spatial and temporal information from the external and internal environments to the brain. These neurophysiological units of messages are coded and stored as programmed. In subsequent identical or similar interactions with the environment, comparable compositions of gnostic units can be retrieved. Guyton described these concepts as follows: "It is primarily in the sensory and sensory association areas that he [the person] experiences effects of motor movements and records 'memories' of the different patterns of motor movements. When he wishes to achieve some purposeful act, he presumably calls forth one of these engrams and then sets the motor system of the brain into action to reproduce the sensory pattern that is laid down in the engram" (15).

Accordingly, under normal circumstances, learning a skill is rarely an entirely new experience. The learner brings to the situation constructs of characteristics that describe objects, conscious or subconscious awareness of external and internal forces to which movements and motor control mechanisms must be adapted, and memory traces of movement compositions that worked previously in interacting with a specific surrounding under given circumstances. Fitts and Posner described the recognition of properties of situations as a prerequisite to positive transfer in learning. Old stimulus-response relationships are recalled as "appropriate cognitive sets and expectancies. 'Set' implies that the learner is prepared in advance for a particular event or class of events. A single name or cue can elicit a whole class of behavior which can be used in the new situation. . . . The degree of similarity between the old stimulus-response relationship and the new one is important" (16).

The various writings cited earlier seem to reflect a common denominator: Engrams from previous contacts with the environment provide a foundation for planning and recruiting appropriate goal-oriented movements for similar situations that arise later (17).

At this point we are forced to recognize how important it is to keep intact those primary and secondary sensory systems (18) that gather, transmit, interpret, and integrate information from within us and around us. Therefore, for successful skills acquisition, the second most important function is the ability to appraise those properties of environmental objects and forces with which movement and motor control must be made compatible.

The neurophysiological functions necessary for such appraisal are the following: (a) memory of the goal selected for achievement; (b) special and general sensory functions for gathering information about environmental events; (c) control of eye, head, trunk, and limb movements necessary for investigation of the environment; (d) recall of past knowledge of characteristic properties of environmental events; (e) judgment that will permit selective attention to the pertinent properties, with disregard for stimuli not important for the task and stimuli that do not interfere with the specific task to be accomplished (19); (f) ability to interpret, compare, integrate, and store, as well as immediately recall, concurrent and successive incoming information; (g) ability to forward sensory information to the cortical and subcortical motor control systems for subsequent motor planning and execution.

A single purposeful movement rarely constitutes an activity. Learning occurs through precise spatial and temporal linking of workable engrams, each of which carries the blueprint of a specific gnostic unit. When fixing a bookshelf, reaching for the hammer on the workbench has a different cognitive-sensory-perceptual-motor stimulus composition than does reaching for nails in the cabinet, and grasping each of these objects establishes different gnostic units than does carrying them to the work area or using them to complete the task. For each of the action components of this endeavor, the sensory-perceptual-motor processes organized and integrated by the peripheral and central nervous systems can be analyzed and defined.

Throughout our lives, and specifically during our growing years, we develop innumerable variations of gnostic units. The variability of these compositions has a direct relationship to the richness of our life experiences. However, in treatment sessions we meet individuals whose potential growth and development cannot be realized, or those whose life activities and expectations have been interrupted by psychosocial or physical trauma or disease. These are the patients or clients who in attempting to learn new skills or adapt old ones may not be able to use the constructs that lead to goal-directed movements. They may have difficulty remembering the purpose of the planned action, or they may be so easily distracted that they cannot pay attention to pertinent details of an activity. They may show symptoms of decreased primary sensory functions or signs of fragmented perceptual skills that prevent them from recognizing the characteristics of objects. Those with cognitive or perceptual deficits may have difficulty in planning the required movements, or they may be unable to control movements because of decreased sensory feedback. Tactile-kinesthetic sensory function also acts as an information-forwarding mechanism for subsequent movements (20). In the presence of any of these problems, learning occurs through negative transfer. This type of learning requires much patience on the part of the learner, because the customary circuits of constructs related to an activity are interrupted, and thus their previous programming is no longer applicable. New circuits must be programmed. Particularly in the case of young patients it must be kept in mind that they may not be amenable to the same thought patterns as the therapist; often they must do things their own way, using their own engrams.

The therapist's professional training facilitates a detailed evaluation of a patient's function-dysfunction status and determination of the cognitive-sensory-perceptual-motor processes necessary for accomplishing each phase of a task. By such determinations the therapist can guide patients toward reaching maximum potential. The following are a few suggestions for assisting patients to structure their experiences as they attempt to acquire or regain the skills necessary to perform specific activities: (a) The therapist should assess the properties of an activity that lead to the formation of groups of gnostic units that are common to most individuals who are in a specific age group and who have similar ethnic-cultural backgrounds. (b) The therapist should determine the patient's educational, cultural, and social history, as well as work and leisure experiences. (c) The therapist should determine the type and quality of constructs and expectations the patient brings to the learning situation. (d) The therapist should structure the learning experience so that the patient will learn to recognize environmental interactions having to do with objects, space, and time, all of which are important to movement planning and execution, as well as any feedback recall during and after the movement (21). (e) The therapist should adapt environmental spaces and highlight those objects appropriate to increase the patient's level of sensory-motor function. Increasing the patient's awareness of environmental factors may constitute treatment in itself, in preparation for building gnostic units. (f) The therapist should steadily increase the complexity of the movement-environment interaction so that the patient will have an opportunity to apply newly developed skills to new, but similar, tasks and later to entirely different life tasks. Through skilled performance the patient "not only interacts with the surrounding environment, but also actively operates on this environment, altering it with respect to particular results" (22).

The process of environmental assimilation and accommodation presupposes that individuals have the ability to recognize the properties of events that occur around them. The level of skills acquisition is reflected in the individual's capacity to reduce such information to concise sensory-motor engrams and to store and encode them in appropriate circumstances. These constructs enable the individual to make swift coordinated movements free of redundant degrees of range of motion (23) that are composed of synchronized, goal-directed components. In the endeavor to perform their selected tasks and implement chosen plans, individuals usually recall past experiences and adapt them to new task requirements. When patients are cognitively or physically disabled, it often takes great expenditure of mental energy to construct new interaction sets or adapt old sets (24,25) in an attempt to reach accommodation between the environment and their redefined goals. Because of their professional training, occupational therapists are well qualified to guide patients in this adjustment process.

PSYCHONEUROPHYSIOLOGICAL PROCESSES OF MOTOR PLANNING

The term "motor planning" appears to be a contradiction in terms. Planning implies cognitive participation in a process (26), whereas motor activity occurs largely involuntarily, reflexively (27). But in neurophysiology motor planning is considered to be a process that has cognitive and reflex-activity characteristics.

Motor planning involves a conception of a movement that will achieve a goal. Achievement of the goal is dependent on sequential sets of events proceeding from a beginning to an end. "A plan is any hierarchical process that can control the order in which a sequence of operations is to be performed" (28). Neurophysiology has not yet explained how an idea of a movement is generated. Cognition theorists have given us descriptions of what they call images, from which we may conjecture what an idea of a movement might be. Miller, Galanter, and Pribram stated that an "image is all the accumulated organized knowledge that the organism has about itself and its world" (29). Applying this thinking to a movement image, we can say that the image is a cognitive picture of a sensory-motor experience of a past environmental contact. This movement image reflects a sequential order of sensory, perceptual, and motor events (30). Therefore it may be said that movement images represent plans of actions that have been carried out and then stored in the memory. They can be retrieved to serve as a basis for planning future actions (31). It is possible that movement images or engrams or both function as blueprints for motor planning during the learning of new skills or the adapting of old skills, or they may act as trigger mechanisms for skilled movements, or they may function as facilitators of the motor control centers that are to generate and control interdependent goal-oriented movements (32).

Thus processes of motor planning are carried out at three levels of consciousness. In learning new skills or in modifying old habits, a plan of action is devised through conscious cognitive processes. Patients either learn for themselves or are taught the interdependent step-by-step procedures required to master each subskill of an activity. In this process they must learn to deal with the environmental factors encountered, such as the properties of objects and the directions and timing of movements. They must learn to accommodate their motions to the factors encountered (33).

Once a skill is acquired, motor planning continues at a subconscious level. Sets of sensory-motor engrams that contain the previously established movement plans are used. These gnostic units are representations of the factors involved: environmental events, sensory-motor transmission patterns, initiating and modulating programs for postural control, and stabilizers, agonists, synergists, and antagonists of successive movement patterns. In short, the memory of previously learned activity-specific movements and their neurophysiological processes can be evoked simply by the intention to perform the activity. An individual does not have to think about how to start a movement or proceed with each phase of the movement. Anticipation of events and subsequent recruitment of appropriate movement patterns occur in an uninterrupted flow, hand in hand with concurrent execution of multiple complex patterns of limb actions. Orienting movements that in the initial phase of skills acquisition were important in gathering information about the environment no longer play an important part. The linkage of engrams that constitutes a train of hierarchically organized movement patterns is the motor plan. This program sets the motor initiating centers and control mechanisms into action (34). During performance of the action, the individual is aware of the sequence progression, and by means of feedback processes any adjustments that the sequence may require are planned and implemented.

The third type of motor planning involves the unconscious processes of initiation and control. The trigger mechanisms that set off motor control programs are different for movements of average speed and movements that involve fast muscle contractions.

During the performance of movements of average speed, activity-related exteroceptive information and feedback from orienting movements conjoin with engrams that match the intended goal. Together they reflexively trigger afferent-fiber circuits belonging to the motor initiation mechanisms of the reticular activating system, the basal ganglia, and the thalamus, whose fibers terminate in the motor cortex (35,36). The cortex elicits motor responses to the prime movers, synergists, trunk and limb stabilizers, and antagonists that participate in a specific movement component at a given time (37). The motor initiation mechanisms also alert the subcortical motor control centers so that subsequent efferent motor impulses can be modulated in response to the intended goal and the motor program of the engram. Feedback from ongoing movements facilitates adjustment (through error-control mechanisms) of tone quality for subsequent movements. Two such error-control centers that function in close association are the cerebellum and the vestibular system (38,39). They send feedback information from muscle spindles, tendon organs, and equilibrium receptors to the subcortical and cortical motor centers, respectively. Motor response recruitment and control processes are quite complex. The types of responses and programs for presetting the motor control mechanisms are different for each muscle that is to participate in the successive movement pattern. This applies to such interdependent movements as reaching, grasping, and releasing.

Motor planning for fast movements involves retrieval of engrams of past similar experiences. These act as advance informers to the motor initiating centers and motor control centers. Fast movements can be executed only if no deliberate planning is required. Fast movements cannot benefit from feedback as an information-forwarding mechanism (40). The performer learns of errors only "after the fact" (41). The reactions of athletes derive solely from a repertoire of accumulated engrams.

Knowledge of the processes of motor planning is fundamental to successful activity analysis. It enables the therapist to identify those movement components that must be learned through conscious motor planning. If the therapist adapts the activity to fit the patient's cultural, educational, and vocational background, the patient will be able to use existing gnostic units or sensory-motor engrams in planning movement strategy for the task. Because of similarity to past experiences, the task will be easier to learn, and ease of learning spurs motivation. Step-by-step learning can be reduced, thus freeing the patient to go on to more creative steps in the process. Thus the patient will see the activity as being more interesting, and progress will be more rapid.

From a therapeutic viewpoint, knowledge of the processes of motor planning can facilitate an understanding of the dynamics of apraxia and determination of the degree of impairment. As stated earlier, the events involved in movement sequences designed to interact with environmental events occur consciously, subconsciously or unconsciously.

An intention to achieve a goal produces movement images and retrieves engrams. Either of these can activate the motor initiating and control centers. Patients who are unable to produce movement images (because of frontal lobe damage or lesion of the motor initiating centers) are incapable of initiating purposeful movements for achieving goals. They may not even be capable of setting goals. Because of the absence of movement images the movement initiating centers are not stimulated to activate the motor cortex. This causes ideational apraxia (42). The actions that these patients do take are conditioned reflexes, such as eating. Gustatory and olfactory sensations trigger these very old motor engrams.

In the attempt to help the patient, the therapist should search for those engrams in the patient's repertoire that were developed very early in life. Activities that involve postural control mechanisms (subcortically controlled) linked with perhaps one strong exteroceptive input (e.g., dancing) may elicit some patient participation. The therapist may also be able to employ simple activities of a vocational nature that a patient has used over many years of adult life. It is to be hoped that such patients will activate deeply rooted engrams that can trigger the movement initiation centers and control mechanisms. Motor planning should then occur subconsciously until the involved brain area has time to recover.

Inability to retrieve sensory-motor engrams applicable to a task at hand causes confusion in motor performance; task-oriented movement plans contained in the engram are not available to guide performance of the current task. In such cases patients have absolutely no idea how to plan their movements in order to interact with the environment, despite the fact that they know their goals, they can identify the characteristics of environmental events, and they have a sense of movement timing. It appears that the sensory engrams have dissociated themselves from the motor engram that contains the movement program for the task to be performed. This disability is called ideokinetic apraxia (43). It is related to lesions of superior temporal and angular gyri (44,45). A milder form of this disability is manifested as clumsiness or confusion regarding handedness. The cause may be that too many motor engrams are attempting to interact with the environment at the same time. In such cases the therapist should highlight environmental cues as reference points to which the patient can seek to subordinate the interaction movement. Also, the therapist should write out a detailed program of step-by-step instructions for movement sequences that coincide with progressive levels of task achievement. The environmental events to which interaction movements are matched must not change until the patient masters the task independently without cues. Patients with ideokinetic apraxia must relearn old skills as if they were totally new skills. They must reintegrate sensory-motor experiences.

Kinetic apraxia appears to be related to ideokinetic apraxia (46), but the focus of the motor planning problem is different. The question the patient faces is not what type of movements to organize, but what sequence of movements to follow. The basic principle of treatment is to provide a structured learning situation in which the proper sequence of actions for the given task can be relearned. Lesions of the somatosensory cortex can cause kinetic apraxia (47).

It is crucial that the therapist analyze all factors that contribute to successful achievement of the patient's goal. The activity must be interesting enough to spur the patient's intrinsic motivation. Better results will be achieved if the environmental events with which the patient is expected to interact are familiar. The patient's interest in the activity and perception of relevant environmental events are the two most important parameters for effective motor functioning, because they are the mobilizers for the conscious and subconscious motor planning processes necessary for coordinated goal-oriented movements related to specific task performance.

In the attempt to match an activity to the patient's level of cognitive-sensory-perceptual-motor functions, the therapist must consider the sensory-motor integrative processes that play important roles in any activity. These may be covert and "must be inferred from the actual performance" (48).

Synchronization of orienting movements of eyes and head is initiated and monitored through the vestibular system. When the head is turned, the vestibular system sends its information regarding head movements to the oculomotor control center for the purpose of synchronizing the eye movements, which have smaller ranges of motion than head movements (49).

Postural adjustments must be made continually during each movement phase of the activity in order to achieve controlled and coordinated limb movements. Appropriate positioning of the body in relation to environmental events assures spatial and temporal matching of the movement component with the engram of a similar past experience.

Characteristics of unfamiliar objects should be explored before training movement matches are initiated.

If conscious motor planning is the treatment objective, the patient must practice interactions with stable objects in the environment. This teaches the use of past and current sensory-motor information that can help predict the possible outcome. If necessary, the environment and the activity can be adapted to the level of the patient's spatial and temporal motor control. An activity that is designed to be carried out in a stable environment is called a "closed skill" (50).

An activity that requires the patient to intercept a moving object in the environment precludes subconscious motor planning. There is insufficient time for prediction and subsequent planning of movements. The mechanisms of the central nervous system must adapt quickly if a moving object is to be intercepted. Such movements are guided by the various engrams available from previous similar experiences. "Practice makes perfect" is not just a behavioral phenomenon; it also works on the neurophysiological level. In situations involving moving objects there are so many possible reactions available to the patient that such an activity is aptly called an "open skill" (51). The therapist can observe that open skills are often less difficult than closed skills for patients with motor planning deficiencies. The speed with which a spontaneous motor reaction is recalled does not give the patient time to stumble over the planning of movements. Catching a ball (open skill) is easier than throwing a ball toward a stable target (closed skill), which requires the planning of an interaction match with specific events in the environment.

ANALYSIS OF ACTIVITY PERFORMANCE

The two most important functions that lead to the execution of goal-oriented movements are goal intentions and recognition of those environmental factors with which movements must be made compatible. These two constructs act as trigger mechanisms for planning the intended movements.

The concept of movement in its many forms has been widely used in philosophy and the natural sciences to describe the flowing energies acting in the universe. Painters, composers, and sculptors often use the term in describing the dynamic processes involved in their work. Thus movement can be analyzed from many frames of reference. This last part of activity analysis involves an understanding of the principles of sensory-motor development, as well as other principles of neurophysiology, kinesiology, and biophysics.

Depending on the limitations and capabilities of individual patients, there is a wide range of activities that may be mastered through occupational therapy. However, because of the complexity of sensory-motor reeducation, particularly for adults, the possibilities often are limited to activities that involve unilateral or bilateral single or multiple joint movements of the arms from a sitting or standing position. This discussion of movement analysis will deal primarily with this most common therapy situation. Also, a descriptive format is not adequate for analysis of activities that involve movements of the entire body. The dynamics of such complex activities (involving eye and head movements, postural adjustments to support multiple limb movements, and internal and external forces acting on the body) can be captured only by means of elaborate electronic technology, and the concomitant perceptual-cognitive processes can only be inferred.

A given activity involves a set of hierarchical events leading to the desired end (52). This concept of activity is used here in describing the sensory-motor processes that occur during each event. The following are some of the basic arm movement patterns involved in this activity analysis: (a) bilateral rhythmic gross movements, with proximal muscle groups acting primarily as agonists and distal muscles performing a holding action; (b) unilateral gross movements of the dominant arm, with the nondominant arm assisting; (c) bilateral concurrent or successive complementary gross or fine movements (the joints move cooperatively, but timing and movement patterns are arhythmic and may not coincide spatially and temporally, e.g., playing a piano); (d) unilateral fine movements involving wrist and finger muscles. Again, it should be emphasized how important postural control mechanisms are to the performance of coordinated limb movements, since the extremities function as pendulums attached to the trunk.

An activity, considered as a sphere of actions, can be analyzed with respect to (a) subskills or tasks to be learned and performed, (b) type and number of processes that compose each subskill or task, and (c) type, number, and sequence of movement components by which each process is accomplished.

An activity is composed of one or more distinct subskills or tasks. These tasks may involve interdependence and time limits and may require proper sequencing. As an example of an activity designed to achieve a specific goal, consider the construction of a bookshelf. The following subskills or tasks are to be performed: (a) selecting and buying the wood, (b) drawing a blueprint or reading and interpreting instructions, (c) preparing the wood surface, (d) applying the design to the wood, (e) cutting the wood, (f) assembling the shelf, (g) finishing the surface. Each of these subskills is a nonrepetitive task. For each of these tasks a number of processes must be carried out. Cutting the wood involves two processes: (a) securing the wood on the workbench, (b) sawing the wood with a handsaw. Each of these processes involves sequentially interdependent cognitive-sensory-perceptual-motor components that require their own unique receptor-effector and feedback processing for achieving the desired purpose. Using the handsaw involves the following environment-interaction matches or components: (a) reaching for the saw (reach phase), (b) grasping its handle (grasp phase), (c) carrying it to the workbench (loaded carry phase), (d) sawing the wood (action phase, here a repetitive movement), (e) returning the saw to its storage place (loaded return phase), (f) releasing its handle (release phase).

When activities are broken down into their many components it becomes obvious that skilled performance is a considerable achievement.

As stated earlier, the learning of a skill involves transposition of previously learned sensory-motor patterns to a new situation (53). What must then be learned is the adaptation and sequencing of movement components. During this acquisition phase, patients are consciously aware of some functions that must be carried out, and they subconsciously employ those controls that have already been mastered. The sequences of the movement components are different for the various processes. In early learning, halts (54) interspersed between components provide an opportunity to assess the environmental events with which the following movement must be compatible and to plan the strategy of its execution (55). Peripheral and central neuromuscular controls of postural adjustments, prime movers, synergists, stabilizers, and antagonists must differ from one component to another in order to deal with the environmental events encountered. During the conscious learning phase of any activity, ocular movements are important for gathering information (scanning) (56), guiding limb movements, providing feedback (tracking), and planning subsequent movements (scanning).

As the activity continues, repetition leads to neurophysiological integration, which facilitates performance of successive components. Convergence of neurophysiological events results in a single sensory-motor engram and motor plan (57) that contains the chain of successive components involved in that activity. These sensory-motor units are coded and stored in the posteriolateral regions of the cortex, in the area of the superior temporal and angular gyri. These regions receive afferent association fibers from all areas of the cortices (58). When recalled, these sensory-motor engrams of specific chains of movement components can trigger the motor initiating and control centers. Thus a movement initiated through engrams alone has the characteristics of being autonomous, self-regulating, apparently requiring no conscious effort for its execution. Bernstein stated that "the automatization of a motor act is the constantly maintained transmission of numerous technical [background] corrections to the lower co-ordinated systems, the sensory syntheses of which are most adequately organized for corrections of the given type and quality" (59). He pointed out that the concept of automated movement arose from the fact that "all component processes in control corrections disappear from the field of consciousness" (60). An automatic or habitual movement is not the same as a skilled movement, with respect to the controlling neurophysiological processes. A controlled habitual movement may be dependent on only a single stimulus to activate appropriate responses, e.g., a factory bell calling the laborer to work. Skilled movements, on the other hand, are what the laborer uses in adapting his actions to the changes and complications that arise in his work environment. Activities that do not require conscious control for their performance can be combined with a task that does require conscious effort. This conception of habitual movement versus skilled movement explains why many patients with cognitive impairments are able to perform routine activities but are unable to learn skilled tasks. One reason for this inability is that these patients cannot assimilate feedback as the activity proceeds. The habitual movement, engram-guided and subcortically regulated, does not bring feedback information to the conscious level. The skilled movement is a deliberate environmental interaction, a movement of choice. Its exteroceptive feedback (and for some patients proprioceptive feedback) is experienced consciously as the activity proceeds. It is coded and stored. Its recall makes possible self-evaluation of performance.

In most situations, feedback influences goal-oriented movements, whether they are being learned or are habitual or skilled movements. An exception to this feedback control is the rapid movement discussed earlier in relation to closed and open skills. Chains of goal-oriented movements are influenced by four functions of feedback information:

Feedback contributes to the development of a motor plan, which is embodied in the engram (61). From the beginning to the end of an activity, afferent information from ongoing movements tends to fix the order to successive neurophysiological events as the chain of environmental interactions proceeds. Thus it is important for learning or relearning a skill that the steps in any activity be carefully planned. Laban inferred this feedback function in his description of habitual movements: "Many movements are, however, done involuntarily, that means without the investigation and guidance of a conscious decision. In the automatic repetitive movements used so frequently in industry, man does not think of the motive, or even the effect of his movements, he simply performs them in the right order after having taken the initial decision to do the work" (62).

Feedback serves as a comparator (63) among intentions, environmental requirements, and step-by-step goal realization. Ongoing feedback from sensory neurons gives the sensory-motor integrative and control centers information on interactions between movements and the environment. It provides information on movement direction and velocity, tensions in muscles, tendons, and skin, and forces acting on the moving and stabilizing structures of the body. This afferent information is correlated with the goal intention and with knowledge of the environmental characteristics with which movements must be compatible. Thus the comparator function of feedback provides a test of the accuracy of motor planning and reveals whether or not intermediate and final objectives are being achieved. Feedback recall provides the signals to go ahead or halt and correct (64).

Feedback subsequently acts as a modulator and adapter of sensory input and motor output. It corrects impulses by adjusting facilitation and inhibition mechanisms (65,66). This accommodation of the spatial-temporal characteristics of the movement to the spatial-temporal requirements of environmental events diminishes the discrepancies among goal, motor plan, and actual output.

Feedback can be a predictor of movement (67), providing the conditioned stimuli for imposing controls on subsequent movement components within an activity process. Extrinsic and intrinsic feedback from an ongoing movement informs the central nervous system of progress; concurrently it tunes in the excitatory and inhibitory mechanisms for subsequent postural adjustments and sets tone requirements for stabilizers, agonists, synergists, and antagonists responsible for executing the next movement. This predictor function of feedback accounts for the fact that learned movements have the capacity to become self-regulating.

Feedback as "afferentation of motor control" (68) is important in any goal-oriented movement, whether it is being learned or is a habitual or skilled movement. Deliberate coordinated interaction with the environment cannot be controlled by the subcortical sensory-motor integrative systems alone. The skilled motor act is always subjected to the consciously determined mode of action, the goal to be achieved; otherwise motor planning and execution would cease to be effective. People occasionally have the experience of going to a closet or cabinet to collect an item only to find when they get there that they have forgotten what they were looking for. Feedback as a comparator will usually enable them to recall their initial goal intentions and readjust their motor plans so that the interaction match will become effective. Laban agreed: "Man is conscious of the efforts bridging the gulf between our intentions and realization of them by our movements and actions" (69).

Not all behavioral responses to information from the external and internal environments are learned reactions. Some purposeful movements have developed phylogenetically and are programmed such that they will be evoked ontogenetically during the growth and development of the individual. Some of these are the following: (a) reflexes and resultant reactive behavior; (b) muscle tone recruitment specific to the task to be performed; (c) multilevel integration of cognitive processes and perceptual information through functional development of associative cortical connections (sometimes interaction with the environment does not occur as overt movement, but rather as symbolic representation; also, nonverbal expression can occur as movement of which the individual is not consciously aware); (d) intrahemispheric and interhemispheric information exchange involving numerous feedback circuits through which sexual behavior, fright behavior, and other reactive behaviors are elicited.

As such unconscious central nervous system functions mature, one's ability to solve problems emanating from within and from the environment steadily increases.

Activity analysis is based on the concept that an activity presents a problem to be solved through a series of sequentially interdependent goal-oriented movements, shaped by the characteristics of environmental events. Each movement in this chain of actions is a product of cognitive-sensory-perceptual-motor behaviors. "The development of skills involves the construction of a hierarchy of behavioral units, each unit guided by its own Plan" (70). This plan is the sensory-motor engram developed during a previous environmental interaction involving feedback, the basis for self-regulation of skilled motor behavior. If cognitive, sensory, perceptual, and motor functions are unimpaired, goal-directed movement capabilities develop ontogenetically to become an integrated system controlled by many centers of the central nervous system. In this context, Luria's hesitancy to consider a voluntary movement a "willed act" is understandable. He saw it as a "complex reflex act carried out under the influence of a group of afferent systems. By regarding efferent mechanisms as only part of the cerebral organization of motor acts, and redirecting attention to those afferent systems taking part in the construction of the motor act, the reflex theory shows, that the voluntary movement is the result of the integrated activity of the whole brain and that as the most highly organized activity, it may be impaired by many lesions of the cerebral hemisphere" (71).

How can occupational therapists, whose objective is to assist patients in increasing their ability to function, promote the learning or relearning of adaptive skills? They can achieve their objective if they apply the following methods of motor learning: (a) Define the subskills and their process units that constitute an activity. (b) Analyze the type and sequential interdependence of subskills and their processes. (c) Determine the cognitive-sensory-perceptual-motor requirements necessary to learn and carry out each component of an activity process. (d) Determine which of the psychoneurophysiological prerequisites of each component need remediation and how this can be integrated into the natural flow of task performance so as not to disturb the meaning and sequence of task performance. (e) Determine the types and characteristics of environmental cues to which the patient can give attention during performance (important to sensory training, multisensory integration, and feedback recall). (f) Determine strategies for structuring, adapting, and upgrading the complex of environmental events to encourage subordination of motor control integration to the subconscious level. (g) Determine the necessary positioning of the patient with respect to objects in the environment so that the patient can elicit engrams of postural adjustment and muscle groups appropriate to accommodate environmental events during the performance of each component of the activity processes. (h) Define the strategy for augmenting feedback to the patient: concurrent, immediate, delayed, and terminal (72). These phases of feedback have reference to goal determination, environmental events, and motor planning for postural mechanisms, single joint movements, joint movement integration, sequencing and timing of movements, and progression of movement execution.

SUMMARY

The life-styles of mature individuals reflect the strategies they have used to organize their tasks and acquire the skills necessary to attain their goals. In this model of activity analysis, task performance is seen as something more than execution of motor acts. Skills acquisition depends on one's capacity to determine one's goals, to receive and transmit external and internal information, to process this information and associate it with information from previous experiences, and to formulate, execute, and readapt responses commensurate with environmental requirements and accomplishment of one's immediate tasks and long-range goals. These parameters of goal-directed movements are mirrored in the structure and problem-solving format of this activity analysis.

Rehabilitation of function can best be achieved when the usual program of joint-movement exercises is combined with life-style-oriented activities and long-range goals. An exercise program without this orientation cannot take advantage of the psychoneurophysiological processes through which a person reaches maturity. Patients in exercise-oriented treatment programs cannot benefit from the richness of their past life experiences. A life-style-oriented rehabilitation program allows the patient to relearn responses that were once meaningful and adapt them to new environmental events.

REFERENCES

1. Council on Standards and Executive Board (1972): Occupational therapy: Its definition and function. *Am. J. Occup. Ther.* 36:204–205.
2. Bernstein, B. (1967): *The Co-ordination and Regulation of Movements,* p. 115. Pergamon Press, Elmsford, N.Y.
3. Gentile, A.M. (1972): *A Working Model of Skill Acquisition with Application to Teaching.* Quest XVII monograph, p. 4.
4. Miller, G., Galanter, E., and Pribram, K. H. (1960): *Plans and the Structure of Behavior,* Chapters 7 and 8. Holt, Rinehart & Winston, New York.
5. Welford, A. T. (1968): *Fundamental of Skills,* pp. 327–328. Methuen & Co., London.
6. Miller et al., op. cit., Chapter 1.
7. Council on Standards, op. cit., pp. 204–205.
8. Legge, D. (1970): *Skills.* Penguin Books, Baltimore.
9. Piaget, J. (1972): *Psychology of Intelligence,* p. 8. Littlefield, and Adams Company, Towa, N.J.
10. Konorski, J. (1967): *Integrative Activity of the Brain, an Interdisciplinary Approach,* Chapter 4. University of Chicago Press, Chicago.
11. Piaget, J., and Inhelder, B. (1967): *The Child's Conception of Space,* pp. 451–454. W. W. Norton & Co., New York.
12. Miller et al., op. cit., Chapter 1.
13. Bernstein, op. cit., p. 37.
14. Piaget, op. cit., pp. 108–110.
15. Guyton, A. C. (1976): *Structure and Function of the Nervous System,* ed. 2, pp. 171–172. W. B. Saunders, Philadelphia.
16. Fitts, P. M., and Posner, M. I. (1968): *Human Performance,* p. 20. Brooks/Cole, Belmont, Calif.
17. Guyton, op. cit., p. 172.
18. Luria, A. K. (1966): *Higher Cortical Functions in Man,* pp. 34 and 85. Basic Books, New York.
19. Gentile, op. cit., pp. 5–6.
20. Guyton, op. cit., p. 169.
21. Gentile, op, cit., pp. 8, 10, 16.
22. Bernstein, op. cit., p. 114.
23. Bernstein, op. cit., p. 127.
24. Miller et al., op. cit., p. 7.
25. Piaget, op. cit., p. 108.
26. Miller et al., op. cit., Chapter 1.
27. Guyton, op. cit., p. 156.
28. Miller et al., op. cit., p. 16.
29. Miller et al., op. cit., p. 17.
30. Piaget, op. cit., pp. 106–107.
31. Luria, op. cit., pp. 165–169.
32. Guyton, op. cit., pp. 171–174.
33. Gentile, op. cit., p. 6.
34. Guyton, op. cit., pp. 173–174.
35. Ibid.
36. Hassler, R. (1975): Interaction of reticular activating system for vigilance and the truncothalamic and pallidal systems for directing awareness and attention under striatal control. In *Cerebral Correlates of Conscious Experience,* edited by P. A. Buser. Elsevier/North Holland, New York.
37. Guyton, op. cit., p. 159.
38. Guyton, op. cit., p. 169.
39. Guyton, op. cit., p. 148.
40. Guyton, op. cit., p. 172.
41. Fitts and Posner, op. cit., p. 109.
42. Luria, op. cit., p. 170.
43. Ibid.
44. Ibid.
45. Guyton, op. cit., p. 201.
46. Luria, op. cit., p. 170.
47. Guyton, op. cit., p. 201.
48. Fitts and Posner, op. cit., p. 112.
49. Bizzi, E. (1974): The coordination of eye-head movements. *Sci. Am.,* 231:100–106; Dichgans, J., Bizzi, E., Morasso, P., and Tagliasco, (1973): Mechanisms underlying recovery of eye-head coordination following bilateral labyrinthectomy in monkeys. *Exp. Brain Res.,* 18:548, 562.

50. Gentile, op. cit., p. 6
51. Ibid.
52. Miller et al., op. cit., Chapter 6.
53. Piaget, op. cit., Chapter 4.
54. Bartlet, F. (1958): *Thinking, an Experimental and Social Study,* p. 16. Basic Books, New York.
55. Luria, op. cit., pp. 166–167, 169.
56. Bernstein, op. cit., p. 117.
57. Miller et al., op. cit., Chapter 14.
58. Luria, op. cit., p. 57.
59. Bernstein, op. cit., p. 136.
60. Ibid.
61. Guyton, op. cit., p. 172.
62. Laban, R., and Lawrence, F. C. (1967): *Effort,* p. 5. MacDonald & Evans, London.
63. Guyton, op. cit., pp. 148, 153, 168.
64. Gentile, op. cit., pp. 8–11.
65. Guyton, op. cit., Chapter 10 and p. 168.
66. Luria, op. cit., pp. 166–168.
67. Guyton, op. cit., p. 169.
68. Bernstein, op. cit., p. 117.
69. Laban and Lawrence, op. cit., p. 5.
70. Miller et al., op. cit., p. 85.
71. Luria, op. cit., p. 169.
72. Holding, D. H. (1965): *Principle of Training,* pp. 21–35. Pergamon Press, Elmsford, N.Y.

APPENDIX

ACTIVITY ANALYSIS
Worksheets

Predominant characteristics of an activity as a whole

A. Role and purpose of the activity: classification related to:

1. Life tasks:
   a. Active engagement ☐ for the purpose of
      - Earning a living ☐
      - Providing services to others ☐
      - Meeting one's own vital needs ☐
      - Meeting one's own nonvital needs ☐
      - Providing oneself relaxation and enjoyment ☐

   b. Passive engagement ☐ for the purpose of
      - Mental and emotional growth ☐
      - Enjoying leisure ☐
2. Social interaction potentials:
   a. It is a solitary activity ____________________
   b. It requires two to four participants ____________________
   c. It is suitable for a group activity ____________________

   ____

B. Description of the activity (type, variations, number of subskills)

____

____

____

____

____

____

____

____

C. Suitability/adaptability of the activity to the background of an individual:

1. Activity related to status:

   a. Age ______________________________

   b. Sex ______________________________

   c. Education ______________________________

   d. Vocation ______________________________

   e. Role in the family ______________________________

   f. Role in the community ______________________________

   g. Socioeconomic background ______________________________

   h. Cultural background ______________________________

2. Activity related to level of function:

   a. Physical strength ______________________________

   b. Physical tolerance ______________________________

   c. Psychosocial function ______________________________

      (identification) ______________________________

   d. Level of intelligence ______________________________

      (imagination, memory) ______________________________

   e. Level of creativity ______________________________

      (initiative, imagination) ______________________________

   f. Approach to learning ______________________________

      (abstract, concrete) ______________________________

   g. Ability to learn ______________________________

      (memory, attention span, perception) ______________________________

   h. Personal interests ______________________________

   i. Personal needs related to status ______________________________

      ____

   j. Personal needs related to personality ______________________________

      ____

   k. Frustration span ______________________________

Analysis of environmental and internal events and their characteristic qualities or properties to which movements must conform

1. Properties of equipment or tools:

- ☐ small
- ☐ large
- ☐ cutting
- ☐ smoothing
- ☐ pounding
- ☐ shaping
- ☐ boring
- ☐ covering
- ☐ marking
- ☐ supporting
- ☐ holding material
- ☐ holding project
- ☐ controlling material
- ☐ controlling action

2. Properties of material:

- ☐ light
- ☐ heavy
- ☐ pliant
- ☐ resistive
- ☐ colored
- ☐ textured
- ☐ small
- ☐ large
- ☐ shaped
- ☐ needs to be shaped
- ☐ assembled
- ☐ needs to be assembled
- ☐ one single structure
- ☐ multiple structures
- ☐ ____________________

3. Properties of processes:

- ☐ rapid
- ☐ slow
- ☐ clean
- ☐ messy
- ☐ long
- ☐ short
- ☐ interruptable
- ☐ noninterruptable
- ☐ structured
- ☐ nonstructured
- ☐ complex
- ☐ simple
- ☐ ____________________

4. Physical requirements for dealing with environmental events:

a. Sensory:

- ☐ light touch
- ☐ deep pressure
- ☐ temperature
- ☐ smell
- ☐ taste
- ☐ vision
- ☐ sound

b. Motor:

- ☐ stability of joints
- ☐ flexibility of joints
- ☐ movements:
  - ☐ gross
  - ☐ fine
  - ☐ light
  - ☐ strenuous
  - ☐ bilateral
  - ☐ unilateral
  - ☐ upper extremity
  - ☐ lower extremity
  - ☐ slow
  - ☐ fast
  - ☐ rhythmic
  - ☐ reciprocal
  - ☐ repetitive
  - ☐ pulling
  - ☐ pushing
  - ☐ rotary

5. Psychosocial properties:

- ☐ constructive
- ☐ destructive
- ☐ structured
- ☐ nonstructured
- ☐ masculine
- ☐ feminine
- ☐ dependent
- ☐ independent
- ☐ ____________________
- ☐ ____________________

6. Properties of dimensions

a. Space allowance for equipment:

width ________________________________

height ________________________________

depth ________________________________

b. Space allowance for range of motion (ROM):

within full range in sagittal plane ☐

frontal plane ☐

vertical plane ☐

beyond full range in sagittal plane ☐

frontal plane ☐

vertical plane ☐

c. Occupation of space:

- ☐ table
- ☐ floor

7. Properties of safety: activity requires

- ☐ maximum precaution
- ☐ moderate precaution
- ☐ minimal precaution
- ☐ no precaution

Analysis of psychoneurophysiological constructs contributing to motor planning of one activity process

I. Description of activity processes

A. Number of processes ______

B. Types ______

C. Major equipment and tools used ______

D. Types of material used ______

E. Mechanics of position (if it is the same for all activity processes)

II. Analysis of one specific activity process

A. Type of activity process ______

B. Description of process ______

______

______

C. Level of function

1. Complexity of performance ______

2. Intellectual ability required ______

3. Physical tolerance required ______

D. Component or phase of activity process

1. Types				
2. Purpose				

E. Analysis of equipment and tool

1. Type of equipment ______

2. Size ______

3. Action used ______

4. Direction of movement used to operate the equipment ______

5. Purpose of movement ______

6. Type of tool or tools ______

7. Size (leverage) ______

8. Shape ______

9. Weight (in lb. or oz.) ______

10. Action ______

11. Direction of movement used to operate the tool ______

12. Purpose of movement ______

F. Description of material

1. Type ______

2. Property ______

Analysis of sensory-perceptual-motor engrams to be developed or recalled for motor planning

III. Psychoneurophysiological constructs contributing to motor planning:	Components of the activity process			
A. Sensory-perceptual-motor functions				
1. Visual perception:				
Recognition of color				
Discrimination of color				
Recognition of form				
Discrimination of form				
Form constancy				
Recognition of object representations				
Visual figure-ground discrimination				
Ability to generalize and classify common elements				
Visual sequencing				
Visual memory				
Visualization				
2. Visual spatial relationships:				
Visual spatial organization of part-to-part relations				
Visual spatial organization of part-to-whole relations				
Judgment of cause-and-effect relationship of events				
Visual spatial orientation (cues for identifying directions)				
Conscious transfer for spatial orientation (reversal or transposition of visual images)				
3. Visual-kinesthetic-motor controls:				
Tracking				
Scanning				
Imitation of movements				
Judgment of direction of movements				
Judgment of distance of movements or objects in space				
Judgment of timing of movements				
Judgment of timing of moving objects in space				
Control of precision of movements with variation of speed				
Control of precision of movements with variation of rhythm				
4. Tactile kinesthetic perception:				
Recognition of form				
Discrimination of form				
Recognition of texture				
Discrimination of texture				
Tactile form constancy				
Recognition of object representations				
Tactile kinesthetic perception				
Tactile kinesthetic memory				
Laterality (body-oriented spatial concepts)				
5. Tactile-kinesthetic-motor control:				
Precision of body parts positioning with respect to events				
Precision of movements (directions and degrees of ROM)				
Control of grasp and/or pinch force				
Control of pressure applied for identifying texture				
Control of pressure applied for shaping materials				
6. Auditory sensory perception:				
Recognition of sound				
Discrimination of sound				

	Components of the activity process			
Sequencing of sounds				
Auditory figure-ground discrimination				
Discrimination of direction of sound				
7. Auditory motor integration (coordination of sound & movement)				
8. Gustatory sensory perception:				
Recognition of taste				
Discrimination of taste				
9. Olfactory sensory perception:				
Recognition of odors				
Discrimination of odors				
Localization of odors				
B. Neuromotor function requirements for each component				
1. Neuromotor requisites for control of head, trunk, legs:				
Control of postural changes: static balance				
dynamic balance				
Control over reciprocal trunk movements: sagittal plane				
lateral plane				
rotation: vertical plane				
Control of rhythm of trunk movements				
Control of speed of head, trunk, and leg movements				
Control of simultaneous gross movements of trunk & legs				
Control of complementary movements of arms & legs				
2. Control of arm movements:				
Control of reciprocal unilateral gross movements				
Control of rhythm of unilateral gross movements				
Control of speed of unilateral gross movements				
Control of timing of bilateral rhythmic movements				
Control of timing of bilateral alternate movements				
Control of bilateral complementary movements (gross)				
Control of unilateral fine movements				
Control of bilateral rhythmic fine movements				
Control of bilateral complementary fine movements				
3. Motor skill required:				
Eye-hand coordination with unilateral or bilateral movements				
Eye-hand-foot coordination				
Slow tension movements, called moving fixation				
Rapid tension (controlled swinging, throwing, catching)				
Unilateral or bilateral movements requiring crossing midline				
4. Muscle strength required:				
Minimal (external forces are eliminated)				
Normal (no resistance except gravitational force)				
Normal (strength to overcome light resistance)				
Very good muscle strength to overcome moderate resistance				
Very good muscle strength to overcome heavy resistance				
5. Muscle power:				
Few minutes of endurance to 20 min				
Moderate endurance (to work 20 to 50 min)				
Long-term endurance (one to several hours)				

Analysis of performance of one activity process

A. Mechanics of postural adaptations and joint stabilization:

1. Fundamental body position ______
2. Worker's proximity to equipment ______
3. Work height ______
4. Body mechanics required to maintain equilibrium:
   a. Level of support ______ b. Size of support ______
   c. Level of gross body movement on stationary support ______
   d. Level of center of gravity in resting position ______
   e. Amount and direction of center of gravity shift during performance ______
   f. Muscle groups that maintain the static or dynamic balance during performance
   1) Lower extremities:
      Left: ______ Right: ______
   2) Trunk:
      Horizontal-frontal axis: anterior: ______
      posterior: ______
      Horizontal-sagittal axis: left: ______
      right: ______
      Vertical axis (rotations): ______
   3) Upper extremities:
      Left: ______ Right: ______
5. Muscle groups that provide joint fixation (proximal/distal) for stabilization or support of body, equipment, or material
   Lower extremities:
   Left: ______ Right: ______
   Trunk: ______
   Upper extremities:
   Left: ______ Right: ______

B. Motion analysis:

1. Use of upper extremities:
   - Right ☐
   - Left ☐
   - Unilateral integrated mov. ☐
   - Bilateral integrated mov. ☐
   - Unilateral localized mov. ☐
   - Bilateral localized mov. ☐
   - Complementary m. ☐
2. Prehension pattern:
   - Reciprocal grasp and release action ☐
   - Holding position ☐
   - Hook grasp ☐
   - Cylindrical grasp ☐
   - Spherical grasp ☐
   - Lateral pinch ☐
   - Palmar pinch ☐
   - Three-jaw chuck ☐
   - Fingertip prehension ☐
3. Starting positions of joints:
   - Trunk ☐
   - Sh. girdle ☐
   - Shoulder ☐
   - Elbow ☐
   - Forearm ☐
   - Wrist ☐
4. Position of the hands:
   - Resting position ☐
   - With fingers in extension ☐

4. Muscle and joint action of performance	Components of activity process											
Contraction/ROM	C	R	C	R	C	R	C	R	C	R	C	R
Trunk:												
flexion												
rotation right												
rotation left												
extension/thoracic lev.												
extension/lumbar lev.												
Shoulder girdle:												
protraction												
retraction												
elevation												
depression												
upward rotation												
downward rotation												
Shoulder:												
flexion												
extension												
abduction												
adduction												
horiz. abduction												
horiz. adduction												
inward rotation												
outward rotation												
Elbow:												
flexion												
extension												
Forearm:												
pronation												
supination												
Wrist:												
flexion												
extension												
radial deviation												
ulnar deviation												
Fingers: MP joints												
flexion												
extension												
abduction												
adduction												
Fingers: PIP joints												
flexion												
extension												
Fingers: DIP joints												
flexion												
extension												
Thumb: CMC joint												
rotation												
Thumb: MP joint												
flexion												
extension/abduction												
volar abduction												
adduction												
opposition												
Thumb: IP joint												
flexion												
extension												

Code:

R: ROM	C: Concentric contr.
F: full ROM	Eccentric contr.
0–¼ ROM	Static contr.
¼–½ ROM	
½–¾ ROM	

APPENDIX 1

Occupational therapy treatment media

A. Metal
- Forming
- Cutting
- Finishing
- Decorating
  - enameling
  - tooling
  - etching
  - copper tooling
  - wire jewelry

B. Leather
- Types of hide and use
- Pattern design
- Cutting
- Construction
  - cementing
  - stitching
  - punching holes
  - lacing
- Decorating
  - carving
  - embossing
  - tooling
  - dyeing
- Findings
- Finishing
- Link belts

C. Plastics
- Cutting
- Smoothing
- Forming
- Construction
- Finishing

D. Woodwork
- Use of hand tools
- Use of power tools
- Design and layout
- Construction
  - cutting
  - shaping
  - joining
- Finishing
  - preparing surface
  - applying finishes
- Decorating
  - veneering
  - parquetry
  - carving
  - wood burning
  - wood turning (lathe)
  - whittling

E. Printing
- Typesetting
- Press operation
  - floor
  - hand

F. Ceramics
- Construction
  - pinch
  - coil
  - slab
  - wheel
  - mold
  - sculpture
- Decoration
  - underglaze
  - glaze
  - carving
  - sgraffito
- Finishing
  - bisque firing
  - glaze firing
- Mosaics
  - design
  - cutting
  - cementing

G. Graphics
- Drawing and sketching
- Painting
- Lettering
- Silk screening
- Block printing
- Stenciling
- Mechanical drawing
- Finger painting

H. Textiles
- Weaving
- Design of pattern and preparation of warp
- Preparation of loom
- Techniques
  - two harness
  - four harness
  - inkle or card weaving
  - braid weaving
  - cord knotting
  - Turkish knotting
  - hooking
  - colonial natting
  - netting
  - "looper"
  - hand-manipulated techniques
- Hand sewing
- Machine sewing
  - garment construction
  - knitting
  - crochetting
  - needlepoint
  - crewel
  - stichery
  - collages
  - huck toweling
  - quilting
- Batic
- Tie-dye
- Macrame
- Upholstery

I. Miscellaneous
- Mosaics
  - shell, seed crafts
  - glass painting
  - tile work
  - sand crafts
- Soap carving
- Cane and reed work
- Papier-mâché
- Plaster of paris sculptures

Documentation and Clinical Research

13

Anne Hiller Scott and Barbara E. Neuhaus

"Our research directions are unlimited in the sense that validation of practice is needed in every aspect of our service to patients with physical and psychosocial dysfunction" (1). This challenge by West is one that we all are urged to meet. In this chapter we shall examine this challenge to enhance the quality and expand the theoretical base of occupational therapy practice by means of improved documentation techniques and exploration of key elements of practice demanding verification through research.

As those involved in occupational therapy attempt to increase its professional stature, there is a crucial need for developing and validating theory and conducting research. Traditional approaches must be put to the test of scientific examination. Recently there has been increasing concern regarding the professional status of occupational therapy, particularly in light of the growing interest in specialization and concern over whether such a move will foster integration or fragmentation (2–4). The future status of occupational therapists (professionals as opposed to technicians) is debated. The lack of a unifying body of theory supported by research is a major developmental delay in a maturing profession. Practice built without a sound theoretical foundation is on shaky ground.

Until occupational therapists can validate through research what West (1) called "the most basic underlying theory of our profession—activity or occupation," the field will continue to carry the label of one of Etzioni's "semi-professions" (5), where research is rather sparse and the workers are more interested in giving service to clients than in mastering professional skills.

In the semi-professions, according to Etzioni, practice does not rest on a firm theoretical base. Gillette (3) has noted that in a technical or paraprofessional field learning is "dependent upon repetition and matching of solutions to problems, as opposed to problem-solving based on the scientific method of inquiry." She proposes a continuum toward professionalism encompassing the model of:

Practice ⟷ Research ⟷ Education

Research is recommended as the linking mechanism that facilitates and underlies practice and education. In this system, practice is based on theory systematically developed through research.

O.T.R.—OBSERVE, THEORIZE, RESEARCH

A unique definition of a practitioner was suggested by Yerxa (6). An O.T.R. represents one who observes, theorizes and researches. In the laboratory of everyday clinical practice, the therapist can apply a scientific approach to analyzing the treatment provided. The goal would be to uncover and clarify the technical and also the theoretical basis of practice. A primary skill in any research or scientific endeavor is critical and objective observing and recording of events. An initial focus for research should be the development of consistent, comprehensive, and accurate documentation. A wealth of clinical research material is available for those with skills to document practice and critically analyze the results. What scientist would formulate hypotheses and make predictions on poorly recorded, incomplete or erroneous data? The report of a Research Seminar (7), sponsored by the American Occupational Therapy Foundation in 1976 cited that "complete and accurate recording of data by all clinicians would provide the foundation for many studies." A suggestion followed (7) that the treatment process be conceptualized as a research model: evaluation, problem identification, intervention hypothesis, treatment plan, treatment implementation, reevaluation of outcome, disposition proposal.

DOCUMENTATION

What are the key elements of documentation? How can clinicians upgrade this critical aspect of practice? It is essential to record a base line of functioning against which to measure the effectiveness of therapeutic interventions. Descriptions of functioning and behaviors during evaluation, during treatment, and during outcome evaluation should be available for scientific inquiry, if they are objectively and systematically recorded. Written records should be clear, concise, objective, and logically organized. Records should document all significant interventions in specific detail and in terminology that will be understood by other team members, auditors, and fiscal reviewers. The Standards of Practice for Occupational Therapy Services for Clients with Physical Disabilities (8) adopted by the representative assembly in May 1978 outline recommended documentation for referral, evaluation, program planning, program implementation, and discharge planning. The following (8) are the essential components of medical records:

1. Identifying data.
2. Referral information.
3. Evaluation of occupational performance: self-care; home, work, and school activities; play and leisure skills; performance components (motor and sensory skills/status, sensory integration, social/interpersonal skills, psychological/intrapersonal skills and cognitive skills), including assessments used, clients goals, functional deficits and abilities, and need for occupational therapy intervention.
4. Treatment plan: indication of long- and short-term goals in achievable and functional terms; methods to reach goals; frequency of service; anticipated duration and outcomes.
5. Progress notes: periodic recording of progress, including treatment and services provided, response to treatment, results of periodic evaluations, and changes in patient's status, goals, or treatment.
6. Discharge summary: overview of course of treatment since initial evaluation, including progress obtained and/or continuing need for treatment, current functional assets and deficits, and plan for home care or aftercare if indicated.

SYSTEMS OF DOCUMENTATION

The Problem Oriented Medical Record (POMR) developed by Weed (9) is one approach that facilitates a consistent, coordinated interdisciplinary approach to documentation. The main components of this system are the following:

1. Data base: Multidisciplinary base-line evaluation includes identifying information, significant current and past history, results of examination, evaluations and laboratory tests, and social, vocational, and family history.
2. Problem list: Problems are derived from the data base and are listed by number; throughout the hospitalization, the problem number remains constant.
3. Problem-oriented clinical notes: Interventions and progress for each problem are recorded

using a subjective-objective-assessment-plan (SOAP) format: (a) subjective (patient and family reports of symptoms); (b) objective (evaluations, reevaluations, treatment and outcome, report on patient's education, and instruction to family); (c) assessment (long- and short-term goals based on functional assets and deficits, effectiveness, and response to treatment); (d) plan (plan for type, frequency, amount, and content of treatment for each problem).

The POMR is readily adapted to occupational therapy treatment, since the occupational therapy process also focuses on systematically evaluating and treating functional problems. This method also provides a logical structure that facilitates evaluation of the sequence and effectiveness of treatment interventions.

All of the elements included in the POMR should be present in any system of charting to ensure thoroughness, continuity of focus, and quality of care. Within the constraints of the policies of each medical records department, therapists should review their current systems of documentation and work toward development of a consistent format that structures material in a logical, clear, and complete sequence. Internal departmental recording mechanisms should also be examined. Well-organized face sheets that summarize identifying data, diagnosis, assessments, and outcomes collected in a standardized, objective, and measurable format can be invaluable if one is interested in retrospectively reviewing a particular aspect of care.

In exploring the potential relationship between documentation and research, there are two specific approaches that the clinician may find beneficial: the Occupational Therapy Sequential Client Care Record developed by Llorens (10) and the Goal Attainment Scaling devised by Kiresuk and Sherman (11). The client care recording system is a model that incorporates POMR with the Occupational Therapy Developmental Evaluation, Analysis, and Intervention Schedule (DEAIS). This system provides a comprehensive theoretical framework for analyzing the developmental parameters associated with occupational therapy in practice. It covers the three bases of practice, research, and education and was developed for the purposes of (a) documenting care sequentially and comprehensively, (b) providing a data base for special studies and research, and (c) providing a teaching tool to enable students to learn the role and process of occupational therapy (10).

A study of this recording system in comparison with traditional recording systems indicated statistically significant differences on variables of completeness, organization, understandability, and usefulness. An individual clinician or several clinicians in one department could effectively use this tool on a select number of clients over time and develop a large enough sample of cases to study. Goal Attainment Scaling (G.A.S.) originally developed for use in mental health has recently been successfully applied to study the results of intervention with neurologically handicapped children (12). Another study, "Goal Oriented Treatment Plans and Behavioral Analysis" (13), has provided an objective measurable program applicable to clinical research. All of these approaches involve specific behavioral definition and measurement of treatment goals and easily lend themselves to improving quality of care, specificity of documentation, and study of potential research problems in the clinical setting.

The Behavioral Objectives Assessment of Scott and Zukmann (14), also developed for psychiatric populations, provides methods for describing clinical goals and observable and quantifiable outcomes.

QUALITY ASSURANCE

It seems important here to focus briefly on quality assurance and assessment of services. Brown (15) said that "if a health professional thinks whatever he does makes a difference in the health of patients, he ought to be involved in improving the quality of care and documenting it." Professional Standards Review Organization (PSRO) review mechanisms provide a tool that is beneficial in assessing quality of care. PSROs were mandated in 1972 by federal legislation requiring nationwide review of health care financed by Medicaid, Medicare, and Maternal and Child Health programs and provided by physicians and other health care practitioners. PSROs operate national, state, and local structures of organizations that review care and determine if it (a) is medically necessary, (b) meets professionally accepted standards of care, and (c) is delivered in the most economical setting for the proper length of time. The spirit of the legislation was to maximize quality of service and shift review to health professionals rather than to fiscal intermediaries. A major concept involved in the assessment is that it is performed on a local level by peer review. Advisory groups that include nonphysician health care providers assist in carrying out PSRO functions.

With support from the American Occupational Therapy Association, occupational therapists nationwide are engaged in developing standards, norms, and criteria for practice and are then conducting patient care evaluation studies aimed at identifying obstacles to quality care and implementation of solutions. There is a network of national and state PRSO liaison persons who serve as resources. *Patient Care Evaluation in Action* (16) is a manual that comprehensively illustrates the nine-step cycle of the evaluation process. Therapists develop criteria for optimal care that are relevant, understandable, measurable, behavioral, and achievable (RUMBA) (16). Review of care is done by chart audit using predetermined criteria. This process stimulates more objective description of services, goals, and treatment outcomes. For third-party payers, these criteria can clearly articulate the specific indications and focus of occupational therapy and appraise the necessity for and quality of practice. In several areas (17) occupational therapists have been successful in obtaining reimbursement for services using standards and criteria developed for practice.

In addition to federal requirements, the Joint Commission on Accreditation of Hospitals also requires review of quality of care by measurement of actual care against specified criteria. "Criteria must be explicit, and measurable, and must reflect the optimal level of care that can be achieved through current medical and related health science knowledge" (16). Much of the focus in evaluating quality care is determined through examination of criteria against documentation. The skills involved in developing measurable, objective criteria are basic skills that can be related to more advanced scientific or research activity.

The Standards for Occupational Therapy Services for Clients with Physical Disabilities (8) require that "Occupational Therapists shall systematically review the quality, including outcomes, of their services using predetermined criteria reflecting professional consensus and recent developments in research and theory." This standard firmly emphasizes the previously mentioned link between practice, research, and education.

CLINICAL RESEARCH

Traditionally, occupational therapists have not been oriented to be researchers. Beginning clinicians have entered the field primarily with practice as their major concern and have directed most of their professional effort toward meeting the needs of their patients and clients. Laudable as such past commitment is, practitioners can neither attain nor maintain professional stature solely through a service-oriented focus.

As recently noted by Yerxa (18), occupational therapy clinical research is needed now as never before to assure the profession's accountability to the public. Increasingly, occupational therapists are being pressured to show tangible results of their services. Without a research base, professional development has been hampered in several other ways, not the least of which is the difficulty in attaining licensure as a profession that can legally define its services as distinct from those of other professions.

Although the mandate for an increase in clinical research has become more urgent in the last decade, similar appeals have been made by concerned colleagues since 1954, when the first research institute was sponsored by the American Occupational Therapy Association (AOTA) for the purpose of stimulating clinical research by practitioners. Since then, several task forces have been set up by the association to focus on research, but it was with the creation of the American Occupational Therapy Foundation in 1965 that research was given a permanent position of importance within the profession. One of the original long-range objectives that is receiving increasing attention from the foundation is to finance and conduct research studies to contribute to the body of knowledge and to the profession. In 1976 the American Occupational Therapy Foundation and the AOTA jointly sponsored a research seminar (7). Twenty professional leaders who were invited to participate in the seminar generated a series of ideas for possible research projects and made recommendations to specific AOTA bodies for implementing those ideas:

1. Develop a battery of evaluative techniques for the components of occupational performance that yield quantitative scores. (A literature review would precede, and the battery would consist of what is already available, as well as new instruments to be developed.)
2. Work out a uniform data collection system to gather a broad base of clinical information regarding the process (perceptual, activity, interpersonal interaction) of occupational therapy and the determination of how that relates to components and areas of occupational performance. (This might provide a systematic way to evaluate occupational therapy processes and outcomes.)
3. Perform a literature search (total, not just occupational therapy) to determine the bases of occupational therapy and ultimately develop a systems theory for practice.
4. Undertake a demographic study to examine the members of the population having or suspected of having performance limitation, for whatever reasons, to determine if there is evidence of central nervous system or sensory integrative dysfunction in order to experiment with the application of purposeful activity to remedy identified problems. (Such a study could be done with a minimum sample size of 400 to 500; ideally, it should be done with 4,000 to 5,000 subjects. An underlying assumption: performance limitation may be due to some unidentified problem.)
5. Compare a developmentally sequenced program of stimulating activities with random activities in counteracting effects of aging on the central nervous system.
6. Initiate a large collaborative study to determine with which groups occupational therapy is most effective. (The variables could include disability, severity of disability, age, sex, and length of treatment. Client outcomes in terms of social, psychological, and cognitive functions could be assessed. The occupational therapy processes that influence client function, including specifically delineated treatment techniques, could be studied. This could be done as a collection of studies.)
7. Determine the effects of occupational therapy versus no occupational therapy on the functional performance of adult hemiplegics (relates to the definition of functional performance).
8. Study the relationship between the development of the vestibular mechanism and functional performance. (Such a study could be initiated with an occupational-therapy-sponsored interdisciplinary investigative seminar to review the literature on the vestibular mechanism.)
9. Establish norms for dominance (eye, hand, foot, ear) for a "normal" cross section of the U.S. population. (This could be coupled with a knowledge of dominance in parents and siblings to suggest a genetic factor.)
10. Compare the effects of medication versus specific kinds of sensorimotor integration techniques on hyperactive children in relation to their academic and social behavior. (This study could be expanded to look at different types of patients.)
11. With persons who have identified limitations in performance of purposeful activities, compare three approaches to treatment: (a) facilitation and/or exercise, (b) involvement in purposeful activity, (c) simutaneous use of a and b.
12. Ascertain the relationship between patients' perceived needs and therapists' views of patients' needs in specific populations of patients relative to diagnosis and age. Assess whether or not a specific occupational therapy treatment technique is effective in meeting those needs.
13. Carry out an electromyographic (EMG) activity analysis to determine the motor components of activity performed by persons with and without central nervous system damage.
14. Investigate and elaborate on the primary care roles of occupational therapy (develop and test a model).
15. With traumatic hand injuries, determine the comparative effect of pure exercise versus occupational therapy on speed of recovery and degree of recovery.

The seminar served to deepen commitment to

the development of research in occupational therapy. The last 3 years have seen encouraging numbers of clinical studies and projects undertaken, but these efforts still fall short of the demand for documentation of the consequences of occupational therapy.

These potential topics stress the need for more consistent standardized evaluation tools and more uniform methods for collecting data. West (1) cited the critical lack of standard evaluation tools. There is much work to be done in this area, and it will require collaborative effort by many therapists.

RESEARCH PROCESSES

The purpose of this section is to introduce the clinician to the rewards and excitement inherent in becoming a consumer of research and a participant in research through (a) introduction to the research process and (b) identification of resources for in-depth information on the various aspects of reading, carrying out, and reporting on research.

Several invisible barriers seem to stand in the way of initiating research. One of these is the dichotomy that has grown up between research and practice. That such a dichotomy should exist is surprising when one considers the similarities between the scientific process and the problem-solving approach used in the therapeutic process. It might be helpful here to show how Dewey (19) outlined the steps in reflective thinking that provide a guide to understand the similarities, which are (a) the occurrence of a felt difficulty, (b) definition of the difficulty in terms of a problem statement, (c) occurrence of a suggested explanation or possible solution, (d) the rational explanation of an idea through the development of its implications, by means of collection of evidence, (e) corroboration of the idea and formation of a concluding belief through experimental verification of the hypothesis. As indicated earlier, the therapeutic process follows the same path, and this type of thinking is reflected in every program plan in occupational therapy. Ethridge and McSweeney (20) suggested a natural flow between practice and research: "Through practice questions are raised to be studied through research, the results of which would hopefully modify and improve practice." Gillette (3) expanded on this natural flow by describing research as "the linking mechanism between practice and education in any professional system of learning and service."

A second barrier that has been allowed to develop is the mystique of the researcher as a person intellectually endowed with special gifts, and occupying a position of respect by virtue of the sacredness of the mission. In addition, the image of the uninvolved, impersonal, unbiased scientist has created a myth in which, according to Mooney (21), the satisfaction must come from *how* things are done, not from the content of what is dealt with. "A person dare not become intrigued or emotionally concerned with the content or he will, in proportion to that involvement, be biased, partial, personal and subjective." In reality, Mooney continued, research is a personal venture that, quite aside from its social benefits, is worth doing for its direct contribution to one's self-realization. Certainly such a view of research not only places it into an achievable realm but, more immediately, presents it as an attractive possibility for every clinician.

Nonetheless, the researcher's enjoyment alone does not justify or validate the results of research. The researcher must also be thorough and meticulous in the use of all available research tools. This includes data collection based on controlled observation of facts in a specific situation (7), reliable and valid instrumentation for measurement, and correct interpretation of statistical results.

Ross (22) defined research as essentially an investigation, a recording and an analysis of evidence for the purpose of gaining knowledge. Payton (23) further described it as a process of looking for a specific answer to a specific question in an organized, objective, reliable way. For the clinician, questions about the behavior of patients or clients that may or may not be influenced through occupational therapy intervention are a prime concern. The goal of finding answers through research is to develop concepts and principles based on observable facts and to develop these to the point of serving as useful predictors of future events. A set of principles based on solid evidence supports the theory.

As seen by Payton (23), "the major purpose of the theory is to stimulate the search for new facts, concepts and principles which will either substantiate the theory or alter it in ways which will make it more accurate, more effective, more predictive or more comprehensive."

Two approaches traditionally used for research are deduction (reasoning from the general to the specific) and induction (reasoning from the specific to the general, or using facts as evidence to prove a conclusion). These have given way to the scientific method, which relies on an inquiry process to search for, find, and substantiate answers to questions. As a clinical researcher following this method, one needs to approach research on three levels: as a consumer of research literature, as an investigator and documentor, and as an interpreter or reporter of study results. Each of these will be briefly discussed, and useful resources and references will be given at the end of this section for further information.

The beginning researcher needs familiarity with the topic of interest. Therefore one must first assume the role of consumer of research literature. As a reader of professional journals, the clinician must accept responsibility for interpreting and evaluating research articles. Crocker (24) prepared a clear, readable outline to follow for understanding and evaluating journal articles without in-depth knowledge of statistics or data analysis. She posed the following seven questions to help readers identify criteria for critically reviewing research articles to assess their importance:

1. What is the purpose of the study?
2. How does this research relate to the current body of knowledge in the professional discipline?
3. What measures are used?
4. Do the sample size and sampling procedures permit results to be generalized to a larger population?
5. What is the design of this study, and what are its inherent limitations?
6. What is the outcome of the data analysis?
7. What (if any) are the implications for practice from this study?

It is recommended that every prospective clinical researcher use Crocker's article as an introduction to the reading of reports of research studies. Understanding terminology is fundamental. Again, it is not necessary (although it is very helpful) to take a course in statistics; however, for all clinicians engaged in any aspect of measurement of behavior or performance, knowledge of basic terms is a prerequisite. There are numerous useful texts in paperback editions that contain glossaries and discuss the most important terms. Hasselkus and Safrit (25) presented basic measurement theory and discussed appropriate methods for estimating validity and reliability of measurement of motor behavior. When such tools are developed, refined, and standardized, therapists must resist the "adaptation syndrome." In a study of motor evaluations used with children (27), findings indicated frequent inappropriate use of evaluations (not age-appropriate or not accounting for limitations or restrictions of the evaluation tools). In addition, the therapists surveyed relied on self-made instruments that borrowed items from a variety of sources that lacked reliability and validity measures. Punwar (26), a critic of this approach, suggested that "rather than spending our time in this counter-productive fashion we would be much better off to critically analyze and study existing published evaluation tools and to improve upon them. Only when we can show that our evaluations can be supported statistically can we be assured of drawing reliable conclusions."

Clinical questions can be answered through a number of different methods or types of research design. Most studies in occupational therapy are descriptive, correlational, or experimental (or quasi-experimental). Each of these asks a question, gathers information, uses a sample population, and interprets the findings or results of the data to answer the question. However, they differ in the types of questions asked, in the degree to which the sample is (or is not) manipulated by the investigator, in the statistical tools used to summarize and/or interpret the data, and in the formal properties of the predictions made on the basis of these data (23).

Descriptive studies collect specific data about a population to show conditions as they exist, without any influence by the investigator. For example, this might include surveys of discharged young adults with quadriplegia, or case studies over long or short periods of time that describe in depth the behavior of autistic children within the family, or studies of the roles of support personnel to determine the need for an increase in supervisory staff. Again, it must be emphasized that one must make every effort to be an unbiased observer in order to collect valid information. For example, results can be biased by the questions selected for inclusion and by the manner in which these questions are phrased.

Correlational research looks at the extent to which two variables are related or the extent to which variation in one factor corresponds to variations in one or more other factors (e.g., a study of the relationship between hand dominance and letter reversal in children, or the extent to which improvement in attention span occurs together with dressing skill).

True experimental research attempts to study cause and effect by exposing one or more experimental groups to one or more treatment conditions and comparing the results to those in a control group not receiving the treatment. In most treatment situations true experimental research is extremely limited, for several apparent reasons: treatment cannot be denied to patients or clients in a therapeutic setting; absolute control by ruling out all other variables (such as other health problems or other interventions) is virtually impossible; finally, in all studies involving human subjects, individual human rights must be protected in the research process. Human investigations committees to screen and evaluate all research proposals have been added to most treatment facilities. Reports addressing the issue of human subjects in research have been prepared by Michels (28) and Stein (29).

This is not to say that patients or clients cannot serve as subjects; however, it is important to be aware of these regulations prior to initiating a study in order to avoid disappointment, delay, or difficulties later on.

Many of the problems of control in experimental studies can be circumvented by using quasi-experimental designs. An entire monograph describing these designs in detail was prepared by Campbell and Stanley (30). Payton (23) described two quasi-experimental designs that are frequently used in clinical studies: time series that are interrupted (e.g., when a client first has exercise, then activity is added to this, then the activity is withdrawn for several days while the exercise continues); sequential clinical trials in which two clients with similar conditions (e.g., limited elbow extension) are matched for sequential trials with two differing forms of treatment.

The following abbreviated outline of steps in initiating a clinical study will serve only as a guide to further information about each of the steps, again with the purpose of bringing the research process into an attainable, achievable realm.

Posing the Research Question

All research begins with a question. Every interaction with a client generates questions for which answers might be found through systematic and careful observation, documentation, and analysis of findings. Asking questions is a useful way to isolate the problem the clinician is attempting to solve. (The word "problem" is used in the sense of "perplexing question"). Schucman (31), in a series of lectures to occupational and physical therapy students in an introductory research course, compared the research question to "the first actor to appear on the empty stage as the curtain goes up. It is his function to announce what the play is about and to set the ground rules for everything that will follow. Your question is the prologue to your study. It directs all subsequent procedures, from the choice of the subjects through the treatment of the data and on to the discussion of the results and their implications."

Once the subject of the study has been selected, the problem needs to be isolated and or specified. As it initially presents itself, the problem may be quite general; it must be refined in order to limit the subject so that there will be a possibility of finding an answer. Although eventually the significance of a study depends on the ability to generalize the findings, for the beginning researcher it is important that the question be suitably limited so that an answer can be found. Ethridge and McSweeney (20) gave three basic considerations for making up a researchable question: (a) Identify the outcome by name; state what will be accepted as evidence that an activity or process has been completed (e.g., improved general appearance, including hair combed or brushed, face clean, hands and fingernails clean). (b) Define the activity or the process through which the desired outcome is to be achieved (e.g., daily charting by the client, or daily practice for 10 min). (c) Specify the criteria within which the research will be confined (e.g., during 2 weeks of self-care practice with 3 depressed patients).

An example of a researchable question is provided by a study in which factors related to accident tendencies in children were addressed. Tower (32) asked, "What is the relationship between a child's performance on a developmental test of visual perception and accident frequency?" "Relationship" is the key word; hence this was a correlational study. The author was looking for statistically significant results. A test of visual perception was used to determine the defect, and the criteria were (a) that the subjects be children capable of performing the test and (b) that they have a past history of accident frequency. In addition to asking the question as specifically as possible, each of the terms used by the author had to be defined clearly, concisely, and precisely. Tower had to specify the study population (age and sex of the children), the procedures, and what constituted "accident frequency." Such operational definitions are part of every study; they refer to phenomena that are concrete, observable, and measurable within the limits of the particular study.

Review of the Literature

When the question has been clearly stated, the clinician-researcher needs to do a thorough search of the literature to review related studies, if available, or to establish that no other studies have been conducted in this area. Frequently this literature review may precede the specification of the question, since it may be necessary to see what has been done to decide if a question is even worth asking the the way one had first thought. There are several useful and relatively inexpensive computer search services (e.g., Medline, Medlars, ERIC) available through major libraries. The researcher provides key words that describe the subject or are related to the subject, and the library sets up a search to generate articles on the subject, frequently with annotations or abstracts. This is a vital first step that must not be omitted, time-consuming though it may appear. It will ultimately prevent unnecessary repetition of research by providing useful information about previous similar studies. This is not to say that a beginning researcher should abandon an idea if similar research is located; there may be a need for replicating the study with another population, or an earlier study may suggest procedures that can be applied to a new study. Finally, the literature review lends credence to a topic if the researcher can establish that experts in the field have investigated similar topics or that no documentation on the topic can be located.

Formulating the Hypothesis

By this time the researcher should be able to venture a guess about the expected results, in the form of a hypothesis or prediction. Ross (22) referred to the hypothesis as a map, chart, or compass, an advancement of a temporary idea that the study will prove or defend. In the previously cited study by Tower (32), the author hypothesized that there was a relationship between test performance and accident frequency and then set out to gather evidence that would or would not support the hypothesis.

Study Design

In the next step, the researcher needs to lay out a design for gathering and analyzing data. This includes the selection of a population of subjects for the study and descriptions of the tools, tests, and activities to be used and any treatments or procedures that will be administered. The design of the study also includes the frequency of use or application of a procedure or performance of an activity. As part of the design, the researcher should begin to consider the type of analysis that will be optimal for verifying the results.

Gathering Data

The development of the study up to this point should have pointed out the most logical ways to gather data. This can be done through systematic observation and through questioning, tests, or performance of a specified activity. A study may include one or several such techniques. Disguised data collection, where the subject is unaware of the purpose of the task, is useful when the researcher believes that the subject's knowledge of being a participant might affect performance.

It is during the planning for data collection that validity and reliability need to be considered. Regardless of which type of data collection, the measuring process or instrument should have both of these distinguishing characteristics. Very simply, validity is the extent to which a test or instrument measures that trait and only that trait it set out to measure. Reliability is the consistency of an instrument to measure a trait in the same way during repeated trials. Both of these terms are defined in greater detail in each of the listed references, including ways to determine and establish validity and reliability.

It is not necessary to be self-reliant in the areas of valid data collection and subsequent statistical analysis; statisticians and statistical consultants are generally available for help with this process. It may be useful to consult with such an expert prior to the data-gathering process in order to assure that all the vital information will be collected in a manner appropriate to the study design. The design of the study must be so clearly stated that anyone with experience in statistical work can suggest a logical plan for data collection. The role of careful documentation has been discussed; its importance is obvious here.

Data Analysis

The researcher must analyze the data carefully when the observation or investigation is completed to see whether or not they support the original hypothesis. The analysis may be done through a system involving coding, tabulation, and statistical techniques and their interpretation. Here again, a statistician will be extremely useful, particularly someone with computer programming experience. The time and effort saved by asking for assistance during this phase are well worth any expense that might be incurred.

Interpretation of Data

Payton (23), in his discussion of clinical research, suggested that "data must be interpreted in light of the question you set out to answer. Is the answer one you had expected, or is it different? What are all of the possible ways in which your research question could be answered on the basis of the data you had gathered? One uses every tool available in working with the data to arrive at their most probable meaning." This step also involves the interpretation of results that may have statistical significance but are of little practical value. For example, in a case where there is a significantly greater increase in performance after treatment A than after treatment B, but performance is still not functional, one must conclude that neither of the treatments, during the time specified by the study, has been effective in changing a nonfunctional state to a functional one. However, this does not lessen the value of the research, since it may suggest not only that other treatment might be more effective but also that treatment might make a difference if one of the conditions (e.g., time, frequency) were to be changed.

Finally, the researcher needs to address not only those questions that the study answered but also those that were left unanswered, including all the new questions raised by the study. Implications of the study also need consideration at this time. What is the meaning of these findings to one's own practice? Can the findings be generalized to a larger group? What do they mean in light of occupational therapy knowledge? Can they contribute to the validation of practice? Do they form the basis for new principles that support or challenge current theories, particularly those that address human behavior and activity performance? These are the kinds of questions that a study may generate and that may form the basis for stimulating further research.

Case Study Research

One extremely promising method of contributing valuable clinical information to the occupational therapy knowledge base is the case study approach. This lends itself ideally to the underdeveloped talents of beginning researchers, since its primary prerequisites are well-developed observational skills and a simple systematic method of comprehensive data collection and documentation.

Rather than carrying out one or a few observations of many subjects, the single case study observes a single subject many times over an extended period of time.

Case studies are primarily descriptive clinical research, although they may also use a quasi-experimental design. A single subject, unit, or event is studied by objective, detailed longitudinal observation in the patient's own environment (this may, of course, include the treatment setting). Since the results of findings are not generalizable by themselves, case studies frequently serve as preliminary tasks to a larger, more formal study or to a replication in another environment.

The specific method used for the case study depends on common sense and the imagination of the person doing the study (33). In gathering data, the researcher must frequently reassess what is important and what is not in order to record only relevant data.

One of the greatest advantages of the case study is that it allows examination of variables that are difficult to quantify such as ability to sort items by color on 1 day out of every 3 or 4 days of observation. The observer (therapist) records the presence or absence of the variable (item sorting) every day over an extended period of time to observe, for example, if there is a pattern to this behavior. It also provides a variety of data that may identify important variables that may be further analyzed. However, certain disadvantages must also be recognized. The length of interaction with the subject may result in loss of objectivity, or a subject (a patient, for example) may no longer be available toward the end of the study. Also, since the observer is merely recording observed behavior, the reason for the behavior is not explained, nor can one always determine a cause-and-effect relationship. However, for recording an individual's response to a specific intervention over a period of time, the case study is eminently useful.

Data may be gathered by the same methods as used for other studies. Analysis of data cannot involve inferential statistics nor statistical significance as a criterion, since the data cannot be comparatively quantified. Instead, one can use descriptive statistics, such as a frequency distribution, or measures of central tendency, such as mean or mode.

Case studies may also use experimental designs with a series of observations of base-line behavior (no treatment) followed by treatment and subsequent observations. The descriptive case study can result in insights about certain behaviors; the experimental study can test and support them.

SUMMARY

As indicated earlier, the purpose of this chapter was to whet the appetite of the clinician to take on the role of the researcher. There are few professional involvements that match the excitement of joining colleagues in finding answers to clinical questions.

REFERENCES

1. West, W. (1979): Historical Perspective. *Occupational Therapy: 2001 AD, Papers Presented at the Special Session of the Representative Assembly,* November 1978, 9–17, American Occupational Therapy Association.
2. Gillette, N., and Kielhofner G. (1979): The impact of specialization on the professionalization and survival of occupational therapy. *Amer. J. Occupat. Ther.,* 33:20–28.
3. Gillette, N. (1979): Practice, education and research, *Occupational Therapy 2001 AD,* 18–25. American Occupational Therapy Association.
4. Fidler, G. (1979): Professional or nonprofessional, *Occupational Therapy: 2001 AD,* 31–36. American Occupational Therapy Association.
5. Etzioni, A. (ed.) (1969): *The Semi Professions and their Organization: Teachers, Nurses, Social Workers.* Free Press, New York.
6. Yerxa, E. (1978): Everything you always wanted to know about research but were afraid to ask, Paper presented at Research Institute, American Occupational Therapy Association Conference, May 5, 1978.
7. Yerxa, E., and Gilfoyle, E. (1976): Research Seminar. *Amer. J. Occupat. Ther.,* 30:509–514.
8. American Occupational Therapy, Manual on Administration, 1978.
9. Weed, L. L. (1970): *Medical Records, Medical Education and Patient Care.* Year Book Medical Publications. Chicago.
10. Llorens, L., and Shuster, J. (1977): Occupational therapy sequential client care recording system: A comparative study. *Amer. J. Occupat. Ther.,* 31:367–371.
11. Kiresuk, T. J., and Sherman, R. F. (1968): Goal attainment scaling: A general method for evaluating comprehensive community health programs. *Commun. Ment. Health J.,* 4:443–453.
12. Maloney, F. P., Mirrett, P., Brooks, C., and Johannes, K. (1978): Use of goal attainment scale in the treatment and ongoing evaluation of neurologically handicapped children. *Amer. J. Occupat. Ther.,* 32:505–510.
13. Gaines, B. (1978): Goal-oriented treatment plans and behavioral analysis. *Amer. J. Occupat. Ther.,* 32:512–516.
14. Scott, A. H., and Zukmann, M. (1978): *A Structure and Evaluation System for Patients and Therapists.* Independent publication by authors.
15. Brown, C. (1974): Remarks at P.S.R.O. Workshop for Occupational Therapists. October 1974.
16. *Patient Care Evaluation In Action* (1978): American Occupational Therapy Association, Inc.
17. Special Task Forces of Kansas City Area: *Criteria for Management of Patients Requiring Occupational Therapy,* American Occupational Therapy Association, Inc.
18. Yerxa, E. (1978): The occupational therapist as

consultant and researcher. In *Willard and Spackman's Occupational Therapy,* 5th edition, edited by H. Hopkins, and H. Smith, J. B. Lippincott Co. Philadelphia.

19. Dewey, J. (1933): *How We Think,* p. 12. D. C. Heath, Boston.
20. Ethridge, D. and McSweeney, M. (1971): *Research in Occupational Therapy,* p. 1. Kendall/Hunt Publishing Co., Dubuque, Iowa.
21. Mooney, R. L. (1957): The researcher himself. *Research for Curriculum Improvement,* Washington, Association for Supervision and Curriculum Development Yearbook.
22. Ross, R. (1974): *Research: An Introduction.* Barnes & Nobel Books, New York.
23. Payton, O. D. (1979): *Research: The Validation of Clinical Practice.* F. A. Davis Co., Philadelphia.
24. Crocker, L. M. (1977): Linking research to practice: suggestions for reading a research article. *Amer. J. Occupat. Ther.,* 31:1.
25. Hasselkus, B. R., and Safrit, M. J. (1976): Measurement in occupational therapy. *Amer. J. Occupat. Ther.,* 30:7.
26. Punwar, A. (1976): A commentary on Dr. Lewko's article. *Amer. J. Occupat. Ther.,* 30:420–421.
27. Lewko, J. (1976): Current practices in evaluating motor behavior of disabled children. *Amer. J. Occupat. Ther.,* 30:413–419.
28. Michels, E. (1976): Research and human rights: Part I. *Phys. Ther.,* 56:407.
29. Stein, F. (1976): *Anatomy of Research in Allied Health.* Schenkman Publishing Co., Cambridge, Mass.
30. Campbell, D. T., and Stanley, J. C. (1967): *Experimental and Quasi-Experimental Designs for Research.* Rand, McNally & Co., Chicago.
31. Schucman, H. (1969): Asking the question—a talk with OT and PT students. Transcript of a lecture in course, *Introduction to Research.* Columbia University, New York.
32. Tower, D. Q. (1976): Relationships between perceptual response and accident frequency. *Amer. J. Occupat. Ther.,* 30:498.
33. Simon, J. L. (1969): *Basic Research Methods in Social Science: The Art of Empirical Investigation.* Random House, New York.

BIBLIOGRAPHY

Campbell, D. T., and Stanley, J. C. (1967): *Experimental and Quasi-Experimental Designs for Research.* Rand, McNally & Co., Chicago.

Ethridge, D. A., and McSweeny, M. (1971): *Research in Occupational Therapy.* Kendall/Hunt Publishing Co., Dubuque, Iowa.

Hersen, M., and Barlow, David H. (1975): *Single Case Experimental Designs Strategies for Studying Behavior Change,* Vol. 56. Pergamon General Psychological Series, New York.

Issac, A. and Michael, W. B. (1971): *Handbook in Research and Evaluation.* Edits Publishers, San Diego.

Payton, O. D. (1979): *Research: The Validation of Clinical Practice.* F. A. Davis, Co., Philadelphia.

Ross, R. (1974): *Research: An Introduction.* Barnes and Noble Books, New York.

Simon, J. L. (1969): *Basic Research Methods in Social Science: The Art of Empirical Investigation.* Random House, New York.

Stein, F. (1976): *Anatomy of Research in Allied Health.* Halsted Press Division, John Wiley & Sons, New York.

Aphasia

14

Damien Martin

Therapy is not just technique. Rather, therapy reflects a theoretical model, the interaction between clinician and client, and, finally, the techniques that constitute the final stage in the evolution of the original thought. In every interaction between clinician and client, the clinician is operating from a variety of models that underlie the therapy. Therefore, if we wish to examine therapy, one way to approach it is to do so by looking at the models which serve as its basis.

I remember that when I was in school and someone would mention the word "model," my eyes would begin to glaze. I would see these little lines and numbers, all arranged in a complex interaction, creating a maze that would challenge Theseus. However, a model is not that complicated. Basically, it is a belief system which is scientific in purpose, reflects a theoretical view, and that involves a shared set if assumptions. It may evolve from observation, from instruction, or from a combination of the two. For example, one model which is basic to our culture involves the relationship between the earth and the sun. For centuries it was believed that the sun revolved around the earth, a perfectly logical conclusion, since one could go outside and see it. But at one point, using a slightly different perspective and different ways to observe, a different model, just the reverse, was proposed: the earth revolves around the sun. The first model was derived by simple observation; the second depended to a large extent on instruction. The model was changed because there was new evidence that challenged the old model.

Hopefully the same thing will occur when you are examining a disorder, or looking at a patient. The clinician begins with a belief system about the patient, about the disorder, and also about what is necessary to help the patient. If the therapist is going to be able to affect any of these, it will be necessary to specify the model that serves as the foundation for your work and to answer the following questions: What is the nature of normal functioning? What is the nature of the disorder? What is the nature of the therapy? (1).

Historically, there have been two basic models of aphasia, the localizationist or loss model and the reduction-of-efficiency model. They express, to a certain extent, directly opposite views about what constitutes the nature of the disorder, although there are certain overlapping areas of agreement. In this necessarily limited discussion we will examine only the sense in which they are incompatible.

The localizationist model arises from concepts first articulated by Gall and developed by other neurologists in the nineteenth century [For a review of this development see Head (2).] They believed that certain areas of the brain served certain specific functions or faculties. In 1801 Gall made the statement that the brain was made up of organs that subserved the vital intellectual and moral faculties of man. Bouillard said that speech was localized in the frontal lobes. At this stage they were still dealing with the nature of normal function. They had not yet defined the disorder. Broca, in 1861, presented two cases that he thought demonstrated that the faculty of language was located in the frontal lobes, specifically at the base of the third left frontal convolution. He said that a lesion at this point would result in a loss of speech.

All these early aphasiologists were good clinicians, which means that they were also good observers. It was soon apparent that what they were seeing did not quite match what they expected to see from their model. There were apparently possible disruptions other than the kind of loss described by Broca. It should be pointed out that Broca, too, noted such differences in types of aphasia, describing first "aphemie," what we now would call a "motor aphasia," and "amnesie verbale," a disruption of the ideas underlying the use of symbols. Wernicke carried the idea of localization of function and its disruption a bit further and postulated four different types of aphasia: motor aphasia, that described by Broca; sensory aphasia, the result of a lesion in the posterior section of the brain; conduction aphasia, a condition that came about because of a lesion in the fibers connecting the anterior and posterior portions; global aphasia, the result of lesions in both the anterior and posterior portions of the brain.

We shall not go into great detail about the various lesions and their possible effects on speech. The important concept here is that a specific lesion can produce a specific problem in the processing of language. An anterior lesion will produce motor problems; a posterior lesion will produce sensory problems. This was seen as an important advance because it gave the physician a valuable tool in diagnosing the site of the lesion.

A major part of the localizationist view has a linear conception of language functioning; that is, language can be viewed as something going in and as something going out (expression). Again, following through on the concept that there can be a specific impairment at a specific point, not only in the brain but also in the processes that are controlled by the brain, it was possible to conceive of a receptive impairment separate from expression, and vice versa, a conception that is prevalent to this day. People still talk about "receptive" aphasics and "expressive" aphasics. Let us say right now that there is no such thing. All aphasics at some level have receptive problems and expressive problems. There is a real danger involved in the use of the terms receptive and expressive aphasia, since they foster the belief that the individual aphasic can "understand everything." This can create problems on the ward, in the therapy sessions, and at home for the aphasic and for those around him.

Pierre Marie (3) was one of the first to demonstrate that the idea of the aphasic who was unimpaired in reception was a function of the way in which the aphasic was tested. He stated that he had not published for a long time because everything he had seen contradicted what he had been taught; he had never seen an aphasic patient who did not have comprehension difficulties. He concluded from this that aphasia was an impairment of comprehension and of intellectual skills.

Freud addressed himself to the problems of the aphasic as well. In a brilliant monograph appropriately entitled "On Aphasia" (4), he suggested that aphasia did not represent specific loss of specific function; rather, it was a "reduction of efficiency" of the total mechanism. He argued that the errors aphasics make are exactly the same as those made by normals whenever the system is not working well. For example, when one is fatigued, one tends to make mistakes in speech. These mistakes are basically the same as those the aphasic makes. Anything that can tend to reduce the efficiency of the total mechanism will affect the output and interactions within that mechanism. Let us take one further example: Suppose you go to class and you are very tired. The teacher is speaking just as loudly as usual and is covering the same material; the material is not necessarily any more difficult than it was in the last class. Yet you have difficulty in comprehension. In a sense, the aphasic is operating in the same way, but all the time.

As mentioned earlier, the two models are basically opposed. This opposition can be seen in the two kinds of speech therapy that have been derived from them. If one holds the view that the aphasic has lost something, such as the ability to name, the use of phonemes or syntax, etc. (or, even more important, if the aphasic has lost those words or sounds or grammatic rules), therapy will be directed toward replacing that lost information. Early therapies with aphasics did just that; they developed what we have called elsewhere a learning approach to therapy (5). This particular approach to therapy arose for several reasons. First and foremost, of course, was the view of what aphasia represented. But a second important factor was the pressing social need created by the Second World War. Prior to this conflict, there had been very little effort directed toward language rehabilitation of aphasic patients. Partially as a result of improved medical capabilities, there were large numbers of young brain-damaged individuals who were going to survive. This, coupled with the moral commitment of several of the involved nations, demanded the development of therapies to serve these men. The first large-scale efforts were set up in Canada in 1939 (6). However, in the United States, the Veterans Administration gave direct impetus to the development of therapy through its commitment to service for the veteran and concern for development of the best help available. Huge amounts of money, time, and effort were devoted to the development of appropriate therapies.

Many of the early clinicians in the field were drawn from the schools and were speech correctionists. The therapeutic techniques they developed were often based on (a) the loss or localizationist view of aphasia (i.e., the aphasic had lost language, that had to be relearned) and (b) the techniques they had developed to correct the defective articulation found in children. The result was what can only be called an "atomistic" regimen (5). For example, the word mother has four sounds. If one were to work on "mother," one would first teach "m" and then "o" to form the syllable "mo." Then one would attack the "th," and when that was mastered, the "er." Then the two syllables "mo" and "ther" could be put together to get "mother." (This is an actual example taken from a book on speech correction.) Martha Taylor Sarno, in a series of studies designed to test this learning approach, found evidence that, at least with seriously impaired patients, it did not work.

One point should be made explicit here. We are not pointing these things out to in any way disparage the early workers in the field. Francis Bacon said that truth arises more readily from error than from confusion. This is very important to remember when we are looking at the work of others and at our own work as well. It is not that important to be correct. It is more important to try to bring some order where confusion exists. When we do that, we have made the first giant step toward "truth."

Even early on, however, there were clinicians who believed that aphasia did not represent a loss of language and that therefore a teaching approach was inappropriate. These clinicians developed what they called the stimulation approach to therapy (7).

If one believes that aphasia represents a reduction in the efficiency of use of the mechanism, then therapy logically will be directed toward stimulation of the mechanism to operate more efficiently. The best-known proponent of this approach was Schuell (7). Schuell presented a series of techniques that were directed toward stimulating the aphasic to use certain underlying processes more efficiently. For example, there has been a great deal of research indicating that the aphasic has more difficulty as the length of the stimulus material increases. Therefore one simple structured task that Schuell developed was the arrangement of stimulus materials in increasing lengths, for the purpose of learning the materials so the aphasic could practice handling the greater complexity and difficulty involved. One might start with a single word, "house," then go to a phrase, "in the house," and graduate to a sentence, "He went into the house."

The same principle can be applied to helping aphasics in their relations with those around them. If they have difficulty with auditory retention span, then those around them can help aphasics understand by varying their phrasing: "I . . . am going . . . to the movies. . . . I will see you . . . later." In this way the aphasic can process the information a little better and easier.

There has been a great deal of research on various aspects of this kind of therapy and on the underlying rationale, but space does not permit us to detail it here. However, there is an interesting article by Wepman (8) that deals with the specific issue of why the aphasic is better able to handle this type of phrasing.

One of the advantages of a "stimulation" approach to therapy is that it can be adapted to many different situations and environments. When I was at the New York Veterans Administration Hospital, the Speech Pathology and Audiology Department worked very closely with the Occupational Therapy Department. There were many tasks and techniques that we were able to adapt in each setting that would supplement and complement the work done by each specialty. However, in order to do this, we had to have many hours of discussion of philosophy, theory, and technique so that we could meet on common ground, not to take over each other's specialties but to share in an efficient manner the realization of our common goal, service to the aphasic. It is important that specialists in all fields who work with aphasics share their theoretical views, therapeutic philosophies, and actual techniques so that we can examine the totality of the service we offer.

REFERENCES

1. Martin, A. D. (1979): Levels of reference in aphasia therapy. In: *Clinical Aphasiology,* edited by R. Brookshire. Brk Publishers, Minneapolis.
2. Head, H. (1926): *Aphasia and Kindred Disorders of Speech, Vol. I.* Macmillan, New York.
3. Cole, M. E., and Cole, M. (1971): *Pierre Marie's Papers on Speech Disorders.* Hafner Publishing, New York.
4. Freud, S. (1953): *On Aphasia* (1891) (translated by E. Stengel). International Universities Press, New York.
5. Martin, A. D. (1978): A critical evaluation of aphasia therapy. In: *Clinical Aphasiology: Collected Proceedings,* edited by R. Brookshire. Brk Publishers, Minneapolis.
6. Huber, M. (1942): Reeducation of aphasics. *J. Speech Hear. Disord.,* 7:289–293.
7. Schuell, H., Jenkins, J., and Jimenez-Pabon, E. (1964): *Aphasia in Adults.* Harper & Row, New York.
8. Wepman, J. (1972): Aphasia therapy: A new look. *J. Speech Hear. Disord.,* 37:203–214.

The Apraxias

15

Renee Okoye

Apraxia, an inability to perform purposeful motor acts, was introduced as a separate neurological disorder by Liepmann in 1900 (1). In his work *Das Krankheitsbild der Aprasie,* Liepmann presented the classic definition of apraxia: inability to perform purposeful movement in the absence of paresis, ataxia, or disturbance of tone.

Apraxias vary in severity from the profound immobility of a patient with an ideational apraxia to the clumsy or awkward attempts at skilled motion of the child with dyskinesia or a developmental apraxia. Apraxias vary in their influence from involvement of the whole body to involvement of only the wrists and fingers. Finally, apraxias vary in their etiology and lesion sites from intracranial tumors and specific lesions in the cerebral cortex to central nervous system dysmaturation syndromes with dysfunction of projection fibers from subcortical structures.

Basic neuropsychological research by Critchley (2), Hecaen et al. (3), and Denny-Brown (4) detailing physiological conditions underlying apraxia has indicated that lesions in the frontal zones of area 4, the precentral region of area 6, and the sensorimotor region of area 3 (Brodmann's classification) contribute to the presence of a variety of apraxias in the adult, even though paresis may mask the manifestation of the disorder. Ayres (5) indicated that dysmaturation of vestibular and somatosensory subcortical systems contributed to the presence of developmental apraxia in childhood.

A redefinition of apraxia, as suggested by Luria (1), would seem indicated in view of the wealth of clinical research findings since Liepmann's articulate but limited definition of 1900. The integration of movement with logical thought and the visual, vestibular, tactile, and most important auditory systems has been clearly documented, thus significantly altering the view that apraxias exist in isolation, apart from other movement disorders and disorders of cognitive perceptual skills.

Statistical documentation pertaining to the incidence of apraxia among brain-injured patients is not readily available. Probable causes for this lack of epidemiologic documentation may stem in part from general disagreement among theorists and researchers as to the definition of apraxia. Another major reason for this lack of documentation arises from inability to develop a sufficiently sensitive tool so as to clearly distinguish apraxia from other movement disturbances. In my clinical experience dealing with patients whose diagnoses have reflected either psychosocial or physical disabilities, I would have to say that many suffered from various types of apraxias. Among the adult population with whom I have dealt whose diagnoses have reflected psychosocial disorders, approximately 20% have appeared to be experiencing apraxia disorders. Among the pediatric population referred for remediation of learning disabilities, where the primary complaint has been behavioral or psychosocial disorders, all have appeared to be experiencing apraxia disorders.

In the adult population with whom I have worked whose diagnoses have indicated brain injury, conservatively 9 of 10 patients have either initially presented with apraxia disorders or given evidence of apraxia disorders once tone has become normalized. Nearly all of the children with whom I have dealt whose severe congenital physical disabilities have precluded involvement in developmental activities have experienced disorders of body scheme, with resultant developmental apraxia.

Since apraxia may be defined as dysfunction in the organization of a motor act, we will review what the organization of a motor act entails before proceeding to discuss various dysfunctions referred to as apraxias.

Initially, movement was believed to originate from the cerebral cortex. However, experiments have shown that the cerebellum and basal ganglia are activated at almost exactly the same time the motor cortex is activated prior to initiation of movement. Also, there is no known mechanism by which the cerebral cortex can conceive the entire sequential pattern necessary for the execution of a motor act. For the present, it appears that the basal regions of the brain are initially responsible for eliciting voluntary motion, although these regions are themselves subject to external control from areas of the brain involved with association of various memories and sensory images.

There are several areas of the cortex that are closely involved with the production of voluntary movement. Destructive lesions or disturbances in these areas lead to various types of apraxias. The frontal lobe of the cortex is closely related to the formulation of voluntary motion. The involvement of the frontal lobe assures preservation, regulation, and correction of voluntary motion. The premotor area provides for both inhibition and modulation of impulses arising from subcortical motor structures and assists in the consecutive organization of movement sequences. The involvement of the premotor area assures smooth transition of movement sequences by providing for inhibition of sequences already completed and feeding forward of sequences to be initiated. The postcentral area of the cortex provides sensory and kinesthetic data necessary for voluntary movement. The involvement of the postcentral zone assures integrity of kinesthetic analysis, synthesis, and feedback into motor effector systems. The parieto-occipital areas of the cortex provide for the integration of visual, vestibular, and kinesthetic input, thus assuring the spatial organization of movement. The basal ganglia are responsible for regulation of muscle tone and smooth changeover from one motor system to another and thus are dynamically involved in the production of purposeful movement. The cerebellum is involved with voluntary motion by way of its complex monitoring of all motion. The cerebellum is responsible for error control and damping of movements already in progress, and it also functions to retrieve engrams for skilled motor patterns. The function of the corpus callosum in connecting symmetrical loci of the premotor and motor zones of each cerebral hemisphere allows for both bilateral movement and bilateral reciprocal movement, important sequences in the organization of purposeful human movement.

When one considers the extent of involvement with movement of these many central structures and the diverse nature of their contributions to purposeful movement, one can begin to predict the symptoms engendered by trauma or disturbance to these regions of the brain.

Current theorists (5–7) propose the possibility that the left cerebral hemisphere is dominant not only for language, but for the cortical organization of movement as well. These theorists have submitted evidence that trauma to specific regions of the left hemisphere, or injury to connective fibers within the corpus callosum, can result in a variety of apraxias. However, there is also documentation contradicting these theories. Nevertheless, the majority of recent research in the etiology of apraxia has indicated that there is an inner language of memories or engrams linking the use of objects, familiar movements, and symbolic questions. The majority of researchers have concluded that the center governing the ordering of this inner language is to be found in close proximity to the speech centers.

ORGANIZATION OF VOLUNTARY MOVEMENT

The organization of purposeful motion centers around four basic premises and may be divided into four major stages of movement. One basic premise of purposeful motion is the development of an intention to move. The intent may arise from integration of sensory input, from a visualized model of a motor task to be performed, or from a desire to fulfill a present or anticipated need. Another basic premise is that the motor task that will satisfy the requirements of the intention represents a constant or invariant task that has been learned. For example, if one intends to catch a large ball, the invariant requirement is to maneuver both arms in such a manner as to grasp the ball between both hands and thus stop the motion of the ball. In order to catch the ball, the requirement remains the same (invariant or constant) whether the ball must be caught overhead, out to one side, or down near the knees. Another basic premise is that the invariant task may be fulfilled by variable programs or sets of movements. For example, the large ball may be caught with shoulders and elbows flexed or with shoulders and elbows extended or with fingers flexed, or with shoulder and elbows extended, or with fingers flexed as opposed to fingers extended. Any of these various sets of movements may be used to fulfill the invariant task demand of catching the ball. The last premise, involving cerebral organization of voluntary motion, is that movement must have a "plastic succession of innervations corresponding to the changing positions of the limbs and to the changing state of the muscular system at each moment."

There are four major stages in the organization of movement: (a) development of an intention to move, (b) selection of an appropriate invariant task that will satisfy the intention, (c) programming of variable movement or efferent impulses that will satisfy the original intention, (d) ongoing analysis and synthesis of afferent impulses to monitor body scheme and motions in progress and to make corrections as needed.

The development of an intention to move presupposes the ability to formalize an action consequence and is a function of the frontal lobes. Selection of an appropriate invariant task from which to pattern movement is believed to originate in the frontal lobe. With the aid of "internal speech" and input from other areas of the cortex, the frontal lobe is able to formulate a program for action and select an appropriate invariant model for the task. The ability to select the appropriate motor task is modified to a great extent by memory of prior experiences and by learning. Persons at extreme ends of the age continuum usually have difficulty with this stage of the motor act. The young or developmentally delayed may have difficulty with this stage because of lack of prior experience, whereas older adults may have difficulty with this stage because of neurological impairment affecting the ability to retrieve memory or learning regarding the invariant model for the task.

The third stage in the organization of movement, the programming of variable movements that will satisfy the original intention of the motor act, is believed to be implemented primarily by the functions of the premotor area and the cerebellum. The cerebellum is involved in this stage in the synthesis of proprioceptive data regarding the location, velocity, and muscular tension each body segment is exposed to and in apprising the premotor area of the coordinates of effort (in time and space) necessary to accomplish the original intention. The cerebellum also anticipates the gamma bias necessary to effect these coordinates and discharges efferent impulses to the gamma system in accordance with the program selected.

The last stage of purposeful movement, ongoing analysis and synthesis of sensory data from visual, auditory, vestibular, tactile, cues and comparison of this incoming data to the original invariant intent, is accomplished by feedback of sensory data through reticular, basal ganglia, and cerebellar subsystems.

ETIOLOGY AND DESCRIPTION

At present there is considerable disagreement concerning apraxia, especially in regard to nomenclature, etiology, and localization of lesions. However, theorists do agree that the syndromes referred to as apraxia may be caused by trauma to any of the structures involved with movement or by trauma to any of the connective neural routes that transmit data from one of these structures to another (1).

Apraxias are characterized by movement disorders other than those due to spasticity, ataxia, and paresis, and they represent disorganization in the intention, sequencing, or analysis of kinesthetic feedback regarding movement.

IDEATIONAL APRAXIA

Movement disorders caused by trauma to the frontal lobes that result in profound difficulties in the development of an intention to move are commonly referred to as ideational apraxias. Other neuropsychological deficits that are frequently manifested along with ideational apraxia include the following: (a) an output language disorder affecting expressive language, oral musculature, or gestural language, or all three; (b) an object agnosia, or inability to recognize objects and their uses by means of vision alone; (c) bilateral apraxic involvement; (d) an attentional deficit.

An ideational apraxia is often characterized by the preservation of isolated idiosyncratic movement, with loss of the ability to formulate or develop an intention to move. Formulation of such an intention requires deliberate sorting and categorizing of data available from sensory associative areas of the cortex, retrieval of pertinent memories previously related to the incoming data, and association of these data with patterns of movement. When ideational apraxia is present, the patient seems either unable to identify the need for such a task or unable to persevere so as to regulate such a task. The patient is frequently unable to associate visual images of objects with the motor patterns required for their use. Once a patient who has an ideational apraxia has been engaged in an activity that involves handling a familiar object, the patient may be able to execute an entire action sequence involving the use of that object. However, once the action sequence has been completed, the patient will be unable to duplicate the sequence or initiate any further consecutive sequences.

A descriptive case is that of Mrs. V, a 63-year-old woman who had suffered a left cardiovascular accident, with resultant spastic hemiparesis on her right side. She was referred to a community-based practice for continued therapy after discharge from a local rehabilitation center 3 months after trauma. Initial findings revealed that she had severe language difficulties in that expressive, receptive, and gestural language modalities were severely impaired. She was hemiparetic and experienced severe spasticity in the flexors of her elbow, wrist, and knee. Contractures and functional changes within the joints were developing despite the presence of a fair amount of active range of motion. Muscles throughout her "unaffected extremities had become hypotonic and somewhat atrophied because of disuse." Joint range was limited slightly throughout the extremities on her left side. The only movements available to Mrs. V were reflexive reactions and occasional automatic movements, such as sitting forward to say something. Further evaluation revealed right hemianopsia, right hemisomatagnosia, oral motor apraxia, and severe sensory loss in her right extremities. Despite complete functional range and strength in the extremities on her left side, she sat entirely immobile unless engaged in a specific activity initiated by a nurse, therapist, or member of her family. She was unable to initiate gestures, use familiar objects, perform familiar motor sequences, or even assist with self-care activities. This clinical picture is consistent with ideational apraxia, although not all patients with ideational apraxia experience aphasia.

An additional common finding associated with the presence of ideational apraxia is inability to perform activities requiring bilateral use of the hands. Activities involving bilateral movement or bilateral reciprocal movement, such as opening a jar, striking a match, or hammering a nail, are extremely difficult for patients with ideational apraxia. Attempts at such activities may be thwarted by improper gripping of tools or by awkward inappropriate movements of the hands. Patients may be aware that their movements are inappropriate for the activity, but they may be unable to retrieve appropriate kinetic engrams for the task, despite attempts to correct movements. Self-care activities requiring bilateral movements, such as soaping up a washcloth, putting toothpaste on a toothbrush, or shaving, are extremely difficult for these patients. They may be well motivated for therapy, but they soon become discouraged as activities requiring bilateral involvement or use of tools prove impossible. Patients with ideational apraxia often tend to be socially and physically isolated from daily activities because of language disabilities and immobility imposed by the apraxia. Routine care for patients with ideational apraxia should include complete passive range of motion for all joints and joint mobilization, where possible, to prevent further disability caused by frozen joints. In addition, aggressive management of social needs may be necessary to maintain appropriate social skills. Sensory integrative approaches to treatment may also be necessary. Methods for remediation of ideational apraxia will be discussed in subsequent sections; they center around facilitation of subcortical patterns of movement and use of a psycholinguistic approach to speech.

IDEOMOTOR APRAXIA

Trauma to the premotor area of the cortex often results in a movement disorder that is clinically referred to as ideomotor apraxia. Ideomotor apraxia is a movement disorder that is characterized by inability to execute a series of goal-directed movements. The involvement may be bilateral or unilateral. Ideomotor apraxia is readily distinguished from ideational apraxia during clinical observation by the relative mobility of the patient. Movement is generally possible, but extremely awkward. Clinical examination of patients with ideomotor apraxia reveals preservation of both the intention to move and the ability to select an appropriate invariant task. Ideomotor apraxia results from inability to program the variable elements of movement (e.g., how far to extend the elbow or pronate the forearm when pouring) that are dependent on ongoing analysis of sensory data. Thus the patient with ideomotor apraxia seems unable to correct or alter the elements of movement once they have been selected and initiated. The patient's movements seem distorted, grossly clumsy, or awkward. Superficially the patient seems to be accident-prone; that is, the patient seems unable to predict that certain movements of his body will result in injury and seems unable to prevent forseeable "avoidable" accidents. The dyskinesia that generally seems to accompany this disorder contributes to the likelihood of accidents in that the patient is unable to appreciate the various positions of the body parts. The body scheme and subskills necessary for skilled movement are impaired with this patient. The involvement usually affects the entire body, gross and fine movements, as well as unilateral and bilateral activities.

It may be of interest to note that at one time ideational apraxia was thought to be a severe form of ideomotor apraxia. This theory has been refuted by many researchers, among them De Renzi (6) and Heilman (7), who have developed more sensitive measures of testing for apraxia. Heilman was able to further document that patients with ideomotor apraxia who have suffered trauma to the left hemisphere consistently experience bilateral apraxic involvement, whereas patients with ideomotor apraxia who have suffered trauma only to the right hemisphere experience only contralateral apraxia. This finding tends to support the current theory of dominance of the left hemisphere in regard to coordination of movement. In this work Heilman referred to aphasia as a disturbance of verbal symbolization and apraxia as a defect in nonverbal symbolization.

The patient with ideomotor apraxia often presents the following clinical findings: (a) absence of primary paresis and primary sensory deficits, (b) dyskinesia, and (c) most notably inability to analyze, synthesize, and monitor body scheme and motions in progress and make corrections.

The absence of primary paresis, or rather the absence of weakness due by atrophy, is a salient feature in the clinical picture of the patient with ideomotor apraxia. The lack of observable defects in the affected limbs is frequently a provocative issue in the clinical management of patients with this type of apraxia. The fact that the appearance belies functional capacities may not be readily understood or believed by nursing staff or family members. Persistent difficulties with grooming and dressing activities, use of ambulatory aids, and even toileting and hygiene tasks spark annoyance and frustration for the novice who is dealing with patients with ideomotor apraxia.

The absence of primary sensory deficits such as the anesthesias and paresthesias common to patients with spastic hemiplegia is notable in patients with ideomotor apraxia. However, these patients are likely to experience deficits in higher cortical functions of haptic and cross-modal perception, such as akinesia, agraphesthesia, and astereognosis. Bilateral diadochokinetic rates are generally also impaired. These additional perceptual deficits are symptomatic of these patients' difficulties with ongoing analysis of somatosensory data. These symptoms further aggravate organization and execution of skilled movement and promote the clumsy and awkward movement sequences characteristic of this disorder. Dyskinesia, marked impairment in cortical analysis and synthesis of proprioceptive data, seems to be another salient finding when evaluating patients with ideomotor apraxia. These patients seem to be unsure of precisely where their body parts are and how they are positioned at any given time. Undue stress to joints and ligaments results. In addition, these patients generally tend to expend a great deal of time and effort to accomplish fairly simple daily tasks (e.g., bed mobility) because of inefficient use of body parts. In certain cases the extent of the dyskinesia poses problems of safety, especially with assistive rehabilitative procedures such as transfer activities. In these cases the patients' performances are quite variable in critical factors such as maintaining proper placement of feet, weight shifting from buttocks to arms and legs, and sequentially ordering movements of body parts so as to effect pushing up to standing. The extent of the dyskinesia in these cases significantly increases the probability of mishap.

A descriptive case is that of Mr. S, a 68-year-old man who had suffered a left cardiovascular accident, with resultant spastic hemiparesis in the extremities on his right side. He was referred to a community-based practice for continued therapy after discharge from the local rehabilitation center 4 months after trauma. Initial examination revealed that he was having moderate expressive and minimal receptive language difficulties. In addition, oral motor apraxia, with dysphagia, was present. His vital capacity was diminished, and breathing was shallow. He also demonstrated mild attentional deficits. The spastic involvement of his right extremities was mild to moderate. However, range of functional motion on the "unaffected" side was limited throughout. His ability to imitate gestures and manipulate objects was unimpaired contralaterally and limited in range because of spasticity ipsilaterally. However, his ability to complete a succession of familiar movements was nil.

Therefore, despite having sufficient functional range, Mr. S was unable to assist even with dressing, hygiene, and transfer activities. He was fairly independent in eating activities, although the dysphagia interfered with his nutritional status. Visual perceptual skills seemed to be intact; however, somatosensory perceptual skills were impaired bilaterally. This clinical picture is consistent with that of patients having ideomotor apraxia, although not all patients with ideomotor apraxia experience aphasic difficulties.

Although no statistics are available detailing the incidences of the various types of apraxia, clinical experience would tend to support evidence suggesting that idea motor apraxia is the most common type of apraxia found in physical rehabilitation centers today. Remedial techniques for management of ideomotor apraxia will be discussed in subsequent sections. However, the majority of the recommended methods center around the use of activities to heighten kinesthetic feedback along with cortical analysis of somatosensory data.

LIMB KINETIC APRAXIA

Limb kinetic apraxia, inability to coordinate wrist and finger movements, has not been a topic of recent investigation among American researchers. European and Russian investigators have discussed this topic in European neurological journals since the late 1950s. However, certain American researchers have expressed the view that the current demarcation of apraxia into various categories is artificial and serve only to confuse an already confusing situation.

Limb kinetic apraxia, when present, is most commonly observed during performance of familiar activities of daily living by brain-injured patients whose gross motor skills are intact. The etiology of limb kinetic apraxia is centered about trauma to the postcentral zones of the dominant cerebral hemisphere. The postcentral zones provide for interpretation and feedback of kinesthetic impulses into motor effector systems. When these zones are damaged, the complex integrative tasks of haptic perception that provide a major afferent basis of movement become impaired. The disorganization of kinesthetic feedback results in inability to differentiate among movements. When the lesion is situated in the middle or upper regions of the dominant postcentral zones, the arms and particularly the hands are affected. When one considers the large area of sensory representation of the hand in the sensory homunculus of the postcentral gyrus, the likelihood of disorganization of movements of the hand, as a result of trauma to this area, is more readily understood. This condition is referred to as limb kinetic apraxia. Similarly, when the lesion is situated in the lower regions of the dominant postcentral zone, the face, lips, tongue, and larynx are affected. The condition is then referred to as oral motor apraxia.

Luria (8) reported findings to support his assertion that with trauma to this region of the cortex, motor patterns lose their selectivity. Although he was quoting unpublished data, he reported finding that motor impulses passed to both agonists and antagonists at the same time in a patient suffering from a meningioma of the postcentral region. He further reported that when the tumor was removed, the diffusion of impulses gradually disappeared.

Since patients with limb kinetic apraxia are unable to differentiate among movements of the hand, finely coordinated tasks that require precision or manual dexterity, such as tying shoelaces or typing, are frequently impossible. One theorist proposed that because of the lack of kinesthetic integration, a type of tactile agnosia results. Consequently the patient is unable to gain sufficient feedback from objects. The organization of motor sequences necessary for manipulation of the hands and objects held by them becomes virtually impossible because of lack of kinesthetic integration.

Patients with limb kinetic apraxia generally present the following clinical picture: (a) absence of primary paresis and primary sensory deficits; (b) akinesia; (c) marked disturbances of fine motor coordination, especially with vision occluded; (d) disorders of imitative and gestural movements.

A descriptive case is that of Mr. B, a 42-year-old man who had suffered a right cardiovascular accident, with resultant hemiparesis in the extremities on his left side. He was referred to a community-based practice for continuing therapy after discharge from a local rehabilitation center. He had experienced good recovery, but he complained of difficulties with activities requiring the use of his left hand. He also experienced "annoying" spasticity in the ankle extensors and invertors. He also exhibited mild visual apperceptive agnosia. The difficulties he encountered in performing routine activities of daily living frustrated him tremendously. During the initial treatment sessions he constantly complained about difficulties inherent in turning doorknobs, rolling up the window in his car, driving his tractor, spading up shrubs, buttoning his cuff buttons, and tying his shoelaces. Although assistive devices were offered, he was determined to regain sufficient use of his hand to become totally independent in self-care.

Evaluation findings with Mr. B revealed that his appreciation of proprioception was intact throughout the extremities on his left side. However, discriminative touch was moderately impaired, and kinesthesia was practically absent. The extremities on his right side were unaffected. However, because of impaired feedback, bilateral tasks were extremely difficult to perform. These findings are consistent with those in patients who have limb kinetic apraxia.

The incidence of limb kinetic apraxia has not been generally discussed in neurological literature. However, approximately 1 in 20 apraxic patients encountered clinically demonstrates limb kinetic apraxia. Clinical management of this disorder will be discussed in subsequent sections. The primary objectives of treatment involve remediation of the kinesthetic disorder and the use of vision to help compensate for discriminative tactile deficits.

DEVELOPMENTAL APRAXIA

The developmental apraxia described by Ayres (5), Gubbay (9), and others is typified by the clumsy-child syndrome. The syndrome is marked by severe disturbances in gross and fine motor coordination. Dysfunction in vestibular functioning is a common finding associated with developmental apraxia.

Developmental apraxia differs from other types of apraxia in three distinct areas: (a) Developmental apraxia is a developmental disability, a childhood disability engendered prior to maturation of the central nervous system. (b) Developmental apraxia is not caused by irritative lesions or other types of trauma to the cortex. It is hypothesized that developmental apraxia is a consequence of dysmaturation within the subcortical systems of the central nervous system. (c) Developmental apraxia is characterized by disorders of somatosensory input to motor effector pathways.

The child with developmental apraxia often presents the following clinical findings: (a) dominating presence of developmental reflexes, (b) vestibular impairment, (c) oculomotor deficits, (d) lack of cerebral dominance, (e) simultagnosia, and (f) presence of various symptoms of somatagnosia (disorders of body scheme, e.g., finger agnosia, tactile agnosia, agraphesthesia, akinesia).

Although it is impossible to localize cortical areas of dysfunction in the child with developmental apraxia, it is usually possible to identify the sensory subsystems that are dysfunctional. Left untreated, developmental apraxia can become molded into disorders of sensory associative perception, and advanced cognitive-perceptual-motor skills such as visual-spatial construction and stereognotic abilities cannot be developed.

It has been documented in studies of United States servicemen that developmental apraxia does not disappear with maturity. Rather, these disabilities, when left untreated, persist through adolescence and adulthood to undermine ego functions and mastery of life tasks. One such study concluded that vocational options as well as psychological adjustment to changing roles in life may be negatively influenced by untreated perceptual motor disabilities.

A descriptive case is that of Christy F, an 8-year-old girl diagnosed as having cerebral dysfunction. Her presenting problems included the dominating presence of tonic neck reflexes, finger agnosia, agraphesthesia, astereognosis, dyskinesia, and simultagnosia. Visual perceptual skills and psycholinguistic skills were intact, but her vestibular responses were hyporeactive. Her legs were a mass of bumps and bruises from various spills, falls, and mishaps. Although she had not broken any bones, she was constantly walking into things, tripping over small obstacles, or stepping into trouble. She was socially immature, her best strategy being to practice teacher-pleasing behaviors, at which she succeeded fairly well.

Careful evaluation revealed that Christy's advanced visual perceptual skills could not compete with multiple incoming haptic stimuli. Skills such as depth perception, construction, and praxia were not sufficiently well developed to be serially integrated with discordant haptic stimuli. The resultant clinical picture as typical for a child with developmental apraxia.

Clinical management of the child with developmental apraxia will be discussed in a subsequent section. Remediation of this disorder centers around developmentally structured introduction of activities that foster integration and maturation of the dysfunctional subcortical sensory subsystems.

CONSTRUCTIONAL APRAXIA

Constructional apraxia has received a fair share of recognition among modern researchers. Constructional apraxia may be generally defined as a motor-executive disorder of visual-spatial perception that results in inability to perform tasks requiring assembly.

Constructional apraxias are caused by retrolandic lesions of the cerebral cortex. When these lesions involve primarily the right cerebral hemisphere, the resulting clinical disorder is dominated by visual-spatial agnosia. When these lesions involve primarily the left cerebral hemisphere, the resulting clinical disorder is dominated by motor-executive constructional disorders (10). Patients having constructional apraxia experience great difficulty when performing activities of daily living that require assembly or construction. Activities such as dressing, cutting meat, and light housework (such as sweeping under furniture) are performed by these patients in an awkward and time-consuming manner. In that these and other similar activities must be performed daily, the disability interferes significantly with the quality of life for the patient and also with the quantity of self-care activities the patient is able to accomplish unassisted.

Constructional apraxia is frequently complicated by the following: hemiparesis, visual associative agnosia, visual apperceptive agnosia, and other types of apraxia.

A descriptive case of contructional apraxia is that of Mr. A, a 63-year-old man diagnosed as having had multiple cardiovascular accidents. He experienced a moderate input and output language disorder, with bilateral apraxic involvement that was more pronounced in the extremities on his left side.

Evaluative findings revealed that Mr. A was able to interpret symbols rather than written communication and voice inflection rather than actual content of auditory input. Verbal output consisted of fluent jargon that was devoid of content. His motor skills were remarkable in that the extremities on his left side were so apraxic as to seem paretic. He was able to perform complex motor tasks spontaneously (even those requiring bilateral reciprocal movements), but he was unable to organize a series of purposeful movements or persist with a motor task apart from the spontaneity of the moment. Sensory findings were unremarkable, with the exception of loss of discriminative touch in the extremities on his left side. He demonstrated left hemianopsia and both visual apperceptive and visual associative agnosias, with moderate dysfunction in visual-spatial perception.

Constructional apraxia became quite evident when Mr. A was cued to duplicate a simple block design. Verbal instructions were omitted because of his moderate language disorder. Although he commenced the construction with flourishing motions of the hand (as though to indicate that the task was far too easy for him), the task was terminated after several attempts at construction ended in head scratching and head shaking, signifying that he was unable to complete the task. He was then presented with a small two-cup coffeepot to assemble, since it was believed that he might be more familiar with this item than with the block design. He visibly "brightened" when he saw the coffeepot and seemed eager to show that he was familiar with it. The examiner slowly took all the pieces apart and then put them together. The coffeepot was then disassembled again, and Mr. A was cued to put it together. He then demonstrated proficient use of both hands, including appropriate grasp patterns for bilateral reciprocal movements. He performed most of the subassembly tasks rapidly, placing and tightening the glass dome in the top and placing the basket strainer with its top on the inner stem of the coffeepot. However, he was unable to put these subassembled parts together correctly or to place them in the coffeepot correctly. He took the subassembled parts apart several times and looked them over carefully, as though to check whether or not they were assembled correctly. He seemed mystified by his inability to put them together in the coffeepot.

Unlike other such patients, Mr. A did not seem to experience frustration with his inability to perform familiar tasks of construction. He was also unable to dress himself. Although this case presented complicating factors, his difficulties with items requiring construction were consistent with those of other patients diagnosed as having constructional apraxia.

EVALUATION METHODS

Review of the literature has produced no documentation of widely accepted standardized procedures used to evaluate the various types of apraxia in adults or children. Rather, all researchers seem to prefer their own evaluative criteria. Since each researcher reviewed considered only one major type of apraxia, there was not one measure available that might be used as a screening tool for all of the apraxias.

This section will deal with those major screening methods that employ documented test criteria currently in use to evaluate patients with apraxia. The purpose is to discuss the possible application of each method as a screening tool for the various types of apraxia. The researchers' reports cited in the references will provide precise instructions regarding the method of application of each method.

Clinical observation and knowledge of the site of the lesion may serve to separate out those patients who have ideational apraxia, from other apraxic patients. As mentioned previously, patients with ideational apraxia present a fairly typical clinical picture of relative immobility, inability to use objects, and aphasia. The condition is usually bilateral, although it may be masked by paresis in the involved side. In addition, if the lesion site is located in the frontal lobes, there is a high probability of ideational apraxia.

Many tests for apraxic involvement that have been developed have incorporated an object-use subtest. The use of this method to assess both psycholinguistic involvement and apraxic involvement has become widespread among medical researchers. Although inability to use objects is only one symptom of ideational apraxia, research has proved this to be a very sensitive criterion for patients with ideational apraxia.

One such evaluative measure that presents standardized criteria of performance that may be used to rate patients with ideational apraxia is the object-use portion of the Porsche Index of Communicative Abilities (PICA). The PICA is a standardized test used to differentiate between various psycholinguistic disorders by specially certified speech pathologists. The object-use portion of the PICA quantifies the ability to use familiar objects such as a cup, match, and cigarette and the ability to pantomime or use gestures, such as pantomiming the use of a toothbrush.

Certainly homespun adaptations of the object-use portion of the PICA and other tests like it would be helpful in any assessment of praxis in brain-injured adults.

Assessment methods used to help differentiate the patient with ideomotor apraxia from other apraxic patients focus on use of the arms to imitate gestures. These methods may also be used to indicate the presence of developmental apraxia in older children. Clinical observation and knowledge of lesion site may also be helpful in determination. Particular aspects of importance in the clinical observation of patients with idea motor apraxia include relative mobility, integrity of purpose for a movement, ability to use objects, and a fumbling or clumsy approach to motor tasks. If the lesion site is known to be in the premotor area of the cortex, the resultant movement disorder may include idea motor apraxia.

Kimura (11) advocated a rather complete series of procedures to be used in the examination of apraxic patients. The procedures were especially designed to rule out the effects that psycholinguistic involvement often has on movement disorders. The movements Kimura suggested are not related to gestural language or object use; instead, they require deliberate isolated motor function. The result is a sensitive tool for examination of apraxic patients. Kimura's work has been cited by other researchers and has served as a springboard for several investigations dealing with patients who have idea motor apraxia.

Kimura detailed procedures for examination of the ability to use objects, unilateral gross and fine movements, and bilateral gross and fine movements. The rating scale used to objectify each performance is designed to separate out those difficulties posed by inability to formulate a plan from those difficulties posed by a lack of precision or a fumbling approach to the task. The assessment also contains a section requiring both simple and complex duplication of positions of the hands. This section can be used for assessment of patients with limb kinetic apraxia.

The Southern California Sensory Integration Tests developed by Ayres (12) contain an imitation-of-postures subtest that has been standardized for use with children. The imitation-of-postures subtest may be used in a gross fashion to indicate the child with developmental apraxia. However, this test, when administered according to protocol, is not sufficiently sensitive to provide conclusive documentation of the disorder. This fact is clearly stated by the principal researcher. Several of the test postures resemble those used for gestural language, thus further handicapping the child with psycholinguistic involvement. In addition, the criteria for rating focus in a general manner on the overall proficiency of the child, rather than separating out motor planning deficits from motor-executive disorders. Ayres suggested that depressed scores on the imitation-of-postures subtest, when coupled with depressed scores on the motor-accuracy and somatosensory subtests, are indicative of apraxic disorders.

Other indices are available from which to rank the motor performance of a child who experiences developmental delays or seems to be extraordinarily clumsy. The Denver Developmental Screening Test (13), the Oseretsky test for motor proficiency (14), and the balance and locomotor-agility subtests of the Cratty perceptual-motor battery (15) are some of the tests currently being used to aid in identification of children with developmental apraxia. Clinical experience indicates that formal observation of the reflexive maturation of each child referred for therapy is quite valuable; most children who are later diagnosed as having developmental apraxia also demonstrate dysmaturation in central nervous system reflexive developmental. A Bobath-style postural assessment (16) seems to work well for preschool children and adolescent children, whereas the Milani-Comparetti model (17) seems to work well with infants and toddlers.

Assessment of limb kinetic apraxia may also be made on the basis of clinical observation and knowledge of lesion site. The motor behavior of patients with limb kinetic apraxia is characterized by difficulties with manual dexterity and precision in movements of the hands. Thus any activities of daily living requiring precise movements of the hands (e.g., folding a letter, opening a padlock, buttoning) may be used as gross measures for assessment of patients who have limb kinetic apraxia. In addition, if the lesion site is known to be in the upper region of the postcentral zone, the resultant movement disorder may include limb kinetic apraxia.

Formal assessment of limb kinetic apraxia may be made by investigation of unilateral fine reciprocal and bilateral reciprocal movements of the hand. Tests described by Kimura (11) and Ayres (12), as discussed previously, may be used. An easily performed series was also offered by Luria (18), with both unilateral and bilateral reciprocal patterns of movement to be performed consecutively. Luria suggested rating the performance on the basis of integrity of the kinetic melody of the motor sequence rather than on the time it takes to execute the pattern. This suggestion appears to have much merit in examination of patients with limb kinetic apraxia.

Informal assessment of patients with constructional apraxia may be made by using common items requiring assembly, such as a coffeepot, flashlight, or shoelaces. Homespun tests for contructional apraxia usually do not quantify the time required for assembly, but simply rate each item on a pass/fail basis.

Formal assessment of patients with constructional apraxia may be made by using Koh's blocks (19) or by using the toothpick construction proposed by Hecaen (20). The block assembly is a common subtest of the Wechsler Adult Intelligence Survey and is highly regarded as an index of intellect and advanced perceptual-motor skills. The toothpick construction developed by Hecaen is a simplified tool requiring minimal intellectual and visual-spatial skills. The test requires two-dimensional duplication of a box, a cube, and other similar items. It is more directly targeted for the assessment of constructional praxis.

Whereas these methods of investigation all call for determination regarding the motor-executive aspect of praxis, the contaminating effects of deficits within psycholinguistic, visual perceptual, somatosensory, and vestibular parameters also need to be considered. Examination of praxis should therefore not be performed in isolation but should be considered an essential portion of a well-integrated assessment battery.

TREATMENT APPROACHES

Substantiative literature regarding remedial approaches and treatment methods for various types of apraxia is virtually nonexistent in rehabilitation medicine. One possible reason for the lack of literature in this area may be the structuring of roles within rehabilitation teams. Historically speaking, it is the role of the physician to diagnose and prescribe medication and treatment; it is the role of the therapist to provide prescriptive treatment once the diagnosis has been made. Whereas there is a historical role for the physician who is involved in pharmacological research, there is no similar role for the therapist involved in functional research regarding physiological and functional aspects of various treatment methods. Empirical research, our traditional method of documentation, is not sufficiently sensitive to be replicated by other professionals dealing with similar case loads. Although the lack of sophistication regarding research methods and use of criteria-referenced documentation is being addressed through education of the therapist, the effects of this aspect of continuing education have not yet been reflected in literature on apraxia.

A study by Taylor (21) attempted to differentiate between treatment outcomes for brain-injured patients based on types of treatment approaches used in therapy. The study, a herculean undertaking, did not sufficiently differentiate among syndromes. Therefore it was not possible to determine whether or not the treatments given were directly related to underlying causative factors of dysfunction. The results of this study cannot be substantiated in the light of current research findings.

Certainly treatment approaches for the various types of apraxia have not been verified in terms of ongoing neurological research supporting the sensory-integrative nature of motor skills. This section will present some approaches to treatment that have been found to be helpful. No attempt is made to suggest that the techniques presented are replicable, although references to the use of these techniques have been made in recent studies dealing with apraxia. The suggestions for treatment are offered only as examples of methods that have been successful with limited number (albeit a wide variety) of brain-injured patients.

Treatment approaches for patients with ideational apraxia are limited because of loss of both speech-related and non-speech-related patterns of movement. The development of effective strategies for treatment of patients with ideational apraxia stems from an appreciation of causative factors. Since these patients remain motionless because of inability to formulate an intention to move, strategies of intervention focus on the use of spontaneous motions or movements that may be elicited from subcortical systems. Neurodevelopmental and neurophysiological approaches to treatment may be effective in maintaining a semblance of integrity of the musculoskeletal system. Because of the transitory nature of the disorder, maintenance of functional motion and joint range and prevention of atrophy are important aspects of treatment when dealing with patients with ideational apraxia. Patients with ideational apraxia frequently recover some degree of motor function as the associated language disorder diminishes.

An ongoing sensory-integrative approach to treatment is usually helpful in stimulating alternate projection fibers around the lesion site, thereby assisting retrieval mechanisms for association of symbolic functions. Sensory-integrative activities for older adults with ideational apraxia include gentle vestibular stimulation and moderate changes in the tactile, auditory, olfactory, and visual inputs associated with the tools and methods of treatment.

Foremost among intervention strategies used to elicit motor responses during the transient period while mechanisms for retrieval of symbolic functions develop alternate routes is the use of spontaneity. It has been documented that patients with ideational apraxia test poorly in artificial clinical environments where objects are presented in isolation, without additional environmental cues. Thus a patient with ideational apraxia may well go through an entire morning routine of oral hygiene when presented with toothbrush and toothpaste at a sink in the washroom, whereas the same patient may be unable to demonstrate the use of the toothbrush in a clinic situation.

Given a familiar environmental setting complete with all its familiar paraphernalia (a perceptual set that constitutes maximal cueing), most patients with ideational apraxia can complete an entire motor sequence that is appropriate and consistent for the setup. Unfortunately, such behaviors represent training for a specific limited motor response pattern. The patients remain apraxic and cannot initiate the activities themselves or generalize the responses to other environments or setups. A descriptive case is that of a young man who suffered aphasia and ideational apraxia following a gunshot wound. He was able to be trained in morning care by the use of maximal cueing. Initially, maximal cueing required sitting him up in bed with a basin and towel resting on the over-bed table. Even with the soaped washcloth wrapped around his hand for him, only a rough scrubbing motion initiated by the therapist accompanied by the sharp command to wash evoked the proper motor response. He would then wash only one part of his body. Cueing was repeated for toweling dry and for washing additional body parts. Within seven treatment sessions this young man was able to persist in washing, drying, and dressing himself with only three distinct sets of cues. However, the motor sequence could not be generalized or used in other environments.

Use of maximal cueing may be helpful in providing a semblance of self-care. However, the patient remains essentially dependent in that the cueing and initiation of the activity must be performed by another person. In addition, each separate activity requires an additional set of environmental cues.

Another strategy that has been useful in retraining adults with ideational apraxia in the use of objects is to present the desired object and encourage the patient to handle it. The use of objects having distinctly textured surfaces is an important consideration. This strategy is particularly effective when the ideational apraxia is dominated by visual agnosia. In these cases, tactile cues, rather than visual cues, assist in object recognition and selection of the appropriate motor response.

These strategies that have been developed, maximal cueing and the use of tactile rather than visual cues to aid in object recognition, are geared only to reduction of the symptoms of ideational apraxia; they offer no remediation of the underlying cause of the condition. In current practice, only the use of sensory-integrative techniques in conjunction with a psycholinguistic approach to the severe language disability offer the long-range objective of remediation of the ideational apraxia.

Treatment approaches for patients with ideomotor apraxia are more expansive than those for patients with ideational apraxia. They also offer remediation of the underlying dysfunction in analysis and synthesis of haptic data.

Effective reduction of idea motor apraxia may be achieved in most cases by persistent use of neurodevelopmental and neurophysiological treatment methods. These methods are commonly employed to aid in muscle reeducation for hemiparetic limbs, but they are not generally applied to the head and trunk or to the noninvolved (but frequently apraxic) contralateral limbs. As mentioned previously, ideomotor apraxia is frequently bilateral, especially when the lesion site is located in the dominant cerebral hemisphere. Application of these methods in patterns that involve the whole body in bilateral reciprocal movement patterns is crucial to remediation of the apraxia.

Combinations of multiple sensory inputs, especially in tactile modalities coupled with subcortical reflexive patterns of movement, seem to be the essential ingredients for reduction of ideomotor apraxia. Neurophysiological techniques that heighten sensory input from affected body parts may be supported by visual cues to foster analysis and synthesis of tactile input. Techniques such as rubbing, scrubbing, kneading, pounding, tapping, vibrating, and icing use a combination of ascending spinal tracts and are routed to many subcortical structures, which then project the sensory data toward the cortex and to other subcortical structures. The likelihood of an appropriate motor response is thus greatly enhanced. Developmental sequences through the use of postures and activities are helpful for patients with ideomotor apraxia, since these positions activate proximal musculature as well as distal musculature in bilateral reciprocal patterns of movement. The subsequent reeducation incorporates repeated stimulation of subcortical mechanisms for movement and relies on lower-level reactions rather than cortical control to provide ongoing shifts in tonus in response to movement of body parts. Since this represents one of the major goals of therapy, use of a neurodevelopmental approach as a guide to treatment implementation is helpful in the remediation of the apraxia.

Treatment of children with developmental apraxia has been reported in rehabilitation literature. However, too few studies have been published that document the efficacy of the sensory-integrative techniques that are widely accepted for use with this population. There have been studies documenting the effectiveness of various methods of administering vestibular stimulation. Clinical studies documenting the effectiveness of various methods of administering olfactory, auditory, tactile, and visual stimulation with this population are simply nonexistent to date. Although most clinicians involved in treating patients with developmental apraxia use carefully selected sequences designed to provide sensory-integrative experiences for apraxic children, these sequences, which are theoretically acceptable, have not been formally validated by clinical research. Empirical documentation supporting the use of these techniques is plentiful; however, formal studies clarifying which sequences and techniques are most helpful for these children are sorely needed.

The developmental approach to treatment of children with developmental apraxia is reflected in the selection of activities that foster gross motor coordination and inhibition of developmental reflexes before those activities for fine visual motor skills are attempted. Examples of gross motor activities that may be used to facilitate vestibular function include the following: swinging in a swing or a suspended automobile tire; using a scooter board in prone, quadruped, and kneeling positions on level surfaces and on low-grade ramps; swaying in a sling hammock; rolling on a ball or barrel. Gross motor activities used to foster bilateral reciprocal patterns of movement include the following: climbing forward and backward on an indoor gym; crawling in foot-placement ladders; rolling over a large beach ball; kicking and throwing large balls; traversing an obstacle course.

In addition, those activities that foster stimulation and integration of the more primitive sensory subsystems (e.g., vestibular and tactile) should be presented before activities based on more highly selective systems (e.g., auditory and visual) are initiated. Many methods of treatment are rapidly being introduced in the professional literature. Journals containing recent studies in the treatment of developmental apraxia include the *American Journal of Occupational Therapy* and the *Journal of Learning Disabilities*.

Methods of remediation of limb kinetic apraxia are limited, but they seem to be effective. Again, only empirical documentation of efficacy is available. Application of neurophysiological treatment techniques that heighten haptic sensation is helpful in the stimulation of alternate routes for projection of sensory stimuli. One intervention strategy is to use visual cues rather than dysfunctional haptic cues to guide finely coordinated movement. Persistent practice in the use of vision to support haptic feedback for motion is an important aspect of treatment. During therapy, the patient may be encouraged to watch the noninvolved limb perform a particular grasp pattern before attempting the pattern with the involved hand (again, using vision to guide the movement). Bilateral activities can be very helpful, providing built-in neural bias for contralateral reciprocal movement through subcortical motor systems.

Limb kinetic apraxia, although one of the milder forms of apraxia, seems to be one of the most frustrating disorders for the patient. In many instances the patient's recovery seems complete (with the exception of limb kinetic apraxia); yet the patient cannot participate fully in either vocational or avocational activities because of lack of precision in movements of the hands. This results in a certain degree of dependence on others for activities of daily living and often distorts the emotional climate of the household in terms of roles, ego functions, and dependence needs within the home. Unfortunately, stroke, the most common cause of limb kinetic apraxia, usually occurs during the middle and latter stages of life when vocational skills and avocational interests have been established for many years. These are not the stages of life in which vocational retraining is easily accomplished.

Because limb kinetic apraxia does tend to diminish with practice, home management programs that complement specific therapeutic goals will not only augment progress but also provide some sense of independence and satisfaction for the patient.

SUMMARY

In conclusion, this review of current rehabilitative theories and practices regarding the neuropsychological disorder known as apraxia has indicated some major issues concerning the nature of apraxia and methods of treatment: There is doubt as to the proper definition of apraxia; there is also doubt concerning the nature of apraxia. Researchers have claimed that paresis or spasticity may mask the appearance of apraxia. Historically, clinicians have been reluctant to use the term apraxia whenever a marked movement disorder has also been present. However, this shift in the definition of the disorder may precipitate a change toward the use of sensory-integrative and neurophysiological treatment techniques when treating apraxic patients, whether or not a marked movement disorder is also present.

Is apraxia a disorder of movement, nonsymbolic language, cortical attention, and sequencing of a plan for movement, or is it simply representative of neurophysiological disruption caused by trauma or dysmaturation in a specific area of the cortex? These are questions yet to be answered by researchers in the field of rehabilitation medicine.

Since precise definition of apraxia is elusive, it is not unreasonable to find a lack of clear direction from clinical researchers in terms of indications for treatment methods or intervention strategies for remediation of the apraxias. Results of neuropsychological research in individual case studies have been helpful in providing new avenues of thought regarding the disorder. These studies have sought to clarify the lesion site and its association with the resultant symptomatology. In so doing they have also provided more sensitive evaluative methods with which to assess the disorder. A summary of clinical research that is needed in the field includes the following: development of one wide-range assessment tool as a measure of the various aspects of praxis for the adult; identification and documentation of which remedial techniques seem to affect which syndromes of apraxia; longitudinal comparative studies of prognoses for rehabilitative outcomes among the various forms of apraxia. Occupational therapists, by virtue of their training in analysis of human activity, would seem to be well equipped for further investigation into these issues regarding the apraxias.

REFERENCES

1. Luria, A. R. (1973): *The Working Brain.* Basic Books, New York.
2. Critchley, M. (1953): *The Parietal Lobes.* Arnold, London.
3. Hécaen, H., Penfield, W., Bertrand, C., and Malmo, R. (1956): The syndrome of apractagnosia following lesions of the minor cerebral hemisphere. *Arch. Neurol. Psychiatry,* 75.
4. Denny-Brown, D. (1958): The nature of apraxia. *J. Nerv. Ment. Dis.,* 176.
5. Ayres, A. J. (1972): *Sensory Integration and Learning Disorders.* Western Psychological Services, Los Angeles.
6. De Renzi, E. (1968): Ideational apraxia: A quantitative study. *Neuropsychologia,* 6:41–52.
7. Heilman, K. M. (1975): Defective motor learning in *ideomotor apraxia. Neurology (Minneap.),* 25:1018–1020.
8. Luria, A. R. (1966): *Human Brain and Psychological Processes.* Harper & Row, New York.
9. Gubbay, S. S. (1978): The management of developmental apraxia. *Dev. Med. Child Neurol.,* 20:643–646.
10. Arena, R. (1978): Constructional apraxia and visual perceptive disabilities in relation to laterality of cerebral lesions. Cortex, 14:463–473.
11. Kimura, D. (1974): Motor functions of the left hemisphere. *Brain,* 97:337–350.
12. Ayres, A. J. (1975): *Southern California Sensory Integration Tests.* Western Psychological Services, Los Angeles.
13. Frankenburg, W. K., and Dodds, J. B. (1967): The Denver Developmental Screening Test. *J. Pediatr.,* 71:181–191.
14. Doll, E. A. (1946): *The Oseretsky Tests of Motor Performance.* Minneapolis Educational Trust Bureau, Minneapolis.
15. Cratty, B. J. (1975): *Remedial Motor Activity for Children.* Lea & Febiger, Philadelphia.
16. Norton, Y. (1972): Minimal cerebral dysfunction in children. *Am. J. Occup. Ther.,* 26:186–199.
17. Milani-Comparetti, A., and Gidoni, E. A. (1967): Pattern analysis of motor development and its disorders. *Dev. Med. Child Neurol.,* 11:625–630.
18. Luria, A. R. (1966): Investigation of motor functions. In: *Higher Cortical Functions in Man,* edited by A. K. Luria, pp. 324–337. Basic Books, New York.
19. Diller, L., Ben Yishay, Y., Wienberg, J., and Goadkin, R.: *Studies in Cognition and Rehabilitation in Hemiplegia.* Project No. RD-2666-P. Department of Health, Education, and Welfare, Washington, D.C.
20. Hecaen, H. (1970): A comparison of constructive deficits following right and left hemispheric lesions. *Neuropsychologia,* 8:289–303.
21. Taylor, M. (1969): *Controlled Evaluation of Percept-Concept-Motor Training Therapy after Stroke Resulting in Left Hemiplegia.* Grant No. RD-2215-M. Department of Health, Education, and Welfare, Washington, D.C.

BIBLIOGRAPHY

Benton, A. (1973): Visuoconstructive disability. *Doc. Ophthalmol.,* 34:67–76.

Black, F. W. (1976): Constructional apraxia in patients

with discrete missle wounds of the brain. *Cortex,* 12:212–220.

Brenner, M. W. (1967): Visuo-motor disability in schoolchildren. *Br. Med. J.,* 4:259–264.

Brown, J. W. (1972): *Aphasia, Apraxia and Agnosia.* Charles C Thomas, Springfield, Ill.

Dee, H. L. (1970): A cross-modal investigation of spatial performance in patients with unilateral cerebral disorders. *Cortex,* 6:261–272.

Dee, H. L. (1970): Visuoconstructive and visuoperceptive deficit in patients with unilateral cerebral lesions. *Neuropsychologia,* 8:305–314.

Dee, H. L. (1970): Apraxia in relation to hemispheric locus of lesion and aphasia. *Trans. Am. Neurol. Assoc.,* 95:147–150.

Gazzaniga, M. S. (1970): *The Bisected Brain.* Appleton-Century-Crofts, New York.

Geschwind, N. (1965): Disconnexion syndromes in animals and man. *Brain,* 88:585–644.

Geschwind, N. (1967): The apraxias. In: *Phenomenology of Will and Action,* edited by E. W. Straus and R. M. Griffith, pp. 91–102. Duquesne University Press, Pittsburgh.

Geschwind, N. (1975): The apraxias: Neural mechanisms of disorders of learned movement. *Am. Sci.,* 63:188–195.

Gordon, E. E. (1978): Neurophysiologic syndromes in stroke as predictors of outcome. *Arch. Phys. Med. Rehabil.,* 59:399–403.

Gubbay, S. S. (1975): Clumsy children in normal schools. *Med. J. Aust.,* 8:233–236.

Hecaen, H. (1962): Clinical symptomatology in right and left hemispheric lesions. In: *Interhemispheric Relations and Cerebral Dominance,* edited by V. B. Mountcastle. Johns Hopkins Press, Baltimore.

Hecaen, H. (1970): A comparison of constructive deficits following right and left hemispheric lesions. *Neuropsychologia,* 8:289–303.

Heilman, K. M. (1973): Apraxia and agraphia in a left-hander. *Brain,* 96:21–28.

Heilman, K. M. (1973): Ideational apraxia—a redefinition. *Brain,* 96:861–864.

Heilman, K. M. (1975): A tapping test in apraxia. *Cortex,* 11:259–263.

Kimura, D. (1963): Right temporal lobe damage. *Arch. Neurol.,* 8:264–271.

MacNeilage, P. F. (1970): Motor control of serial ordering of speech. *Psychol. Rev.,* 77:182–196.

Nielsen, J. M. (1946): *Agnosia, Apraxia, Aphasia.* Hoeber, New York.

Piercy, M. F., Hecaen, H., and Ajuriaguerra, J. (1960): Constructional apraxia associated with unilateral cerebral lesions—left and right sided cases compared. *Brain,* 83:225–242.

Shane, H. C. (1978): The effect of auditory rhythmic stimulation on articulatory accuracy in apraxia of speech. *Cortex,* 14:444–450.

Amputation and Impaired Independence

16

Ruth E. Dickey and Linda Stieritz

This chapter is concerned with the problems of decreased independence experienced by the individual who has undergone amputation of one or both arms. The information presented will focus on the principles and processes of evaluation and training necessary for the arm amputee to attain maximum independence in all activities of daily living, both with and without prosthetic equipment. The phrase "activities of daily living" (ADL), which is used throughout this chapter, applies to all of an individual's functional activities, from self-care through vocational pursuits. The discussion will begin with postoperative care and continue through basic prosthetic training with conventional prosthetic equipment, emphasizing the needs of the adult unilateral amputee. Additional sections will deal with specialized training for the individual with a myoelectric prosthesis, the unique problems faced by the bilateral arm amputee, and selection of special devices and adaptation of equipment.

The outline follows a recommended prosthetic clinical procedures format (1), highlighting the role of the therapist in that process. This framework is an ideal vehicle for emphasizing a clinical team approach. This approach in the evaluation, treatment, and prosthetic training of the arm amputee is in contrast to the traditional clinical approach, which attempts to prescribe a prosthetic device in a setting where relevant information is very difficult to obtain.

Directed by the physiatrist, the professional team should include the prosthetist, occupational and physical therapist, vocational counselor, social worker, and psychologist. Equally important team members are the amputee and the amputee's family and friends. The successful combination of a prosthesis, technical factors, acceptance, and skilled functional use requires a collection of all pertinent information. In addition to gathering technical data, the team must employ short private evaluations to obtain from the amputee valuable impressions that will aid in deciding on a proper course of action (2).

PREPROSTHETIC MANAGEMENT

Training of the arm amputee begins immediately after surgery. Preprosthetic management includes postoperative therapy and the process of preprosthetic evaluation. The emphasis of treatment is directed first toward physical care of the residual limb and second toward information that will provide a base line for directing future treatment and selection of proper equipment (both prosthetic and special devices). All equipment is provided based on the patient's medical status (diagnosis and prognosis), age, sex, intellectual and psychological functioning, social and cultural values, economic status, and general personal goals (3).

Postoperative therapy is directed toward the physical care of the stump, residual motions that will be used for control of prosthetic equipment, and substitutions for lost motions. The following areas of treatment are essential in this period.

Maximum active range of motion must be maintained or increased in all remaining arm joints so that there will be adequate excursion for operating prosthetic or assistive equipment. Bilateral mobility of the scapula and shoulder is important for all arm amputees. For the below-elbow amputee, maximum elbow range in extension and flexion is necessary, as well as maximum supination and pronation, in order to ensure proper distal placement of the terminal device.

Strengthening and conditioning exercises are necessary for motions that are used to power and stabilize prosthetic equipment. Progressive resistive exercise can be used for increasing strength, coordination, and endurance. Specific areas of weakness can be strengthened using proprioceptive neuromuscular facilitation. The ability to voluntarily vary stump volume in the socket is necessary for maintaining prosthetic socket stability. Isometric exercises are used to increase this ability to stabilize the prosthesis. For example, the patient with an above-elbow amputation depends on the external rotators and biceps to prevent internal socket rotation while performing activities involving shoulder flexion and abduction. The patient with a below-elbow amputation uses the residual muscles of supination and pronation, if present, for socket stability (4).

Exercises to correct problems of posture may be necessary in cases where amputation has led to changes in body alignment. Also, exercises may be required to improve poor body mechanics that have led or could lead to postural or other complications such as decreased endurance (5).

Massage of the stump is beneficial in (a) increasing circulation, (b) reducing edema, (c) increasing skin mobility, (d) toughening the stump for use in functional ways, and (e) reducing the patient's apprehension about having the stump handled (6).

Stump shrinkage is used to ensure proper stump-to-socket contact by (a) achieving maximum shrinkage of stump volume before socket measurements are made, (b) preventing edema and hematoma, and (c) decreasing the possibilities of infection. Stump shaping for the below-elbow stump is used to produce a tapered or "screwdrive" shape that will decrease forearm rotation in the socket and thereby retain maximum supination and pronation. Shaping of the above-elbow stump encourages a conical tapered shape. One common method of stump shrinkage is to use an elastic shrinker (Fig. 1). The arm amputee can usually use a below-elbow shrinker. This method produces a consistent form of pressure, and it is the safest because of its easy application. However, care must be taken to see that the shrinker does not slide down the arm and produce a proximal tourniquet effect and distal edema (7). It is possible to adapt the figure-of-8 harness as a suspension system for the shrinker on a standard or short above-elbow stump. This method allows the patient to don the shrinker independently, whereas the elastic bandage technique that will be described next is not amenable to independent application, since it is wrapped around the body for adequate stability.

The elastic bandage technique gives the therapist more control over both pressure and shaping. Figures 2 and 3 demonstrate this method of wrapping for below-elbow (BE) and above-elbow (AE) stump shrinkage. The same care must

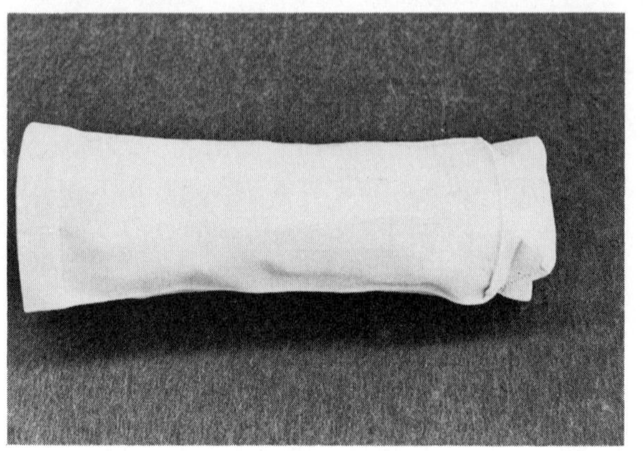

FIG. 1. Elastic stump shrinker.

ABOVE-ELBOW SHRINKAGE WRAP

Materials—same as for the BE wrap.

Position of the Patient
With the patient either sitting or standing: the humerus should be flexed to 90° and midway between internal and external rotation.

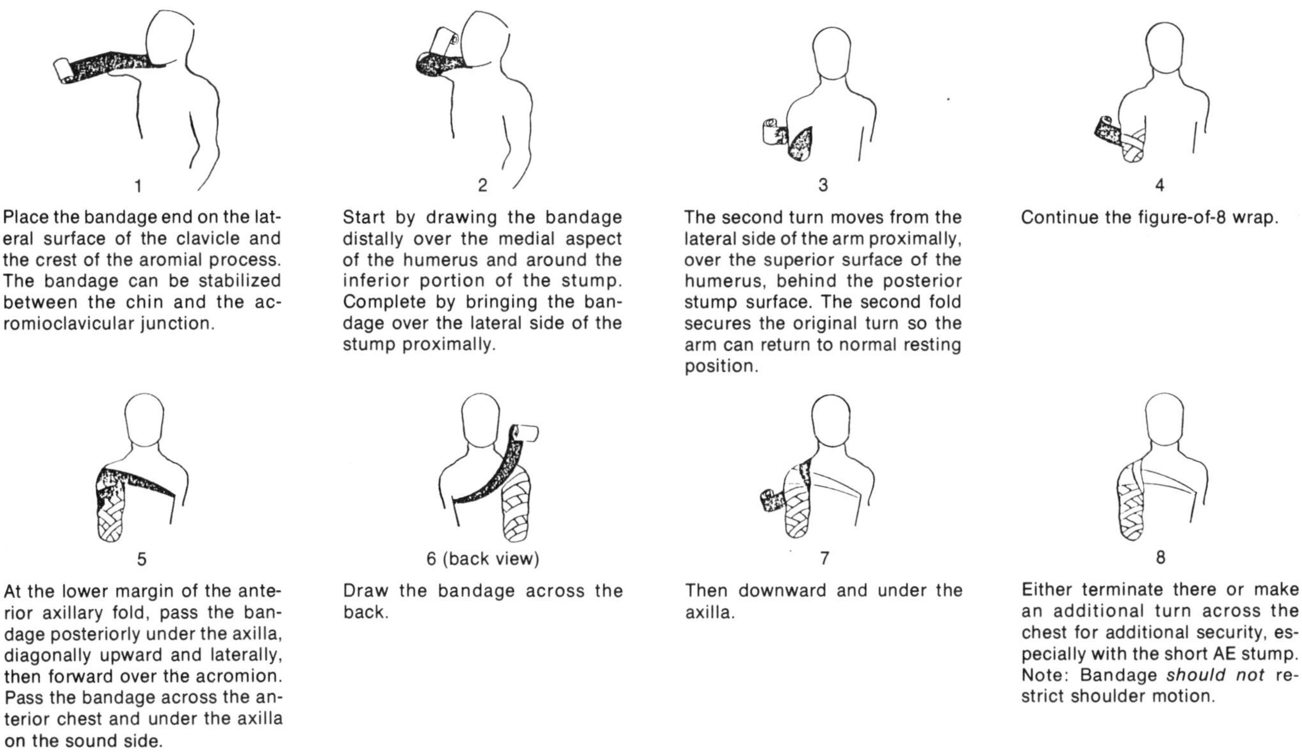

FIG. 2. AE shrinkage wrap. (Reproduced by permission of NYU/IRM Occupational Therapy Department.)

be exercised in wrapping to prevent excessive proximal pressure on the stump.

A third method of shrinkage and shaping uses plaster-of-Paris bandage and is good for fatty or edematous stumps. A conventional harnessing system is used to suspend and hold the plaster socket in place. As edema is reduced, the socket is replaced (8). The advantages of this technique are the same as those cited for the early socket fitting done immediately postoperatively.

Volume measurements of the stump are taken every 2 weeks at 2-inch intervals beginning 1 inch from the stump tip. Shrinkage rates vary for individuals; however, constant shrinkage applied for a period of 6 to 8 weeks is generally adequate. Proper shrinkage has been achieved when the stump circumference measurements are less than those for the sound extremity and when there is no more cutaneous or subcutaneous edema. Wrapping is continued until the patient is regularly wearing the prosthesis (9).

Immediate or early postoperative prosthetic fitting is carried out only infrequently. However, the amputee who has had early or immediate fitting deserves some discussion. This technique involves the application of a rigid dressing with a harness suspension system and terminal device. Immediate postsurgical prosthetic fitting is defined as the fitting of a functional socket immediately after surgery while the sutures are still in place. Early fitting is defined as the fitting of an unfinished functional arm replacement to be worn for a period of time to facilitate wear and use. Early fitting is done immediately after suture removal (10).

The advantages of this technique include (a) reduced pain, (b) earlier and more rapid prosthetic use, which decreases dependence, (c) easier psychological adjustment (11), (d) reduced postsurgical edema, (e) facilitation of the desensitization process, and (f) decreased healing time (12).

With these techniques the training process precedes the fitting of the permanent prosthesis and often reduces the time required for the entire

BELOW-ELBOW SHRINKAGE WRAP

Materials
1. Two rubber-reinforced elastic compression bandages. Bandages are 11½ yds. stretched length by 3 in. or 4 in. wide.
2. Bandage clips.

Position of the Patient
With the patient either sitting or standing: place the humerus in slight flexion, abduction and external rotation, the elbow in about 110° flexion and the forearm midway between supination and pronation.

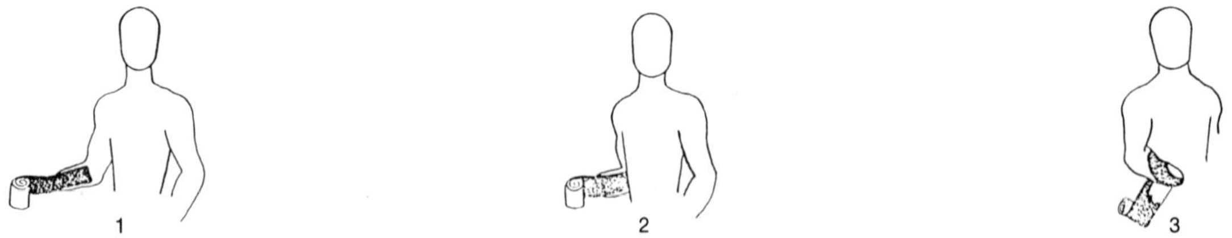

1. Place the bandage end on the medial epicondyle and the immediately superior epicondylar ridge.
2. The bandage is held in place by asking the patient to abduct the humerus. With increased proficiency this step can be omitted.
3. The first turn draws the bandage along the medial aspect of the forearm and around the ulnar half of the distal stump end. Continue by bringing the bandage over the radius and down the medial aspect of the stump.

4. The second turn draws underneath the ulna and over the lateral side of the stump.
5. Then over the radial half of the distal stump end.
6. Have the patient extend the elbow and continue the figure-of-8 weave.
7. Terminate the bandage above the elbow joint with bandage clips. Note: The bandage *should not* restrict elbow motion.

FIG. 3. BE shrinkage wrap. (Reproduced by permission of NYU/IRM Occupational Therapy Department.)

training process. Other advantages that have been cited include (a) making socket and harness adjustments on trial equipment rather than on the final prosthesis, (b) decreased need for adapted devices, and (c) decreased likelihood of the prosthesis being rejected because the patient has gone for a long period of time depending only on the intact extremity (13).

ADAPTIVE METHODS FOR ADL

Alternative methods for carrying out ADL can also be provided by (a) using the residual limb for function and (b) using assistive and adaptive equipment to provide some substitution for loss of function. For the unilateral amputee, most functions can be performed with the sound arm. Frustration can be reduced by providing solutions for object stabilization and work simplification.

PREPROSTHETIC EVALUATION

The preprosthetic examination brings together information from the entire team that updates everyone on the current status of the patient. It also provides information that will determine the kind of treatment still needed and the choice of proper prosthetic equipment. The occupational therapy preprosthetic evaluation should include information related to the following areas: demographic data, diagnostic data, physical status, stump descriptors, ADL status with and without equipment, equipment expectations, and recommendations. Appendix 1 shows a sample evaluation form.

Treatment prior to fitting is usually done concurrently with the fabrication process, unless the results of treatment would radically change the selection of the permanent prosthetic equipment.

PROSTHETIC COMPONENTS

Arm prosthetic components are chosen primarily to meet specific functional needs, with emphasis on replacement of prehension, especially for vocational pursuits.

BE Prosthetic Components

The conventional BE prosthetic components are pictured and labeled in Fig. 4. The socket for

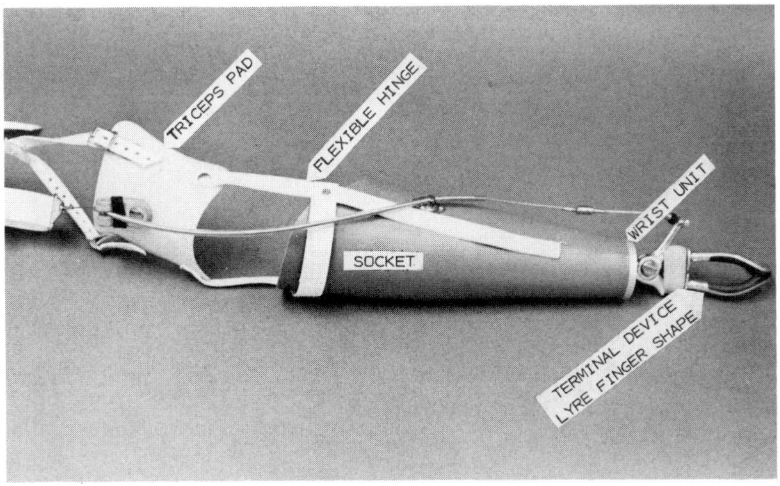

FIG. 4. BE prosthesis.

the long or medium-length stump is made of plastic laminate, as are all arm sockets. It is constructed to preserve maximum supination and pronation. The flexible elbow hinges also allow maximum use of forearm rotation. A triceps cuff provides an attachment point for the Bowden control cable and the front suspension strap of the harness. The harness system configuration is a figure-of-8 with a Northwestern ring providing a single control system for terminal device (TD) operation. The wrist unit is either an interchangeable friction-controlled unit (Fig. 4) or a quick-change rotation unit.

Prosthetic fitting for the short or very short BE stump frequently involves a prosthesis of the Muenster type (Fig. 5) because of its control and increased weight-carrying ability. This socket fits over the olecranon process and biceps tendon, eliminating the need for the triceps cuff and elbow hinges. The harness system is a figure-of-9 with a single cable control running through the crossbar assembly that attaches directly to the socket. This socket limits both full elbow flexion and extension (which is generally not of any significant disadvantage to the unilateral amputee) and eliminates the need to use step-up hinge or split socket with half cuff. Step-up hinges and split sockets do allow full 135° elbow flexion; however, they are bulky and less cosmetic.

AE Prosthetic Components

The conventional AE components are shown in Fig. 6. Socket length depends on residual stump length, but the design is essentially consistent for

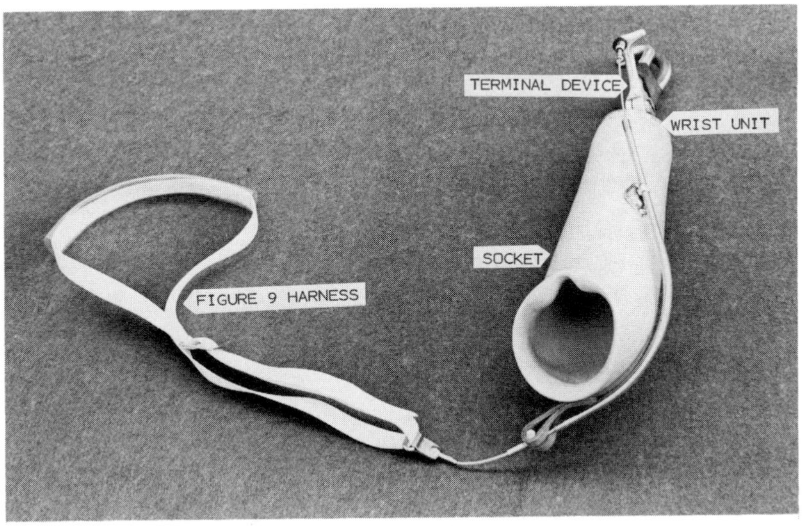

FIG. 5. Muenster prosthesis.

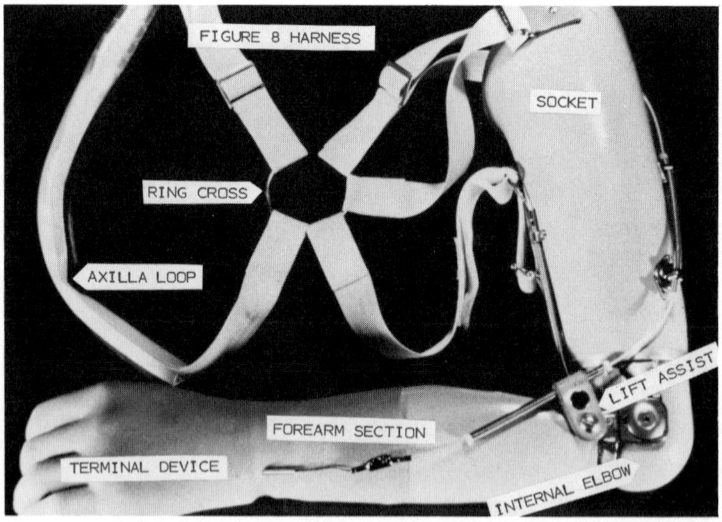

FIG. 6. AE prosthesis. (Reproduced by permission from a slide provided by NYU/IRM Orthotics and Prosthetics Department.)

all AE prostheses, except when the stump length is very short, which requires stabilization over the acromion and anterior and posterior stabilization to resist internal and external rotation.

Except in the case of elbow disarticulation where there is residual internal and external rotation, the elbow unit has a turntable that allows passive rotation. The elbow unit has an internal locking mechanism that can be alternately locked, at one of 11 different positions, and unlocked with the same motion. When unlocked, the elbow unit allows forearm flexion and extension; when locked, the terminal device operates constituting a dual control system.

The harness system is the figure-of-8 configuration, with an additional lateral support strap added to increase socket stability and prevent slippage when carrying heavy loads. A lift assist may be added to decrease the effort during elbow flexion.

Shoulder Disarticulation Components

The conventional shoulder disarticulation (SD) components are shown in Fig. 7. Here the socket covers the scapula and the pectoralis major areas. The shoulder units can be either free-motion abduction joints (Fig. 7) or friction joints for abduction or flexion. The elbow and forearm units are as described earlier. The chest strap harness system controls elbow and terminal device function by scapular abduction, with assistance sometimes necessary from an excursion amplifier, which is a mechanical device on a lever or movable sheave that converts a large force with small excursion into a lesser force with increased excursion. It is usually an extension of the control attachment strap, but it can be internally mounted inside the arm section. A waistband strap attaches to the elbow lock control, which is actuated by elevation.

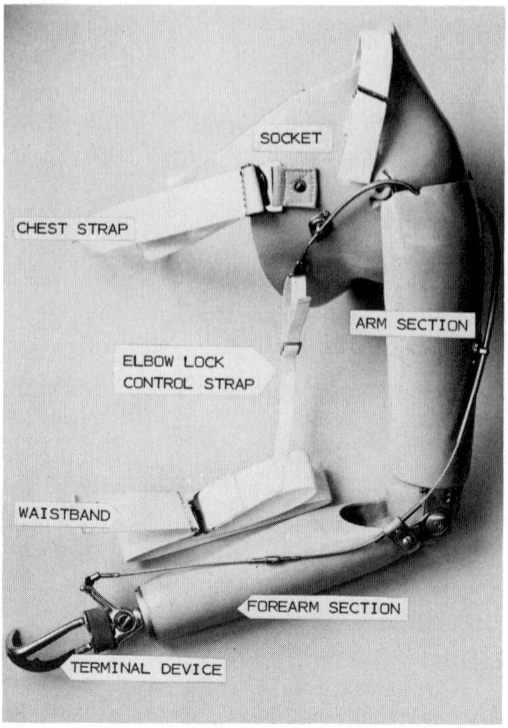

FIG. 7. Shoulder disarticulation prosthesis.

An alternative elbow lock control is the nudge control activated by the chin or sound extremity. A perineal control strap is another option for elbow positioning and terminal device operation.

Because of loss of body control motions necessary for functioning, the patient who has undergone forequarter scapulothoracic amputation is usually fitted with a cosmetic replacement that has a light shoulder cap and passive arm. Functional fitting is more feasible with external power, as will be discussed in the section on myoelectric control.

Terminal Devices

Terminal devices fall into two categories: hands and hooks. The hook is generally more functional than the hand, although the hand function provided by myoelectric control is an improvement. Final functional value is determined by the specific task or tasks to be performed as well as by the patient's desire to appear more normal. There has been a definite trend in the past 20 years among adult arm amputees toward preference for the hand over the hook, even if this results in somewhat less functional capacity. The desire of the amputee should certainly weigh heavily in the final prescription. Child amputees have also been requesting hand replacements more frequently.

Among the functional TDs, both hooks and hands can be either voluntary-closing or voluntary-opening. The voluntary-opening hook is most frequently provided because of its simplicity of operation. The Dorrance 5XA hook (Fig. 8) is the most popular. Made of aluminum, it has a neoprene finger lining to increase friction and a canted (toward body midline) finger shape, which allows better visual contact with objects being held or manipulated. The lyre finger shape, allowing a straight approach, is used more frequently if stabilization is necessary. These shapes are sometimes combined on a bilateral prosthesis using the lyre shape on the nondominant arm, where holding stability is needed.

The voluntary-closing TD has an alternating locking device that allows long-term grasp at any aperture without maintaining muscle tension. The voluntary-closing device is usually considered for the blind amputee because prehension can be predetermined and set. The bilateral amputee is sometimes fitted with a voluntary-closing TD on the dominant arm and a voluntary-opening TD on the nondominant arm.

Most arm amputees receive both hook and hand TDs. Figure 9 shows the Otto Bock hand, which is a voluntary-opening mechanism. In general, all glove materials continue to be easily damaged by stain and tearing.

Figure 10 shows a new TD, the Accru-Hook system. It has a positive locking feature that combines with adaptors attached to hand, power, recreational, and household tools to make the tools extensions of the hook. Finger opening and closing remains free while the tool is safely locked in the proximal end of the stable finger.

Two new units available are the HR (humeral rotator) unit (Fig. 11) for the elbow, which permits 220° of movement with nine positive locking positions, and the rotation wrist unit (Fig. 12),

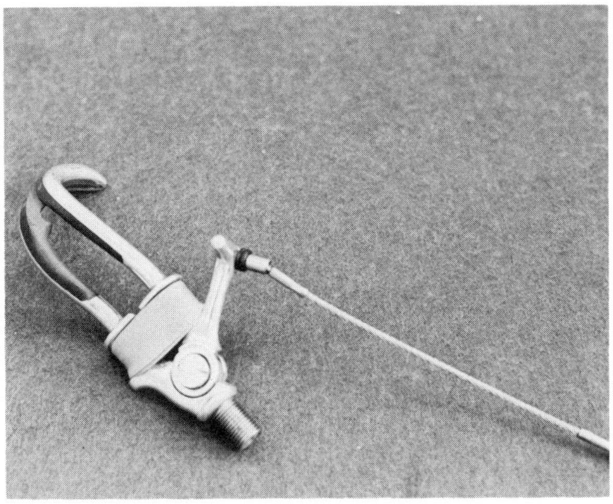

FIG. 8. Dorrance 5 A hook, canted finger shape.

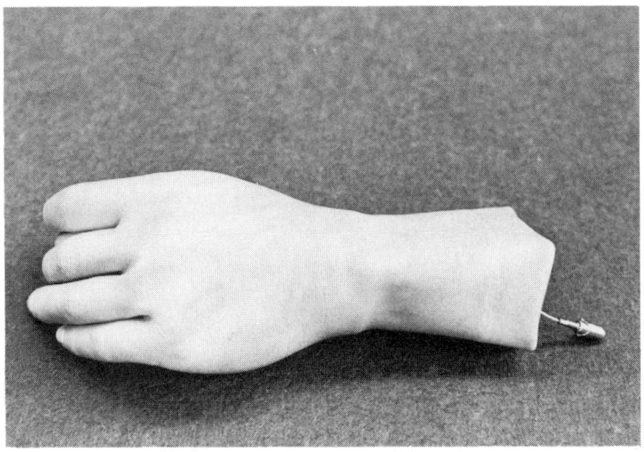

FIG. 9. Otto Bock hand.

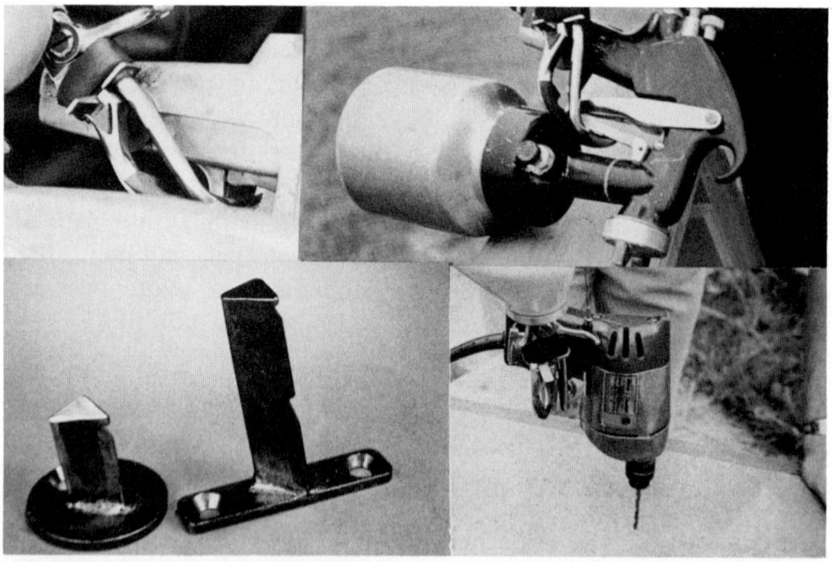

FIG. 10. The Accru-Hook system and universal adaptors. (Reproduced by permission of Pope Brace.)

which permits TD rotation without passive assistance. They are useful to the unilateral amputee, but they may be of greater functional value to the bilateral amputee.

PROSTHETIC TRAINING

Early fitting and proper training are crucial factors in the difference between the amputee who successfully uses the prosthesis and the amputee who leaves the prosthesis hanging on a hook in a closet. As stated previously, the overall aim of training is to provide maximum independence in all activities of daily living. Training involves the process of skills acquisition, from basic prosthesis control to working out solutions for special needs. Training also provides time to effectively evaluate prosthetic equipment, both mechanically and functionally, and make revisions if necessary.

Motivation for training is usually generated by a desire for independence, cosmetic replacement, vocational success, and participation in leisure pursuits. Training allows the therapist and the patient to clearly outline goals and monitor progress. The therapist's skill in directing and motivating during this period is also important. Four areas of training will be discussed: orientation and initial checkout, control training, skills training, and functional activities.

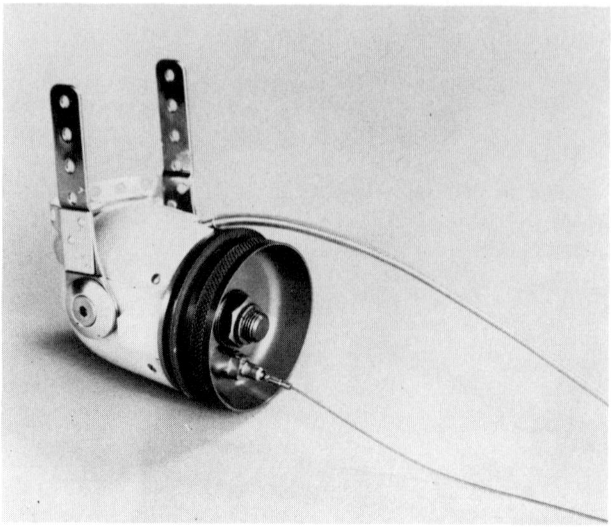

FIG. 11. Hr (humeral rotator) unit. (Reproduced by permission of Pope Brace.)

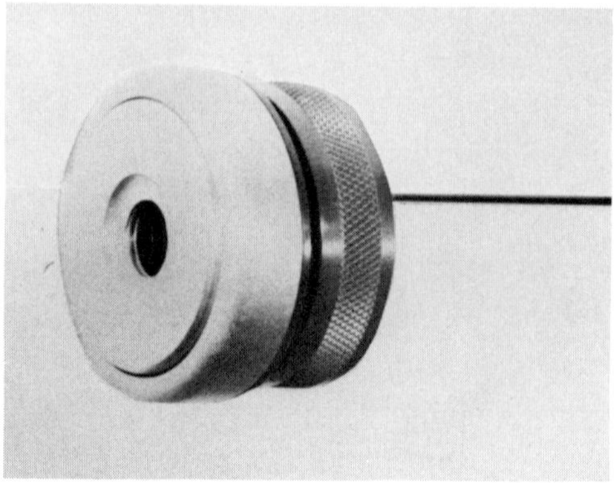

FIG. 12. Rotation wrist unit. (Reproduced by permission of Pope Brace.)

Orientation and Initial Checkout

The orientation should begin with a clear explanation of the entire training process. Goals must be established. Instruction should be given on equipment nomenclature, skin and stump hygiene as it relates to the prosthesis and harness system, and how to care for the prosthesis. Stump socks, tubular stockinette in cotton, nylon, or wool, are recommended to protect the skin from the socket and to absorb perspiration. Written instructions and labeled drawings of the patient's prosthetic equipment and harness must be provided.

The initial checkout is done to ensure maximum comfort and mechanical functioning of the prosthesis. This evaluation includes three areas: The fit evaluation includes harness system placement and socket comfort. The mechanical function evaluation covers range of motion, cable system operation, control system efficiency, and wrist unit and terminal device operation. The craftsmanship evaluation covers factors that will reflect the kinds and amounts of stress the amputee will put on the equipment over a period of time that will reduce long-term durability. Any changes that will increase mechanical efficiency or comfort should be completed before the training begins. A sound working relationship between the occupational therapist and the prosthetist facilitates exchange of information about the function of the prosthesis and assures revisions when necessary. Informal checkout proceeds throughout the training. Appendix 2 shows the current NYU/IRM initial checkout form for BE prostheses.

Control Training

Control training involves teaching (a) the methods of donning and doffing the prosthesis and (b) the control motions required for operating the prosthetic equipment.

The BE prothesis is donned either by the coat method (where the stump is inserted into the socket first, and the sound arm reaches around through the axilla loop, as in putting on a coat) or by the over-the-head method (where the sound arm is placed through the axilla loop, the stump is inserted under the Y strap, and both arms are lifted over the head, allowing the ring-cross to drop behind). The BE prothesis has a single-cable control system. One body control motion, humeral flexion of the amputated side, produces TD opening (voluntary-opening TD).

The AE prosthesis is donned in a similar manner, either the coat method or the over-the-head method. In the over-the-head method, the elbow is locked at 90°, and the forearm section is held by the sound arm, which has first been inserted through the axilla loop. The AE control is a dual control. One body control motion, humeral flexion and/or scapular abduction, produces forearm flexion with the elbow unlocked and TD opening with the elbow locked.

The shoulder disarticulation prosthesis is usually donned with the prothesis stabilized against or on a surface while the sound arm is used to attach the chest strap harness. The control system is dual. The elbow lock and unlock control is attached either to a waist belt or to a perineal belt controlled by scapular elevation or a manual or chin nudge control. Biscapular abduction produces forearm flexion with the elbow unlocked and TD opening with the elbow locked.

The conventional forequarter prosthesis is so deficient as a functional prosthesis that it is generally given only as a cosmetic replacement. Functional replacements are best managed prosthetically through the use of external power. If nothing is available in the way of external control, the conventional prosthesis is fitted with the nudge controls and perineal straps described previously.

The more complicated the control motions, the more time needed for this training. Training of control motions begins in the standing position and progresses to sitting. Special emphasis is placed on having the patient learn the various kinds of sensory information received from the socket and harness in relation to the position of the prosthesis. Auditory cues are helpful for the AE amputee in the elbow locking and unlocking sequencing. Visual cues are discouraged, as they tend to make the user dependent on them and tend to slow the process of moving into functional activity.

To begin skills training, basic reliable and consistent operation and prepositioning of the terminal device, forearm, and elbow are necessary. Exaggerated body motions and energy expenditure should be minimal, although much refinement can be accomplished in skills training.

Skills Training

Skills training shifts the focus of activity from learning the basic controls to learning how they are used by introducing the principles of prepositioning, operation of the prosthesis in space, and object stability, both static and dynamic. Proper prepositioning of the prosthesis and the ability to stabilize the prosthesis are the keys to ultimate skillful prosthetic use. The overall goal is to have the amputee use the equipment in as normal a manner as possible (14).

In order not to attach too much initial significance to how well the patient performs a functional task, the use of graded training devices separates skills practice from the actual attempt to perform functional activities. These devices are helpful for all levels of amputees learning skills, but they are especially useful for working with amputees who have dual control systems.

For proper prepositioning and approach, two goals must be met: (a) correct TD positioning and (b) stabilization of the stump in the socket. Figure 13 shows a simple basic exercise with a ruler that allows the therapist to vary the position and angle of the object, allowing the amputee to practice predicting the correct prepositioning of the TD. Socket stability exercises are incorporated by adding resistance at the grasp phase, particularly where the socket would have a tendency to rotate during functional skills (e.g., on external rotation with the AE prosthesis). Figure 14 shows a multiobject training box for practicing the principles of optimum grasp and release. Aspects that can be covered relate to (a) judicious use of cable, (b) proper aperture for grasp, (c) maximum object stability, (d) proper finger position, and (e) consistent cable tension.

Further training begins to increase in complexity and emphasize bilateral tasks using the prosthesis as an effective assist. The therapist's judgment must control the kind and amount of these drills based on the needs of the patient. There are some guidelines (15) that can be used to determine when work toward specific functional skills can begin: (a) How skillfully are the principles of operation applied? (b) How near normal are the motions? (c) Is the energy being expended commensurate with the complexity of the task? (d) How much time is required to complete the task? There are no rigid guidelines. Usually, some functional tasks can be started soon after basic skills are learned. The therapist can shift back and forth to help the amputee see progress and help establish new goals.

Functional Activities

Obviously, the unilateral amputee will be able to do most things with the sound arm. Just how useful the prosthesis will be depends on the instruction and encouragement the amputee receives, as well as on the motivation and ingenuity applied to its use beyond basic training. All ADL should be discussed, with specific emphasis on the needs and concerns related to the patient's specific life-style and vocation. The following list should be reviewed:

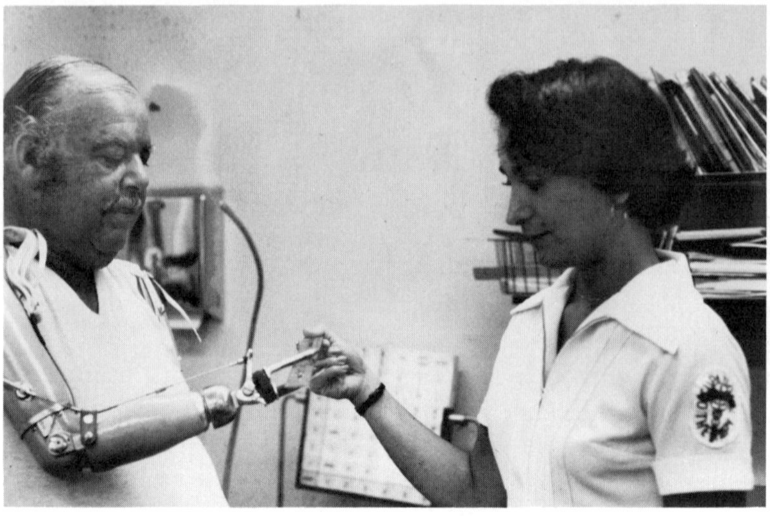

FIG. 13. Early exercise used in practicing TD prepositioning.

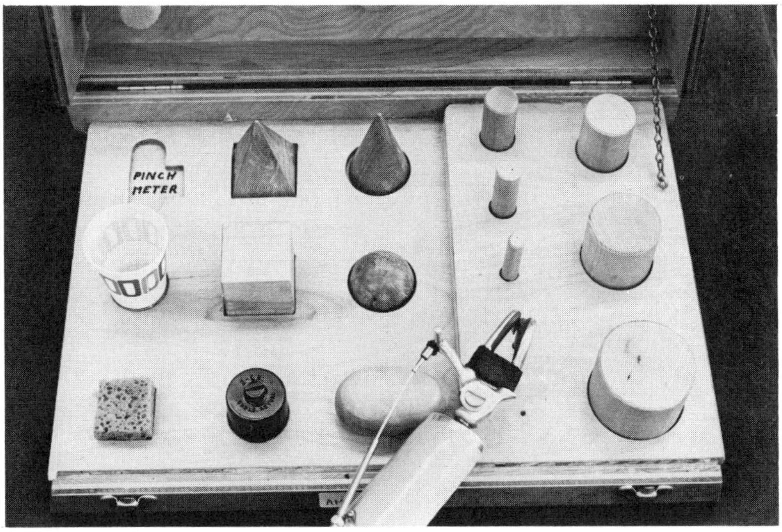

FIG. 14. Multiobject training box used for practice in approach, grasp, and release of the TD.

1. Self-care: Eating, grooming, dressing, personal hygiene.
2. Communicating skills: Writing, telephone use, general office tasks.
3. Homemaking: Housekeeping, cooking, cleaning, washing, ironing, child or baby care.
4. Social and avocational skills: Areas of concern involve device cosmesis, former avocational interests, and knowledge of commercially available recreational devices. Figures 15 and 16 show two of these devices for bowling and baseball.
5. Prevocational and vocational skills exploration: Evaluation relates to previous work and exploration of new vocational possibilities. The vocational counseling and psychosocial services have specific input here. Their expertise is necessary throughout the entire team process (16). If necessary, follow-up and on-the-job evaluation can be useful here. Three general courses of action are possible: (a) return to the previous job in the same or a related capacity, (b) receive new on-the-job training, (c) receive new vocational education and placement.
6. Mobility: Public and private transportation aspects are covered. Figures 17 and 18 show two driving devices.

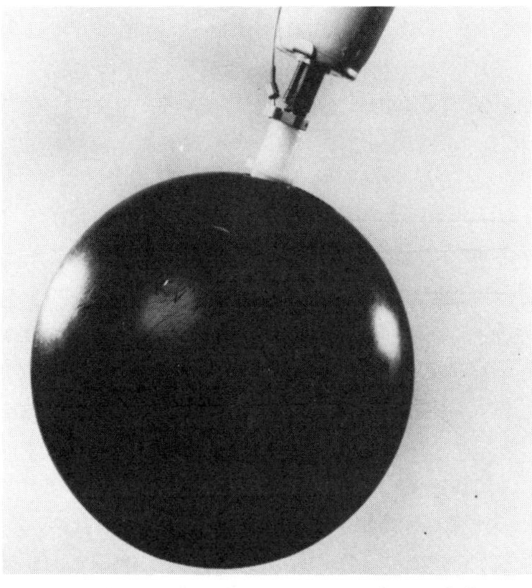

FIG. 15. Bowling device. (Reproduced by permission of the Hosmer Dorrance Corp.)

A checklist including the tasks in the previous list can be useful to help ensure complete coverage of all ADL, both general and unique. The final checkout reexamines mechanical functioning and evaluates use effectiveness. A summary of final function, special devices, and follow-up recommendations should also be included.

BILATERAL ARM AMPUTEES

Prosthetic fitting and training for the bilateral arm amputee require special consideration. Since the bilateral amputee is more dependent on the prosthetic equipment, the following general matters should be considered:

1. The harnessing and socket construction should allow ease and independence in donning and doffing.

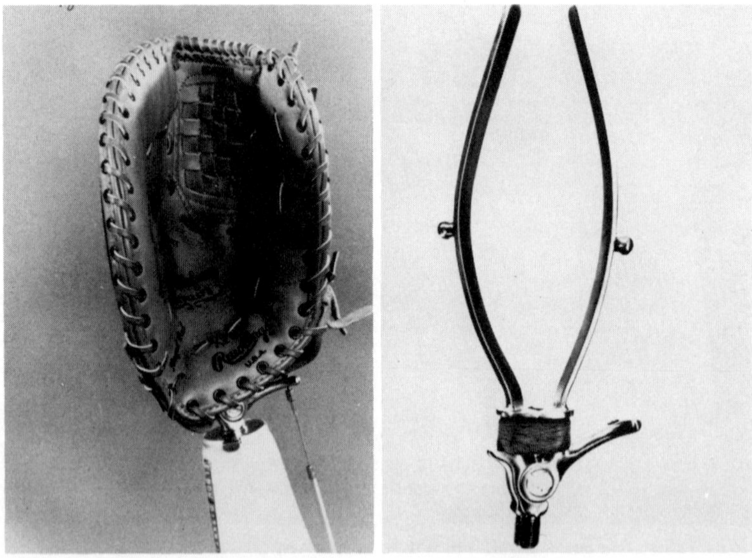

FIG. 16. Baseball glove device. (Reproduced by permission of the Hosmer Dorrance Corp.)

2. Maximum reliability and safety must be incorporated into the design. Choice of materials and construction of the prosthesis are important, since overall wear and tear is significant.
3. Components, socket design, and alignment must allow for maximum range of motion. Almost all bilateral amputees need wrist flexion units to reach close to the body for ADL such as personal hygiene and eating. Figure 19 shows a wrist flexion unit used for a dressing task.
4. When providing terminal devices, general and specific functional use must be taken into consideration, e.g., heavy-duty or recreational devices. Cosmetic hands are generally discouraged because of their limited functional value.

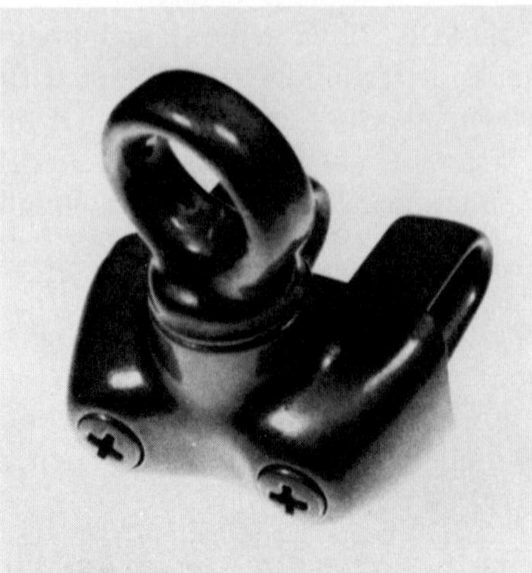

FIG. 17. Driving device. (Reproduced by permission of the Hosmer Dorrance Corp.)

5. Fit and comfort must be maximized for long-term wear.
6. Loss of sensory feedback must be considered, although little can be done to compensate. In some instances construction of the prosthesis can allow for an open-ended socket exposing the distal end of the stump (Fig. 20). More realistic compensation is achieved by learning the kinds of sensory feedback obtained from the socket and harness in relation to the various positions of the prosthesis in space (17).

After adequate prosthetic equipment has been provided, the degree of independence achieved by the bilateral amputee will depend on (a) motivation, (b) the residual lengths of the arms, (c) age, (d) body build, (e) ability to use the feet to some extent, (f) kind and degree of other medical problems, and (g) training.

The advantages of immediate or early fitting are obvious for the bilateral amputee. It can reduce dependence and the feeling of frustration. Even unilateral fitting with a temporary prosthesis can provide some independence for such self-care activities as toileting, personal hygiene, and eating.

The occupational therapist involved in training the bilateral amputee should be familiar with unilateral training. The process followed is essentially the same, with more emphasis on some or all of the following areas: (a) general body condi-

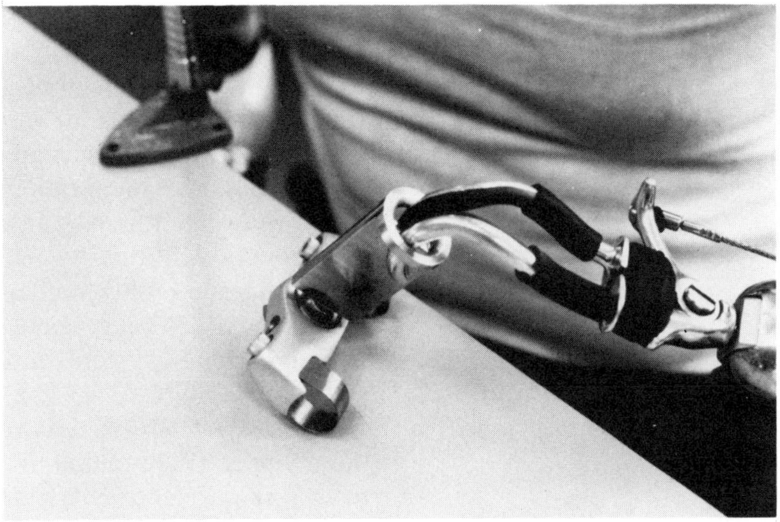

FIG. 18. Driving device. (Designed by Jiri Sipajlo, NYU/IRM Driver Education Program, Physical Therapy Department, and reproduced with his permission.)

tioning and endurance, (b) development of joint hypermobility and range of motion, (c) development of good body mechanics and posture, (d) use of residual arms and use of the feet, and (e) use of prefabricated or specialized assistive or adaptive devices.

EXTERNALLY ENERGIZED PROSTHESES: MYOELECTRIC CONTROL SYSTEMS

The development of external power and control mechanisms for operating artificial arms, hands, and hooks has markedly changed the options available to the amputee. The future of prosthetics management may well lie in externally powered prostheses, whether they are myoelectrically (EMG) controlled, switch-controlled, or computerized pattern recognition systems. The occupational therapist will be increasingly responsible for understanding the complexities of these new systems and for training patients effectively in their use so as to provide optimal functioning in all aspects of daily living.

Before dealing with the specifics of the evaluation and training process, it is essential to acquire a basic understanding of the mechanics of externally powered prostheses. Presently, the greatest benefit from these devices is gained by the unilateral BE amputee. The literature describes successful research into myoelectric control of mo-

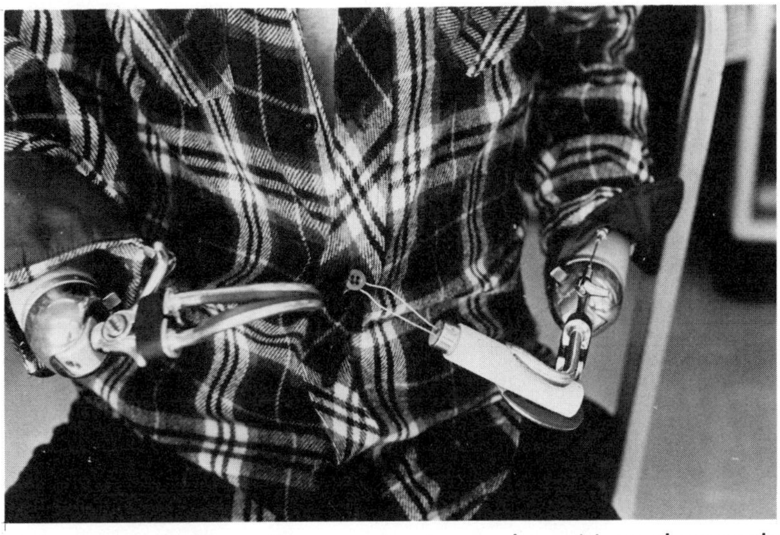

FIG. 19. The wrist flexion unit allows the amputee to reach positions close to the body for ADL.

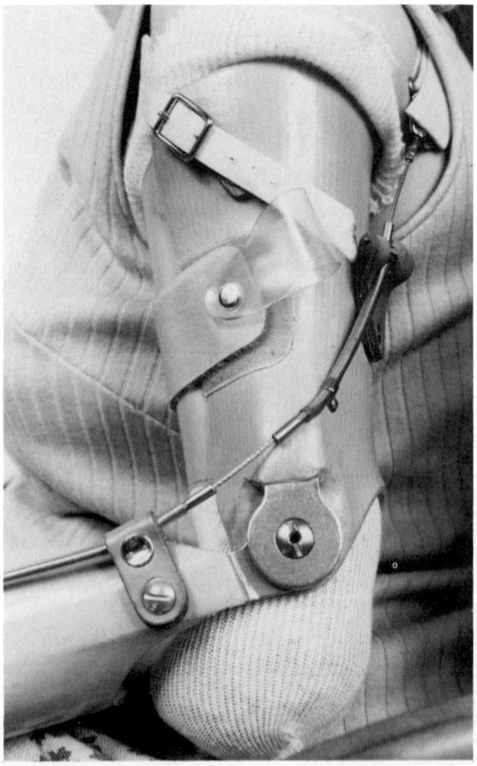

FIG. 20. Open-ended socket exposing the stump distal end. (Reproduced by permission from a slide provided by the NYU/IRM Orthotics and Prosthetics Department.)

tion in three areas (hand, wrist, and elbow) (18–20) using both hook and hand terminal devices. It is believed that the greatest functional advantages and the greatest patient acceptance are found among unilateral BE amputees. For a prosthesis replacing more movements, myoelectric or switch control of powered elbow units needs further refinement to provide maximal function. For example, the lifting force of the presently available electric elbows is limited to only 3 pounds at the terminal device. For this and other reasons, the AE amputee is customarily treated conventionally. The bilateral amputee needs the fine prehension ability, better visibility of manipulated objects, and durability offered by a conventional system with hook terminal devices.

The myoelectrically controlled prosthesis uses the myoelectric potential of a contracting muscle to trigger an electrically powered hand terminal device. Myoelectric electrode sites are determined by use of a myometer, as shown in Fig. 21, to measure surface EMG potentials of intact muscle bellies on the residual arm distal to the last intact joint. It is fundamental that the control mechanism of the prosthesis be located on the same side as the amputation and does not involve muscle groups that will be required during normal use and positioning of the arm.

The myometer is used to determine the point of maximal muscle contraction, i.e., the greatest EMG output reading. Two sites are preferred, responding to the two motions supplied by the hand terminal device: opening and closing of the index and middle fingers, with the thumb moving simultaneously to provide a three-jaw chuck. Commonly, the residual wrist/finger extensors on

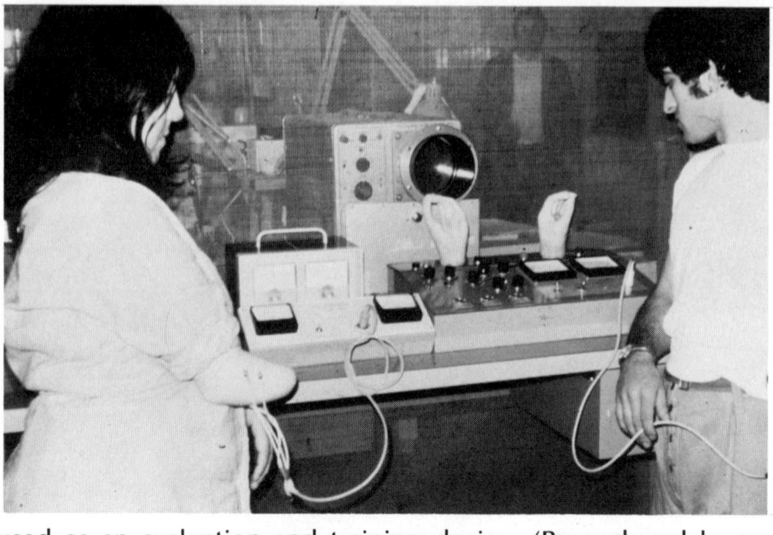

FIG. 21. Myometer, used as an evaluation and training device. (Reproduced by permission from a slide provided by the NYU/IRM Orthotics and Prosthetics Department.)

the forearm (stump) are used to trigger opening, and the wrist/finger flexors are used to operate closure and to achieve grasp. To operate the hand successfully, the patient must be able to execute isolated contractions producing a minimum of 50 μV with no interference of the opposing muscle group. With greater EMG output (e.g., 125 μV), a proportionately larger amount of interference can be accepted. If one site is unavailable because of nerve injury, insufficient muscle bulk, or more commonly the abnormalities found with congenital absence of the arm, a tri-state control system is available that uses only one electrode site. The patient must be able to produce and distinguish between slight contractions (e.g., 50–100 μV to open the hand at a proportional rate) and stronger contraction (e.g., 100 μV or more to reverse the motor for closure).

After determination of the EMG sites, a double-wall Muenster-type socket is constructed with the surface electrodes and a ground electrode permanently placed in the predetermined position within the socket (Fig. 22). As the amputee contracts the proper muscle group, the myoelectric potential is picked up by the electrodes and initially amplified 25 to 40,000 times by an integrated-circuit differential amplifier. An amplifier circuit further increases the signal to the level of 12 V. Regulation of the myoelectric output is achieved by use of a potentiometer. When the strength of the myoelectric signal reaches a predetermined level (controlled by the potentiometer), an electronic switch closes, allowing electricity to flow from the 12-V battery to the electric motor in the Otto Bock hand terminal device (21,22). When two separate muscles are used to open and close, the hand operates at a set speed with digital control. With the tri-state control, forward speed is proportional to the strength of muscle contraction. Usually, all electronics are contained within the prosthesis (Fig. 23).

The prosthesis battery must be charged daily. The battery charger, which is the size of a cigarette pack, is plugged into the prosthesis and into a standard 125-V or 220-V electrical outlet, and charging occurs overnight. A full charge lasts approximately 12 hr with normal use.

There is a passive constant-friction wrist unit. A cosmetic glove covers the hand and wrist to midforearm.

This is a simplistic explanation of the mechanical functioning of only one system. Myoelectric control is also being explored for use by the unilateral forequarter amputee. The hand terminal device is myoelectrically controlled using any residual muscle potential on the amputation site, e.g., upper or middle trapezius, platysma, rhomboids, erector spinae, etc. (Fig. 24). All motions of the shoulder, elbow, and wrist are produced passively. To reduce the total weight of the forequarter prosthesis, an endoskeletal design is provided, rather than the heavier plastic laminate. An aluminum tube is used for the forearm and humeral sections. The socket needs to be

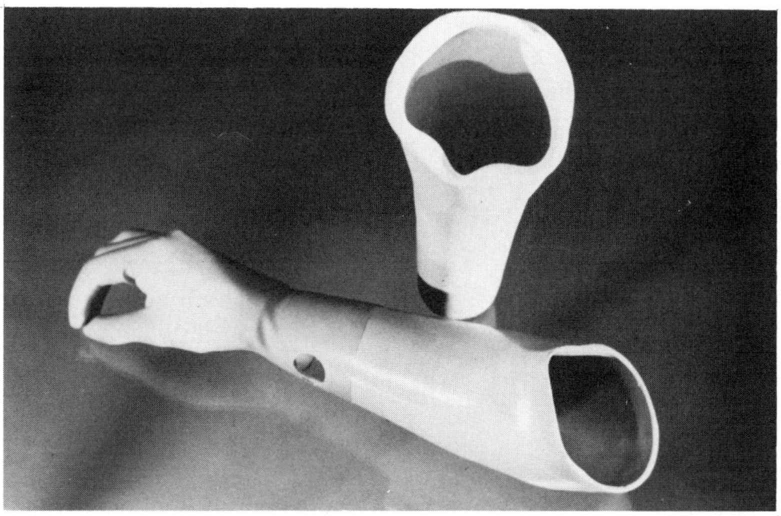

FIG. 22. Myoelectric Muenster prosthesis. (Reproduced by permission from a slide provided by the NYU/IRM Orthotics and Prosthetics Department.)

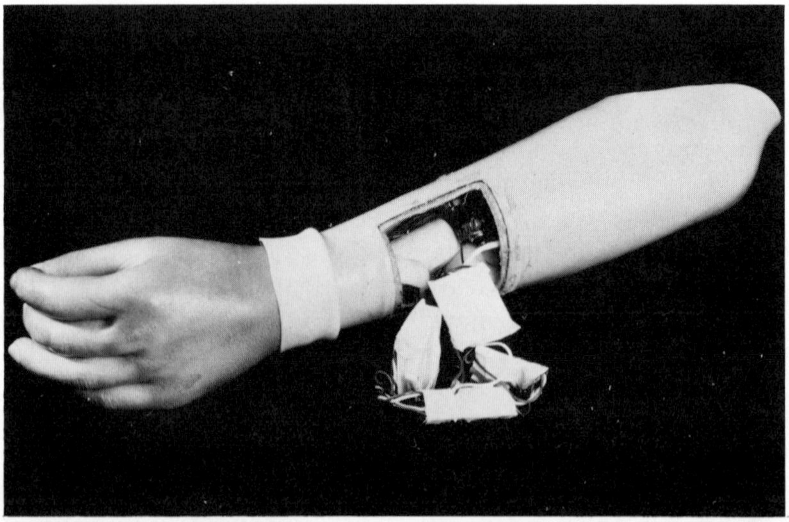

FIG. 23. Placement of electronics in prosthesis. (Reproduced by permission from a slide provided by the NYU/IRM Orthotics and Prosthetics Department.)

rigid for secure placement of electrodes; so this part is constructed of molded plastic laminate. The passive friction shoulder joint, manual locking elbow, and arm sections are then covered with foam, contoured to match as close as possible the sound arm. A flesh-tone sleeve then encases the arm. Despite obvious limitations, most patients thus far fitted and trained have responded positively to the added functional abilities provided by the prosthesis, especially the grasp and release of the electric hand (Fig. 25).

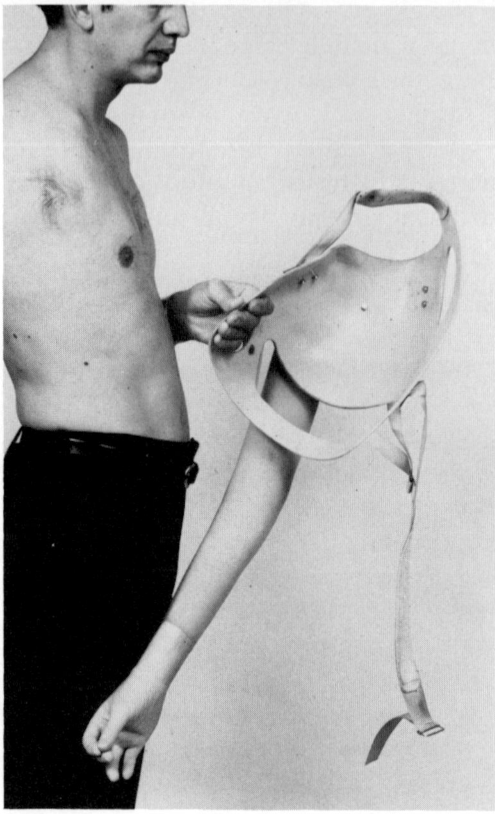

FIG. 24. Myoelectric forequarter prosthesis. Note electrode placement. (Reproduced by permission from a slide provided by the NYU/IRM Orthotics and Prosthetics Department.)

Team Considerations

The prosthetic team must weigh all factors in the attempt to fulfill the patient's specific needs and desires. Because of increasing sophistication in prosthetic technology, even greater attention must be paid to the multiplicity of factors that may contribute to success or failure in prosthetics use (23). There are numerous advantages, disadvantages, and special considerations to be discussed before opting for a myoelectric prosthesis. Most will be directed to BE amputation, but they can also pertain to amputation at any other level.

The cost and weight of the myoelectric prosthesis appear to be its most serious drawbacks. The approximate weight of a BE conventional prosthesis with hook terminal device ranges from 1 to 1.5 pounds, whereas a myoelectric device weighs 2 pounds. With a short or very short BE stump, this difference becomes a significant factor in patient acceptance or rejection. A long stump or wrist disarticulation may necessitate placement of the electronics or battery outside the socket (e.g., on a belt or in a pocket). Other occasional problem factors are excessive noise,

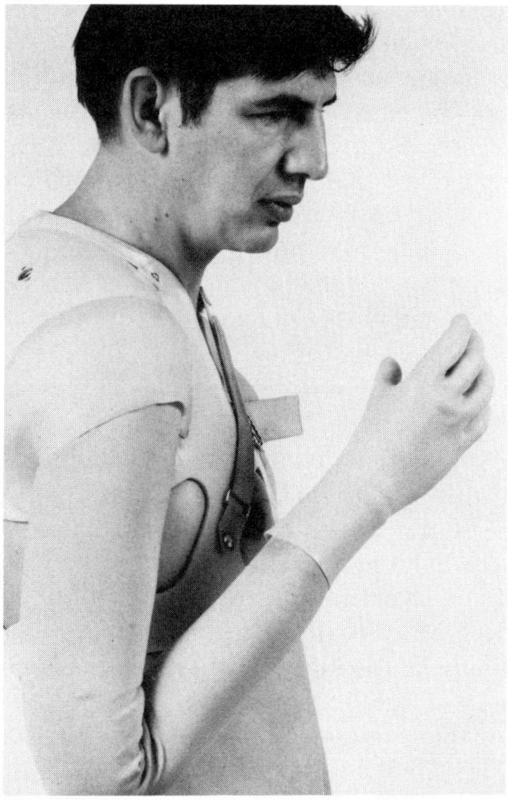

FIG. 25. Endoskeletal design of myoelectric forequarter prosthesis. (Reproduced by permission from a slide provided by the NYU/IRM Orthotics and Prosthetics Department.)

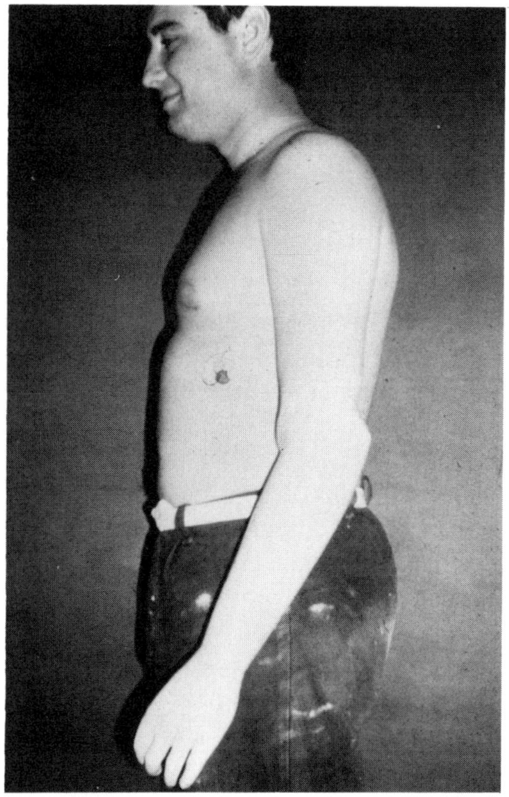

FIG. 26. Myoelectric BE prosthesis illustrating improved cosmesis. (Reproduced by permission from a slide provided by the NYU/IRM Orthotics and Prosthetics Department.)

slow response, involuntary operation, interference (inadvertent operation), frequent repairs and servicing, obtaining adequate control sites, decreased sensory feedback, muscle fatigue, and restricted elbow movement because of the Muenster socket design when used by the BE amputee (24).

However, the advantages can (and in most cases do) outweigh the disadvantages. Of primary importance to most patients is elimination of the harness, allowing more freedom of movement and operation of the terminal device in positions behind the back or over the head (Fig. 26). Also, there is greater physical ease of operation, improved cosmesis, control that is psychologically more "natural," decreased compressive force at the end of the stump, and ease of learning myoelectric control. Especially significant is the available prehension strength of the myoelectric prosthesis (up to 22 pounds, versus 3–5 pounds for a conventional prosthesis). Maximal opening of the myoelectric hand is 10 cm; that of a conventional prosthetic hand is 6 cm, a range inadequate to close on and stabilize a can of soda. The cosmetic glove is the same for either type of prosthesis.

Phantom Sensation

If amputation occurs after a patient is 8 years of age (sometimes even younger), there is usually the phenomenon of phantom sensation, as if stimuli were still being received from the amputated limb. Those parts (e.g., the hand) with the greatest sensory representation in the cerebral cortex are the phantom sources of the strongest sensations (25). Phantom sensation usually diminishes, in a telescoping fashion, as time elapses following amputation.

During the preprosthetic evaluation, the amputee should be asked to describe the phantom limb in terms of position and movability of the parts. A patient who can perceive and "move" a phantom wrist, for example, may be able to learn the control muscle contractions for the myoelectric prosthesis more easily. A small percentage of patients may report painful phantoms with burning, cramping, or shooting pain that may require medical intervention. Bilateral exercise of the phantom limb and the sound limb, massage, and desensitization techniques may also relieve the phantom pain.

Evaluation

Occupational therapy preprosthetic considerations are essentially the same for a myoelectric prosthesis as for a conventional prosthesis, with a particularly thorough examination of ADL status being required. A job that demands fine bilateral skill or one that involves an environment with a lot of electronic equipment (sources of interference) may require a conventional approach. In some cases a patient may obtain both types of prostheses, depending on specific vocational or avocational needs. It is also vital that the patient's expectations regarding any externally energized prosthesis be realistic. In contrast with a conventional prosthesis, a myoelectric prosthesis may be regarded as a "bionic" replacement of the lost hand, and this belief may later cause rejection.

Initial Checkout

The therapist must first check to see if the myoelectric prosthesis has been adequately charged and which electrodes have been chosen for which actions. This is accomplished by running the fingertips lightly over both sets of electrodes; static electricity will trigger opening or closing. The patient then dons the prosthesis in a manner similar to that for a regular Muenster socket, except that the stockinette is moistened with water to provide a good conduction medium. The stockinette is removed; perspiration later replaces the water. The patient is then requested to fully open and close the hand at various positions of the arm.

Training

Skills and functional training techniques and modalities are the same as for conventional prosthetic devices. If the patient is unable to operate the hand in a specific position, the cause is usually inadvertent contraction of the opposing muscle, which causes interference. Another cause may be too high a gain setting of the potentiometer of the opposing muscle or insufficient gain of the contracting muscle site. The lowest possible potential setting necessitates a stronger muscular contraction and is preferable, for it reduces the chance of inadvertent operation of the terminal device, caused either by the patient during an activity or by an external source (e.g., strong radio waves, certain machinery).

Control training is specifically geared toward having the patient learn controlled closure and timing of release. By using a pinch meter, the

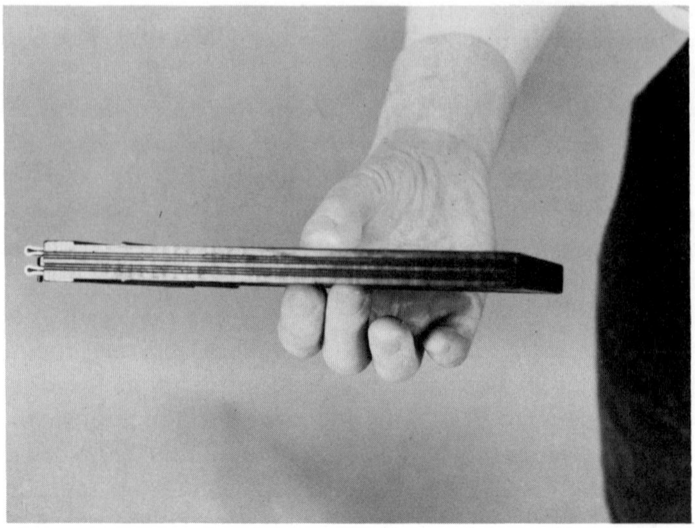

FIG. 27. Otto Bock electric hand. (Reproduced by permission from a slide provided by the NYU/IRM Orthotics and Prosthetics Department.)

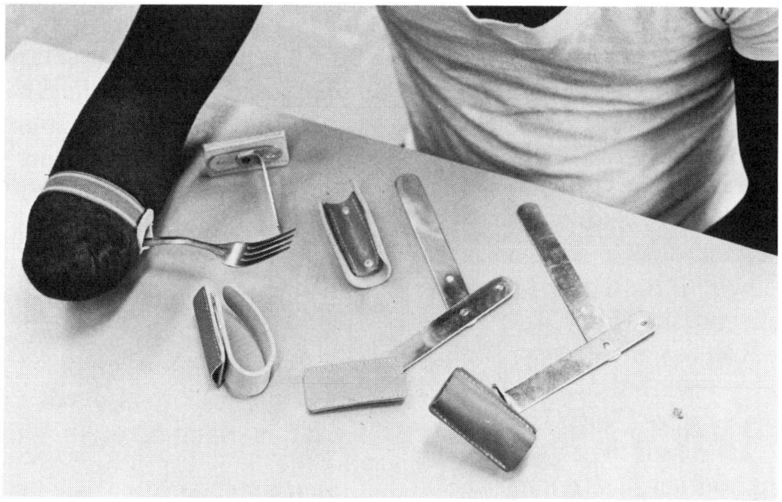

FIG. 28. Universal component system.

patient can learn to approximate and sensorially appreciate the difference between a "light" or "quick" contraction producing less force than a "strong" or "prolonged" closing contraction utilizing total prehension force. Thus the patient can control grasp on a heavy block or a paper cup (Fig. 27). Visual and auditory cues are important for learning good control. A feedback system is available that consists of a small motor set in the socket that vibrates proportionately to the force of the grasp applied to an object. This can provide the patient with a sensation of "gripping harder" on an object.

Training proceeds to skilled and functional activities, unilateral to bilateral, one-handed training, and use of adaptive equipment. Barring any mechanical or fitting complications, occupational therapy training of the BE amputee with a myoelectric prosthesis should take 8 to 10 hr. For the patient with a prosthesis replacing more joints and actions, all training takes significantly longer.

SPECIAL DEVICES

The provision of specialized devices falls into two categories: (a) specialized selection of commercially available or prefabricated equipment; (b) construction of special devices to meet special needs.

The matching of appropriate equipment to specialized needs is increasingly less dependent on

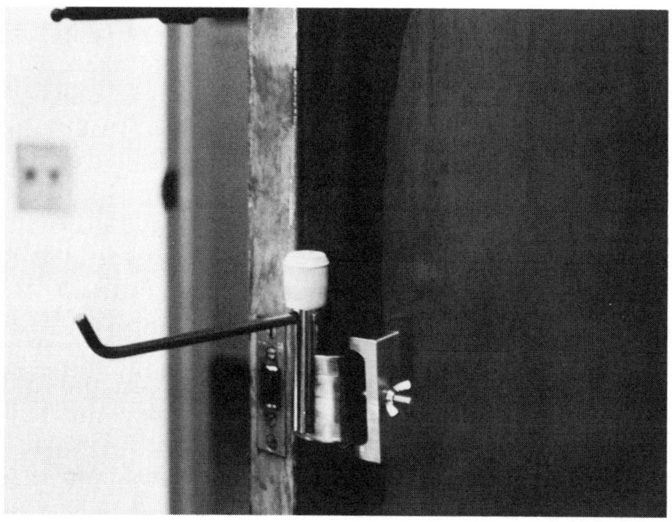

FIG. 29. Multipurpose door clamp with interchangeable sections for a buttonhook, chest-strap hooking aid, and aid for T-shirt removal.

the old trial-and-error methods for several reasons. Methods of evaluation are more sophisticated (e.g., use of the functional motion test to delineate individual function). There is increasing availability of commercial technical aids that meet specific needs (e.g., aids that increase stabilization, allow one-handed use, or substitute for lost function). There have also been many advances in the development of these aids and in the materials used in their construction (24).

The role of the therapist is fourfold in providing these devices:

1. To determine by evaluation the patient's limitation and what activities will require assistance or substitution.
2. To provide commercially available technical aids (Fig. 28 shows a universal component system) that can be used to substitute for hand function before the prosthesis is ready or as an alternative means of independence (25).
3. To design, construct, and fit special devices for special needs (Fig. 29 shows a clamp attached to a door with interchangeable units used to assist with shirt buttoning, undressing skills, and donning of the prosthesis).
4. To train the patient in the use of these devices, incorporating the principles of energy conservation and work simplification in environmental organization and specific task setup. A general guideline for selecting any equipment is to provide maximum independence with the least number of devices, least amount of time, least number of steps, and least energy expenditure.

More recently, electronic technology has added another dimension by providing devices for the severely disabled: environmental control systems (ECS). With the ECS it becomes possible to operate any piece of electrical equipment (e.g., a door lock, telephone, light, etc.) in a living or work area by using sensitive microswitches, pneumatic switches, and voice-activated or other wireless controls. Of particular importance is the possibility of independence for the patient who has undergone high-level bilateral amputation who is not a candidate for a prosthesis or who gains only limited independence with a prosthesis (26).

SUMMARY

Activities are an essential part of man's being. In using activities therapeutically, the occupational therapist is able to help patients respond to the demands of their environment, both physically and psychologically. We have tried to present some of the many situations in which occupational therapy has something valuable to contribute to the evaluation, treatment, and training of the adult arm amputee. We have also attempted to emphasize the importance of the clinic team in meeting individual needs and helping the patient reach maximum potential as a total human being.

REFERENCES

1. New York University, Post-Graduate Medical School, Prosthetics and Orthotics (1971): Upper-extremity prosthetics. p. 13.
2. Sarno, J. E. (1979): Amputee clinic or clinic team? *Prosthetics and Orthotics Clinic Newsletter,* 3:2.
3. Lehneis, H. R., and Dickey, R. (1980): The bilateral upper limb amputee. In: *Atlas on Limb Prosthetics; Surgical and Prosthetic Principles,* edited by N. C. McCullough III. C. V. Mosby, St. Louis.
4. Gullickson, G., Jr. (1961): Exercise for amputees. In: *Therapeutic Exercise,* edited by S. Licht, p. 626. S. Licht, New Haven.
5. Gullickson, G., Jr. (1961): Exercise for amputees. In: *Therapeutic Exercise,* edited by S. Licht, p. 637. S. Licht, New Haven.
6. Friedman, L. W. (1968): Rehabilitation of amputees. In: *Rehabilitation and Medicine,* edited by S. Licht, p. 303. S. Licht, New Haven.
7. Bender, L. F. (1974): *Prostheses and Rehabilitation after Arm Amputation.* Charles C Thomas, Springfield, Ill., p. 12.
8. University of California (Los Angeles) School of Medicine (1958): *Manual of Upper Extremity Prosthetics,* edited by W. R. Santschi and M. P. Winston, p. 19. UCLA, Los Angeles.
9. Bender, L. F. (1974): *Prostheses and Rehabilitation after Arm Amputation.* Charles C Thomas, Springfield, Ill., p. 12.
10. Wilson, A. B., Jr. (1976): *Limb Prosthetics.* Robert E. Krieger Publishing, Huntington, N.Y., p. 25.
11. Sarmiento, A., McCullough, N. C., III, Williams, E. M., and Sinclair, W. F. (1968): Immediate postsurgical prosthesis fitting in the management of upper extremity amputees. *Artificial Limbs,* 12:14.

12. Reyburn, T. V. (1971): A method of early prosthetics training for upper-extremity amputees. *Artificial Limbs,* 15:1.
13. Loughlin, E., Stanford, J. W., and Phelps, M. (1968): Immediate postsurgical prosthesis fitting of a bilateral below-elbow amputee. A report. *Artificial Limbs,* 12:17.
14. New York University, Post-Graduate Medical School, Prosthetics and Orthotics (1971): Upper-extremity prosthetics. p. 133.
15. New York University, Post-Graduate Medical School, Prosthetics and Orthotics (1971): Upper-extremity prosthetics. p. 121.
16. Sarno, J. E. (1979): Amputee clinic or clinic team? *Prosthetics and Orthotics Clinic Newsletter,* 3:2.
17. Lehneis, H. R., and Dickey, R. (1980): The bilateral upper limb amputee. In: *Atlas on Limb Prosthetics; Surgical and Prosthetic Principles,* edited by N. C. McCullough III, AAOS. C. V. Mosby, St. Louis.
18. Schmidl, H. (1977): The I.N.A.I.L. experience fitting upper-limb dysmelia patients with myoelectric control. *Bull. Prosthet. Res.,* 10:17–42.
19. Schmeisser, G., Seamone, W., and Moshall, C. H. (1972): Early clinical experience with the Johns Hopkins externally powered modular system for upper-limb prostheses. *Orthotics and Prosthetics,* 26:41–52.
20. Dankmeyer, C. H., Sr., Dankmeyer, C. H., Jr., and Massey, M. D. (1972): An externally powered modular system for upper limb prostheses. *Orthotics and Prosthetics,* 26:36–40.
21. Schmidl, H. (1973): The I.N.A.I.L. CECA prosthesis. *Orthotics and Prosthetics,* 27:6–12.
22. Bender, L. F. (1974): *Prostheses and Rehabilitation after Arm Amputation.* Charles C Thomas, Springfield, Ill., pp. 67–69, 74–76, 130–135.
23. Sarno, J. E. (1979): Amputee clinic or clinic team? *Prosthetics and Orthotics Clinic Newsletter,* 3:2.
24. Zimmerman, M. E. (1957): Analysis of adapted equipment. *Am. J. Occup. Ther.,* 11:4.
25. Zimmerman, M. E. (1977): The role of special equipment in the rehabilitation of the spinal cord injured. In: *Physical Medicine and Rehabilitation Approaches in Spinal Cord Injury,* edited by J. G. Cull and R. E. Hardy, p. 225. Charles C Thomas, Springfield, Ill.
26. NYU (1979): Environmental control systems and vocational aids for high level quadriplegics (rehab monograph #55). Institute of Rehabilitation Medicine, New York University Medical Center.

BIBLIOGRAPHY

Bailey, R. B. (1970): An upper extremity prosthetic training arm. *Am. J. Occup. Ther.,* 24:5.

Friedman, L. W. (1978): *The Surgical Rehabilitation of the Amputee.* Charles C Thomas, Springfield, Ill.

Friedman, L. W. (1978): *The Psychological Rehabilitation of the Amputee.* Charles C Thomas, Springfield, Ill.

Leavy, J. D. (1980): It can be done: An upper extremity amputee training handbook. Cascade Orthopedic Supply, Westwood, Calif.

Omer, G. E., Jr. (1978): Amputation. In: *Rehabilitation of the Hand,* edited by J. M. Hunter, L. H. Schneider, E. J. Mackin, and J. A. Bell, pp. 541–573. C. V. Mosby, St. Louis.

Prior, R. E., Lyman, J., Case, P., and Scott, C. M. (1976): Supplemental sensory feedback for the VA/NU myoelectric hand. Background and preliminary designs. *Bull. Prosthet. Res.,* 26:170–191.

Spencer, E. A. (1978): Amputations. In: *Occupational Therapy,* ed. 5, edited by H. S. Willard and C. S. Spackman, pp. 593–608. J. B. Lippincott, Philadelphia.

Wellerson, T. L. (1958): *A Manual for Occupational Therapists on the Rehabilitation of Upper Extremity Amputees.* Kendall/Hunt Publishing, Dubuque, Ill.

Wirta, R. W., Taylor, P. R., and Finley, F. R. (1978): Pattern-recognition arm prostheses: A historical perspective—a final report. *Bull. Prosthet. Res.,* 30:8–35.

Wright, S. (1978): Prosthetics, the upper extremity amputee—prosthetic training programs. In: *Rehabilitation of the Hand,* edited by J. M. Hunter, L. H. Schneider, E. J. Mackin, and J. A. Bell, pp. 574–588. C. V. Mosby, St. Louis.

APPENDIX 1

Institute of Rehabilitation Medicine
New York University Medical Center

OCCUPATIONAL THERAPY SERVICE
UPPER-EXTREMITY PREPROSTHETIC EVALUATION

SERVICE DR. ______________________

REPORT DATE ______________________

THERAPIST ______________________

NAME ______________ CHART # ________

ADDRESS ______________________

AGE ______________ SEX ________

DIAGNOSIS ______________________

ETIOLOGY OF AMPUTATION ______________

DATE OF AMPUTATION ______________

SURGICAL REVISION DATE ______________

OCCUPATION ______________________

DOMINANCE ______________________

I. MEDICAL STATUS (any information that could affect overall prosthetic training or use) ______________

____

II. PHYSICAL STATUS

LEFT (circle amputated side) RIGHT

LOSS OF ROM	FUNCTIONAL MOTION STRENGTH		FUNCTIONAL MOTION STRENGTH	LOSS OF ROM
	(grading on a O–N basis)	SCAPULA ELEVATION		
		DEPRESSION		
		ABDUCTION		
		ADDUCTION		
		SHOULDER ABDUCTION		
		ADDUCTION		
		FLEXION		
		EXTENSION		
		INT. ROTATION		
		EXT. ROTATION		
		ELBOW FLEXION		
		EXTENSION		
		FOREARM		
		SUPINATION		
		PRONATION		
		WRIST FLEXION		

LEFT (circle amputated side)			RIGHT	
LOSS OF ROM	FUNCTIONAL MOTION STRENGTH		FUNCTIONAL MOTION STRENGTH	LOSS OF ROM
	(grading on a O–N basis)	EXTENSION		
		HAND GROSS GRASP		
		PREHENSION LATERAL #		
		PALMAR #		

GENERAL COORDINATION ______________ DEXTERITY ______________

ENDURANCE (Etiology may be a medical problem, which would decrease endurance, i.e., diabetes, cancer.)

III. STUMP DESCRIPTORS

CLASSIFICATION BY LEVEL OF AMPUTATION ______________

SHAPE (conical, screwdrive, edematous)

SKIN CONDITION (Note presence of skin diseases, scarring, unhealed areas, abrasions, discoloration, allergies esp. to stump socket materials or plastic laminate.)

VOLUME MEASUREMENTS (Has maximum shrinkage been attained?) SHRINKAGE TECHNIQUE (shrinker, elastic bandage)

FOR HOW LONG USED (Data shrinkage was begun. Is it presently done?)

TONE OF MUSCULATURE (normal, decreased tone)

CIRCULATION (Is stump cold, warm, moist, dry?)

SENSORY STATUS

TACTILE SENSIBILITY (STUMP) (tested using Semmes Weinstein pressure aesthesiometer)
(SOUND) ______________

PAIN OR TENDERNESS (Specify areas of pain or tenderness.)

PHANTOM SENSATION (Describe residual limb parts, positions, ability to move.)

PHANTOM PAIN ______________

IV. ADL STATUS

PRIOR PROSTHESIS (If patient had or has a prosthesis, is it worn? Describe all components: harness and modifications, socket, elbow unit, hinges, wrist unit, terminal devices, and controls.)

CURRENT LEVEL OF INDEPENDENCE ______________

____

____

WITH PREVIOUS PROSTHESIS OR ADAPTIVE DEVICES (Specify adaptive devices if used.)

____

WITHOUT EQUIPMENT ______________________________

____

PREVIOUS ADL RESPONSIBILITIES (SELF-CARE, AVOCATIONAL, HOMEMAKING) (Describe all patient's home, work, recreational responsibilities; what activities take too long now.) ______________

____

V. EXPECTATION OF PROSTHESIS

GENERAL FUNCTION (what patient expects the prosthesis to do)

VOCATIONAL ______________________________

COSMETIC ______________________________

VI. DISCUSSION OR REMARKS

____

____

____

VII. RECOMMENDATIONS

TREATMENT: (stump wrapping techniques, exercise to increase ROM and/or strength, coordination)

TYPE OF PROSTHESIS (Describe components.)

TYPE OF ADAPTIVE EQUIPMENT: (any assistive/adaptive equipment to increase ADL, energy conservation)

FURTHER EVALUATION: ______________________________

____

Reproduced by permission from the NYU/IRM Occupational Therapy Department.

APPENDIX 2

Institute of Rehabilitation Medicine New York University Medical Center OCCUPATIONAL THERAPY PROSTHETIC CHECKOUT BELOW-ELBOW PROSTHESIS Date:	Name: ______________ Address: ______________ Age: ________ Chart No. ________ Disability: ______________ Occupation: ______________

DATE OF FINAL SURGERY: ______________ SIDE OF AMPUTATION: Right: ____ Left: ____

PERCENTAGE LENGTH OF STUMP:

$$\text{Unilateral BE} = \frac{\text{stump length} \times 100}{\text{sound forearm length}} = \underline{\qquad\qquad} \%$$

$$\text{Bilateral BE} = \frac{\text{stump length} \times 100}{\text{height (inches)} \times 0.14} = \underline{\qquad\qquad} \%$$

AMPUTEE TYPE (based on percentage length of stump): ______________________________

DESCRIPTION OF PROSTHESIS:

Harness: Figure 8 or 9 ____ Shoulder saddle ________________ Other ________

Harness modifications: ____________________________

Harness material: Dacron ____________ Cotton ____________ Other ________

Control System: Single ____ Dual ____ Biceps cineplasty ____________ Other ________

Cuff: Full ____________ Triceps pad ____________ Other ________

Elbow hinge: Rigid: Single pivot ________ Polycentric ________ Step-up ________ Flexible ________

Other ________

Socket: Double wall ________ Single wall ________ Split ________ Muenster ________

Socket material: Plastic laminate ________________ Other ________

Wrist unit: Manual friction ________ Quick change ________ Wrist flexion ________

Constant friction ________________ Other ________

Terminal devices: Hooks ________ Hands ________

Reproduced by permission from the NYU/IRM Occupational Therapy Department.

CHECKOUT

Initial C.O.	Final C.O.	I. FIT:
		HARNESS
		1. Is *axilla loop* padded or covered and is it comfortable to amputee?
		2. Is *axilla loop* small enough to keep cross of figure-8 harness well below seventh cervical vertebra and slightly to unamputated side?
		3. Is *control attachment* strap below midscapular level and does it remain low enough to give adequate cable travel?
		4. Can any additional harness straps be justified?
		5. Does *front support* strap pass through delto-pectoral groove?
		CUFF OR TRICEPS PAD
		6. Does the *cuff* fit snugly without gapping during forearm flexion and terminal device operation?
		ELBOW HINGE
		7. Does the *elbow hinge* function smoothly without pinching flesh or otherwise causing discomfort?
		SOCKET
		8. Is the *socket* comfortable (especially when compressive force or torque is applied)?
		9. Is the patient's *stump* free from abrasions, discoloration, etc., within 10 minutes after prosthesis is taken off?
		DIMENSIONS AND WEIGHT
		10. Is prosthesis the *correct length?*
		11. Is the *weight* of the entire prosthesis satisfactory?

II. FUNCTION:

	Initial C.O. Prosthesis		Final C.O. Prosthesis		
	on	off	on	off	
A. RANGE OF MOTION 1. Stump rotation (total range)					Total rotation with prosthesis on should be half that with prosthesis off.*
2. Elbow flexion					Active flexion with prosthesis on should be within 10° of range with prosthesis off.

* This standard applies to medium, well-formed stumps, but is often exceeded with wrist disarticulation and long B/E stumps. Short or fleshy stumps may not be able to attain the 50% standard.

B. CABLE SYSTEM

Initial C.O.	Final C.O.	
		3. Is control cable free from sharp bends?
		4. Is cable housing proper length between distal and proximal retainers, neither too loose nor too tight, so that TD operates with full opening and closing?
		5. Are control cables arranged so that they do not touch amputee's flesh?
		6. If hook is to be interchanged with hand, is hook-to-cable adapter the proper length?

C. CONTROL SYSTEM EFFICIENCY

	Initial C.O. Hook	Initial C.O. Hand	Final C.O. Hook	Final C.O. Hand	
7. Force applied at TD	____ lb	____ lb	____ lb	____ lb	
8. Force applied at hanger	____ lb	____ lb	____ lb	____ lb	
9. Efficiency $= \frac{\text{force at TD}}{\text{force at hanger}}$	____ %	____ %	____ %	____ %	75% or greater
D. TENSION STABILITY 10. Displacement of socket on stump with 50-lb axial load					Prosthesis should not slip on stump more than 1 inch

E. WRIST UNIT AND TERMINAL DEVICE

Initial C.O.	Final C.O.	
		11. If FM disconnect is used, is operating button placed in the anterior-medial quadrant of the prosthetic wrist?
		12. If wrist flexion unit is used, does the patient operate it quickly and easily?
		13. Does compression on wrist unit prevent involuntary rotation of terminal device on active opening?
		14. If length adapter is used, is hand or hook fairing installed?
		15. If APRL hand is used without length adapter, is back shell of hand faired to prevent sharp bend in operating cable?
		16. If cosmetic is used, is it pulled completely onto hand and is it undamaged and properly color-matched?
		17. Does TD function properly in all respects?

F. TERMINAL DEVICE OPENING AND CLOSING

	Initial C.O. Hook	Initial C.O. Hand	Final C.O. Hook	Final C.O. Hand	
18. Mechanical range					Full opening and closing should be obtained with forearm at 90°.
19. Active range (forearm at 90°)					
20. Active range (fly)					100% opening and closing should be obtained at mouth and fly.
21. Active range (mouth)					Note: Children may have less than 100%.

III. Craftsmanship

Initial C.O.	Final C.O.	
		1. Have all *cut edges* on cable housing been filed smooth or tipped with ferrules?
		2. Is harness firmly sewn?
		3. Are all *strap ends* sealed to prevent fraying?
		4. Is neoprene lining on hook firmly bonded?
		5. Are all *rivets* properly peened and all screws securely fastened?
		6. Are all soldered *joints* strong, neat, and workmanlike?
		7. Is *cuff* made of good-quality leather, lined and finished in a workmanlike manner and coated with nylon solution overall?
		8. Have all *trimmed edges, rough spots, starved* or *uncured areas* been sealed?
		9. Is arm *color* satisfactory and consistent?
		CONFORMANCE WITH PRESCRIPTION 10. Is the prosthesis as *prescribed*? If a re-check, have previous recommendations been accomplished?
		THE FOLLOWING SECTIONS APPLY AT FINAL ONLY TRAINING 11. Has the patient completed a *training program* in the use of his prosthesis?
		12. Can the patient demonstrate *effective use* of terminal device and wrist unit?

INITIAL CHECKOUT: Date:	FINAL CHECKOUT: Date:
Pass ( ) Provisional pass ( ) Fail ( )	Pass ( ) Fail ( )
Patient needs further attention in the following area:	Patient needs further attention in the following area:
Medical-surgical ( ) Training ( )	Medical-surgical ( ) Training ( )
Prosthetic ( ) Other ( ) (vocational, psychological, other)	Prosthetic ( ) Other ( ) (vocational, psychological, other)
COMMENTS & RECOMMENDATIONS:	COMMENTS & RECOMMENDATIONS:

PATIENT'S OPINION OF PROSTHESIS: ______________________________

Examiner: ______________________

Cancer and Impaired Independence

17

Annette Bieringer

As more accurate diagnostic tests detect more cancer patients each year, and as modern medical techniques prolong their lives, it becomes important to provide treatment that will improve the quality of life for these patients with cancer related disabilities.

In this chapter, we shall describe an occupational therapy program in an acute inpatient cancer center and discuss cancer-related disabilities and their causes, special problems that affect rehabilitation of cancer patients, indications for and expected outcomes of occupational therapy, and ways in which staff members can learn to deal with the stress involved in working with cancer patients.

Rehabilitation is usually thought of as being an aspect of living, but cancer is commonly linked with dying. Consequently, before discussing rehabilitation for patients with cancer, it is important to dispel at least some of the mystique surrounding the word "cancer" and put it into a perspective that will make rehabilitation for cancer patients as reasonable as rehabilitation for patients disabled by other causes.

The common conceptions about cancer involve an exaggerated sense of finality. The word itself has considerable impact. Evidence of lengthening life-spans for cancer patients has neither reduced this impact nor produced wider acceptance of the idea of rehabilitation. As one social worker wrote in describing the impact of the word "cancer" on most people, "When I think of the word 'impact' and couple it with a word as loaded as 'cancer' I have an image of the buckling, collapsing, and grunting that one experiences when being punched in the stomach by someone as powerful as Muhammad Ali" (1). It is this impact that profoundly influences attitudes regarding cancer rehabilitation.

Rehabilitation programs for disabled cancer patients are relatively new, having been developed within the past 15 to 20 years. Before that time, a diagnosis of cancer was thought to mean imminent death, and, in fact, not too long ago that was generally true. Today, however, the life-span for a patient with disseminated lymphoma or widespread breast cancer or Hodgkin's disease may be as long as or longer than that for patients with many forms of cardiovascular disease. Because of improved methods of diagnosis and treatment, both the numbers of patients known to have cancer and their life-spans have increased.

As a consequence, there are more patients in the clinic with cancer, many of whom have some kind of temporary or permanent disability and need to learn to function independently. Although surgical techniques, more sophisticated use of radiation therapy, and wider use of chemotherapy have resulted in increased longevity, their side effects sometimes cause disabilities that can be overcome or diminished by means of rehabilitation programs. These disabilities vary widely. In addition, because of the particularly severe form of psychological stress that accompanies a diagnosis of cancer, cancer patients seem to have greater difficulty in adjusting to their handicaps than do patients handicapped by other causes.

Although many disabilities resulting from cancer are similar to those that result from other conditions, there are subtle differences. It is these differences that make working with cancer patients unique. Just as each area of occupational therapy has its special quality, so does this one.

In terms of rehabilitation, chronic diseases and life-threatening diseases have much in common. Usually, both are controlled rather than cured. Disabled patients become depressed, they tend to feel that what is happening to them has never happened to anyone else, they suffer many losses (e.g., privacy, independence, familiar surroundings), they may be forced to change their lifestyles. They become debilitated from prolonged bed rest. They undergo changes in body image, they suffer from postoperative pain. They need emotional support and appropriate reassurance.

There are also subtle differences between chronic diseases and life-threatening diseases. There is the special stress that accompanies a diagnosis of cancer. Patients are frightened, and families are immobilized by fear and uncertainty. Patients with cancer vary in emotional and physical status from day to day, or even from hour to hour. Many are subject to pathologic fractures. Physical defects are often extensive, the consequences of radical surgery. Body image disturbances arise from this and from other causes, such as the hair loss caused by radiation therapy and chemotherapy. These treatments may also cause nausea, vomiting, numbness, and tingling. Many patients suffer remote effects of cancer on the nervous system and develop muscular weakness and wasting, which come and go without apparent reason. Each of these special problems will be covered in this chapter, and their implications for evaluation, goal setting, and treatment planning will be discussed.

FRAME OF REFERENCE

It is important for the occupational therapist to develop a frame of reference, a philosophy that will serve as a guide. For most patients whose disabilities are related to causes other than cancer, rehabilitation is not started until the patient's medical condition has stabilized and rehabilitation becomes the main focus. The therapist evaluates the patient and establishes a base line, then sets short-term and long-range goals. With cancer patients in an acute hospital setting, things are different. Patients are admitted primarily for diagnosis and treatment of their diseases, and rehabilitation is often started during the time that diagnosis and treatment are taking place.

As a result, there are some special factors that must be considered: (a) Occupational therapy may be started before the sequelae of disease are known. (b) Patients are often discharged as soon as medical treatment is finished, whether or not rehabilitation goals have been achieved. (c) Most treatment is conducted at bedside, and this limits the types of activities. (d) Evaluation becomes a daily ongoing process, since there is seldom time for complete, detailed initial evaluations. (e) Rehabilitation sessions are often interrupted or postponed because other matters (e.g., radiation therapy or chemotherapy or diagnostic procedures) take precedence. (f) Occupational therapy sessions may not be possible if patients are suffering from the side effects of other treatments. (g) Probably most important, rehabilitation is not foremost in the minds of patients who are worried about death and the disease process of cancer or patients who are incapacitated by side effects such as nausea and vomiting.

All these factors demand much interdisciplinary teamwork. They demand that goals be set that are important to the patient, that the therapist help plan postdischarge rehabilitation, that the therapist, while being involved, avoid overidentification. They demand common sense.

It is helpful, when setting common-sense goals that are realizable and achievable, to select goals in the context of prognosis. One way of doing this is to think in terms of restorative, supportive, and palliative goals. A restorative goal is a goal selected for a patient who is expected to return to a previous state of function without a remarkable residual handicap (e.g., a patient who has had early diagnosis and treatment of breast cancer or lung cancer). Goals for these patients are geared to enable them to be fully functional and to resume previous life-styles.

Supportive goals are for patients with residual permanent disabilities (e.g., amputees who need treatment to offset as much of the disability as possible). Also in this category are patients with ongoing but controlled disease, patients who are expected to live many years but who may face increasing disability during those years. For patients in this group, physical and occupational therapists often work together to teach wheelchair independence along with ambulation.

Perhaps an example is in order: The patient was a 50-year-old man with lymphoma that had been diagnosed many years earlier. When referred for physical and occupational therapy while in the hospital, he was receiving chemotherapy, and as a result he had severe neuropathies, most pronounced in the distal musculature. This meant that he had difficulty with ambulation and self-care. He could barely hold a toothbrush or a fork, and he was only partially independent in dressing. The rehabilitation goals were to encourage him to use a walker, to provide activities to increase hand function, and to develop an exercise program to prevent the joint stiffness and muscle atrophy that accompany disuse. These were the short-term goals. Although it was expected that once the course of chemotherapy was finished, the patient would improve functionally, it was apparent from his history that, as time passed, he would probably become increasingly disabled and might need a wheelchair. Goals had to be selected on two levels, some for the present and some for the future. It is in this area more than any other that both occupational therapy and physical therapy involve more art than technique. For a patient who is ambulatory, however poorly, accepting the idea of a wheelchair is difficult; yet knowing how to manage a wheelchair often increases the chance of acceptance of one if and when it is needed. Reconciliation between patient goals and therapist goals calls for the application of psychological expertise as well as physical expertise and requires skillful use of each.

The third goal-setting classification, palliative, involves patients with increasing disabilities caused by progressive disease and patients with limited life-spans. The objective of therapy in this area is not rehabilitation of the patient but adaptation to circumstances in which no rehabilitation is possible. Such patients must be permitted to set their own goals, goals meaningful to them (1). During this period, many patients also fear abandonment by friends, family, and staff; continuing treatment helps negate that sense of abandonment through human contact (2). Self-help devices or techniques that increase independence in personal hygiene help maintain a sense of self-esteem. Great flexibility on the part of the therapist is needed so that a patient can be helped to set realistic and achievable goals. Working with terminally ill patients can be a painful experience, but it need not be. Reward comes from the realization that a dying patient was made physically and psychologically more comfortable through a program of activities scaled to the patient's needs and interests.

SPECIAL PROBLEMS

In addition to having to cope with a diagnosis of cancer, these patients face other problems. As stated earlier, the disabilities that stem from the cancer itself and those that result from the various treatments present unique difficulties. An occupational therapist must be aware of these in planning treatment and setting goals.

One problem concerns the remote effects of some cancers, neuropathies arising far from the site of the cancer. They are believed to result from the way cancer cells alter nutrition, resulting in muscular weakness and wasting, with weakness being most common in the proximal rather than the distal musculature. Such weakness waxes and wanes and may last for an hour, for a day, or even for months. Often, there are long periods of remission. There seems to be no relation to the course of the tumor or to other treatments. Sometimes a patient who is barely able to come to a sitting position in the morning is walking with ease that same afternoon. Thus the therapist must be ready to adjust treatment plans daily.

The main goal for patients who suffer muscular weakness from remote effects or from other treatments is to prevent the effects of disuse, decrease in range of motion, and too much bed rest by a program of graded activities. Planning such a program involves finding ways to motivate the patient who is weak, frequently discouraged, and often frightened. It requires a therapeutic relationship as well as teamwork between disciplines so that a patient can be encouraged to continue planned activities at other times during the day and evening.

Pathologic fractures constitute another special problem. These occur when bone has been replaced and weakened by a neoplastic lesion, a lesion that is usually a focus of metastasis. All bones can be affected, but most such fractures occur in the long bones, the spine, the pelvis, and the ribs. They sometimes occur from the most innocuous movements, and patients have reported breaking an arm while picking up a glass of water or rolling in bed. This means that activities must be selected carefully in order to minimize the risk of further fractures. Progressive resistive exercise (PRE), for example, is contraindicated.

A third difficulty faced by cancer patients stems from surgery. Surgical procedures for cancer often are necessarily radical and usually leave extensive deficits. For example, an affected limb is usually amputated one joint above the lesion. Thus a humeral lesion would necessitate an interscapulothoracic (IST) amputation rather than an above-elbow amputation or shoulder disarticulation. An IST amputation involves excision of the distal third of the clavicle and all or part of the scapula, in addition to the entire arm and shoulder. Because so little muscular support remains, there is at present no satisfactory prosthesis. Some prosthetists are experimenting, but for now patients who have had this surgery must rely on thorough training in one-handed accomplishment of ADL. They also will need psychological counseling.

A fourth problem concerns the side effects of chemotherapy. Methotrexate, one common chemotherapeutic agent, usually causes proximal weakness, whereas Vincristine, another such agent, may cause paresthesias of the fingers and ankles, diminished reflexes, and ataxia. Although these side effects usually disappear in the months following treatment, they cause severe ADL problems while they exist. Another drug, 5-Fluorouracil, causes emotional lability. The implication of this for the therapist is that a crying patient may not necessarily be depressed. Procarbazine commonly decreases the platelet count, and when this count approaches 50,000/mm^3, activities must be modified in terms of time and energy, as a low platelet count combined with exercise may cause bleeding into the joints or elsewhere.

Radiation therapy is another form of treatment with iatrogenic side effects. Malfunction of the central nervous system may occur soon after radiation therapy, and fibrosis and formation of scar tissue can occur after a year or more.

More detailed listings of these side effects and their relevance to occupational therapy can be found in Table 1 and Appendix 1. These were compiled by the occupational therapy staff at M.D. Anderson Hospital and Tumor Institute, Houston, Texas, with advice from the medical staff, based on studies reported in the literature and on direct observation. The suggested safe activity periods for anemic patients are not hard and fast rules, but guides in treatment planning.

There are also side effects involved in the use of steroids. These often are used to reduce edema following resection of the brain. Steroids have so many side effects that their use must be tapered as soon as possible following surgery. Because the amount of edema in the brain affects neurological status and degree of lethargy, occupational therapists, by noting a patient's functional level and activity tolerance each day, can help the medical staff determine if steroids are being tapered too quickly and can help determine adequate minimal dosages.

One other significant problem that affects activity programs is the exhaustion experienced by many patients following lengthy and involved diagnostic and treatment procedures. It is important for therapists to be aware of this and to be prepared to postpone or modify planned treatment programs.

OCCUPATIONAL THERAPY

In an acute care setting with inpatients only, where the average hospital stay is less than 3 weeks, occupational therapy is geared toward helping patients achieve as much ADL independence as possible. The major treatment areas are as follows:

1. Self-feeding problems: (a) poor grasp because of decreased sensation or endurance or the presence of apraxia or pain; (b) limited range of motion; (c) muscle weakness.
2. Dressing problems: (a) perceptual difficulties; (b) decreased range of motion; (c) change in body structure requiring clothing adaptations or assistive devices; (d) poor balance; (e) poor endurance; (f) pain.
3. One-handed functioning techniques, along with the fabrication of cosmetic soft shoulder caps following IST amputations. These improve appearance and help support clothing on the operated side. They must be soft so as not to irritate a fresh wound and are temporary. Caps that are more durable and better fitting can be obtained once the wound is healed and medical clearance is given.
4. Redominance training, if needed.
5. Activities to increase strength, range of motion, dexterity, and coordination.
6. Splinting: (a) protective positioning for peripheral nerve palsies; (b) prevention of contractures; (c) mechanical substitution for lost motion.
7. Provision of adaptive equipment.

Because an average hospital stay is 3 weeks, a detailed and lengthy initial evaluation is precluded. However, a base line must be established before treatment planning and goal setting can even be considered. Thus treatment must begin with a careful reading of the patient's chart, followed by observation of the patient's functional status. What a patient can do and cannot do, mental status, cognition, gross muscle strength, range of motion, balance, and activity tolerance are some of the areas included in an initial functional evaluation.

Evaluation does not end here, but continues right along with daily treatment sessions. Day-to-day patient responses may reveal problem areas that require more detailed evaluation. Adjustments and changes in treatment planning and goal setting may be required. Evaluation is a daily ongoing process that requires flexibility on the part of the occupational therapist.

Another facet of the evaluation process concerns the patient's view of the disability. It is not possible to overemphasize that a diagnosis of cancer creates a special stress that is compounded by the presence of physical disability, thus making adjustment to the disability even more difficult. This can be the greatest disabling factor of all. Couple this with the hope that treatment will eliminate the disability, and it creates a barrier against the patient's acceptance of the need for a rehabilitation program.

Whereas treatment may wholly or partially alleviate many disabilities, the time between diagnosis and initiation of treatment is crucial. It can be used effectively by the patient and therapist to establish the trust that will enable them to agree to a contract that sets mutually acceptable goals. Such a contract can mean the difference between goal achievement and nonachievement. It provides one means by which patients who since diagnosis have had little control over their own lives, can exert some control. It is one area in which patients can have a voice in their treatment by being allowed to set realistic and meaningful goals. It is in the giving of this control to the patient that the therapist's goals are more easily achieved.

STAFF REACTIONS

Working with patients with cancer can be extremely stressful. To work effectively in such an environment, therapists need to find means to reduce this stress and to facilitate the development of an intelligent awareness of what is happening to them so that their emotions will not interfere with good judgment.

Frequently the therapist identifies with the patient. This is a normal tendency. For example, the death of a patient may trigger memories of losses the therapist has experienced, such as loss of a family member. It is necessary for the therapist to understand what is really causing sadness or anger so that these feelings can be placed into perspective and defused. Work-related stress can be debilitating to the therapist, but it can also be put to use to produce growth. One way to facilitate this growth is to provide an opportunity for therapists to express feelings of frustration, anger, or sadness in a peer group that meets regularly and is directed by a trained leader who can keep discussions purposeful and focused.

The basic premise in the development of such a group is that staff members have and should have feelings and reactions when working with extremely sick, debilitated, and sometimes disfigured people. Unless these reactions are explored, understood, and put into perspective, they interfere with optimal patient care. Such group meetings promote growth and improve the quality of patient care. They permit the sharing of experiences and reactions. No feelings are considered inappropriate or unspeakable. There is an opportunity to air and to solve intradepartmental and interdepartmental problems. Feelings of warmth develop among group participants, and an atmosphere is created in which professionals in various disciplines (occupational therapy and physical therapy, etc.) can work together harmoniously and without professional rivalry. Participants get to know one another's personalities and work behavior. They develop awareness of behavioral clues that indicate problems, and thus support can be offered when the need arises. There is opportunity for professional growth as the therapist gains insight into the kinds of events that stimulate these anxieties.

In such meetings the discussions are usually wide-ranging. Beginning from the focus of how patient care can be improved, therapists discuss their own feelings about illness and death and often discover that their own life crises affect patient treatment. Some issues that frequently arise are (a) avoidance of some patients, (b) emotional involvement with others, (c) the anger, sadness, and relief involved in leaving and being left, and (d) the risk of getting involved and caring, then losing patients. Some themes continually run through these sessions: Are we filling patients' needs or our own? How far should we go in dealing and working with patients' feelings?

SUMMARY

Generally, occupational therapy with disabled cancer patients is not unlike occupational therapy with patients disabled by other causes. "The challenge in rehabilitation of the cancer patient lies in the extent and the variety of disease-related and treatment-related disabilities presented" (3). Therapists must understand the causes of these disabilities in order to treat patients appropriately and effectively. They must understand the stress produced on the patient by the concept of cancer. They must understand what it is in the patient that triggers emotional reactions in themselves.

These considerations apply to a multitude of other diseases that also produce long-term stress and anxiety (e.g., heart disease, multiple sclerosis, renal failure), but life expectancy following diagnosis is steadily increasing. As new medical techniques prolong life, it becomes more important to provide treatment that will improve the quality of life. "Most people want to live longer but they also want to live as fully as possible. While neither we nor the patient has control over the limitations imposed by a disease process and its treatment we [therapists] have the ability to affect how these limitations are perceived and managed" (2).

Occupational therapists, as well as workers in all other rehabilitation disciplines, can and should play increasingly important roles in helping patients to live fuller lives. Once therapists understand their own needs and fears and patients' needs and fears and they are put in perspective, treatment becomes easier and more effective.

REFERENCES

1. Botsford, T. (editor) (1968): *Cancer: A Manual for Practitioners,* ed. 3. American Cancer Society, Massachusetts Division, Boston.
2. Dietz, J. H., Jr. (1969): Rehabilitation of the cancer patient. *Med. Clin. North Am.,* 53:607–624.
3. Asher, R. A. J. (1947): The dangers of going to bed. *Br. Med. J.,* 2:967–971.

BIBLIOGRAPHY

Euster, S. (1978): A system to meet the psychosocial needs of the chronically ill. Paper read before the National Conference on Social Welfare, Los Angeles, Calif. Rehabilitation Service, Memorial Sloan-Kettering Cancer Center, New York (mimeograph).

Golden, S., Harwich, C., and Lokich, J.: *Chemotherapy and You,* U.S. Public Health Service bulletin 78-1136. U.S. Department of Health, Education, and Welfare, Washington, D.C.

Purtillo, R. (1972): Don't mention it: The physical therapist in a death-denying society. *Phys. Ther.,* 52:1031–1035.

Dietz, J. H., Jr. (1974): Rehabilitation of the cancer patient: Its role in the scheme of comprehensive care. *Clin. Bull.* 4:104–107.

Rusk, H. A. (editor) (1977): *Rehabilitation Medicine,* ed. 4, Chapter 31. C. V. Mosby, St. Louis.

Trachtenberg, J. (1973): The impact of cancer on the patient, the family, and the community. Paper read before a meeting at Downstate Medical Center, New York, March 3, 1973. Rehabilitation Service, Memorial Sloan-Kettering Cancer Center, New York (mimeograph).

Trachtenberg, J., and Dansky, S. (1978): Professional staff reactions to patients with catastrophic illness: Modification through psychosocial rounds. Memorial Sloan-Kettering Cancer Center, New York (unpublished report).

Villanueva, R., Drane, J. B., Gunn, A., Brandon, B., Knight, N., and Bell, K. (1976): Rehabilitation of the cancer patient. In: *Cancer Patient Care at M. D. Anderson Hospital and Tumor Institute,* edited by R. L. Clark and C. D. Howe, pp. 671–691. Year Book Medical Publishers, Chicago.

Winick, L., and Robbins, G. (1977): Physical and psychological readjustment after mastectomy; an evaluation of Memorial Hospital's PMRG program. *Cancer,* 39:478–486.

APPENDIX 1

Side-Effects of Chemotherapeutic Agents

Chemotherapeutic agents may be administered as primary treatment or as an adjuvant to radiation therapy or surgery. The mechanism of action of some anticancer agents can be explained at the cellular level. Certain drugs are antimetabolites (i.e., inhibit the biosynthesis of nucleic acids), while others may interfere with the structure or function of DNA, or inhibit mitosis or protein synthesis. Chemotherapeutic agents may be *phase-specific* (i.e., kill dividing cells during a specific phase of the cell cycle), or *cycle-specific* (i.e., destroy proliferating cells more effectively than resting cells), or *non-cycle specific* (i.e., equally toxic to resting or proliferating cells).

The toxicities of different drugs vary, and are based on the type of drug, dose, and individual sensitivity. One should check the PDR or an Investigational Drug Book for side-effects and contraindications of specific drugs.

Listed on the next page are possible side-effects that are common to many chemotherapeutic agents, and that should be considered when formulating Rehabilitation treatment plans or progressing treatment programs.

Myelosuppression (bone marrow depression)

Since the bone marrow is one of the main blood-forming organs, this depression results in decreased production of all the blood components. It is important to obtain a complete blood count (WBC, platelets, HCT, or HGB) before each rehabilitation session, since vigorous resistive exercise or activities requiring sharp tools may be contraindicated if blood counts are low.

Thrombocytopenia (low platelet count). Normal value: 200,000–500,000/cu mm between 30,000–50,000/cu mm: a resistive exercise or ambulation program should be changed to active exercises without resistance, due to risk of internal hemorrhage. Below 30,000/cu mm: gentle exercises at bedside. Below 20,000/cu mm: Minimal exercises.

Please keep in mind that the treatment limitations for the above platelet values are not absolute. The activity level of different patients with the same platelet count may vary, depending on such factors as acute versus chronic thrombocytopenia, or a stable versus a hemorrhagic condition.

Leukopenia (low white blood count). Normal value: 5,000–10,000/cu mm Since leukopenic patients are extremely susceptible to infections, contact with other persons should be limited and strict hygiene procedures observed.

Anemia

Normal Values	Male	Female
Hct (packed cell volume)	approx. 45-47%	approx. 40-42%
Hgb (g/100 ml)	approx. 15-16	approx. 13-15
RBC (million/cu mm)	approx. 5.0	approx. 4.5

Anemic patients may have elevated pulse and respiration rates due to the body's effort to maintain an adequate oxygen supply. The therapist should carefully monitor pulse, and often blood pressure, before and after an exercise or activity. Patient may also be easily fatigued with minimal exertion, so that a maintenance, bedside exercise program is recommended.

Cardiac toxicity
Adriamycin or Daunomycin may cause irreversible cardiac damage. Complications such as congestive heart failure can develop, so check vital signs frequently.

Pulmonary fibrosis
Bleomycin may cause this side-effect, with resulting restrictive lung disease and impaired gas exchange.

Peripheral neuropathy
Vincristine, particularly, may cause weakness (distal greater than proximal) and paresthesias. Loss of strength in the intrinsics of the hand, wrist drop, and foot drop may result in varying combinations and degrees.

Cock-up splints, dorsiflexion assists, and strengthening exercises are indicated.

Fibrosis
In infiltration of an intravenously administered drug occurs, cellulitis may develop. This results in hard edema and fibrotic tissue limiting ROM. These patients may require splinting and ROM exercises to prevent contractures.

Gastrointestinal toxicity
Moderate to severe nausea, vomiting, diarrhea, and ulceration of the mucosal lining may occur. Therapy to maintain strength and endurance should be continued, if possible.

Alopecia (hair loss)
This is a temporary side-effect of certain drugs. Although the texture and color may be slightly altered, regrowth of the hair always occurs either during or after the chemotherapy treatment.

Emotional Reactions
All of the above side-effects may cause a variety of emotional reactions such as depression, anxiety, withdrawal, and hostility. Emotional reactions are also *direct* side-effects of certain drugs.

Side-Effects of Radiation Therapy and Their Importance for Physical and Occupational Therapists

Radiation therapy is used frequently in the treatment of cancer and can be administered in a number of ways.

External radiation therapy or radioactive implants may either be curative or palliative, and may be used alone or with chemotherapy, immunotherapy, or surgery. Radiation can be used in the treatment of inoperable tumors; to decrease tumor mass prior to surgery or as a primary treatment modality. Prior to treating patients with implants, therapists should contact the hospital Department of Radiation Safety for specific guidelines and instruction in precautionary measures.

Radiation therapy is believed to affect the nucleic acids, such as DNA, RNA and vital enzymes. These are the targets for biologic injury, and result in chromosomal aberrations and cell death. The ideal is to eradicate as much tumor as possible with maximal preservation and minimal irradiation of surrounding normal tissue.

Reactions to radiation therapy are determined by the type, quantity, duration, and site of exposure. Effects may be immediate, or may appear a number of months or years following treatment. Often it is difficult to differentiate between the effects of the treatment and the disease. Some of the side effects of radiation may actually be due to poorly planned treatment.

Listed on the next page are possible negative side-effects of radiation.

1. Myelosuppression (i.e., bone marrow depression), particularly leukopenia.
2. Fatigue and decreased endurance.
3. Erythema, mild burning or tanning, pigmentation of the skin.
4. Moist or dry desquamation, ulcerations of skin and mucous membranes; mucositis.
5. Pneumonitis from external irradiation of lungs followed by fibrosis. Radioactive implants in lungs may cause blood-tinged secretions.

6. Fibrosis and atrophy in soft tissues, causing decreased ROM.
7. Decreased vascularity and lymphedema, causing delayed healing and decreased ability to disseminate heat and cold from irradiated tissues.
8. Alopecia (hair loss).
9. CNS effects: CNS tissue is more radiosensitive than peripheral nerves. "Radiation myelitis," or inflammation of the spinal cord may occur as a delayed reaction and will be manifested by paresis or plegia.
10. "Radiation sickness": systemic illness, usually caused by abdominal irradiation and often manifested by anorexia, nausea and vomiting, and weakness.
11. Bone and joint necrosis, delayed or impaired growth in immature bone (infrequent).
12. Radiation induced neoplasia in the irradiated area (rare).
13. Emotional reactions, including:
    fear of pain or of being burned.
    negative body image caused by alopecia, skin changes, and visible dye markings.
    depression and withdrawal behavior caused by disruption in lifestyle, economic hardships, or physical changes and discomfort.

Dysphagia: Evaluation and Management

18

Nancy H. Wasserman

Dysphagia is a disorder of swallowing or impaired deglutition that can result from a variety of pathological processes. Major causes of dysphagia in adults are central nervous system damage and disease, including stroke, brainstem or cranial nerve disturbances, and degenerative neuropathic diseases (such as amyotrophic lateral sclerosis, multiple sclerosis, and myasthenia gravis), resulting in muscular atrophy, paresis, spasticity, or incoordination of the swallowing mechanism.

Swallowing difficulty frequently interferes with the patient's ability to obtain adequate nutrition and may lead to the serious medical hazards of aspiration pneumonia or asphyxiation. Consequently, patients who have serious difficulty in chewing or swallowing are generally fed parenterally by intravenous infusion, nasogastric tube, or syringe. Intravenous feeding is at best a temporary measure because of its nutritional limitations and the problem of venous breakdown. The limitations of nasogastric tube feeding include reflux esophagitis and nasal and pharyngeal irritation, and syringe feedings are generally time-consuming and may result in aspiration. Moreover, in terms of comfort and social acceptability, none of these above methods is desirable as a permanent solution to the problem of impaired swallowing.

It is the purpose of this chapter to discuss diagnostic and therapeutic management procedures that can enable many dysphagic patients to resume adequate alimentary functioning or maintain a maximum level of functioning under conditions of progressive neuromuscular deterioration.

PHYSIOLOGY OF DEGLUTITION

Swallowing is a complex act that is initiated voluntarily and completed reflexively. It is routinely divided into three stages (Fig. 1) oral, pharyngeal, and esophageal (1,2). The shortest stages are the oral and pharyngeal, which take approximately 1 sec each; the esophageal stage takes 3 to 7 sec on the average.

Oral stage. After food has been introduced into the mouth, acted on by the articulators, and formed into a bolus, the oral stage of swallowing begins. The tongue is drawn upward and backward against the hard palate by contraction of the mylohyoid muscle, projecting the bolus into the pharynx. Concomitantly there is a slight elevation of the larynx. The bolus then stimulates nerve

SWALLOWING

ORAL STAGE

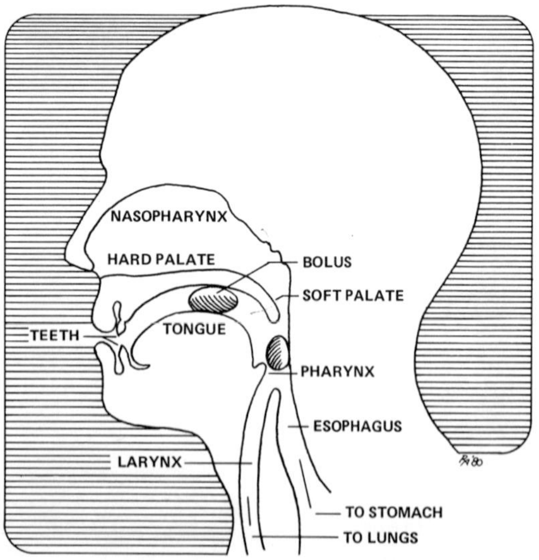

Function

* Food formed into bolus
* Tongue moves upwards and backwards against the hard palate
* Bolus projected into pharynx
* Slight elevation of larynx
* Respiration inhibited

Dysfunction

* Drooling
* Oral leakage
* Oral retention
* Food packing in cheek
* Biting of lip, tongue or cheek

PHARYNGEAL STAGE

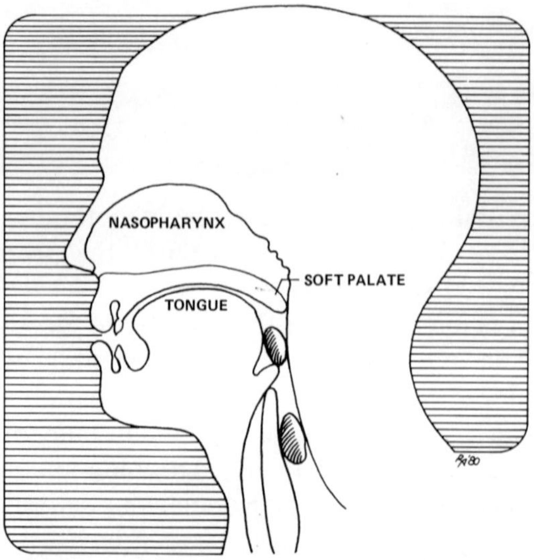

Function

* Bolus stimulates contraction of pharyngeal wall
* Bolus squeezed into esophagus
* Soft palate elevates to prevent nasal reflux
* Vocal folds close
* Base of tongue is forced against posterior pharyngeal wall
* Pharynx empties
* Larynx descends

Dysfunction

* Nasal reflux
* Coughing
* Choking
* Aspiration

ESOPHAGEAL STAGE

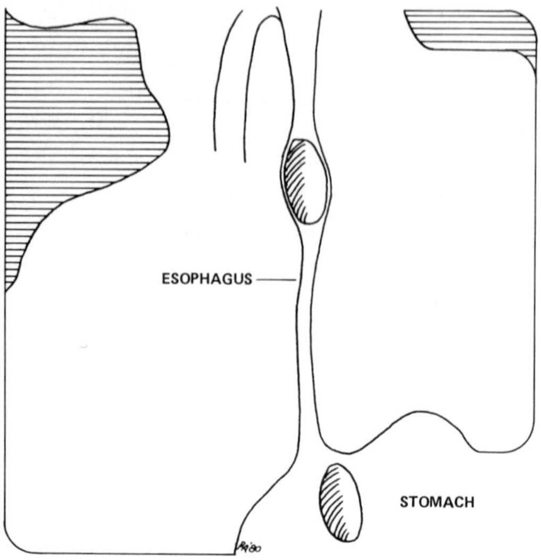

Function

* Respiration resumed
* Peristaltic action and relaxation of lower eosphageal sphincter

Dysfunction

* Oral reflux
* Pain

FIG. 1.

endings at the back of the tongue and throat. Respiration is temporarily inhibited. The oral stage is under voluntary control.

Pharyngeal stage. The pharyngeal stage is an involuntary stage in which the bolus stimulates contraction of the pharyngeal wall, which squeezes the bolus into the esophagus. The soft palate is elevated and brought forward during the beginning of this phase to prevent food from entering the nose. The vocal folds close, and the base of the tongue is forced against the posterior pharyngeal wall, creating increased pressure in the pharynx, followed by contraction of the pharyngeal constrictors that empty the pharynx. The larynx descends, and respiration resumes.

Esophageal stage. The esophageal stage is characterized by peristaltic action and relaxation of the lower esophageal sphincter, an involuntary function.

Aspiration of food is prevented chiefly by the elevation and forward movement of the larynx, with simultaneous closing of the vocal folds. It is no longer believed that the epiglottis is a vital structure in the prevention of aspiration (2).

Bolus formation and chewing. During bolus preparation, the tongue and buccinator muscles keep the food between the molars, where it is ground by the muscles of mastication. The styloglossus and the intrinsic tongue muscles are responsible for alternate side-to-side mixing of saliva with food, sorting of food particles, and formation of the bolus.

At rest, the jaw is held lightly closed. During chewing, closure is inhibited by the tactile stimulation produced by pressure of the food against the teeth, gums, and palate. Opening of the jaw is followed by rebound closing, which continues in a rhythmic manner while food remains in the mouth to provide the necessary stimulation. Chewing stimulates the flow of saliva, which in turn stimulates swallowing. The chewing process continues involuntarily, but it is subject to higher neural control in terms of speeding up or slowing down. The swallowing center in the medulla oblongata is innervated partially by mechanical stimulation and partially by neural receptors in the mouth that pick up sensations of taste, texture, and pressure (3).

EVALUATION OF DYSPHAGIA

Evaluation of dysphagia includes the gathering of historical information, a medical or neurological examination to determine specific causes, direct oral examination, and cineradiographic studies where indicated. From the clinician's perspective it is essential to obtain the patient's description of the problem, collect information relevant to dietary management, and evaluate the feeding and swallowing mechanisms by examination of structure and function (see Appendix A).

Report of the Patient's Problem

Dysphagic patients complain of a variety of symptoms that can provide a useful index for determining the dysfunctional phase of swallowing as well as the mechanism involved. Drooling, oral leakage, and oral retention are generally related to the oral phase, indicating lip and tongue dysfunction. Nasal regurgitation and nasal speech imply palatal involvement, and coughing, choking, and aspiration reflect pharyngeal phase dysfunction. Reflux and pain occur frequently when there is esophageal phase dysfunction (4). Food packing between the teeth and buccal surfaces generally occurs on the paretic side and indicates tongue or cheek dysfunction. Biting of the cheek, tongue, or lip occurs mostly when there is flaccid tonus or sensory deficit. Patients with neurologic dysphagia usually have greater difficulty in swallowing liquids than solids; however, these patients may not be able to masticate solids because they lack the finite coordination required of the tongue, cheek, and palate.

Examination of the Oral Mechanism

It is advisable to make an assessment of the integrity of the mechanism prior to evaluating the patient's ability to swallow fluid or food. Evaluation is conducted with tongue depressors, cotton-tip applicators, and an oral flashlight. Wherever possible, the patient is examined in an upright position with midline confrontation.

Structure

The lips, cheeks, tongue, and palate should be examined for evidence of paresis or paralysis. The lips may be pulled to one side (the unaffected side). The tongue may bulge or fasciculate (involuntary twitching of muscle fibers indicative of atrophy). The tongue may protrude at rest. The cheeks may have a hollow or slack appearance typical of hypotonicity. The palate may droop on one side, with uvular deviation toward the normal side (5).

The teeth should be examined for integrity; one should look for absence of a tooth or spaced teeth, malocclusion, and loose dentures. In the presence of unilateral paresis one often encounters loose dentures, possibly resulting from a change in muscle tone.

Reflexes

One should next examine the oral protective reflexes, including the palatal and gag reflexes. These reflexes are present at birth and persist throughout life. The palatal reflex consists of velar elevation in response to touch; one should test bilaterally and note asymmetry. The pharyngeal, or gag, reflex is stimulated by touching the posterior portion of the tongue, the fauces, or the posterior pharyngeal wall; this evokes elevation of the velum, constriction of the lateral and posterior pharyngeal wall, and reflexive swallowing. The gag reflex is considered hyperactive if it can be elicited by tactile stimulation to the anterior half of the tongue (6), hypoactive if it can be elicited only after multiple stimulations or if it can be elicited only partially or on one parameter, and absent if it cannot be elicited by stimulation of any parameter.

Often in cases of neuropathic dysphagia where there is known to be bilateral damage or degenerating neuropathy, there may be release of primitive or infantile reflexes by lower brain control. All or any of these reflexes may be found in adults when there is brain injury, and they often interfere with feeding as well as with speech production (5). Therefore it is advisable to examine for these primitive reflexes.

Mouth-opening reflex. A visual stimulus presented to the mouth may effect reflexive mouth opening.

Lip reflex or mouth phenomena. Tapping near the angle of the mouth may evoke involuntary movements of the lips and eventual lip closure and pouting.

Biting reflex. A stimulus placed between the gums or teeth may evoke mouth closure and holding behavior.

Sucking reflex. Placing a tongue depressor or finger in contact with the lips, the front of the tongue, the gums, or the hard palate may produce a suckling response that consists of forward, upward, and backward movement of the tongue, followed by swallowing. The suckling reflex is not to be confused with sucking, in which the stimulus is held between the lips while creating negative pressure within the mouth. The tongue-thrust swallow (visceral swallow or reverse swallow) is believed to be a retained swallow pattern from the suckling reflex exhibited in infancy. This swallow pattern is frequently seen in adults, and when seen in the absence of other released infantile reflexes it probably reflects a retained pattern rather than a neuropathological symptom.

Rooting reflex. Gently stroking away from the corner of the lips and stimulating the middle of the upper and lower lips may cause movement of the lips, tongue, jaw, or head in the direction of the stimulus.

Chewing reflex. Stimulating the gums or teeth with a finger may elicit reflexive chewing (7).

Oral Function

An examination of the strength, range of movement, and coordination of the lips, tongue, jaw, and palate should be conducted. There is a great deal of individual variation in normal function of articulators. Since no standardized method exists for determining strength and there is no method of definitively measuring range or coordination of the articulators, examination of oral function requires the judgment of an experienced clinician, preferably one who has conducted hundreds of oral mechanism examinations.

Lip function. Examination of lip function involves assessing the patient's ability to produce lip elevation (sneering), depression (pouting), protrusion (pursing), and retraction (voluntary smiling). One should also assess the ability to perform smooth and rapid alternated lip movements, as in protrusion-retraction, and the ability to differentiate lip movement from jaw and tongue movement.

Tongue function. One should examine the range of movement of the tongue for protrusion, lateralization, elevation, and retraction. Protrusion is necessary for lip clearing; the minimum range is to protrude the tongue beyond the lips.

Elevation and retraction are used in forming and propelling the bolus; the minimum range for elevation is to extend the tongue tip to the gum line behind the central incisors; the minimum range for retraction is to pull the tongue back in the mouth, clearing the inner surfaces of the teeth. Lateralization is used for directing food between the teeth and clearing the buccal surfaces; the minimum range is to extend the tongue tip to the right and left angles of the lips.

Coordination of tongue movement is examined by assessing the patient's ability to rapidly and smoothly alternate tongue protrusion-retraction, left-right lateralization, and elevation-depression. During isolated and alternated movements the patient should produce the expected movements independent of any extraneous lip and mandible movement (8).

Palatal function. Bilateral elevation of the palate may be observed during production of the vowel "a." Sustained vocalization of "a" is required to assess maintained palatal function. Although it is possible to observe palatal elevation, it is not possible to determine velopharyngeal valve competence by direct observation, as it is obscured by the inferior margin of the soft palate (8). The presence of nasal speech of nasal regurgitation indicates reduced competence of the mechanism. Cineradiographic studies during swallowing may be indicated to determine the competence of palatal valving.

Jaw and cheek function. One should assess lateral jaw movement and rapid jaw clicking. The strength of the masseter and temporalis should be assessed by placing the hands along the sides of the patient's face, with the patient being requested to bite down with force and maintain biting pressure. Muscle contraction can be palpated at the level of the temporalis and masseter muscles; the forces should be the same on both sides. The patient should be able to execute jaw movements independent of extraneous lip or tongue movement.

Laryngeal-glottal function. One should observe the larynx during swallowing for deviation from the midline and for laryngeal excursion. Glottal function is examined indirectly on the basis of volitional control in halting respiration and alternated on-off phonation at a minimum rate of one shift per second (5).

Oral Sensation

Reduced sensation is a frequent contributing factor in dysphagia. This is assessed by applying a light touch periorally with a wisp of cotton loosened from a cotton-tip applicator while the patient's eyes are closed; the patient is instructed to indicate the stimulated area with a fingertip. Lips, tongue, inner cheek, and palate should be examined for sensory deficits.

Feeding and Swallowing Examination

After the initial oral examination, the patient should be given small quantities of liquids and solids so that functional limitations may be observed. Any patient who exhibited severe deficits of tongue and mandible control should not be given solids during this examination.

Lip function. One should assess the adequacy of lip seal during sucking and swallowing. Leakage or inability to maintain seal during sucking indicates impaired function. One should assess the ability of the upper lip to remove food from a spoon.

Tongue function. One should assess the patient's ability to use the tongue to localize and retrieve food placed between the dental surfaces. Food packing indicates deficiencies in lateral tongue movement and buccinator muscle control. Tongue biting occurs with reduced tonus or sensation. Tongue pumping or continuous forward repetitive movements of the tongue suggest incoordination of muscular control or reduced ability to build sufficient intraoral breath pressure.

Jaw and cheek function. Cheek flapping (puffing out), poor sucking ability, and food packing suggest flaccid tonus of the buccinator muscle. Functional chewing consists of rotary as opposed to vertical jaw movement. Hyperextension of the jaw during mouth opening, with mandibular subluxation, may suggest abnormal tone in the muscles that open the mouth, rather than weakness (6); hyperextension will interrupt the normal rebound closure necessary for rhythmic chewing.

Palatal, pharyngeal, and laryngeal function. Nasal regurgitation and, in some cases, weak sucking ability imply palatal dysfunction. Coughing, choking, and aspiration are signs of pharyngeal paresis, reduced laryngeal excursion, or poor glottal closure. In addition to the organic symptoms presented, the patient may experience limitations caused by fear of aspiration and pain. After extended intubation feeding, the mucous membranes may become irritated, causing pain during the swallowing process, especially in the pharyngeal stage. This can lead to voluntary interruption of swallowing during the oral stage and may produce an adequate but static swallowing pattern.

MANAGEMENT OF DYSPHAGIA

Medical Compensatory Methods

Alternate methods of feeding, such as syringe, orogastric and nasogastric tubes, and intravenous infusion, are frequently employed means of medical management. As mentioned earlier, these are temporary measures that may be used simultaneously with therapeutic techniques to rehabilitate the patient's feeding and swallowing ability.

Surgical Methods

Surgical reconstruction may be achieved through a number of bypass procedures chosen after careful consideration of the patient's problems and needs. Esophagostomy is often the procedure of choice; it provides a low-visibility permanent stoma in the lower neck through which a feeding tube is passed at mealtime. A pharyngotomy provides a stoma high in the neck that is highly visible and often presents difficulties when changing the tube. With gastrostomy a tube is placed through the lower abdomen to the stomach; this requires partial undressing for feeding. A jejunostomy is useful in cases of esophageal reflux; it provides bypass to the small intestine, often increasing the problem of diarrhea. Several reversible procedures have been developed that separate the alimentary and respiratory tracts, thus allowing the patient a safe means of feeding while dysphagia rehabilitation is being conducted. If the patient improves, the surgical procedure can be reversed. These include the epiglottic arytenoid flap, vocal cord closure, and laryngeal diversion. Finally, in cases of extreme drooling, decreased salivary flow can be achieved through tympanic neurectomy and parotid duct ligation (4).

Therapeutic Methods

There is a paucity of information in the literature concerning rehabilitation techniques for adult neuropathic dysphagia. Larsen (9) and Griffen (10) reported treatment programs that stressed maximum use of assets, capitalizing on conscious volitional control to support reflexive swallowing behavior. Buckley et al. (11) published guidelines for dysphagia stressing sensorimotor reflex positioning and stimulation techniques designed to increase muscle tone, encourage normal sensory feedback, and heighten motor control.

The management approach described in the remainder of this chapter emphasizes a combination of symptom and compensatory techniques that stress inhibition of negative symptoms and excitation of oral sensation, increased muscle tonus, and oroneuromotor control. It is important to keep in mind as the principles of swallowing management are discussed that there is an emphasis on symptom alleviation to provide better support for the underlying mechanisms that are used in swallowing and feeding. Many of the techniques may not be applied indiscriminately; they require the expertise of an experienced therapist who has adequate knowledge and training in principles of neuromuscular facilitation and proprioceptive feedback. The exercises listed here by no means exhaust the possibilities; they provide a sampling of the methods that can be selected and adapted for effective treatment of dysphagia.

Positioning. One general rule to be followed when feeding a dysphagic patient is that the patient should be sitting upright at a 90 degree angle with the head and chin tilted slightly forward and down. This position facilitates swallowing by taking advantage of gravitational force and affords the best protection against aspiration of food because the larynx is protected by the back of the tongue (9). The head position must be maintained throughout, despite the natural tendency to throw the head back in an attempt to force food back into the pharynx. The upright position should be maintained for 15 to 30 min before and after eating (11). Patients who can are encouraged to feed themselves. Those who require assistance are fed with the therapist sitting slightly lower than the patient to encourage good head posture.

Environmental considerations. Whenever possible, the environment should be kept pleasant and quiet, free from distractions that might heighten anxiety and interfere with the patient's concentration. This caution should not be taken lightly, as certain aspects of the oral phase and control of respiration during the pharyngeal phase may require conscious voluntary effort.

Food considerations. A pureed diet provides a limited taste range and minimal pressure stimulation to the oral receptors. Soft, slightly chewable food is often preferred. Food that has more texture triggers sensory receptors, provides some resistance for increased tone, increases saliva flow, and is more palatable. Some dietary considerations for a soft chewable diet are listed in Appendix B. Liquid, especially water, has a tendency to trigger coughing and choking. There are some minor differences of opinion regarding temperature considerations. Larsen (9) and Dobbie (4) suggested hot or cold liquids rather than tepid liquids, claiming that they increase sensory input, whereas Buckley et al. (11) contended that liquids that are too hot or too cold have an anesthetic effect and diminish subsequent taste sensation. He favored room-temperature foods.

Patients who are at high risk of aspiration may require initial swallowing training with lemon glycerine swabs or fruit juice popsicles to stimulate saliva swallowing prior to the introduction of food. Substitute chewing practice can be conducted with "tea-bag" foods; i.e., food is placed in a piece of cheesecloth and is firmly tied and attached to a string, which is held by the therapist. The bag is then used for chewing practice and stimulation of the oral swallowing stage.

Oral sensation. Food that is attractive and palatable will help stimulate the flow of saliva and increase the desire to eat. If evaluation has revealed sensory deficits, then it will be necessary to determine the tongue receptor areas that have the strongest sensation. Small amounts of food (including sweet, salt, sour, and bitter) are placed on the center of the tongue and then on either side, anteriorly and posteriorly, to be identified by the patient. When the strongest receptor areas have been located, amounts and textures are increased. Storey (12) indicated that tactile receptors are responsible for initiating the swallowing reflex. Rood speculated that mobility of the tongue was facilitated by taste stimuli (13). She determined that bitter solutions were useful in activating tongue protrusion, whereas sweet and pleasant stimuli were responsible for activating tongue retraction in preparation for swallowing. McCracken (6) speculated that swallowing may be facilitated by increased tactile perception, which is brought about by any therapy to the oral area.

Oral reflex control. The palatal and gag reflexes are protective functions that are present from birth and are retained throughout life. Hypoactive reflexes may be activated and strengthened by increased sensation. An attempt to excite the palatal and pharyngeal reflexes to evoke a more normal rate of swallowing (approximately twice per minute) may be made by stimulating the back of the tongue with a tongue depressor or brush, by velar stroking, or by directing a stream of water from an eyedropper against the posterior pharyngeal wall (6,7).

Hyperactive or exaggerated reflexes require desensitization. The gag reflex is desensitized by applying strong pressure with the fingers walking back on the tongue and stopping just prior to excitation of the reflex. This procedure is continued gradually, increasing the parameters until the reflex is elicited only by stimulation to the posterior portion of the tongue. During feeding, the gag reflex is diminished by applying firm pressure down on the tongue with the bowl of the spoon when inserting food (14).

Primitive reflexes are brought under control by providing appropriate stimulation and preventing the expected reflex pattern. For example, the rooting reflex is elicited by tapping the angles of the mouth or stroking the cheek outward from the angle; the anticipated response is aborted by asserting strong pressure on the lip angle and lower lip (15). The mouth-opening reflex is elicited by presentation of a visual stimulus to the mouth; the response is aborted by holding the lips closed. For oral reflex control it is advisable to allow the patient to provide self-stimulation when possible; this is believed to be more tolerable. The jaw control techniques outlined by Mueller (14) may be necessary in feeding adults who exhibit released infantile oral reflexes.

Increased oral muscle tone. A general technique that involves coordinated control of the lips, tongue, cheeks, and palate is resisted sucking. The patient who has severe limitations in oral muscle strength and control should begin with low-resistance fluids. Fluid is trapped in a straw by placing a finger over one end and dipping the other end in a glass of liquid. The straw is placed between the lips, and the fluid is sucked out while resistance is maintained. The fluid can be released suddenly; this, when combined with the increased intraoral pressure, will cause the fluid to spurt to the posterior pharyngeal wall, triggering contraction of the pharyngeal constrictors and swallowing. When this task has been mastered, higher-resistance substances (diluted applesauce, yogurt, thick milk shakes) may be used. Strengthening of lip closure can be facilitated by the addition of a disc, through which the straw is placed, held firmly against the lips. Fast brushing, icing, or vibration of the orbicularis oris may be a necessary prerequisite to stimulate mouth closure (6).

Nonfeeding techniques may be developed that use the same skills. For example, in resisted sucking a Ping-Pong ball or large bean may be substituted for the fluid, with the patient sucking the object up against the end of the straw and maintaining it there for progressively longer periods of time. A nonfeeding technique designed to strengthen lip closure is to place a button, held firmly by a string, between the patient's lips in front of the teeth; steady resistive pressure is obtained by pulling the string while the patient maintains the seal. Smaller buttons are substituted to develop more finite control.

Resistance techniques can be applied to increase tongue tip elevation and lateral movements. For tongue tip elevation, a tongue depressor is placed horizontally across the superior surface of the protruded tongue tip, with mild resistance; the patient is requested to push the depressor up to the upper lip. For resisted lateralization, the broad surface of the tongue depressor is placed against the lateral surface of the tongue; the patient is asked to push the depressor to the inner surface of the cheek.

Increased glottal control. Intact glottal closure is essential for temporary cessation of respiration and to protect from aspiration. Pushing or lifting techniques, designed primarily to increase laryngeal tonus and vocal fold approximation for voicing, have a secondary effect of temporarily halting respiration to allow for the buildup of thoracic pressure. The patient should be sitting in a chair with palms placed against the under surface of a solid table, then instructed to push up against the table while holding the breath (5).

Increased oral coordination. Suppression of the primitive reflex patterns mentioned earlier is vital to reinstate the oral control and coordination necessary for feeding as well as for speech. A pattern frequently observed with severe limitation of oral coordination is reduced differentiation of oral movement. Differentiation work is done to improve control of the articulators for isolated voluntary movements. Sample differentiation exercises are suggested in the book by Mysak (5). The patient is asked to extend the mandible to a half-open position and then spread and pucker the lips while keeping the tongue and mandible still. Then, with the mandible at a three-quarter-open position, the patient is asked to move the tongue tip up behind the upper teeth and then down behind the lower teeth, continuing the alternation while maintaining no movement of lips or jaw. Then the patient is asked to flex and extend the mandible while inhibiting any movement of the lips or tongue. If the patient does not manifest sufficient control on a voluntary level, assistance may be provided with stabilizing devices. A jaw block or thick rubber eraser may be placed between the teeth during tongue or lip alternating exercises, or the patient may be asked to stabilize the tongue against the alveolar ridge while performing alternated jaw movements.

Special problems. When swallowing is delayed or when incomplete swallowing occurs and food remains in the mouth, the chin should be pressed downward toward the sternum; frequently this will cause a counteracting response, with oppositional elevation of the larynx. Another technique is to press the larynx gently from the lateral borders, with side-to-side action and upward movement.

Chewing and swallowing may require extreme

effort and concentration, and this can fatigue the patient before nutritional needs have been met. Nursing and dietary staffs should be consulted to provide smaller and more frequent feedings throughout the day.

Feeding a patient with a tracheostomy tube requires extreme caution. If the patient has a cuffed tracheostomy tube, temporary inflation of the tube will provide some protection against aspiration but will not totally prevent it. The tracheostomy tube generally interferes with laryngeal elevation, thus adding to the dysphagia (4).

CONCLUSION

No controlled studies of adult central nervous system dysphagias have been reported in the literature. Furthermore, there is an alarming lack of information regarding evaluation and management of these patients. Questions of patient selection, nature and amount of treatment, and prognosis are virtually unanswered. The issue of who should treat swallowing disorders remains unclear. Traditionally, occupational, speech, and physical therapists have attempted to provide therapeutic intervention; however, the limited information available and the lack of clarity regarding roles have more often resulted in no treatment for these patients.

Dysphagia stems from various neuropathological processes that result in many forms of dysfunction: muscular atrophy, paralysis, spasticity, and hyperreflexia, dysfunction of oral sensory mechanisms, release of infantile oral reflexes. Still not much is known about dysphagia symptom complexes as they relate to specific causes. Brain and Walton (1) reported that in lower motor neuron diseases such as progressive bulbar palsy, amyotrophic lateral sclerosis, and progressive muscular atrophy, there is initial tongue wasting and lip paresis followed by palatal involvement and eventually pharyngeal and laryngeal muscular atrophy, whereas in upper motor neuron disease (pseudobulbar palsy) there is muscular spasticity, with exaggeration of jaw jerk, palatal and pharyngeal reflexes, and release phenomena. Also, commonly seen are mixed upper and lower motor neuron dysphagias in which symptoms of atrophy, paresis, and spasticity are combined. Identification and analysis of these and other dysphagia symptom complexes would aid in the development of specific treatment programs for the various symptom complexes. Careful assessment of abilities and dysfunctions will allow for symptom-specific treatment, as opposed to symptom-composite treatment, and will permit maximum use of assets to assist in the alleviation of dysfunction as well as in the development of compensatory function.

REFERENCES

1. Brain, W. R., and Walton, J. (1969): *Diseases of the Nervous System.* Oxford University Press, London.
2. Zoethout, W. D., and Tuttle, W. W. (1955): *Textbook of Physiology.* C. V. Mosby, St. Louis.
3. Davenport, H. W. (1961): *Physiology of the Digestive Tract.* Year Book, Chicago.
4. Dobbie, R. A. (1978): Rehabilitation of swallowing disorders. *Am. Fam. Physician,* 17:84–95.
5. Mysak, E. D. (1976): *Pathologies of Speech Systems.* Williams & Wilkins, Baltimore.
7. McCracken, A. (1978): Drool control and tongue thrust therapy for the mentally retarded. *Am. J. Occup. Ther.,* 32:79–85.
7. Mysak, E. D. (1968): *Neuroevolutional Approach to Cerebral Palsy and Speech.* Teachers College Press, New York.
8. Johnson, W., Darley, F. L., and Spriestersbach, D. C. (1963): *Diagnostic Methods in Speech Pathology.* Harper & Row, New York.
9. Larsen, G. L. (1972): Rehabilitation for dysphagia paralytica. *J. Speech Hear. Disord.,* 37:187–194.
10. Griffen, K. M. (1974): Swallowing training for dysphagic patients. *Arch. Phys. Med. Rehabil.,* 55:467–470.
11. Buckley, J. E., Addicks, C. L., and Maniglia, J. (1976): Feeding patients with dysphagia. *Nurs. Forum,* 15:69–85.
12. Storey, A. T. (1967): Extra-trigeminal sensory systems related to oral function. In: *Symposium on Oral Sensation and Perception,* edited by J. F. Bosma, pp. 83–97. Charles C. Thomas, Springfield, Ill.
13. Stockmeyer, S. A. (1967): An interpretation of the approach of Rood to the treatment of neuromuscular dysfunction. *Am. J. Phys. Med.,* 46:900–956.
14. Mueller, H. A. (1972): Facilitating feeding and prespeech. In: *Physical Therapy Services in Developmental Disabilities,* edited by P. H. Pearson and C. E. Williams, pp. 283–310. Springfield, Ill.
15. Mysak, E. D. (1963): Dysarthria and oropharyngeal reflexology: A review. *J. Speech Hear. Disord.,* 28:252–260.

BIBLIOGRAPHY

Ardan, G. M., and Kemp, F. H. (1970): Some important factors in the assessment of oral pharyngeal function. *Dev. Med. Child Neurol.*, 12:158–166.

Ingram, T. T. S. (1962): Clinical significance of the infantile feeding reflexes. *Dev. Med. Child Neurol.*, 4:159–169.

Kabat, H., and Knott, M. (1953): Proprioceptive facilitation techniques for treatment of paralysis. *Phys. Ther. Rev.*, 33:53–63.

Kawamura, Y., and Morimoto, T. (1973): Neurophysiological mechanisms related to reflex control of tongue movements. *Symp. Oral Sens. Percept.*, 4:206–217.

Ogg, H. L. (1975): Oral-pharyngeal development and evaluation. *Phys. Ther. Rev.*, 55:235–241.

Pitcher, J. L. (1973): Dysphagia in the elderly: Causes and diagnosis. *Geriatrics*, 28:64–69.

Rood, M. (1954): Neurophysiological reactions as a basis for physical therapy. *Phys. Ther. Rev.*, 34:444–449.

Semans, S. (1967): The Bobath concept in treatment of neurological disorders. *Am. J. Phys. Med.*, 46:732–785.

Sheppard, J. J. (1964): Cranio-oropharyngeal motor patterns in dysarthria associated with cerebral palsy. *J. Speech Hear. Res.*, 7:373–380.

APPENDIX A: DYSPHAGIA EXAMINATION

I. *Report of patient's problem*

A. *Dietary management*

____intravenous____nasogastric tube ____syringe____other. Foods tolerated by mouth:____fluids____puree ____solids

B. *Symptoms*

____drooling (saliva/food)____oral retention____nasal reflux____oral reflux ____food packing (right/left)____biting (lip/tongue/cheek)____coughing ____aspiration

II. *Oral mechanism examination*

A. *Reflexes*

1. Protective reflexes:
Palatal:____normal____hyperactive ____hypoactive____absent____; gag:____normal____hyperactive ____hypoactive____absent
2. Primitive reflexes (check if present):
____mouth-opening____lip____ biting____suckling____rooting ____chewing____

B. *Lip strength and coordination*

1. Symmetry:____right____left
2. Range:____elevation____depression____pursing____retraction
3. Coordination:____alternated pursing/retraction____moves independent of jaw/tongue

C. *Tongue strength and coordination*

1. Symmetry and tone:____deviates right____left____fasciculations ____protrudes at rest
2. Range:____protrusion____retraction____elevation____depression ____lateralization right____left
3. Coordination:____alternated protrusion/retraction____alternates elevation/depression____alternates lateralization____moves independent of lips/jaw

D. *Cheek and jaw strength and coordination*

1. Symmetry and tone:____cheek____ jaw deviation right____left____palpation masseter____temporalis
2. Range (jaw):____lateral____extension
3. Coordination:____rapid jaw clicking ____moves independent lip/tongue

E. *Palatal movement*

1. Symmetry:____deviation at rest ____during movement
2. Elevation:____production "a"____ sustained "a"____absent
3. Function:____nasal speech

F. *Laryngeal excursion and glottal closure*

1. Symmetry:____deviation right____ left
2. Closure:____holds breath____ breathy voice____on-off "a"

G. *Oral sensation*

1. Perioral (light touch):____lip____ tongue____palate____cheek

III. *Swallowing Examination*

A. *Lip function*

____closure____leakage____seal for sucking____removal/spoon

B. *Tongue function*

____directs food between teeth____localizes/retrieves food_____tongue pumping_____biting_____tongue-thrust swallow

C. *Cheek and jaw function*
_____cheek flapping_____straw sucking _____rotary chewing_____vertical chewing_____hyperextended jaw

D. *Palatal, pharyngeal, and laryngeal function*
_____nasal regurgitation_____coughing _____choking_____aspiration

E. *Swallowing function*
_____static swallow_____continuous swallow_____delayed_____incomplete _____oral retention fluids/foods

APPENDIX B: SOFT CHEWABLE FOOD SUGGESTIONS FOR DYSPHAGIC PATIENTS

Dairy

Avoid all milk products, when possible, as they tend to increase production of mucus, which will cause an increase in coughing/choking syndrome in many patients. Introduce milk products slowly; start with hard cheeses or potted cheeses. Eggs: scrambled or soft boiled (avoid hard-cooked yolks).

Meats

Ground meats, meatballs, stews, soft fish (not flaky or dry); avoid tough-fiber meats; no pureed meats. Gravy and tomato sauces are advisable to moisten meats.

Starches

Mashed potatoes, fat noodles (avoid thin spaghetti or rice); moisten with gravy. Bread with butter, moistened soft toast (with jam or butter). Avoid cake textures and crackers.

Vegetables

Any soft chewable vegetable such as cooked carrots, squash, spinach, beans, etc. (avoid small pieces, such as peas).

Fruits

Canned fruits such as chopped or slightly mashed peaches, pears, fruit cocktail, stewed apples, prunes, cooked cherries (no pits); progress to fresh fruits such as raw apples, pears, bananas, ripe peaches, peeled whenever necessary.

Fluids

Diluted mild juices (apple or cranberry), juice nectars, soups (avoid cream soups initially), coffee or tea as tolerated; avoid carbonated colas.

All food selections should be planned in conjunction with a dietitian unless the patient has no dietary restrictions and nutrition is already under controlled supervision. The preceding food choices are suggestions only. Adaptations should be made in keeping with the patient's food preferences and ease in swallowing.

Adult Perceptual Motor Evaluation and Management

19

Nina Wold-Tortelli, Sophia Chioteli, Susan Miron-Bernstein, and Laurie Kalb-Ritter

A person in the act of perceiving engages in an active process that involves locating and extracting information from the environment, then evaluating, processing, and organizing that information; hence perception is a basic process that is used to acquire cognition or knowledge and cannot be dissociated from any aspect of human organization, including development, learning, thinking, creativity, personality, and social interaction (1). Beginning from this holistic view of the perceptual process, this chapter will be concerned with the management of patients who have experienced a breakdown in this process and who are faced with the functional deficits that accompany brain damage. The discussion will focus on (a) current evaluation procedures used in occupational therapy to assess deficits and their interpretation and (b) approaches and treatment techniques used in training patients to compensate for or diminish such deficits in order to facilitate functional recovery.

To provide some perspective, a brief description of the treatment facility will be given. The Institute of Rehabilitation Medicine (IRM) is an acute rehabilitation center located in New York City. On the average, services for 117 adult inpatients ranging in age from 17 to 80 years are provided. Of these patients, 50% to 60% are brain-damaged, primarily as a result of cerebral vascular accident. The average hospitalization is 3 months, after which some patients are followed as outpatients. Every brain-damaged patient undergoes a comprehensive evaluation of sensory, motor, perceptual, and cognitive systems by a multidiscipline team. This interdisciplinary collaboration continues throughout the patient's therapy, with program assessment monthly. In addition, the institute has a research and training program for the study of brain damage that is carried out by the Behavioral Sciences Department. This program is made possible through research funding and is primarily concerned with development and testing techniques used in training patients with specific cognitive perceptual deficits. Because of experimental design considerations, patients must meet specific criteria to be eligible for this program. Several techniques whose efficacies have been demonstrated experimentally have been incorporated by the Occupational Therapy Department as part of clinical practice for treatment of brain-damaged patients (2). During the following discussion, two fundamental concepts should be kept in mind: (a) In this program, no single theoretical principle of treatment is preferred. Rather, a combination of techniques is used, and these are constantly being adapted, elaborated, and structured as needed. (b) Activity is the stimulus underlying all occupational therapy treatment, and that activity must be selected because of its inherent qualities and anticipated effect on the response of the patient (3). It should be kept in mind that this program involves a team approach, as much as possible, and that at times it is necessary to have overlapping of interdisciplinary roles.

EVALUATION

In these evaluation procedures for brain-damaged adults, specific tests have been selected that focus on the impairments that occur most frequently and that cause the greatest interference with optimum functioning. As a general rule, an evaluation procedure should undergo periodic revision to meet the changing demands of the program. Revision takes place by application of new knowledge one gathers from clinical experience, from the literature, and from the results of research. The evaluation procedure that will be discussed here was developed and revised over a period of several years. This evaluation procedure has been used in its current state for approximately 1 year with an adult population.

The evaluation procedure involves three parts: physical assessment, sensory-perceptual-motor assessment, and integrated function summary. The procedures of the individual tests are carried out according to test directions and are scored accordingly. Procedures for administration and key are available from IRM. For the most part, the tests are not standardized for adults, but an attempt has been made to decrease subjectivity by establishing specific methods of administration and measurement. It is hoped that in future endeavors the currently recorded data can be quantified and validated and thereby used to develop standards.

The results of each test are not viewed singularly; rather, results are interpreted as a whole in such a way that the therapist considers the interrelationship of all findings, along with the patient's observed behavior. The patient's behavior is observed throughout the evaluation, since it does influence the method of administering the evaluation and may affect the reliability and interpretation of the results. Lack of orientation, the presence of impulsivity, lability, motor impersistence, and perseveration are all informally indicated, if present. Other behaviors informally observed are attitude, frustration tolerance, endurance, attention span, ability to follow directions, awareness of errors, and ability in self-correction (Appendix A).

Individual differences among patients and their levels of functioning must be kept in mind during testing so that certain tests can be eliminated or elaborated in order to best understand a particular patient's limitations and capabilities. The following is a brief description of each of the sections of the evaluation procedure and its functional significance.

Physical Assessment

Physical assessment is usually carried out first, with the patient in the sitting position. During physical assessment, both the impaired and nonimpaired extremities are tested, the patient being essentially passive. The time spent in conducting this part of the procedure provides an opportunity for the therapist and patient to establish rapport so that they will feel comfortable with each other. The therapist can begin to determine the best method of giving directions and can observe any behaviors and problems that will require specific testing later. Physical movement is assessed according to Brunnstrom's six stages of recovery (4).

Physical factors such as impaired balance, impairments in sitting position and in mobility, decreased range of motion, and spasticity decrease the patient's body awareness, thus inhibiting normal sensory input. Such deprivation significantly influences the patient's sensory-perceptual-motor functions (5).

Sensory-Perceptual-Motor Assessment

Sensory Status

Primary sensations (touch sensation, hot/cold sensitivity, kinesthetic awareness, and static position sense) are tested throughout the upper extremities. Pressure touch sensitivity in the hands is measured using the Semmes-Weinstein pressure esthesiometer (6). Decreased sensibility significantly influences coordination in the involved extremity. Intact sensibilities are important in accurately interpreting one's environment for proper motor output and accurate perceptual functioning.

Perceptual-Motor Status

Stereognosis is an integrative ability based on synthesis of elementary tactile and kinesthetic sensations and cognition. It is tested by having the patient identify by means of touch an object placed in the hand (7). The significance of astereognosis for the patient's function is limited; testing of stereognosis is done investigatively rather than to determine implications for treatment.

Sensory neglect involves extinction of stimuli when double simultaneous stimulation (DSS) is administered to both the face and hands, whereas sensibility is intact when hands and face are tested separately. The rationale for this extinction phenomenon is discussed by Bender (8).

Patients who have extinguished stimuli on DSS, with no primary sensory loss, are frequently observed to disregard their involved extremity and even those who have the physical potential for functioning neglect to use that arm when performing tasks.

Investigation of *visual fields* is done through the confrontation test. The patient is instructed to look directly forward; then the therapist presents a stimulus at each periphery. A primary visual field cut is usually indicated when the stimulus is given on the involved side and unobserved by the patient. However, even when the visual fields are intact, visual neglect of stimuli on the involved side may be observed when visual stimuli are presented to both sides simultaneously (8). Functionally, patients with either a visual field cut or visual neglect will be recognized by the fact that they do not respond to a portion of the visual environment.

Oculomotor pursuit involves having the patient visually track a moving target. Lack of oculomotor control may be caused by weak eye musculature, resulting in diplopia, or it may be caused by motor impersistence, resulting in impaired visual attention (9).

Visual scanning is an integrative process in which an image is briefly fixed on the fovea as the eyes scan a given surface of the environment. Impairments are determined with a simple search task such as letter cancellation, which has been standardized for adults by the IRM Behavioral Psychology Research Department. Their studies indicate that scanning is an essential information-gathering process involved in all activities. Scanning impairments may be informally observed during testing and in functional tasks. The consequences of scanning impairments are various degrees of lack of awareness (visual inattention) of the environment, depending on severity (11).

Determination of spatial relationships involves the capacity to receive and interpret sensory stimuli from all modalities (e.g., sight, hearing, touch) to build up postural sensation and awareness of the body and its image and parts. Although determination of spatial relationships is an integrative ability incorporating all senses, most methods of evaluation involve object manipulation in space or multiple-choice responses to visual-spatial tasks. At IRM the Ayres design copying test is used to evaluate this function; it involves copying line drawings ranging from simple to moderately complex (5). Results from the design copying test are interpreted in combination with those from purely visual multiple-choice tasks such as the Vanguard school program (10). Deficits in visual-spatial abilities often cause problems with dressing, maneuverability in the environment, and general orientation and organization on all tasks.

Figure-ground discrimination involves selective responses to given stimuli, focusing on the essential and ignoring the irrelevant. Accurate responses in a figure-ground test exercise the patient's capabilities in visual scanning, attention to detail, spatial relationships, and ability to concentrate on a task. The Ayres figure-ground test is used (5).

Tests of eye-hand coordination measure the patient's ability to coordinate sight with hand movements to produce precise skilled actions. The Purdue pegboard is used for evaluation of eye-hand coordination. This test has been modified and standardized for brain-damaged adults at IRM. Impairments in this area may be evident when the patient is required to perform skilled activities such as writing.

Praxis involves the ability to skillfully perform

voluntary movements. A disturbance or disintegration of the dynamics of the motor act, despite the presence of adequate motor power, sensation, and coordination, is termed apraxia (7). Three general categories are evaluated: kinesthetic praxis, ideational praxis, and constructional praxis.

Imitation of postures is used to evaluate gross *kinesthetic praxis*. Disturbances (e.g., misplacement of extremity, incoordination of movement, hesitation) may be observed when the patient understands the concept and purpose of the requested action but cannot carry out the act, implying that the relationship between the idea of the movement and its motor execution is disrupted. It has been hypothesized that the patient has difficulty in selecting or is unable to select the required kinesthetic modulated program for bringing about the requested movement (7). A modified version of Luria's fist-and-finger test is used for testing praxis of finer motions. Examples of kinesthetic apraxia include difficulty in coordinating hand and leg movements for propelling a wheelchair, unusual difficulty in coordinating steps for a transfer, difficulty in following demonstrated directions, and awkward manipulation of objects, such as a pen for writing.

Ideational apraxia is impairment in the processes that occur between language comprehension and motor encoding (12). It has been speculated that in performing normal voluntary movement, the anticipation of the movement produces the desired movement by evoking the proper kinesthetic engram. Heilman (11) suggested that the deficit in ideational apraxia is in the "verbal mediated motor sequence selector." Evaluation of ideational praxis begins with requesting the patient to use objects that are presented (e.g., an electric razor or a toothbrush). One can also observe the patient's performance on any task in which sequencing is required while using an object. Deficits are observed when movements are irrelevant or inappropriate (misuse of object, incorrect sequence) and the patient appears not to understand the command: A patient might persevere in putting an electric razor to the hair, a pencil to the mouth, or, in less severe cases, incorrectly sequencing the steps while participating in tasks such as grooming. In ideational apraxia the ability to handle objects is preserved.

Constructional praxis involves the ability to properly coordinate the spatial properties of the visual fields with the motor or constructional responses. The patient performing a constructional task has to analyze the following components: the idea of the completed task, the design or image of the work when the job is begun, the mental picture of the various fractionated activities in their temporal sequence and the manual technique (13). Benton's three-dimensional constructional praxis clinical test is used which involves constructing three wooden models. It is often observed that patients with left hemiplegia display impairment resulting from visual-spatial deficits and patients with right hemiplegia have difficulty with the motor (praxis) components of a task.

The functional portion of this evaluation procedure consists in observing the patient's performance during the activities of daily living (ADL) (Appendix A). There may not be adequate time for a complete functional evaluation during the first few sessions. Some complex tasks, such as dressing, are often postponed until later, since current deficits can create considerable difficulty and frustration for the patient.

Integrated Function

Assessment of integrated function includes a summary of actual or predicted ADL status. Perceptual testing alone will not allow determination of the functional significance of certain deficits. Functional evaluation alone will not provide enough information for an understanding of the specific nature of a patient's difficulties. Therefore it is necessary to do both types of testing in order to obtain comprehensive information regarding the patient's functional status. In interpreting the results of testing, the therapist must consider all behavioral factors, the interrelationship of deficits found during task performance, as well as specific test outcomes. The integrated function portion of the evaluation incorporates all information necessary for arriving at a final summary of actual or predicted performance in functional activities and developing a treatment plan.

TREATMENT PROCEDURES

After the evaluation is completed and key problems have been identified, a therapeutic intervention program is formulated to diminish the deficits and use the patient's residual capabilities to relearn skills. Therapeutic planning is developed by considering the following: (a) Key problems are examined as they relate to the patient's physical and perceptual function and functional life activities. (b) Short- and long-term goals are established. (c) Appropriate approaches and therapeutic activities are analyzed and selected to best ameliorate the deficits (3). Periodically, goals are reassessed, and approaches are adjusted or changed accordingly.

The IRM treatment approaches can be termed (a) active sensory processing, (b) skill generalization, and (c) functional integration/adaptation. Their application in treatment is guided by the needs of the patient and the skill of the therapist. These approaches are often used in combination, and the emphasis of each may vary during the patient's treatment. Inherent in all three is a cueing system that will be outlined later.

Active sensory processing. This approach involves the appropriate use of sensory input (kinesthetic, vestibular, tactile, visual, and auditory) to effect change while the patient is engaged in purposeful activity (5). For example, an effective change might be increased awareness of the impaired side of the body, which could result in improvements in sitting position, balance, body scheme, praxis, etc., and improved visual awareness of the environment.

Skills generalization. This approach uses structured generic tasks presented in a systematic way, depending on the severity of the patient's deficits and the purpose of the task, that provide the patient with the optimum atmosphere for learning. The tasks presented are primarily paper-and-pencil and table-top activities, such as parquetry and block designs, constructional projects, and academic worksheets. Having successfully learned certain skills, the patient can then use those skills and this system of learning in other functional activities.

Functional integration/adaptation. This approach involves the patient's actual practice of functional skills, such as eating, personal hygiene, dressing, homemaking, prevocational activities, and leisure activities. Again, according to the patient's problems, functional activity is structured and guided by the therapist. The patient will integrate or adapt the techniques necessary for the activities of daily living.

Fundamental to all three approaches is the use of a cueing system; this is the key to all these

TABLE 1. *Cueing system*

Behavior	Treatment
1. Patient will not recognize errors when they are pointed out.	1. Not amenable to saturation cueing.
2. Patient is able to recognize errors but cannot self-correct. Patient is not consistent in locating specific errors.	2. Cues are given to help patient locate errors.
3. Patient finds errors but cannot self-correct. Patient may attempt to self-correct, but is not often successful.	3. Cues are given to assist patient in self-correction.
4. Patient finds all errors and can self-cue for correction of errors.	4. Patient continues to err; however, therapist no longer gives cues to indicate errors or to self-correct.
5. Patient consistently performs with no errors.	5. No cues are given.

Note: A new higher-level task can be given when patient's behavior is at stage 5. Therapist returns to the stage of cues needed, depending on patient's behavior (approach) on the new task.

therapeutic intervention techniques, whether applied to generic skills development or functional skills development. Diller and associates (2) have developed some principles of cueing. Saturation cueing, with spotting and continuous feedback and validation as part of the cueing system, begins with the patient following a programmed cueing system devised in a decreasing order, from the most structured condition to the least structured condition of patient performance. Spotting consists in the therapist designating for the patient the order of execution of the maneuvers. Continuous feedback and validation occur as the patient monitors performance. This programming was conceived to form a continuum: training, cueing, learning, and internalization of problem solving.

In our programmed cueing system the term

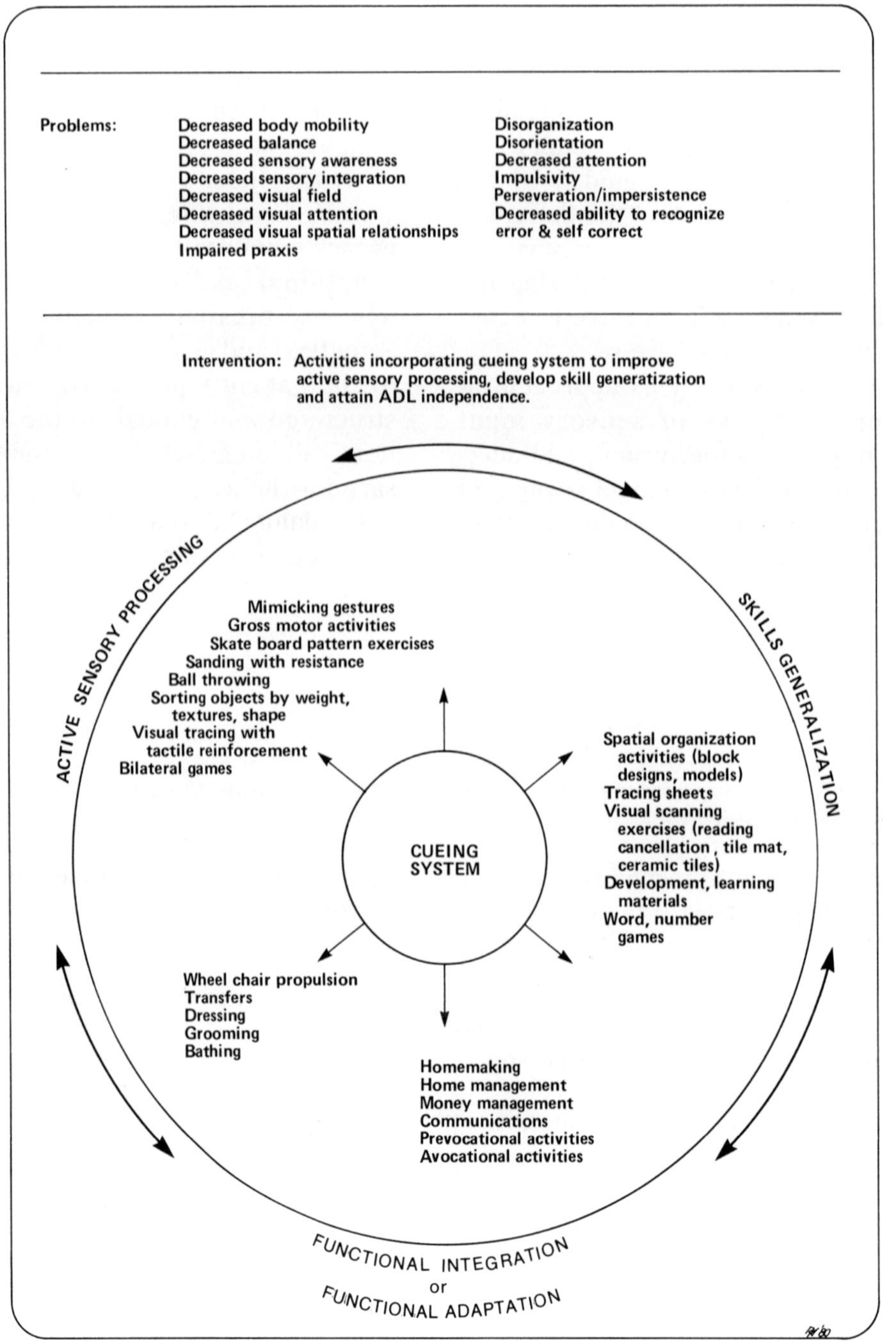

FIG. 1. IRM treatment model.

"cues" is used in a broad sense to include verbal, visual, tactile, manual, and auditory input or any combination of these given to the patient during treatment. This cueing system as used in occupational therapy requires appropriate selection of the activity, whether it be throwing a ball, copying a block design, or putting on a shirt, appropriate structuring of that activity, and finally appropriate use of cues. To understand the patient's level of performance and potential to learn, the therapist must determine the patient's awareness of error. Patients who deny their errors often are not amenable to treatment and do not profit from cues (7). Initially, cues should help patients identify their errors if they are unable to do this on their own. The therapist should intervene if patients are unable to cue themselves. Cues should be consistent in quality and quantity from session to session and should be taught to staff and family members for reinforcement. Patients are expected to be active participants in the cueing system. During performance of activities, the therapist will be taking note of patients' abilities to recognize errors, correct themselves, and carry over learning. Patients who do not integrate cues and carry over learning are best treated with a purely functional approach, where the environment or functional task is adapted to allow for optimum performance. Table 1 illustrates the method of cueing that applies to most patient-therapist relationships in this system.

SUMMARY

The IRM treatment model is summarized in Fig. 1. It is hoped that this description of these evaluation procedures and approaches to treatment will lead to increased collection of data for research studies in the evaluation and management of brain-damaged adults.

ACKNOWLEDGMENTS

The authors wish to thank the occupational therapy staff at IRM for their assistance throughout the years, and a special thank you to Carol Seplowitz for her major contribution in the development of the evaluation form.

REFERENCES

1. Forgus, R. H. (1966): *Perception of the Basic Process in Cognitive Development*. McGraw-Hill, New York.
2. Diller, L., et al. (1974): *Studies in Cognition and Rehabilitation in Hemiplegia*. Rehabilitation Monograph No. 50, Institute of Rehabilitation Medicine, New York University Medical Center, New York.
3. Llorens, L. A. (1973): Activity analysis for cognitive perceptual motor dysfunction. *Am. J. Occup. Ther.*, 27:453–456.
4. Brunnstrom, S. (1970): *Movement Therapy in Hemiplegia*. Harper & Row, New York.
5. Ayres, A. J. (1972): *Sensory Integration and Learning Disorders*. Western Psychological Services, Los Angeles.
6. Semmes-Weinstein Pressure Aesthesiometer, Research Media, 4 Midland Ave., Hicksville, N.Y. 11801.
7. Luria, A. R. (1966): *Higher Cortical Functions in Man*. Basic Books, New York, pp. 354–355.
8. Bender, M. B. (1952): *Disorders in Perception*. Charles C Thomas, Springfield, Ill.
9. Ben-Yishay, Y., et al. (1968): *Neurology, Vol. 18: The Relationship Between Impersistence, Intellectual Function and Outcome of Rehabilitation in Patients with Left Hemiplegia*. Lancet, Boston, 852–861.
10. Vanguard School Program, Teaching Resources Corp., Boston.
11. Heilman K. M. (1973): Ideational apraxia—a redefinition. *Brain*, 96:861–864.
12. Benton, A. L., and Fogel, M. L. (1962): Three dimensional constructional praxis: Clinical test. *Arch. Neurol.*, 7:347–354.

BIBLIOGRAPHY

Chedru, F., Leblanc, M., and Lhermitte, F. (1973): Visual searching in normal and brain-damaged subjects (contribution to study of unilateral inattention). *Cortex*, 9:94–111.

De Renzi, E., and Scotti, G. (1970): Autotopagnosia: Fiction or reality? *Arch. Neurol.*, 23:221–227.

Lorenze, E. J., and Cancro, R. (1962): Dysfunction in visual perception with hemiplegia: Its relation to activities of daily living. *Arch. Phys. Med. Rehabil.*, 43:514–517.

Sanquet, J., et al. (1971): Disturbances of the body schema in relation to language impairment and hemispheric locus of lesion. *J. Neurol. Neurosurg. Psychiatry*, 34:496–501.

Siev, E., and Freishat, B. (1976): *Perceptual Dysfunction in the Adult Stroke Patient—A manual for Evaluation and Treatment*, Charles B. Slack, Thorofare, N.J.

APPENDIX A

INSTITUTE OF REHABILITATION MEDICINE
OCCUPATIONAL THERAPY SERVICE
CENTRAL NERVOUS SYSTEM EVALUATION

Patient's Name ______________________

Diagnosis

I PHYSICAL ASSESSMENT	Date		
A. Body attitude 1. Sitting position			
2. Balance			
3. Facial paralysis			

B. UNINVOLVED EXTREMITY R L	ROM	Functional Strength	ROM	Functional Strength	ROM	Functional Strength
Shoulder flexion						
Shoulder abduction						
Shoulder ext. rotation						
Elbow flexion						
Wrist extension						
Finger flexion						
Finger extension						
Grasp						
Lateral prehension						
Palmar prehension						
Dexterity						
C. INVOLVED EXTREMITY R L						
1. SUBLUXATION						
2. EDEMA						
3. PASSIVE MOTION						

a./Range of motion/b. Spasticity/c. Pain	ROM	Spas.	Pain	ROM	Spas.	Pain	ROM	Spas.	Pain
SHOULDER:									
Flexion to 180°									
Extension									
Abduction to 180°									
Adduction									
External rotation									
Internal rotation									

ELBOW:									
Flexion									
Extension									
FOREARM:									
Supination									
Pronation									
WRIST:									
Flexion									
Extension									
FINGERS:									
Flexion - MCP									
- PIP									
Extension - MCP									
- PIP									
THUMB:									
Flexion									
Extension									
Abduction									
Adduction									

4. ACTIVE MOTION: gross to isolated

Date:				COMMENTS:
a. SCAPULAR elevation				
retraction				
protraction				
b. ARM MOTION				
1) Flaccidity				
2) Synergies/components appearing				
3) Synergy/components initiated				
Flexor: Elevation				
Retraction				
Abduction				
Hyperextension				

External rotation			
Elbow flexion			
Supination			
Extensor: Adduct./int. rot.			
Elbow extension			
Pronation			
4) Beginning deviation from synergy			
Hand to same shoulder			
Hand to opposite shoulder			
Forward reach			
Pronation/supination			
Hand to lumbar region			
5) Beginning of independent motion			
Side reach			
Overhead reach			
Forward reach: ext./int. rot.			
6) Total recovery from synergy			
c. WRIST MOTIONS			
1. No voluntary motion			
2. Flexion			
3. Extension			
d. HAND MOTIONS			
1. No active motion elicited			
2. Semivoluntary mass grasp			
3. Voluntary mass grasp			
4. Voluntary mass extension			
5. Thumb motions: flexion			
extension			
abduction			
opposition			

e. ISOLATED PREHENSION PATTERNS	√	Pounds	√	Pounds	√	Pounds
Gross grasp & release Lateral prehension & release Palmar prehension & release Wrist stabilization						

Date:						
5. UNILATERAL SPEED TEST	R	L	R	L	R	L
a. Hand from lap to chin						
a. Hand from knee to opposite knee						

6. RECIPROCAL MOTIONS Date:			
a. Alternate drumming fists			
b. Alternate opening and closing fists			
c. Alternate pronation and supination			
d. Alternate touching shoulder/knee			

Date:						
7. SPONTANEOUS USE OF INVOLVED EXTREMITY	√	Total Perf.	√	Total Perf.	√	Total Perf.
a. Nonfunctional						
b. Gross assist						
c. Semifunctional						
d. Adequate						
e. Fully functional						

II SENSORY-PERCEPTUAL-MOTOR ASSESSMENT

Date:						
A. **SENSORY STATUS**	R	L	R	L	R	L
1. *Tactile sensation*						
a. Pressure touch						
b. Pressure sensitivity						
c. Hot/cold sensitivity						
2. *Kinesthetic awareness*						
Shoulder						
Elbow						
Wrist						
Fingers						
3. *Position sense*						
Shoulder						
Elbow						

Wrist						
Fingers						

B. SENSORY-PERCEPTUAL STATUS

1. *Stereognosis*						
2. *Double simultaneous stimulation*	R	L	R	L	R	L
L hand R hand						
L hand R cheek						
L cheek R cheek						
L hand L cheek						
R hand L cheek						
R hand R cheek						
L hand R cheek						
L hand R cheek						
L hand L cheek						
R hand L cheek						
L cheek R cheek						
R hand R cheek						

3. *Visual hemianopsia* or *Visual field neglect* a. Confrontation			
b. Bisecting line			
4. *Oculomotor control* a. Pursuit			
b. Convergence			
5. *Visual scanning*			
6. *Visual-spatial perception*			
a. Ayres design copying test			
b. Vanguard Part 4 spatial relations			
7. *Figure-ground visual perception*			
a. Ayres Test 1 8. *Eye-hand coordination*			
Purdue pegboard			

9. *Praxis*			
a. *Kinesthetic motor*	intact/impaired	intact/impaired	intact/impaired
Gross hand to same sh. (90° sh. flex.)			
hand to oppos. knee, palm up			
hand under chin, palm down			
hand behind head			
hand to opposite ear			
Fine palm down, extend index & middle			
palm up, fist closed, extend thumb			
palm down, extend index & 5th			
palm down, extend 5th & thumb			
palm up, extend index & middle			

Date:

b. *Ideational praxis*	P/F	Comments	P/F	Comments	P/F	Comments
1) comb						
2) electric razor						
3) toothbrush						
4) key						

c. *Constructional praxis*			
1) sample			
2) first model			
3) second model			
III INTEGRATED FUNCTION **A. Functional Activities** 1. Self-care feeding grooming dressing			
2. Communication skills writing reading			
3. Wheelchair mobility			
4. Leisure-time activities			

B. Behavior Orientation a. time			
b. place			
Attitude			
Anxiety/frustration			
Attention span			
Following instructions			
Self-correction			
Carry over			
Perseveration			
Motor impersistence			
Impulsivity			
Lability			
Fatigue/endurance			
Unilateral neglect			
Denial			
Learning potential			

Respiratory Problems and Impaired Function

20

Joanne De Scherer

This chapter will present only a brief overview of an extensive subject. It is not intended as an exhaustive treatment of the topic, but only as an introduction to provoke interest and further study. It is intended to provide an idea of what the field of pulmonary rehabilitation encompasses and what it has to offer to whom.

Any health professional who deals with the respiratory system must have a basic knowledge of its normal anatomy and physiology, as well as the various pathological processes to which it is susceptible. References for further study can be found at the end of the chapter.

The respiratory passages that carry air from the atmosphere to the alveoli include the nose and mouth, the pharynx (nasopharynx, oropharynx, laryngopharynx), the larynx, the trachea, and the two main bronchi and their branches within the lungs. The nasal cavities are lined with columnar ciliated epithelium on a membrane that also contains goblet cells and mucous and serous glands. Their secretions trap foreign particles and bacteria that the cilia propel toward the nasopharynx to be swallowed or expectorated. This is an important defense mechanism protecting the lower airways from infection.

The components of the pharynx and larynx aid the nose in filtering and humidifying the inspired air. The larynx is composed of cartilages and cords moved by muscles. Rapid closure of the glottis prevents food, liquids, and foreign objects from entering the lower airways. The glottis controls airflow, and it can close so that thoracic pressure can be raised and the upper airways cleared by a propulsive cough when it opens. All but one of the intrinsic laryngeal muscles are innervated by the recurrent laryngeal nerve (a branch of the vagus nerve). Damage to this nerve can facilitate aspiration of food or liquids into the lower airways and compromise pulmonary status by causing blockage or infection.

The trachea is a cylindrical tube (Fig. 1), with cartilaginous support, extending from the larynx downward to its bifurcation into the two main bronchi. Its mucous membrane has ciliated epithelial cells whose cilia beat in a coordinated fashion to propel a sheet of mucus and foreign particles from the lower respiratory tract to the pharynx, from where it is swallowed or expectorated. This "mucociliary escalator" is essential. When cilia are paralyzed (by smoke, alcohol, dehydration, anesthesia, starvation, or hypoxia), mucus begins to accumulate in distal gravity-dependent airways, causing infiltrates and atelectasis.

The trachea is basically a gas-conducting tube that divides at the carina into the right and left main-stem bronchi. The right main-stem bronchus divides into three lobar bronchi, one for each of the three lobes of the right lung. The left main-stem bronchus divides into two lobar bronchi. Each lobar branch divides into segmental bronchi, and each segmental bronchus together with the part of the lung it supplies is called a bronchopulmonary segment. The segments can be identified on a model of the lung, and the direction of each segmental bronchus can be determined. This knowledge is the basis for postural drainage of the lungs.

The bronchi of the airways continue to divide until there are approximately 23 generations of airways, including the trachea, main bronchi, lobar bronchi, segmental bronchi, small bronchi, bronchioles, and alveolar ducts and sacs. These and their structural characteristics are listed in Table 1, and a diagram of the tracheopulmonary tree is shown in Fig. 1.

The trachea, bronchi, and bronchioles through the terminal bronchioles are only gas conduits, containing in the adult approximately 150 cc of air. This area is known as anatomic dead space, which implies that because of the structure of the tubes ventilation does not take place. It is to be distinguished from physiologic dead space. The latter includes the anatomic dead space in addition to whatever tissue in the lower airways,

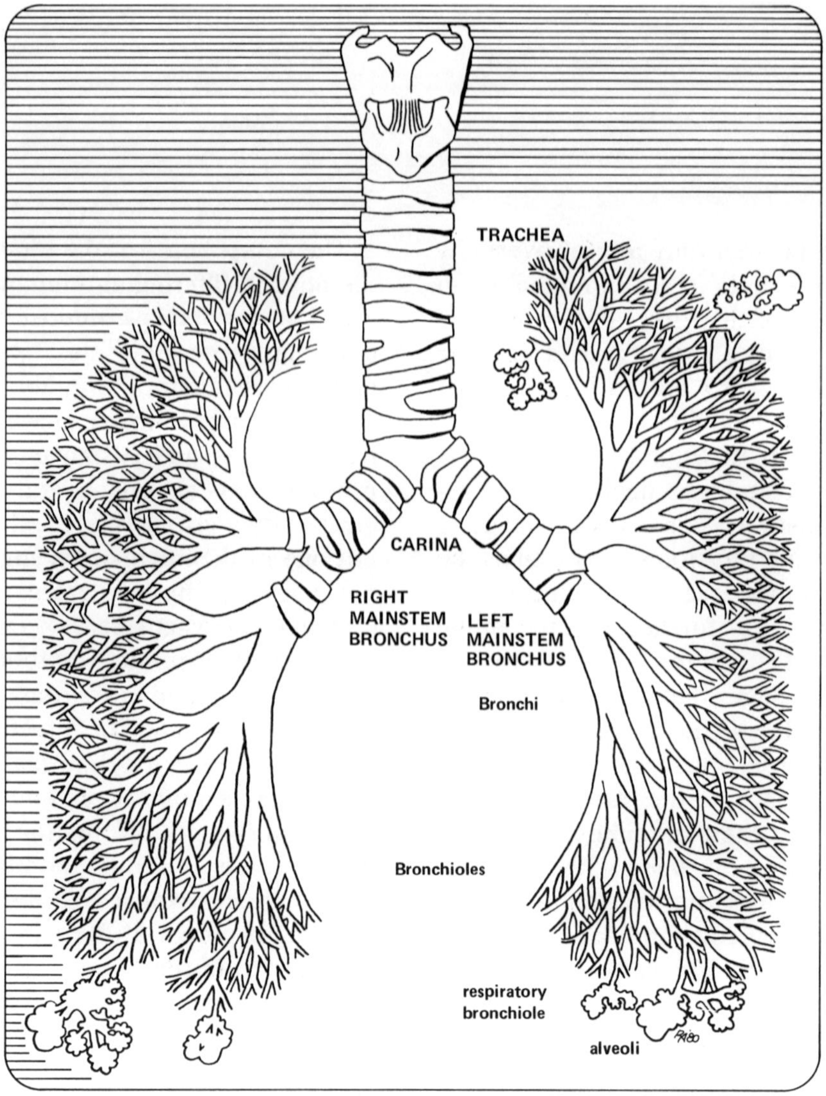

FIG. 1.

TABLE 1. *Structural characteristics of the air passages*

	Generation	Number	Mean diameter	Area supplied	Cartilage	Muscle	Location
Trachea	0	1	18	Both lungs	C-shaped cart.		
Main bronchi	1	2	13	Individual lungs			
Lobar bronchi	2 ↓ 3	4 ↓ 8	7 ↓ 5	Lobes	Irregular shaped and helical plates of cartilage	Helical muscle bands	Within connective tissue sheath alongside arterial vessels
Segmental bronchi	4	16	4	Segments			
Small bronchi	5 ↓ 11	23 ↓ 2000	3 ↓ 1	Secondary lobules		(Smooth muscle)	
Bronchioles and terminal bronchioles	12 ↓ 16	4000 ↓ 65,000	1 ↓ 0.5			Strong helical bands	Embedded directly in the lung parenchyma
Respiratory bronchioles	17 ↓ 19	130,000 ↓ 500,000	0.5	Primary lobules	None	M. bands between alveoli	
Alveolar ducts	20 ↓ 22	1,000,000 ↓ 4,000,000	0.3	Alveoli		Thin m. bands in alveolar septa	Forms the lung parenchyma
Alveolar sacs	23	8,000,000	0.3				

Morphology of The Human Lung, E. R. Weibel, reprinted with permission from Springer-Verlag, New York.

normally functioning in gas exchange, cannot be used because of destruction or the presence of pathological processes.

The airways that participate in gas exchange include the respiratory bronchioles and alveolar ducts with their alveoli. The pulmonary capillaries closely line the alveoli, and it is through the alveolar-capillary membrane that gas exchange occurs by means of diffusion.

An excellent description of respiratory physiology is provided by West (1). Only those aspects directly applicable to chest physiotherapy will be presented here.

Briefly, for optimal gas exchange and respiratory function there should be a matching between ventilation and perfusion in the lung. Both are greatest at the lung bases, or the most dependent areas; they decrease in higher lung segments, perfusion more than ventilation. Blockages (by mucus plugging, airway spasm, destructive lesions, pulmonary emboli, etc.) in either the capillaries or the airways interfere with gas exchange and respiratory function. By understanding the mechanisms of the pathological processes involved, the chest physiotherapist can help compensate for or correct ventilation-perfusion mismatches through specific positioning, segmental breathing and mobilization techniques, controlled breathing, and mechanical drainage maneuvers.

In both normal and abnormal respiratory activity the muscles of respiration must be considered. The diaphragm is the principle muscle of respiration; it is used in the active inspiratory cycle. The diaphragm is normally dome-shaped, but it is flattened in the presence of obstructive lung disease. With inspiration, it descends against the abdominal contents, intrathoracic pressure decreases as lung and thoracic volumes increase, and air flows into the lungs. Movement of the muscular diaphragm can be controlled to some extent voluntarily. In some cases of restrictive and obstructive lung disease, this is the basis of the chest physiotherapy regimen.

The external intercostal muscles help to increase the volume of the thoracic cavity during inspiration. Other inspiratory muscles, usually used as accessory muscles of respiration, include the sternocleidomastoid, scalenes, serratus anterior, pectorals, trapezius, and erector spinae. They may help to stabilize or enlarge the thoracic cavity; they are visibly used in dyspneic patients and in those with chronic obstructive pulmonary disease.

Expiration is typically a passive process, occurring when the intercostals and diaphragm relax. Their relaxation allows the ribs to drop to their preinspiratory positions and the diaphragm to rise. This compresses the lungs, raising intrathoracic pressure above atmospheric pressure, thus allowing air to flow out of the lungs. In pathological states, where air has difficulty in leaving the lungs, as in chronic obstructive pulmonary disease (COPD), or where coughing must be strengthened, a more active expiratory phase may be stressed. The rectus abdominis, internal and external obliques, and transversus abdominis may be contracted slowly or expulsively to accomplish whichever goal the therapist is working toward.

Nervous system control and chemical control of respiration, reflexes, mechanical factors in breathing, lung volumes, gas transport, etc., are all important to the chest physiotherapist, and they can often be manipulated to advantage, but extensive examination of these factors is beyond the scope of this chapter. The types of disabilities seen by the chest physiotherapist, and their appropriate treatments, will be considered here.

PULMONARY DISABILITIES

Pulmonary diseases are often classified as restrictive, obstructive, or mixed. They are classified on the basis of pulmonary function tests, X-rays, clinical observation, history, and subjective feelings of the patient.

Restrictive diseases are characterized by inability to fully expand the lungs. Restriction can be caused by any one of numerous factors: impairment of the bony framework caused by trauma (rib fractures), kyphoscoliosis, or ankylosing spondylitis; obesity (Pickwickian syndrome) and ascites that limit diaphragmatic movement; neuromuscular or CNS disorders such as quadriplegia, stroke, drug overdose, or coma; decreased elasticity of the lung parenchyma, as in interstitial fibrosis, sarcoidosis, and scleroderma; pleural abnormalities that compress the lungs, such as pleural effusion; blockage of airways, as in pneumonia and mucus plugging; aftereffects of thoracic or abdominal surgery that inhibit respiratory movements; collapsed or unexpanded lung tissue, as in atelectasis.

Obstructive diseases are characterized by increased airway resistance, typically on expiration. There may be chronic cough with increased mucus production and expectoration, poor exercise tolerance, hyperinflated lungs, wheezing and other evidence of airway obstruction, impairment of gas exchange, a flattened diaphragm, or an enlarged right ventricle caused by increased pulmonary artery pressure. The different entities of COPD may occur by themselves or in combinations.

Bronchitis is characterized by excessive mucus secretions of the bronchial tree manifested as a chronic productive cough. The mucus glands increase in size, and there is goblet cell hyperplasia, ciliary dysfunction, bronchiolar narrowing, and inflammation. When secretions are retained, their pooling blocks the airways, causing further obstruction and infection. By definition, bronchitis involves expectoration on most days for at least 3 months in the year for 2 consecutive years.

Emphysema is characterized by abnormal enlargement of the airspaces distal to the terminal bronchioles, with destruction of their airways. There are different types of emphysema, and they may be described anatomically or clinically. The "pink puffer" and the "blue bloater" are examples of the latter. Pink puffers have the most emphysematous type of COPD, and demonstrate increasing shortness of breath, little mucus production, quiet and diminished breath sounds, and overexpanded chest. Blue bloaters have a more bronchitic COPD, and they may demonstrate productive and purulent cough, cyanosis, noisy breath sounds, fluid retention, dyspnea, and decreased exercise tolerance. The amount of mucus production depends on the bronchitic component present. Understanding the difference between these two clinical types is essential for formulating a physiotherapy plan.

Asthma is a disease characterized by increased responsiveness of the trachea and bronchi to various stimuli. It is manifested as widespread spasms and narrowing of the airways. The lumina of the airways are narrowed or occluded by the combination of bronchial smooth-muscle spasm, inflammation of the mucosa, and overproduction of a thick sticky mucus. The disorder usually appears as "attacks" and may be completely reversible between episodes.

Bronchiectasis is usually a localized defect, an abnormal dilation of medium-size bronchi and bronchioles that is often preceded by an acute respiratory infection. The infection causes excess mucus production and destroys parts of the mucosa of bronchial walls. This leads to permanent dilations, pooling of secretions, chronic infections, and further destruction. Bronchiectasis is very often a component of other types of COPD, notably cystic fibrosis.

Physiotherapy in both restrictive and obstructive diseases is aimed at clearing excess mucus secretions and instituting breathing and mobility patterns that will improve ventilatory efficiency.

EVALUATION

A patient is referred for chest physiotherapy after diagnosis by a physician. The diagnosis is based on some or all of the following factors: patient history, clinical findings, X-rays, pulmonary function tests, blood gas determinations, bronchoscopy, and tomograms. The physician's diagnosis serves as a guideline for the therapist, but no diagnosis entails a predetermined recipe for treatment, only suggestions of what to look for and what to expect. A full clinical evaluation by the physiotherapist is required before beginning any kind of rehabilitative treatment. The therapist must treat the symptoms of the diagnosis.

It is a point of controversy whether or not a chest therapy program should involve a formal evaluation report. Whereas the condition of an acutely ill patient may change too rapidly for meaningful documentation, chronically ill patients may benefit from careful base-line measurements and follow-up. In any case, certain evaluative techniques must be carried out.

By inspection the therapist is able to determine the general condition of the patient. The overall structure of the thoracic cage must be checked, as well as the ranges of motion of the extremities, to determine if there are any bony deformities. The therapist must check for symmetry of chest wall movement. Gross differences between left and right can indicate underlying pathological conditions such as atelectasis, pneumonia, or trauma. The breathing pattern at rest must be observed. Shallow respirations and rapid respiratory rate may be indicative of pain, fear, or COPD. Extensive use of accessory muscles indicates that the work of breathing is increased, possibly because of congestion, airway destruction, or spasm. The therapist will also note the presence of cyanosis (caused by decreased oxygen saturation of the blood), fingernail clubbing (indicative of chronic pulmonary disease), posture, scars or adhesions that could impede breathing, breathlessness, and jugular vein distension (indicating congestive heart failure). It is important to note the apparent frame of mind of the patient; in some cases anxiety can be an important impediment to controlling the disease manifestations (e.g., asthma).

Palpation involves assessment of chest movement and the quality of the underlying tissues. Vocal fremitus can be detected when the patient says "ninety-nine" and vibration is felt over the chest. Tactile fremitus is felt normally on breathing, but it may be interfered with by atelectasis, pneumothorax, or pleural effusion. Rhonchal fremitus can be felt when air passes a bronchial obstruction like mucus, and it must be differentiated from the other kinds of fremitus.

Percussion may also aid in evaluation. With one hand flat against the patient's chest, a knuckle is struck with a finger of the other hand, and the subsequent tone can be indicative of the underlying pathological process. A dull sound will be heard over a tumor, pleural effusion, or atelectatic area, whereas a hyperresonant note will be heard over emphysema or pneumothorax.

During auscultation the patient is asked to breathe deeply through the mouth, and the therapist uses a stethoscope to evaluate the sounds from the lungs. All parts of the lungs should be auscultated in order to localize abnormal findings. Vesicular breath sounds are normal over most of the chest and are characterized by long inspirations and tapering expirations. Bronchial breath sounds are harsh, especially over their prolonged expiration. They may be heard over areas of consolidation, pleural effusion, and tumor. Rales and rhonchi are evidence of wet congestion, usually mucus accumulations, heard in smaller and larger airways, respectively. They are classified into different gradations of sound, from fine crackles (rales) to bubbling or rattling noise (rhonchi). Wheezing is caused by airway narrowing or obstruction, usually in asthma or emphysema.

Additional indications may be obtained from voice sounds. Normal voice sounds are heard all over the chest, although they are muffled and indistinct. A patient with consolidation, pneumothorax, or tumor who whispers "ninety-nine" will produce very clear and distinct sounds over the chest. This is termed whispered pectoriloquy. Egophony, or "E-to-A change," occurs over a pleural effusion and distinguishes it from consolidation.

By understanding the nature of the pathological process involved, the therapist can better select realistic goals and methods for the therapy program.

More active evaluation can be made by taking a thorough history and watching the patient's activities. It is helpful to know the patient's smoking history and previous pulmonary problems, as well as how the patient functions in daily life. It is necessary to know if the patient experiences shortness of breath, dyspnea on exertion, orthopnea, dizziness, periods of confusion, somnolence, or headaches. The therapist should also make other determinations about the patient: whether or not it is possible to walk without dyspnea, whether or not it is possible to climb stairs, how often rest is necessary during daily functions, which activities present the most difficulty. The therapist should then, if possible, watch the patient walk and perform any convenient ADL activities in order to get the most complete base-line measure of the patient's current capability.

During rest and activity the therapist should record pulse and respiratory rates for the patient, as well as blood pressure. This will give an idea of the patient's tolerance for therapy.

The patient should be thoroughly evaluated on the therapist's first visit: history, observation, inspection, palpation, percussion, auscultation, activity tolerance. Any auxiliary tests, such as pulmonary function tests and X-rays, must be reviewed. With a thorough understanding of the patient's pulmonary status and associated cardiac, neuromuscular, and skeletal factors, the therapist can begin the active rehabilitation process.

MANAGEMENT OF PULMONARY PROBLEMS

Frownfelter (2) has summarized the goals of chest physiotherapy:

1. Prevent the accumulation of secretions
2. Improve mobilization and drainage of secretions
3. Instruct patients in home bronchial hygiene programs
4. Promote relaxation to avoid muscle splinting
5. Maintain and improve chest wall mobility
6. Regain the most efficient breathing pattern
7. Instruct and retrain in the use of respiratory muscles
8. Develop respiratory muscle endurance
9. Prevent venous stasis
10. Improve cardiopulmonary exercise tolerance

Not every therapeutic program will need to meet all of these goals. The knowledgeable and skillful therapist will choose goals specific to the patient's problems and will continually vary the treatment plan to meet them.

In acute pulmonary illness where mucus secretions have overwhelmed the respiratory system, or where other factors have acted to compromise it, the primary function of physiotherapy is to mobilize and remove the secretions and reestablish a patent airway. "Postural drainage is a physical means of forcing secretions from the lung toward the trachea so that they can be removed by expulsive coughing or aseptic suctioning. The aim of postural drainage is to promote more efficient clearing of the bronchial tree in less time and with less energy expenditure and stress for the patient than is otherwise possible" (3). The patient may be placed in different positions, often with head down, to facilitate gravity drainage of mucus from the lungs. Most textbooks dealing with pulmonary care contain diagrams of postural drainage positions (see Figs. 2–10). Patients with severe cardiac or pulmonary disease cannot tolerate the tipped position, and treatment may be modified by positioning the patient on one side, prone, or supine on a flat bed.

A mechanical means of loosening secretions is manual percussion or vibration over the chest wall. The percussion with cupped hands should produce a resonant sound. It should not be done over bare skin, and care should be taken to work within the patient's tolerance. Percussion may be performed for 2 min, followed by shaking or vibration of the rib cage through four or five expirations, with this sequence being repeated until coughing is to be attempted. If coughing or expectoration is difficult, it can be facilitated by various measures: a "tracheal tickle" (stimulation of the cough reflex by pressing over the trachea in the area between the larynx and sternal notch), drinking water, deep breathing, upper extremity range of motion, changing positions, or abdominal splinting and/or suctioning.

Nasotracheal suctioning may effectively remove mucus secretions that the therapist has mobilized, but this should be done only by a therapist skilled in the technique. It can be traumatic and dangerous, and it should be performed only when coughing techniques have failed and there remains significant mucus accumulation. On the other hand, congested patients who must be suctioned should not be treated until a suctioning apparatus is readily available. Loosening secretions and leaving them may only result in increased airway obstruction and respiratory failure.

In alert patients, incentive spirometers are often employed to encourage deep breathing patterns. Sustained maximal inspirations afford more time for gas exchange. They also fully inflate alveoli, allowing adherent mucus to "peel off" the alveolar walls and be expelled during expiration. Spirocare and Triflow™ incentive spirometers are widely used for patients in various conditions: congested, atelectatic, hypoventilating, postoperative, immobile. Intermittent positive-pressure breathing, ultrasound nebulizers, and other respiratory therapy equipment may also help to loosen secretions and should be followed by chest physiotherapy.

Modified postural drainage and percussion techniques are important (sometimes lifesaving) modalities in pulmonary medical care. The primary indication for their use is the presence of airway secretions (cystic fibrosis, bronchiectasis, bronchitis, emphysema, pneumonia, asthma, spinal cord injuries, etc.). Major contraindications to percussion include osteoporosis, rib fractures, cardiac instability, major gastrointestinal bleeding, excessive pain, untreated pneumothorax, and hemoptysis, as well as a recent meal. Vibration or deep breathing techniques alone may often be used where percussion is not feasible. Segmental breathing patterns can be used, in which an attempt is made to force air into specific lung segments with the help of proprioceptive pressure cues. To aid in the expansion of an atelectatic or hypoventilated area, the patient can be positioned lying on the side, with the affected area uppermost, and given pressure cues over that area of the chest wall to facilitate expansion. To afford the best ventilation-perfusion ratio of the same area, the patient should then be positioned so that the area is most dependent.

In all acute care the breathing pattern is of great importance. The pattern used for a restrictive pulmonary defect is different from that used for obstructive disease. The latter should be slow and deep in an attempt to decrease the work of breathing and the use of accessory muscles. The patient with a restrictive defect has no choice but to breathe rapidly. It is not feasible to do any breathing retraining. The goal of therapy will be to maintain the integrity of the airways through the use of postural drainage (Figs. 2a, 3a, 4a, 5a, 6a, 7a, 8a, 9a, and 10a), percussion, and spirometry.

COPD is encountered more often than restrictive disease in the hospital setting. It is usually possible to follow COPD patients through several admissions, as this problem usually worsens. Therapy attempts to maintain optimal pulmonary and functional status for as long as possible by clearing excess mucus secretions and by teaching energy conservation measures to the patient. The treatment of COPD will be considered from here on. Petty (3,4) is an acknowledged expert in the field of pulmonary rehabilitation, and his writings should be consulted for extensive coverage of the subject.

COPD has an insidious onset, not being clini-

Figures 2–10: postural drainage positions.

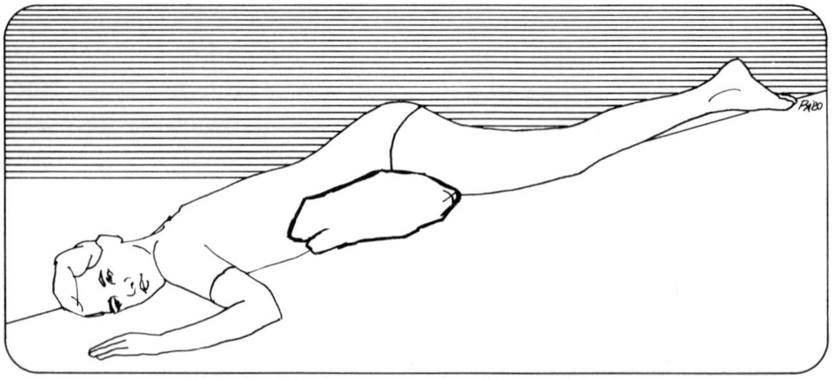

FIG. 2. Drains posterior lower lobes.

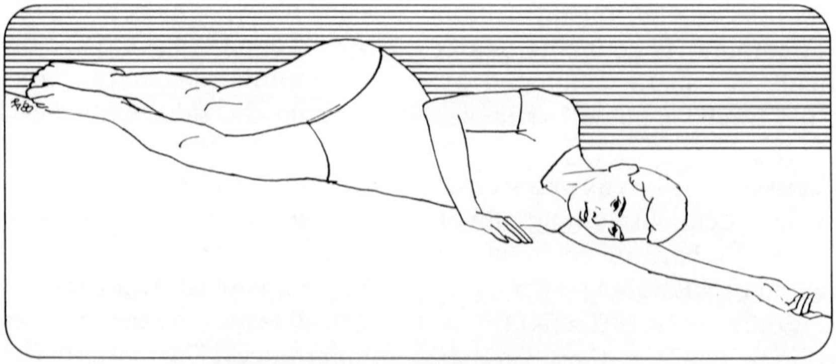

FIG. 3. Drains right lower lobes.

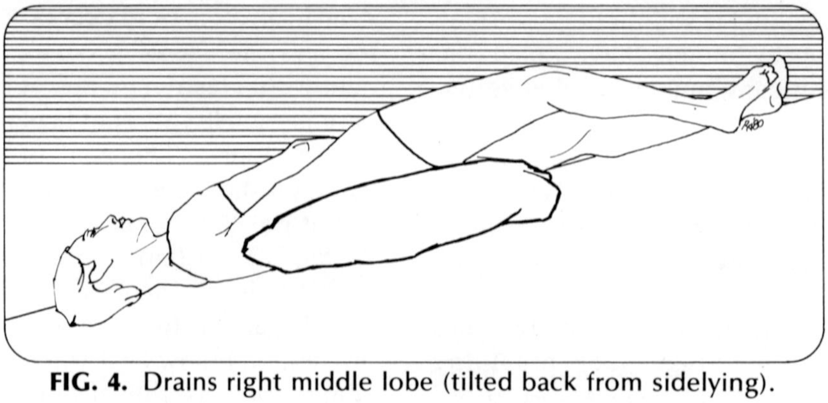

FIG. 4. Drains right middle lobe (tilted back from sidelying).

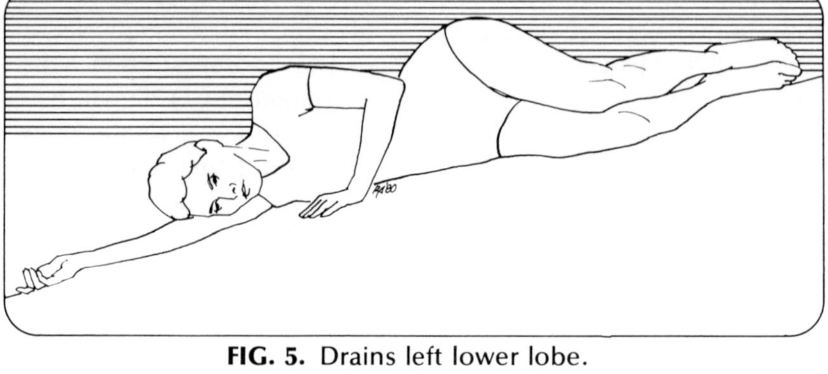

FIG. 5. Drains left lower lobe.

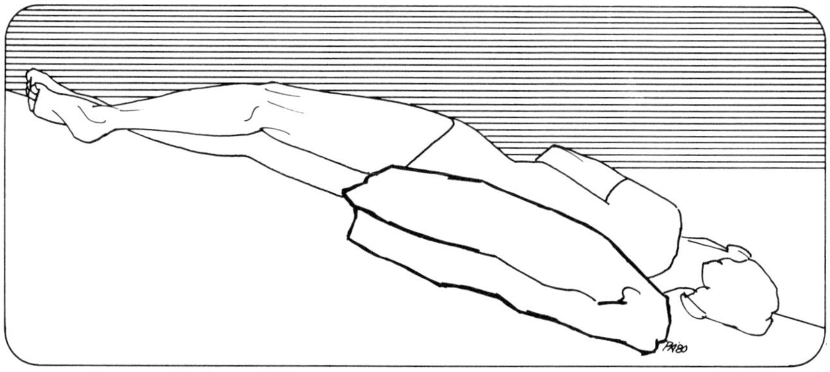

FIG. 6. Drains left middle lobe (lingular) (tilted back from sidelying).

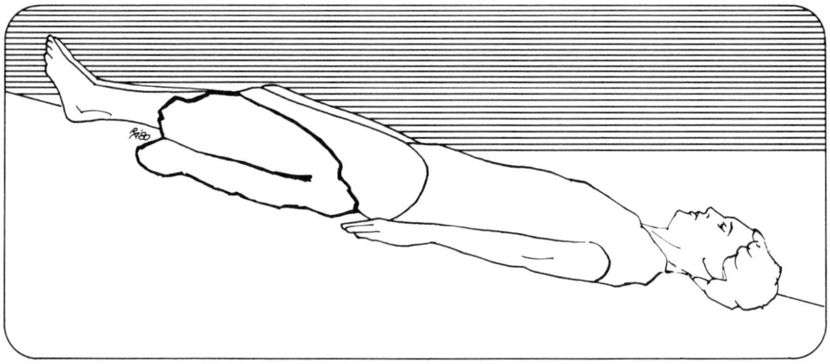

FIG. 7. Drains anterior lower lobes.

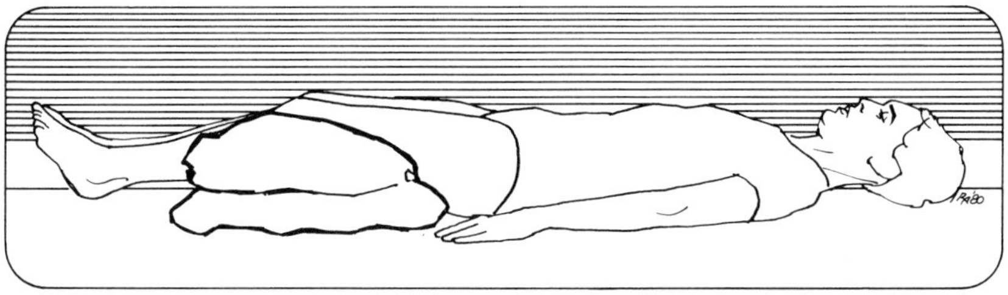

FIG. 8. Drains anterior upper lobes.

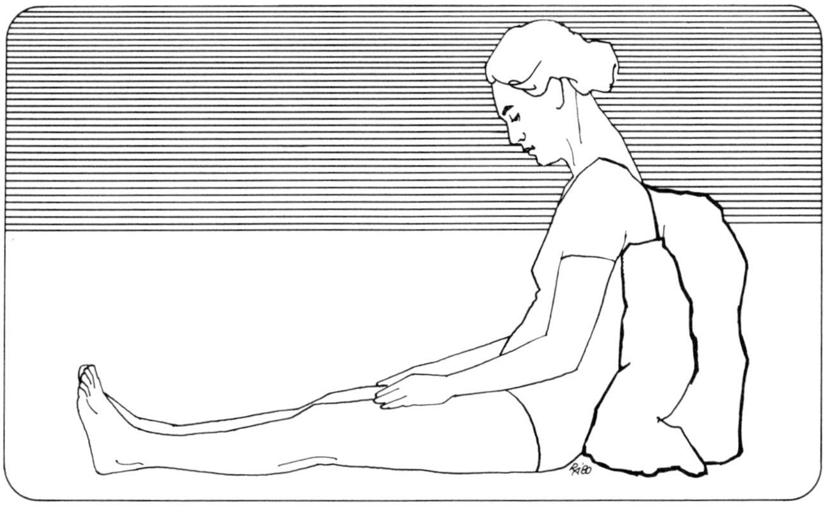

FIG. 9. Drains anterior upper lobes.

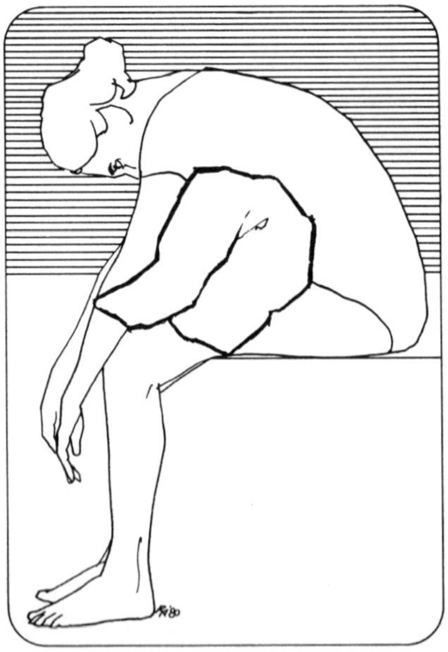

FIG. 10. Drains posterior upper lobe.

cally evident until there has already been a good deal of lung tissue destruction. The surface area of the lung is great, and the pathological process may be extensive before the patient becomes symptomatic. Once it begins, the disease may run a slowly or rapidly progressive course; the victim becomes more debilitated with time, often ending as a respiratory cripple dependent on oxygen and ventilator. Functional independence is severely compromised because of dyspnea and fatigue. The patient is periodically plagued by acute exacerbations of the condition necessitating hospitalization. If diagnosis and treatment, medical and rehabilitative, can be accomplished early in the course of the disease, it is possible that its progress can be slowed or that its manifestations can be better controlled.

On admission, it is imperative to clear excess mucus from the lungs. For better ventilation and pulmonary hygiene, the patient is often intubated by endotracheal or tracheal (in tracheostomy) tube and placed on a ventilator. Airway tubes are irritating and create their own secretions. Modified postural drainage, percussion, and suctioning are the treatments of choice.

Once the patient is extubated, postural drainage may continue, but the emphasis of treatment may shift to teaching the patient to cope with the disability. Included in the regimen will be relaxation techniques, diaphragmatic breathing, breathing retraining techniques, mobility exercises, ADL and ambulation activities, and physical conditioning with or without oxygen.

By placing the patient in positions in which little or no energy is being expended, the accessory muscles of respiration are more prone to relax, and the diaphragm is in a better position to perform its normal function. When short of breath or in respiratory distress, patients should assume a semi-Fowler or high side-lying position in bed, lean forward on a table or prop themselves on their knees while sitting, or lean the back or side against a wall and bend forward slightly while standing. With the abdominal muscles slack and the diaphragm potentially able to traverse its full excursion, the therapist and patient can attempt to train it to do so. Local hand pressure on the abdomen facilitates greater use of the diaphragm during inspiration and less use of the accessory muscles. There is controversy whether this training is designed to actually strengthen the diaphragm or whether it is more a sensory cue to call attention to diaphragmatic and abdominal sensations during breathing. Diaphragmatic breathing is best taught to the patient in the semi-Fowler position, when little energy is being expended to maintain posture. It can then be applied to the sitting, standing, and walking positions.

While learning to use the diaphragm during inspiration, the patient may be taught to splint or compress the abdominal region during expiratory maneuvers to aid in huffing, expulsive coughing, or active expiration. Active expiration can be taught.

Pursed-lip breathing is a retraining technique taught to the patient very early in the recuperative phase and continued throughout rehabilitation. Whereas some patients normally develop this pattern, others must be taught to expire against the resistance of pursed lips. In this way the patient makes use of a positive pressure reflected back to the bronchial passageway. In severe COPD, where much of the fibroelastic support of airways has been destroyed, the airways tend to collapse on expiration, trapping air behind them. Pursed-lip breathing appears to maintain the patency of the airways longer and allow the air to be expelled, thus decreasing dyspnea and decreasing the use of accessory muscles of respiration. Pursed-lip breathing was the precursor for the development of PEEP (positive end-expiratory pressure) on the ventilator.

Along with pursed-lip expiration, the patient is instructed in slow and deep inspirations. This is a nonobstructive breathing pattern that allows more time for gas exchange; it can improve blood gases if done by habit, and it can decrease the work of breathing.

While patients are learning the diaphragmatic and pursed-lip breathing patterns, they must be encouraged to incorporate these patterns into various mobility exercises. The aims of these exercises are to maintain adequate posture and joint position (stretching, range-of-motion exercises), expel air from the lungs (bending, twisting, abdominal compression exercises during expiration), increase thoracic volume (arms raised, stretching and reaching during inspiration), and maintain or increase endurance in physical activities. The exercises teach the patient that work is decreased when inspiration is performed in a fairly erect position with arms expanded, and expiration is augmented by a compressed or bending-over position. The methods and repetitions of the exercises should be thoroughly explained. It should be stressed that some shortness of breath during exercise is not a contraindication; a training effect cannot be obtained without stressing the system.

Naturally following and complementing the learning of breathing patterns and mobility exercises is their incorporation into ADL. The acts of eating, talking, washing, dressing, walking, and climbing stairs are among the most fatiguing and dyspnea-producing. Energy conservation methods and materials should be stressed. The patient must be taught to space out activities and do them all slowly. There are energy conservation materials on the market (e.g., long shoehorns, raised toilet seats, railings), but the therapist and patient must rely a great deal on their own ingenuity in determining the most conservative methods of functioning.

Exercises and ambulation are often begun with the use of low-flow oxygen to enrich the atmosphere and decrease breathlessness. The oxygen may be decreased as the patient develops endurance for physical activity. The bending-forward position (10–20 degrees) and pursed-lip breathing should be stressed. During ambulation, patients may be taught paced breathing (i.e., breathing in for two steps and blowing out for four). This often results in forced expiration and dyspnea toward the end; so patients are frequently instructed just to breathe in and blow out comfortably during ambulation. The expiratory phase is usually prolonged in any case; so the same goal is achieved with less stress. Ambulation should begin slowly, often with assistive devices like a high walker (shoulder level), with distance being increased as indicated.

Physical training for patients with COPD is indicated to develop the muscles employed in locomotion as well as to develop or improve use of the diaphragm. The trained system appears to use oxygen more efficiently, and this will decrease the energy expended in walking and climbing stairs. Patients can work with abdominal weights in the supine and head-down positions, whichever is more easily tolerated, and they may attach weights to their ankles for resistive work with ankle, knee, and thigh muscles.

It is not realistic to expect all COPD patients to be able to climb stairs. Those who attempt it must be instructed to do so slowly and with rest stops. For patients with severe COPD it is easiest to avoid the step-over-step pattern, breathing in while both feet are on one step and blowing out as a step is mounted. Some patients will not accept this adaptation; they should at least be encouraged to breath in and blow out through pursed lips rhythmically and regularly.

Regular exercise on a treadmill or bicycle is

suggested for patients who are home-bound or oxygen-dependent. COPD patients are like athletes; they must continually train to maintain themselves in optimal condition to help ward off further pulmonary complications. The families and friends of COPD patients should be instructed in home-care techniques to help these patients with pulmonary hygiene.

CONCLUSION

Pulmonary rehabilitation involves teaching patients to adapt their treatment to meet their life-styles, rather than adjusting their life-styles to the demands of the disease. Inpatient hospital care may aid in clearing acute exacerbations of COPD and can give the patient an opportunity to learn about the disease and techniques for easing its symptoms. These techniques of breathing control and energy conservation must be continued religiously through outpatient therapy and at home until they are a normal part of living.

Some of the problems associated with COPD (excessive mucus secretions, dyspnea, poor exercise tolerance, limited ADL) can be managed by the techniques discussed in this chapter. Patients have reported that they feel better and can function better after acute and chronic rehabilitation. Progress can be measured by objective tests (arterial blood gases, pulmonary function tests), but whether or not intensive rehabilitation can actually forestall advancement of the disease is still to be determined.

The therapeutic methods presently available to victims of COPD are helpful. COPD patients should begin to learn them as soon as the diagnosis is made. It is the responsibility of those actively engaged in rehabilitation to conduct research and develop further therapeutic techniques to complement the medical knowledge that is continually being added to the field of obstructive lung disease.

REFERENCES

1. West, J. B. (1975): *Respiratory Physiology*. Williams & Wilkins, Baltimore.
2. Frownfelter, D. (1978): *Chest Physical Therapy and Pulmonary Rehabilitation*. Year Book, Chicago.
3. Petty, T. L. (editor) (1978): *Chronic Obstructive Pulmonary Disease*. Marcel Dekker, New York.
4. Petty, T. L., and Nett, L. (1967): *For Those Who Live and Breathe with Emphysema and Chronic Bronchitis*. Charles C Thomas, Springfield, Ill.

BIBLIOGRAPHY

Bates, D., and Christie, R. (1971): *Respiratory Function in Disease*. W. B. Saunders, Philadelphia.

Cash, J. (editor) (1975): *Chest, Heart, and Vascular Disorders for Physiotherapists*. Faber & Faber, London.

Cherniack, R., Cherniack, L., and Naimark, A. (1972): *Respirations in Health and Disease*. W. B. Saunders, Philadelphia.

Comroe, J. (1974): *Physiology of Respiration*. Year Book, Chicago.

Gaskell, D. V., and Webber, B. A. (1973): *The Brompton Hospital Guide to Chest Physiotherapy*. Blackwell, London.

Glenn, W., Liebow, A., and Lindskog, G. (1975): *Thoracic and Cardiovascular Surgery with Related Pathology*. Appleton-Century-Crofts, New York.

Lough, M., Doershuk, C., and Stern, R. (1974): *Pediatric Respiratory Therapy*. Year Book, Chicago.

Miller, W. (1967): Rehabilitation of patients with chronic obstructive lung disease. *Med. Clin. North Am.*, 51:239–251.

Mitchell, R. S. (1978): *Synopsis of Clinical Pulmonary Disease*. C. V. Mosby, St. Louis.

Proctor, D. (1978): The upper airways: Nasal physiology and defense of the lungs. In: *Lung Disease—State of the Art 1976-1977*, edited by J. F. Murray, pp. 25–58. American Lung Association, New York.

Proctor, D. (1978): The upper airways: Larynx and trachea. In: *Lung Disease—State of the Art 1976-1977*, edited by J. F. Murray, pp. 59–86. American Lung Association, New York.

Reinisch, E. (1978): Functional approach to chest physical therapy. *Phys. Ther.*, 58:972–978.

West, J. B. (1977): *Pulmonary Pathophysiology*. Williams & Wilkins, Baltimore.

Young, J. A., and Crocker, D. (1976): *Respiratory Therapy*. Year Book, Chicago.

Spinal Cord Injury

21

S. Elaine Bennethum

There are eight major categories of causes of vertebral injury and spinal cord compression: accidents, degenerative conditions, neoplasms, toxins, vascular diseases, iatrogenic causes, infectious diseases, and congenital disorders (1).

Following heart disease, cancer, and stroke, accident is the fourth leading cause of death in the United States, accounting for 50 deaths per 100,000 population. Of these, 3% are caused directly by traumatic spinal cord (SC) injury, with an additional 2% being caused by SC injury in conjunction with multiple systemic trauma (2). Ducker and Perot reported in the national spinal cord injury (SCI) registry that 40% of SC injuries are caused by vehicular accidents, 20% are caused by falls, and 40% are caused by gunshot wounds, sporting accidents, industrial accidents, and agricultural accidents, in order of decreasing importance. Approximately 85% of SC injuries are sustained by males, with a peak age range of 15 to 28 years. Ducker and Perot found that the most common time of occurrence of SC injuries is between midnight and 5:00 a.m. There is a rise in the incidence of SC injuries caused by automobile accidents in the summer and a similar rise caused by skiing and snowmobile accidents in the winter (3). The most commonly encountered injury is the middle-to-low cervical lesion (C5-6). The thoracolumbar junction (T12-L1) has the next highest incidence because of the hypermobility of these areas of the spinal column. The SCI registry reported that 43% of these patients have complete neurological deficits below the level of injury, 18% have partial deficits, 3% have central cervical cord syndrome, 12% have nerve root injury only, and 23% have vertebral fractures. The SCI registry estimated that there are approximately 200,000 patients with SC injuries presently living in the United States, with 10,000 to 12,000 new cases occurring each year (3). The cost of supporting a patient incurring SC injury during the prime of life may exceed $1 million over the patient's lifetime (1).

SC injuries may affect bladder, bowel, and sexual functioning, as well as nerves, bones, and the autonomic nervous system, to say nothing of the emotional state. These complex problems necessitate a team approach to their solution.

Patients who have sustained SC lesions have either complete or partial transection of the cord. If transection is complete, there is total loss of (a) voluntary movement below the level of the lesion, (b) sensation below the level of the lesion, (c) normal sensation and control of bladder, bowel, and sexual functioning, and (d) normal control of the sympathetic nervous system, which can affect heart, blood pressure, and temperature control (4). If incomplete transection has occurred because of compression or trauma, as in stabbing or gunshot wounds, multiple levels may be affected, with any combination of the symptoms described previously. It is possible to have lesions at two totally separate levels affecting the two sides of the body differently.

An upper motor neuron injury is diagnosed when damage occurs to the brain or spinal cord; this is manifested as hyperreflexia, spasticity, and involuntary muscle control. The spasticity is believed to occur because of hyperactivity of the gamma motor neurons to antigravity muscles. The hyperactivity is presumably occurring as a result of being released from inhibitory influences of the alpha system (1). A lower motor neuron lesion manifests itself as hyporeflexia, flaccidity, and absence of involuntary movement. This will occur when the level of injury is at the cauda equina, nerve, nerve root, or anterior horn cell of the spinal cord.

All patients who sustain SC injuries will go through a period of "spinal shock" immediately following the injury. This term was coined in 1850 by Hall; it refers to the total absence of reflexes following a severe SC injury. This may occur when the spinal cord is disconnected anatomically or physiologically or when the spinal cord is cooled or anesthetized. Spinal shock may last from a few days to several weeks. Clinically it has been observed that a patient with incomplete transection of the spinal cord will experience a return of deep-tendon reflexes within a few days. This indicates some remaining function below the level of the lesion. When spinal shock has subsided, reflex activity may return. In many cases violent withdrawal movements accompanied by autonomic discharge (profuse sweating, evacuation of bowel and bladder) will occur; this is called "mass reflex." This is indicative of automatic activity in the isolated segment of the spinal cord (1).

Spinal shock is also accompanied by other autonomic changes: decreased blood pressure, hypothermia, and bradycardia. There is some evidence that after transection of the spinal cord occurs, posterior root fibers in the area of injury develop new collaterals and produce more synaptic connections with more motor neurons and interneurons. Such a development might increase the magnitude of reflex response to peripheral stimulation, causing a hyperactivity known as spasticity (1).

Probably most critical in the care of SC injury is the emergency management at the time of injury. If possible, the patient should be left in the position that results from the accident, unless other lifesaving procedures must be carried out. Any movement of the patient should await a trained team, so that the spine will not be flexed or extended. The patient should be firmly positioned on a spinal board for transportation to the nearest medical facility. Respiration should be watched closely. When the patient arrives in the emergency room, monitoring of respiration and blood pressure must be continued. A tracheostomy will be done if necessary. A quick neurological examination will reveal the location of any pain described by the patient, the level of sensory and motor function, and the degree of reflex activity. Base-line laboratory studies should be carried out: blood sugar, blood gases, blood count, urinalysis, and electrolyte levels. An intravenous infusion should be started to increase circulating volume to keep blood pressure up and provide a means of administering medication. The patient may be catheterized at this point. If indicated, X-rays of spine, abdomen, chest, and extremities should be made. Further evaluation will be carried out over the next several months. As soon as the patient is medically stable, a decision will be made regarding any surgical intervention. The patient will still be in spinal shock. During this period the injured area will be stabilized either by traction or by laminectomy and/or fusion. The neurologist and/or orthopedist will observe all other bodily functions and provide supportive measures until the injury site becomes stable enough to permit a diagnosis of the kind of injury and selection of a rehabilitation program. In cases involving C3-4 injury the physician will watch the respiratory system closely for signs of anoxia and to determine if tracheostomy and artificial respiration are required. The phrenic nerve originating at C4 innervates the diaphragm, and if one side of the cord is pressured, respiration may be inadequate. It must be remembered that it is possible with a traumatic stab or gunshot wound to have two different levels of function for the left and right sides of the body. C1-2 quadriplegics will always require respiratory aids such as the MA-1, LP-3, or bantam respirator. A portable respirator (e.g., bantam or LP-3) will allow for mobility when the patient is able to use a motorized wheelchair, thus providing relief from a confined environment. The recovery period after the initial injury may continue for as long as 18 months, unless the lesion was complete, in which case no return of function is expected.

On arriving in the emergency room, patients are usually catheterized with an internal or Foley catheter inserted directly through the urethra to the bladder. At a later date the appropriate type of catheter or urinary device will be determined. After the patient has become stabilized and is sitting, intravenous pyelography and cinecystography will probably be carried out to determine what type of urinary procedure, if any, is needed. There are also other tests for determining bladder function. If the patient has a very spastic bladder, a Foley catheter may be left in place. After prolonged use of a Foley catheter, a fistula can develop in the urethra leading directly into the scrotum, causing a serious problem. In many such cases a suprapubic procedure is carried out to create an opening in the abdominal wall so that a catheter may be inserted directly into the bladder. This will remain until the fistula has closed; then the suprapubic opening will be closed, and another type of external or internal device or method may be chosen. If there is not a large amount of residual urine left in the bladder after it is emptied, an external condom drainage device may be used. A maneuver similar to the Credé method may be used if the patient can exert sufficient external pressure over the abdominal wall with the hand to empty the bladder manually. Today many hospitals are using intermittent catheterization. With this method the patient is taught the procedure of inserting an internal catheter and then removing it. This is done throughout the day on a very rigid schedule. Liquid intake must be carefully monitored. This procedure has worked well for some, but it has the disadvantages of inconvenience and rigid scheduling.

The ileum loop may have to be chosen if all other methods fail. This procedure involves diverting the urethra to an artificial bladder (made from a section of the intestine) that has a stoma or external opening to the lower quadrant of the abdominal wall. This stoma then drains into a removable pouch. This procedure will be chosen only as a last resort.

If any method other than the ileum loop is chosen, it is important that the washable or disposable leg bag be kept lower than the bladder at all times.

If a patient has a suprapubic catheter, it may leak when the patient is exercising in a supine position. There is no cause for alarm, as urine from the bladder may build up and be forcefully ejected when the patient is exercising. The seal of the bag may be broken if the patient is wearing an ileum type of collection bag. It is best to check with each patient's urologist or physician to determine why the specific procedure was selected.

Both patients and staff often ignore the matter of sexual function. Fear of sexual dysfunction is a major cause of severe depression and lack of motivation for many patients. Those who fear that they may never be able to please a partner or themselves in sexual activity can feel very inadequate. They should be reassured from the beginning that they are still sexual beings and that they can indeed share sexual activity with other persons, although roles, methods, and positions may have to be altered to compensate for the disability. The general rule for the male is that the higher the lesion the more likely it is that a reflex erection is possible. The lower the lesion the more likely it is that ejaculation can occur. A patient with a cauda equina lesion in the S2-3-4 area will have great difficulty in achieving an erection or ejaculation, since the sacral reflex arc has been damaged. If an incomplete lesion has occurred in this area, it will be difficult to determine sexual potential until some time has passed. Also, sexual potential cannot be determined until the spinal shock caused by the initial trauma has subsided.

As soon as possible, patients need to become aware of the new and altered sensations they will be receiving. Clinical experience has shown that patients experience increases in their normal sensations above the lesion. Either parts of the body stimulated above the lesion can cause excitation or erogenous zones stimulated through vibration, pressure, or light touch below or above the lesion can cause pleasurable sensation above the lesion.

The patient who wants to be a sexual partner must follow a good bowel and bladder program to reduce the potential for accidents during intercourse. The bladder should be as empty as possible, but the catheter can be left in place in the man during intercourse by removing the tubing and bag and folding the rubber catheter behind the penile shaft. A condom can then be slipped over the penis, and intercourse can proceed. The woman can tape the catheter tubing to the abdomen or thigh until intercourse is finished. In either case, intercourse should not be prolonged because of the danger of internal abrasions caused by the catheter.

Sexuality can also be maintained by means other than direct genital stimulation or intercourse. The most important ingredient is communication; each partner must make an effort to understand the other's needs and frustrations.

The woman will resume menstruation shortly after the injury and will be sexually fertile. She must be instructed to use birth control methods if she does not want to become pregnant. Birth control pills are not usually recommended because of the potential for blood clots in the lower extremities. IUDs are not usually recommended because there may be an absence of the sensation of pain should the device malfunction or cause infection. Diaphragms, foams, and condoms are most frequently recommended. Every patient should be thoroughly checked by a gynecologist, and birth control should be discussed with the patient and her primary physician. If a woman with SC injury becomes pregnant, she can usually carry a fetus to full term, but she may experience complications such as urinary tract infections or thrombophlebitis. In many cases a woman will be admitted to the hospital at the end of the eighth month or the beginning of the ninth month, since she may not be aware of the onset of labor. Sometimes labor will be induced. The majority of such babies are born without complications and are delivered healthy.

Both men and women can still contract venereal disease, and they must be mindful of this because of the serious nature of any infection in patients with SC injuries.

EVALUATION

There are several points to consider when evaluating a patient with SC injury. (a) How did the injury occur? Was it caused by trauma, disease, infection, stab wound, or gunshot wound, or was it congenital? (b) What is the prognosis? The prognosis will vary depending on the cause. (c) The age of the patient must be considered in the rehabilitation program in order to estimate tolerance, endurance, general body condition prior to injury, and avocational and vocational potentials. (d) Motivation, endurance, and mobility should be considered in determining equipment requirements. (e) The patient's own sexual role identification must also be considered in planning the rehabilitation program. In general, each program will have the standard basic goals.

The importance of a thorough history cannot be overemphasized. It will be of assistance later in planning a realistic treatment program and helping the patient begin to accept the disability. Next, the chart must be read thoroughly, and the therapist must collect as much information as possible about the patient, medically, socially, and psychologically. There are several items to be specifically checked in the chart:

1. Medication record. What medications is the patient taking and why? This can have a direct bearing on attentiveness, wakefulness, mood, physical behavior, and general behavior. For example, diazepam may cause drowsiness, flaccidity, fatigue, and severe mood swings.
2. Temperature and blood pressure records. Is the patient stabilized?
3. Nursing notes. Are there consistent complaints, behavior or physical problems such as reddened skin areas, sweating, or nausea?
4. Physician's orders. Notes and orders provide information on past and present physical problems. The therapist must be aware of these problems when treating a patient and report results to the physician or nurse.
5. Consultation reports. What specific problems have been diagnosed or will need evalu-

ation by a specialist (e.g., urologist, orthopedist, cardiologist)?

6. Respiratory reports. For the quadriplegic with high SC injury who is using a respirator, a sheet in the chart reports daily levels of functioning on and off the respirator, the type of machine, and the machine settings for rate and volume.
7. Laboratory reports. Laboratory reports reveal blood count, infection, CO_2 levels, and other medical problems that may drastically change the patient's behavior during treatment.
8. X-ray reports. X-ray studies will show any specific joint or bone problems that exist.
9. Social history. This section may contain the crucial elements for motivation. Is there a family, home, or job to which the patient will be returning? What is the patient's work history? What formal education has the patient had? This information can play a vital role in treatment planning and in determining how to handle the patient psychologically.
10. Insurance information. This may help to determine whether or not to introduce equipment or devices into the treatment program when the patient may be unable to afford these items following discharge.

After reading the chart, the therapist must next determine what rehabilitation goals the patient has in mind. It is crucial to listen to the patient at this point and try to follow through. This is where trust and motivation begin. The patient must also receive an explanation of the formal evaluation necessary and how it will help. The therapist must always keep the patient informed. Fear and anxiety can arise from lack of knowledge about what has already happened and what to expect. The therapist must be as honest as possible from the beginning.

The formal evaluation begins with a manual muscle test to determine the levels of injury on both sides of the body. This also may indicate what improvement is to be expected, and it serves as a reference point.

Next, a sensory evaluation helps to determine the level of the sensory lesion, which may be different from that of the motor lesion. All types of sensations should be tested: temperature, pain, vibration, light touch, and deep pressure. One or more nerve tracts may have been spared, and these can be used in treatment to educate the patient about the disability. When patients become attuned to their bodies, they often become more sensitive above their lesions to compensate for lack of sensation below the lesions. For example, just before the bladder or bowel empties, a patient may have a strange tingling sensation of the face, shoulder, or some part of the body above the lesion. The treatment plan should make provision for enhancing such awarenesses, since they can be used for learning good body positioning and bladder and bowel control and for dealing with sexual activity or possible pressure problems.

Goniometry should be carried out to detect any joint restrictions or contractures, as well as spasticity and its degree. Spasticity is often the reason that patients do not achieve their potentials of motor functioning.

For C7-8 lesions and lower lesions, the Jebsen hand function test can be used to determine the residual function in the hands. Also tests to measure grasp, pinch, coordination, and sensation should be done. The information obtained can be used in treatment planning for functional activities as well as vocational activities.

At this time the therapist should consider potential or immediate splinting needs. The therapist should evaluate only basic functional skills relating to feeding, grooming, and washing and what devices may be needed. There may be other skills present, but a discrepancy exists between physical ability and psychological capability. When these skills are mastered, the therapist can determine from the initial evaluation what functions the patient is physically capable of carrying out. This ability may differ from the patient's emotional capability.

It is important to get a vital capacity reading from the spirometer during physical therapy, respiratory therapy, or occupational therapy. This reading must be compared with the average vital capacity reading for a nondisabled person. If the reading is much below normal, this can be the cause of the patient's decreased endurance, ashen or cyanotic color, inability to remember things, sweating, nightmares, or lack of concern and constant fatigue. The patient may need respiratory exercises, which can be done manually by physical therapy or mechanically with a respiratory aid used two or three times a day for 10 to 15 min. This keeps the chest wall flexible, induces deeper inspiration, and prevents severe fibrosis from developing because of acute infection or disuse. Patients with a high lesion that requires monitored respiratory equipment or carefully controlled equipment must be totally evaluated and treated by a pulmonary function laboratory and respiratory therapy.

A wheelchair evaluation is usually done by the occupational or physical therapy department and the patient will be evaluated for an appropriate wheelchair and for positioning in the wheelchair and in bed. The patient will use a manual wheelchair first, often with a semireclining or fully reclining back, until the blood pressure is stabilized. Respiratory patients and high quadriplegics should remain in full recliners. Patients with T3 injuries and lower injuries will use standard-back wheelchairs unless they are unusually tall or have other medical problems warranting a recliner. A tall patient may not be able to bend sufficiently to get into a van if the wheelchair doesn't recline. Also, there is 1 inch more seat depth in a full recliner. A motorized wheelchair may be considered, and the choice of a particular model may be determined at this time.

Later, after the patient has become emotionally and physically adjusted, other evaluations for ADL, home barriers, driving adaptations, and vocational activities must be carefully considered.

Throughout the whole rehabilitation process, from the initial meeting on, it is extremely important to be honest with the patient at all times.

TREATMENT

If the patient has a C1-3 lesion, little head motion, if any, will be possible. Such a patient is truly limited in function, except for electronic devices and equipment. Bed positioning should be considered first to maintain neutral head alignment, shoulder abduction and external rotation, elbow extension, good hand positioning to help maintain arches and web spaces, moderate hip abduction and neutral rotation, neutral ankle alignment and dorsiflexion. Adaptive positioning devices made of foam, sheepskin, Kodel, webbing, or other material may be needed to assist in maintaining good body alignment. This will help in preventing pressure sores and later in positioning the patient in the wheelchair. Contractures in the lower extremities and scoliosis are the primary problems in wheelchair positioning. If it is at all feasible for the patient to use a motorized wheelchair with specially adapted controls, this should be selected, as it is the only real form of independence the patient will have. The controls must be compatible with the full-time respiratory equipment. No device can be expected to work without proper supervision of its use. What may work for one patient in a particular situation may not work for another. Equipment for wheelchair positioning might include lapboards, commercial or specially designed and fabricated by the occupational therapist. Special cushioning for buttocks, back, and feet may be necessary. Trunk supports can be purchased or fabricated by the occupational therapist and attached directly onto the lapboard. Leg straps or foam abduction cushions may be made by the occupational therapist. It is extremely important to keep the body as flexible and as evenly aligned as possible. The straighter the patient sits, the better the pulmonary function. Different devices may be required for day and night use. It is important to prevent contracture whenever possible and to maintain good skin care and cleanliness.

Electronic devices that permit control of various factors in the immediate environment (e.g., lights, TV, radio, alarm) are appropriate for patients with lesions at this level, assuming that the necessary funds are available. There are many types of units commercially available with varying degrees of control. They range from a simple single-input switch requiring minimal movement to panels of switches requiring complex movements. Patients with injuries at this level will always require full-time attendant care. An alarm system that permits the patient to call for help is a necessity. A unit that plugs into a wall socket is better than a battery-operated unit.

These patients will probably be tracheostomized, with a positive-pressure respirator attached to the tracheal tube. This usually causes problems with speech; so a communicator may be required also. Following careful assessment by a speech therapist, a device can be chosen that will be compatible with wheelchair and respiratory devices.

These patients will always have to use respiratory devices. The small portable units fit onto a wheelchair. The positive-pressure system blows air directly into the lungs to inflate them; when the blowing stops, the lungs deflate, and air is forced out. The bantam respirator is most frequently used in such cases. It consists of a mechanism housed in a Samsonite cosmetic case that can be set by a dial to blow air out of a tube directly into the patient's mouth or tracheostomy. There are dials for setting the force and frequency of respirations. The tube may be held between the patient's teeth or connected to an adapter fastened directly to the tracheostomy tube. The tube is held up by microphone goosenecks and clamped to the wheelchair push handle with No. 10 radiator hose clamps. Two tool clips are attached to the goosenecks with No. 7 hose clamps so that the tubing from the machine can be held adjacent to the tracheostomy tube or in the correct position for the mouth. To provide negative pressure, the bantam respirator may be attached to a pneumatic belt worn around the chest. As the belt fills with air, it exerts pressure on the chest that forces air out of the lungs. When the pressure is released, air rushes into the lungs. The Iron Lung and Cuirass work on the same principle. The most critical factor is to keep the CO_2-O_2 ratio balanced. If the CO_2 level gets too high, the patient becomes drowsy, often has nightmares, becomes forgetful, has a hard time concentrating, and could potentially go into coma and die. There are machines that can monitor the CO_2 level immediately on insertion of a piece of tubing into the patient's nose. Thus blood gases need not be determined from blood samples, which can take hours of laboratory analysis. The new LP-3 respirator is a portable volume respirator much like the bedside MA-1, which is used for most patients with SC lesions during the acute-care period in the hospital. The LP-3 provides the desired amount of air directly through the tracheostomy. An alarm sounds if the desired amount of air is not being provided or if the power source is low. Both the LP-3 and bantam machines may be run from direct-current and alternating-current power sources.

The C4-5 quadriplegic will remain dependent on the respirator unless a phrenic pacemaker has been installed and is functioning. Not all phrenic pacemakers are successful. These patients should have the same modifications for bed and wheelchair positioning as C1-3 quadriplegics. These patients should have good neck movement, and they can usually use mouthsticks or headsticks to operate many devices. Mouthsticks and headsticks can be made from wooden dowels, Plexiglas or aluminum tubing or rods. Rubber tubing may be directly attached to objects like pencils, pens, and paint brushes to be held in the mouth. The major considerations are the length and weight of the stick, 12″-14″, and its function. For example, if an elevator button is to be pushed, a Plexiglas rod may be too flexible to accomplish the task without a lot of unnecessary effort. Mouthsticks can be made with mouthpieces fitted by a dentist, or easily molded materials can be applied directly to the patient's teeth to take an impression for fabricating a mouthpiece. Sometimes a piece of rubber tubing over a solid Plexiglas stick (to be held by the back teeth and maneuvered by the tongue and lips) can be used for dialing a telephone or turning pages. Ideally, a mouthstick or headstick should be designed to serve as many functions as possible. The positioning of the patient will determine its length. Adjustable mouthsticks can be designed with aluminum tubing and extensions made of aluminum rod. A transmission climax collar can be used to hold the two pieces together. This can then serve a patient in a wheelchair or bed.

Some type of commercial or fabricated reading rack should be provided for those patients interested in reading, painting, drawing, or writing. An electric typewriter with an on-off switch on the keyboard is a useful item. An aluminum mouthstick or headstick with a slight bend at the end will permit faster typing and require less energy. Some patients can type as fast as 14 to 17 words per minute after they have been correctly set up and have practiced. By using a mouthstick, patients with SC lesions can independently operate remote-control TV, tape recorders, pushbutton radios, typewriters, telephones, elevator buttons, intercom buttons, and calculators, as well as turn pages, paint, and draw and do many other tasks.

When these patients are being prepared for

school or employment, there must be a thorough evaluation in regard to necessary equipment and the structural barriers that will be encountered. The more opportunity a patient has to practice using the equipment, the less anxiety will be experienced in actually attending school or going to work.

The C4-5 quadriplegic can be brought to the clinic to work on developing mouthstick and headstick control to the maximum. It is important to deal with the psychological difficulties involved in using an object rather than the hands to perform a task. Some patients will resent adaptive devices and refuse to use them. Others will want everything available. Both behaviors must be controlled. The goal of the therapist is to have the patient succeed at as many tasks as possible with the least amount of equipment. Craft and game activities may fulfill avocational needs and develop skills and strength with adaptive equipment (e.g., leather lacing using the teeth can increase the range of motion and strengthen the neck muscles).

The C4-5 quadriplegic will be most independent in a chin-control motorized wheelchair. Some centers prefer to use a sip-and-puff control for the wheelchair.

The C6 patient can use devices attached to an ADL splint or universal cuff. By using a combination of shoulder movement, elbow flexion, supination, and some wrist extension, the patient can reach objects and grossly manipulate them. Injuries at this level cause a frustrating and controversial problem: If no triceps is present to oppose the function of the biceps, strengthening of the biceps can cause severe elbow flexion contractures. In some cases the arm can be splinted in extension so that movement and friction cannot occur. Often there is moderate to severe spasticity in the biceps, which reduces the chances of preventing elbow flexion contractures. The therapist and physician must resolve such problems on an individual basis.

If spasticity is not a limiting factor, the patient may be able to use a mobile arm support for all types of activity, from eating to controlling a hand-operated motorized wheelchair. Theoretically, these patients should be able to push a manual wheelchair with projections; however, the amount of energy needed for this function may be excessive. If a patient is going to school or to a job, a motorized wheelchair will provide more mobility and conserve energy. Again, it is important to consider the patient's total life-style and preferences.

Bed mobility must be considered as soon as the SC injury is stable. The patient must learn to roll using whatever help is available: head, shoulder, and arm motions, side rails, pull straps, or other devices. Special soft mattresses and positioning devices may hinder the patient's efforts to move. Positioning devices will be required, depending on spasticity and skin conditions.

The degree of spasticity in the arms and the patient's motivation will largely determine how many functional ADL skills can be mastered. Hand positioning is important. With tension in finger flexors and strength in wrist extensors, a tenodesis grasp is possible and may be very functional for gross grasp activities. An opponens splint may be enough to position the hand if the wrist extensors are strong enough and the tension in the finger flexors is tight enough to allow for positioning the hand and grasping an object. If the finger flexors are overstretched and no arch remains in the palm of the hand, a flexor hinge splint may be necessary. Utensils with built-up handles can enable the patient to carry out feeding, grooming, and vocational and avocational activities.

If spasticity in the biceps is minimal, body transfer by means of a sliding board is possible. By using external rotators in the shoulders, the patient can lock the elbows to lift the body weight.

On an exercise mat these patients can be taught to use the shoulders and head for turning, moving, and extending the elbows by use of the rotator cuffs. At first this is very frustrating because of reduced strength and flexibility. However, patients will begin to learn the key roles the shoulders and head play in activities such as maneuvering in bed. Activities performed while sitting at the side of a mat, table, or bed can assist patients in readying themselves for transfer activity. Learning sitting balance and learning to shift the body weight with extended elbows and body movements are important pretransfer activities. Use of a mirror during such movements can assist patients in learning orientation of the body in space. This is a good opportunity to work with body awareness with regard to changed body sensations while patients see themselves in a mirror. This experience tends to be neglected unless it is brought to the patients' attention. This experience can also be of assistance in the prevention of decubitus ulcers by showing patients the importance of movement. Again, this helps patients become more actively responsible for their own care. This process should also be used with patients who have SC lesions at other levels.

The C6 quadriplegic will most likely require some degree of attendant care. It is necessary to choose with the patients those activities they will seek to carry out independently. For instance, some patients may choose not to feed themselves because it is exhausting; they may prefer to use their energy turning pages during reading. Initially all patients should be taught self-care skills and then given the choice of continuing with them. C6 patients can turn pages, type, and feed, wash, and partially dress themselves with adaptive equipment attached to their hands, but someone must attach the equipment to their hands or set up the activity. Psychologically, some patients feel that they are not independent anyway.

Prevocational testing should be carried out with C6 patients. It is necessary to determine their levels of skills, motivation, and responsibility. Tasks not requiring fine finger dexterity are important. These patients are good candidates for further schooling, especially in office activities.

Treatment of C7-8 quadriplegics involves many added dimensions because they have functioning wrist flexors, latissimus dorsi, and triceps. When the extensors are strong, the patient can begin tenodesis action with the hand to grasp objects, and the extensors allow for transfer activity and more independence. Treatment should involve bed mobility so that the patient can move from one position to another to prevent decubitus ulcers. Then, with the aid of bedrails, pull straps tied to the foot of the bed, or a trapeze, the patient can be taught the process of long sitting in bed. This is in preparation for dressing and bathing activities. Short sitting on the edge of the bed can be used for grooming and dressing, assuming that trunk balance is sufficiently stable; this is often the easiest method for a side transfer, although long sitting with a trapeze can also be used, in which case the lower extremities are moved last instead of first as in short sitting. Bathing at bedside can begin with a wash mit made of terry cloth, with Velcro attachments to prevent dropping of the cloth. To stabilize a bar of soap, a rubber octopus or a wrung-out washcloth can be placed under the soap. A light or medium terry cloth towel is recommended, as too much weight can hinder the patient's grasp or cause fatigue. After these skills are thoroughly mastered, as well as transfer from bed to wheelchair, the learning of bathtub or shower transfer may begin. Usually a bathtub bench, chair, or seat will be tried first, if sitting balance is stable; if not, a commode shower chair with removable arms may be necessary. Since it is usually difficult for C6 quadriplegics to move up from the bottom of the tub, a bench or chair of the same height as the wheelchair is recommended. The patient must be taught to dry in the tub as thoroughly as possible in order to prevent slipping while getting out. Mats and rubber stick-ons also help prevent slipping. Nonslip grab bars can also be of assistance. A hand-held showerhead, if it can be grasped by the patient, or an extended showerhead may also help.

Grooming may require many adaptive devices, built-up handles for comb, toothbrush, mirror, brush, razor, etc. Some type of stabilizing device may be necessary for makeup and other routine tasks.

Simultaneously with the development of hygiene and grooming skills, other activities should be going on. Would tenodesis splints be helpful, and would the patient use them? The therapist must be careful not to overstretch the finger flexors. Slight tightness can allow for a better grasp. A tenodesis splint fabricated from easily molded material can be tried before an expensive metal tenodesis splint is fabricated. In occupational therapy the patient should practice picking up different shapes and weights. Activities such as woodworking, leatherworking, copper tooling, tile work, and writing can be used. Any project set up in muscle testing positions can be attempted. For example, if the wrist extensors are weak, place the work object in such a position that the hand and wrist can be lying on their sides.

It is important to develop avocational and leisure activities as well as functional activities. A game of checkers or cards can be as therapeutic as picking up pegs. Motivated patients will often guide the therapist toward what they want to accomplish. This can require ingenuity on the part of the therapist to fabricate the adaptive equipment needed.

Lesions at the C6 level often necessitate more adaptive equipment to offset weak grasp than do injuries at other levels. If the wrist extensors are too weak, the patient and therapist may choose to use an ADL cuff. The ADL cuff has a pocket in the palm of the hand to hold feeding, grooming, and functional tools; such a cuff can be purchased or made by an occupational therapist. Some commercial cuffs have a wrist extension assist. A wrist extension assist allows the hand to be held in a more functional position for grasping objects.

These patients should be capable of propelling their own wheelchairs by means of pegs or rubber rim covers. They must be constantly encouraged because they will fatigue rapidly until their shoulders, elbows, and wrists become strong. If a patient plans to be a full-time student or to hold a full-time job requiring much mobility, a motorized wheelchair may be considered. These patients may still require high-back or semireclined wheelchairs. Their posture is very important, as respiratory problems can still be dangerous. A lapboard or side positioners may be of help in maintaining good posture, but they will limit movement. It is best if these patients can shift position in the wheelchair to change the weight distribution, but the lapboard may not allow for such movement. These patients should be evaluated for proper wheelchair cushioning. Many products are available, and a trial of various cushions may be necessary before determining the best one. The cushioning qualities and life expectancies of cushions vary, and the choice should be reevaluated immediately if any redness occurs after the patient sits for a period of time.

During ADL training patients should be thoroughly educated about skin care and inspection to minimize skin breakdown. It is important that some type of written communication be taught, handwriting, if possible, or typing.

Patients can learn some household activities from the wheelchair, such as cooking simple meals. To ensure success in such activities, equipment must be set up to maximize functioning. This will require a home visit by the therapist to arrange utensils and increase efficiency. C6 patients may also drive automobiles if they have achieved stable sitting balance and if their shoulders are strong enough. Many patients with C6 lesions will require some attendant care.

There are many reasons that patients do not reach maximum potential in terms of independence: (a) lack of education about their disabilities; (b) severe spasticity; (c) lack of significant other persons to help motivate them; (d) fear of the unknown; (e) anger about their situations; (f) fear of rejection by others; (g) lack of employable skills; (h) depression; (i) rejection of their sexuality; (j) a nonsupportive community. Many more could be listed.

It takes a lot of ego strength and identity for patients to accept their disabilities and work to their fullest potential. It is difficult for many patients to accept the fact that changes will be necessary if they are to accomplish the same things they were doing before their injuries.

T1-8 paraplegics have functioning hands, and this allows total independence if these patients are willing to make the effort. They are physically capable of caring for all their own bowel and bladder needs. Usually the nursing department will institute a training program to care for these problems. These patients should be able to transfer easily. When rehabilitation begins, such things as bed mobility, positioning, and ADL skills will still need to be taught. This is an opportune time to begin educating these patients about their newly limited physical states. Their tolerance and endurance will be decreased. These can be slowly increased by exercise, good positioning, awareness training, and supportive therapy. Because of disuse and consequent weakness of the intercostal and abdominal muscles, these patients will have lowered endurance, and they must be encouraged to increase endurance by means of a regular exercise program. Sports can help with this problem. If these patients are well motivated, they should be physically capable of functioning independently, requiring little, if any, attendant care. They can usually hold full-time jobs. They should be taught homemaking skills whether or not they will be living alone.

T9-12 paraplegics should have total wheelchair independence and should have good trunk stability. These patients should be able to transfer from wheelchair to floor and back, be able to drive with hand controls, and be able to get a wheelchair in and out of a car. They should be capable of doing household tasks such as cleaning and cooking, as well as shopping and all self-care. Much planning and preparation will be needed to ensure that they achieve their potential. Therapy for these patients should include meal planning, shopping, cooking, recreation endeavors, and wheelchair skills (curbs, ramps, distance, etc.). Minimal equipment should be required: a good wheelchair, bathroom equipment, inspection mirror for the skin, and a few simple household items such as a one-handed mop, a long-handled bath brush for cleaning the tub, and a long-handled dustpan and broom. The therapist should make a home visit to see if any changes in organization, furniture placement, or architectural changes can make functioning more efficient.

These patients may choose to ambulate with braces and crutches part of the time, but this will probably require too much energy to be used on a regular basis. Standing and ambulation help to minimize decalcification of the long bones, increase circulation, and assist kidney function.

L1-5 paraplegics have pelvic stability and can ambulate full time on long leg braces and crutches if they choose. Again, many patients find that this requires too much energy and choose the wheelchair for part of the day.

These patients also need education about their disabilities and limitations. The male patients may have greater difficulty with their bowel, bladder, and sexual function because of sacral reflex problems (S1-3). These men will be flaccid. These L1-5 paraplegics can be totally self-sufficient, but they need training in planning and organization. Since they can be totally independent, it is extremely important to teach them skills of survival in the community and how to plan ahead so that they will not be frustrated.

S1-3 paraplegics should be capable of ambulating in short leg braces with crutches or canes. They also need general education about their disabilities and limitations. Patients with lumbar and sacral lesions need strengthening exercises and endurance training. Careful vocational guidance is important to help them select careers not requiring more physical strength and endurance than they can master.

All patients with SC lesions (except C4 lesions) should begin with bed mobility and mat activities, progressing to ADL skills and homemaking, if indicated. At any time after a patient is sitting, vocational training can be considered, and prevocational testing can be done. It is important to encourage those patients who are good candidates for school to pursue this possibility, since additional schooling will prepare them for jobs involving less strenuous physical demands.

It is important to remember that these are only a few guidelines to be used in directing treatment of patients with SC lesions. Much depends on the emotional state of the patient when rehabilitation begins. This will establish a motivational level. It is important to provide patients with tasks at which they are sure to succeed, interspersed with more difficult tasks. Sessions should begin and end with success-oriented tasks that the patients can accomplish. No one likes to be left frustrated, with no gratification.

It is important to have several possibilities in mind when beginning a new task, especially if adaptive equipment might be required. The therapist should always ask patients if they have any ideas on how to accomplish the task. This helps to involve patients from the beginning and gives them a sense of responsibility for their own care. No adult likes to be constantly told what to do and how to do it. Offering a number of alternatives and allowing patients to select the method is often helpful in motivating patients to be active participants in their rehabilitation. Very seldom will a patient's injury be precisely identifiable, as on a functional chart. Nowhere in such charts are medical complications taken into consideration in providing the therapist guidelines to independent functioning. All patients must go through a mental process of accepting their disabilities before the maximum potential rehabilitation can be achieved. All patients who reach this level will go through a period of depression, then work through this stage and move on. This may take a week, or it may never happen. Many patients are not physically ready for rehabilitation during the acute stage. Some require a period of 2 to 3 years to accept their disabilities and the associated limitations. Only then may they want to take responsibility for their actions.

Many times patients are not ready or willing to see what they can do; they require motivation by the therapist. In occupational therapy, patients are required to be active participants, and often they do not like that role. They may refuse to attend. In physical therapy, patients can be treated passively; this is less threatening. To reduce the threat in occupational therapy, it may be sufficient for patients to talk with the therapist until trust develops and they decide that they want to get better and care for themselves.

During the time that patients just want to talk, there is an excellent opportunity to educate them about their disabilities and reassure them that all patients with SC lesions go through the same feelings and process. The therapist is there to help them become as independent as possible, but the therapist cannot do it for them.

Some patients have very strong religious or spiritual feelings; these must not be ignored. In some cases it may be desirable to ask the clergy to come to a patient's assistance. This and all other aspects of this devastating experience must be considered in order to rehabilitate the total patient. A full team approach is truly necessary. If each discipline works separately, patients will tend to see themselves as fragmented and will find it more difficult to function as total persons who must now adjust to new life-styles. Finally, it is important that the therapist be empathetic, but not sympathetic, which would not be effective.

REFERENCES

1. Weber, D., and McKenzie, M.: *Spinal Cord Injury: A Treatment Guide for Occupational Therapists.* Charles B. Slack, 6900 Grove Ave., Thorofare, N.J. 08086.
2. Ford, G. R. and Duckworth, B. (1974): *Physical Management of the Quadriplegic Patient.* F. A. Davis, Philadelphia.
3. Hardy, A., and Elson, R. (1976): *Practical Management of Spinal Injuries.* Churchill Livingstone, New York.
4. Duttarer, J., and Elberg, E.: *Quadriplegia after Spinal Cord Injury, A Treatment Guide for Physical Therapists.* Charles B. Slack, 6900 Grove Ave., Thorofare, N.J. 08086.

BIBLIOGRAPHY

Becker, E. F. (1978): *Female Sexuality Following Spinal Cord Injury.* Accent Special Publications, Bloomington, Ill.

Bell, F., Fernie, G. R., and Bar Benel, G. C. (1974): Pressure sores: Their causes and prevention. *Nurs. Times,* 70:740–745.

Carlos, S. (1978): Importance of communication in counseling the spinal cord injured patient. *Paraplegia,* 16:206–211.

Charney, K. J., Juler, J., and Comarr, A. E. (1975): General surgery problems in patients with spinal cord injuries. *Arch. Surg.,* 110:1083–1088.

Cole, T. (1973): A new program of sex education and counseling for spinal cord injured adults and health care professionals. *Paraplegia,* 11:111–124.

Cole, J. M. (1975): Sexuality and physical disabilities. *Arch. Sex Behav.,* 4:389–403.

Comarr, A. E. (1966): Observations on menstruation and pregnancy among spinal cord patients. *Paraplegia,* 3:263–271.

Comarr, A. E., and Vigue, M. (1978): Sexual counseling among male and female patients with spinal cord or cauda equina injuries, part II. *Am. J. Phys. Med.,* 57:215–227.

Conine, T. A., Disher, C. F., Gillmore, S. L., and Fisher, B. A. (1979): Physical therapists' knowledge of sexuality of adults with spinal cord injury. *Phys. Ther.,* 59:395–398.

Conine, T. A., Christie, G. M., Hammond, G. K., and Smith, M. F. (1979): An assessment of occupational therapists' roles and attitudes toward sexual rehabilitation of the disabled. *Am. J. Occup. Ther.,* 33:515–519.

Copp, L. A. (1974): Pain series. *Am. J. Nurs.,* 74:489–519.

Craver, P. N. (1975): Typing splints for the quadriplegic patient. *Am. J. Occup. Ther.,* 29:551.

Crigler, L. (1974): Sexual concerns of the spinal cord injured. *Nurs. Clin. North Am.,* 9:703–716.

Cruikshank, H. S. (1973): Wheelchair adaptations for self-propulsion by a patient with elbow flexion contracture. *J. Am. Phys. Ther. Assoc.,* 53:398–399.

Daily, G. and Michael, R. (1977): Non-sterile self-intermittent catheterization for male quadriplegia patients. *Am. J. Occup. Ther.,* 31:86–89.

Denholm, D. H. (1974): The hair dryer treatment for decubiti. *Can. Nurs.,* 70:33–34.

Evans, R. L., Halar, E. M., De Freece, A. B., and Larsen, G. L. (1976): Multidisciplinary approach to sex education of spinal cord injured patients. *Phys. Ther.* 56:541–545.

El Ghatit, A. Z. (1978): Variables associated with obtaining and sustaining employment among spinal cord injured males. *J. Chronic Dis.*, 31:363–369.

Gachkeim, K. and Runge, M. (1967): Self-dressing techniques for patients with spinal cord injury. *Am. J. Occup. Ther.*, 21:367–375.

Gregory, M. F. and Ferguson, M. (1974): *Sexual Adjustment: A Guide for the Spinal Cord Injured.* Accent on Living Publications, Bloomington, Ill.

Griffith, E. R., Tomko, M. A., and Timms, R. G. (1973): Sexual function in the spinal cord injured: A review. *Arch. Phys. Med.*, 54:539.

Hilleary, O. O.: *Buildings for All to Use: The Goal of Barrier-free Architecture* (publication A222, 1172). National Easter Seal Society for Crippled Children and Adults, Chicago.

Huggins, K. (1977): Simple alarm for quadriplegic patients. *Anaesthesia,* 32:177–178, 679–680.

Kahn, E. (1969): Social functioning of the patient with a spinal cord injury. *Phys. Ther.*, 49:757–782.

Lawson, N. C. (1978): Significant events in the rehabilitation process: The spinal cord patient's point of view. *Arch. Phys. Med. Rehabil.*, 59: 573–579.

Macauley, C. A. (1978): Spinal cord injuries in an inner city hospital. *Arch. Phys. Med. Rehabil.*, 59:76–79.

Manninga, J. B., and Rosen, J. (1975): Problems associated with the use of external urinary collectors in the male paraplegic. *Paraplegia,* 13:56–61.

McGee, M. and Hertling, D. (1977): Equipment and transfer techniques used by C6 quadriplegic patients. *Phys. Ther.*, 57:1372–1375.

McKenzie, M. W. (1970): Role of occupational therapy in rehabilitating spinal cord injured patients. *Am. J. Occup. Ther.*, 24:257–263.

Mooney, T. O., Cole, T. M., and Chilgren, R. A. (1975): *Sexual Options for Paraplegics and Quadriplegics.* Little, Brown, Boston.

Montero, D. and Feldman, D. J. (1967): Effects of glossopharyngeal breathing on respiratory function after cervical cord transection. *Arch. Phys. Med.*, 48:650.

Morley, M. H. (1973): Decubitus ulcer management—a team approach. *Can. Nurs.*, 69:41–43.

O'Flynn, J. D. (1974): Early management of neuropathic bladder in spinal cord injuries. *Paraplegia,* 12:83–86.

Orton, S. J. (1974): Simplified wheelchair measure form. *J. Am. Phys. Ther. Assoc.*, 54:149–152.

Pollock, D. and Sell, H. (1978): Myallectric control sites in the high-level quadriplegic patient. *Arch. Phys. Med. Rehabil.*, 59:217–220.

Rogers, J. C., and Figone, J. J. (1978): The avocational pursuits of rehabilitants with traumatic quadriplegia. *Am. J. Occup. Ther.*, 32:571–576.

Rogers, J. C., and Figone, J. J. (1979): Psychosocial parameters in treating the person with quadriplegia. *Am. J. Occup. Ther.*, 33:432–439.

Rossier, A. B. (1974): Neurogenic bladders in spinal cord injured patients of Geneva, Switzerland and West Roxbury, Massachusetts. *Urol. Clin. North Am.*, 1:125–138.

Sidman, J. M. (1977): Sexual functioning and the physically disabled adult. *Am. J. Occup. Ther.*, 31:81–85.

Smith, B. (1978): Adapted bed controls and the quadriplegia patient. *Am. J. Occup. Ther.*, 32:322.

Singh, S. P., and Magner, T. (1975): Sex and self—the spinal cord injured. *Rehabil. Lit.*, 36:1–10.

Safilios, A. and Rothschild, C. (1970): *The Sociology and Social Psychology of Disability and Rehabilitation.* Random House, New York.

Torelli, M. (1973): Topical hyperbaric oxygen for decubitus ulcers. *Am. J. Nurs.*, 73:494–496.

Van Steen, H. (1975): Treatment of a patient with a complete C1 quadriplegia. *Phys. Ther.*, 55:35–38.

Yashon, D. (1978): *Spinal Injury.* Appleton-Century-Crofts, New York.

APPENDIX

The following organizations may be contacted for additional information.

Recreation

Committee on Recreation and Leisure, President's Committee on Employment of the Handicapped, Washington, D.C. 20210

Kenneth Perry, Southern California Wheelchair Aviators, 7426 Elk Trail 57P, Yucca Valley, Calif. 92284

Handicapped Artists of America, Inc., 8 Sandy Lane, Salisburg, Mass. 01950

National Association of the Physically Handicapped, 124 W. S. Boardway, Perrysburg, Ohio 43551

American Wheelchair Bowling Association, Inc., 2635 N.E. 19th Street, Pompano Beach, Fla. 33062

National Wheelchair Basketball Association, Box 100, Rehabilitation-Education Center, Oak Street at Stadium Drive, Champaign, Ill. 61820

Activities and Politics

American Coalition of Citizens with Disabilities, 1224 Dupont Circle, Room 308, Washington, D.C. 20036

Magazines and Subscriptions

Paraplegia News, 5201 N. 19th Avenue, Suite 108, Phoenix, Ariz. 85015 (monthly)

Accent on Living, P.O. Box 700, Bloomington, Ill. 61701 (quarterly)

ADL Materials

Center for Independent Living, 2539 Telegraph Avenue, Berkeley, Calif. 94704

Institute of Physical Medicine and Rehabilitation, New York University Medical Center, New York, N.Y. 10016

National Easter Seal Society for Crippled Children and Adults, Inc., 2023 Ogden Avenue, Chicago, Ill. 60612

Education for the Disabled

National Paraplegia Foundation, 333 N. Michigan Avenue, Chicago, Ill. 60601

Office of Education, Department of Health, Education and Welfare, Washington, D.C. 20202

Physical and Occupational Therapy Department, Rancho Los Amigos Hospital, 7601 Imperial Highway, Downey, Calif. 90242

Subject Index